Global Outlook on Stem Cells Research

Volume I

Global Outlook on Stem Cells Research
Volume I

Edited by **Samantha Granger**

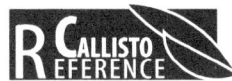

R CALLISTO REFERENCE

New York

Published by Callisto Reference,
106 Park Avenue, Suite 200,
New York, NY 10016, USA
www.callistoreference.com

Global Outlook on Stem Cells Research: Volume I
Edited by Samantha Granger

International Standard Book Number: 978-1-63239-362-3 (Hardback)

Printed in the United States of America.

Contents

Preface

The phrase 'stem cell' is being regularly used in today's world. What are Stem Cells? Stem cells are a type of undifferentiated cells which are able to differentiate or divide into specialized types of cells. Stem cells play an important role for living organisms. They have unique regenerative abilities that offer new potentials for treating diseases such as diabetes, and heart disease. In some cases, such as bone muscle, brain and marrow, discrete groups of stem cells generate replacements for cells that are lost through normal wear and tear, injury, or disease. Stem Cells have the potential to treat many diseases and illnesses, including Parkinson's disease and Alzheimer's as well as cancer. Thus, stem cell research is one of the most intriguing and exciting fields of biology, such that often research on stem cells raises scientific questions as fast as it generates new discoveries. Although the advancements in the applications of stem cells are great, a lot of work remains to be done in the laboratories and clinics to grasp how to use these cells for cell-based therapies to treat disease, which is also referred to as regenerative or reparative medicine. This results in a demand for more efficient and skilled research scientists who can take this field further

This book attempts to compile and collate the research and data available in the field of stem cells. I am grateful to those who put in effort and hard work in this field. I wish to thank my publisher for considering me worthy of such a potential task and supporting me at every step.

Editor

1

Neural Crest Stem Cells from Dental Tissues: A New Hope for Dental and Neural Regeneration

Gaskon Ibarretxe, Olatz Crende, Maitane Aurrekoetxea, Victoria García-Murga, Javier Etxaniz, and Fernando Unda

Department of Cell Biology and Histology, Faculty of Medicine and Dentistry, University of the Basque Country (UPV/EHU), 48940 Bizkaia, Leioa, Spain

Correspondence should be addressed to Fernando Unda, fernando.unda@ehu.es

Academic Editor: Sabine Wislet-Gendebien

Several stem cell sources persist in the adult human body, which opens the doors to both allogeneic and autologous cell therapies. Tooth tissues have proven to be a surprisingly rich and accessible source of neural crest-derived ectomesenchymal stem cells (EMSCs), which may be employed to repair disease-affected oral tissues in advanced regenerative dentistry. Additionally, one area of medicine that demands intensive research on new sources of stem cells is nervous system regeneration, since this constitutes a therapeutic hope for patients affected by highly invalidating conditions such as spinal cord injury, stroke, or neurodegenerative diseases. However, endogenous adult sources of neural stem cells present major drawbacks, such as their scarcity and complicated obtention. In this context, EMSCs from dental tissues emerge as good alternative candidates, since they are preserved in adult human individuals, and retain both high proliferation ability and a neural-like phenotype *in vitro*. In this paper, we discuss some important aspects of tissue regeneration by cell therapy and point out some advantages that EMSCs provide for dental and neural regeneration. We will finally review some of the latest research featuring experimental approaches and benefits of dental stem cell therapy.

1. Stem Cells: Neural Differentiation and Regeneration

The human body possesses several sources of stem cells that remain active during adult life. These stem cells are responsible for renewal of differentiated cell pools in the adult organism, and are particularly enriched in tissues that present a high cell turnover, like the hematopoietic bone-marrow and the skin, among others. Stem cell transplantation has been successfully tested at the clinical level to cure several diseases, confirming the big hopes that were placed upon this emerging technique [1, 2]. These accomplishments encourage further research on stem cells for their use in cell therapy. However, several issues need to be fully addressed before the clinical use of stem cells becomes generalized, such as the control of their cellular physiology and their long-term safety [3]. Another important point concerns the discovery of highly accessible tissue sources which may provide a sufficient amount of stem cells for use in autologous cell therapies, or "patient-specific" cell transplants, which is most interesting from the view of graft immunotolerance. Intensive research will be needed to properly evaluate, over the next decades, which will be the true power of cell therapy to repair diseased or damaged tissues on demand. Research on new sources of human stem cells, controlling the differentiation potential of these stem cells and assessing their safety *in vivo*, will be all fundamental to ultimately reach that goal.

The nerve tissue constitutes a particular case where a big social demand for new therapies aimed at its restoration exists. Currently, there is no effective treatment for many devastating diseases and conditions that involve a destruction of nerve tissue, such as brain or spinal cord injury, stroke, Alzheimer's disease, Parkinson's disease, or amyotrophic lateral sclerosis, among others. As the nervous system controls the rest of bodily functions, these neural damages end to be, both physically and psychologically, highly invalidating for the affected patients, representing a huge social burden for both them and their relatives [4, 5]. In spite of the great interest in neural restoration therapies for brain diseases, nerve tissue presents inherent difficulties for its effective regeneration. The central nervous system in an adult human individual contains billions of neurons. Each neuron in turn can receive hundreds of synaptic connections. From the medical point of view, regenerating this complex pattern of neuronal circuitry constitutes an extraordinary challenge. As an additional complication, when nerve tissue is destroyed, glial cells around tend to accumulate and form a fibrous glial scar that prevents growing nerve fibers from penetrating and thus reinnervating the affected area [6].

A major research effort is being currently undertaken to devise new strategies to aid growing nerve fibers to overcome the glial scar. Some approaches relying on cell therapy have been notably successful, including the transplantation of glial cells from the olfactory bulb, which boosts functional recovery in rodent and primate models of spinal cord injury [7, 8]. Nevertheless, if this kind of regenerative approaches was to be translated to the clinic with human patients, efficient methods to provide a sufficient amount of stem cells should be devised. Neural stem cells (NSCs) in the adult human body are found in two main locations: the subgranular zone of the dentate gyrus of the hippocampus and the subventricular zone of the lateral ventricles [9]. Both of them are highly inaccessible areas, only reachable by invasive brain surgery. Furthermore, the amount of neural stem cells that might be obtained from these areas would arguably be very reduced, unless they were harvested from postmortem brain [10], thus discarding autologous cell therapy.

Probably some of the most available and best-characterized human stem cells to date are the multipotent mesenchymal stem cells (MSCs), which can be isolated from the umbilical cord, the bone marrow, and adipose tissue, among others [11]. MSCs have a mesodermal origin, and they are the forming precursors of the majority of connective tissues in the organism, therefore constituting ideal candidates for their use in connective tissue regeneration strategies. Given their availability, abundance, and well-established methods of isolation, the potential of MSCs to generate neural cell phenotypes has been extensively tested. Although this neural differentiation step involves breaching a major cellular differentiation barrier, the one that separates mesoderm from neuroectoderm lineages, this extent has been reported to be possible in numerous studies; for some examples, see [12–17]. However, very serious doubts were raised as to whether the cells obtained in this way correspond indeed to genuine functional neural/glial cells or are just artefactual [18, 19]. Some neural differentiation procedures involve permanent genetic manipulation of MSCs by gene transfection, which would be undesirable from a clinical point of view [20]. More seriously, a lot of the so-reported neural differentiation protocols were subsequently proven to induce merely cytoskeletal shape changes and/or cell death [18, 19, 21]. Additionally, the expression of neural markers, especially when it is only assessed after very short periods (several hours) after application of neural differentiation protocols, appears very weak and unreliable as a sole criterion

to define neural transdifferentiation [19]. Therefore, mesodermal MSC transdifferentiation to neural fates has yet to solve important issues before being widely accepted by the scientific community [22, 23]. Finally, up to date, we lack definite evidence that transplanted MSCs whether or not transdifferentiated, are able to form functional synapses with neurons of the host, to integrate, and to effectively replace neural components within a functional brain network.

Although evidence that mesodermal MSCs can indeed transdifferentiate to neurons and integrate in an existing neural network is still to be provided, transplanted MSCs and other stem cells may contribute to nerve tissue regeneration by other mechanisms, such as the secretion of anti-inflammatory cytokines [24, 25], and a big array of growth factors promoting cell survival and angiogenesis [26, 27]. Transplantation of MSC to neural tissue has succeeded in ameliorating the functional outcome in several animal models of brain injury, stroke autoimmune and neurodegenerative diseases [28–33]. Cell fusion and transfer of mitochondria between MSCs and host cells has been demonstrated [34–37], and similar mechanisms could contribute to the healing activity of MSCs *in vivo*. At the present time, we do not certainly know which of the three mechanisms: (i) transdifferentiation, (ii) factor secretion, or (iii) cell fusion, plays the most critical role with regard to the neural function improvement in MSC transplantation experiments [22]. However, these results overall invite to optimism. Whatever the mechanisms underlying it, brain function recovery by stem cell transplantation is possible, and it might not be long before such therapies are broadly available for their use in patients. Moreover, transplanted cells possess a significant advantage over other vehicles for trophic factor delivery, in that they are live dynamics entities capable of interacting with and adapting to their environment [38].

2. Neural Crest Stem Cells from Dental and Periodontal Tissues

Dental and periodontal tissues constitute a relatively recently discovered source of neural crest stem cells (NCSCs) [39]. The majority of craniofacial connective tissues, including those of the dental pulp and periodontal ligament, are formed by an special type of mesenchymal tissue, derived from the neural crest during embryonic development, thus termed ectomesenchyme [40]. Ectomesenchyme contributes to the generation of craniofacial structures, such as oral muscles, bones, tongue, craniofacial nerves, and teeth, and dental ectomesenchymal stem cells (EMSCs) therefore share a common origin with neural crest cells [41] (Figure 1).

One important feature of dental EMSC is that a substantial amount of these are maintained in the dental pulp and periodontium of both deciduous and permanent teeth [42]. These EMSCs function in the dental pulp *in vivo* to renew populations of dental pulp fibroblasts, and also when needed, to replace injured odontoblastic cells and create a protective layer of reparative dentin [39]. Additionally, EMSCs are also enriched in periodontal tissues, which need a continuous fibroblast cell supply and collagen fiber remodeling to adapt to strong masticatory forces [43].

(a)

(b)

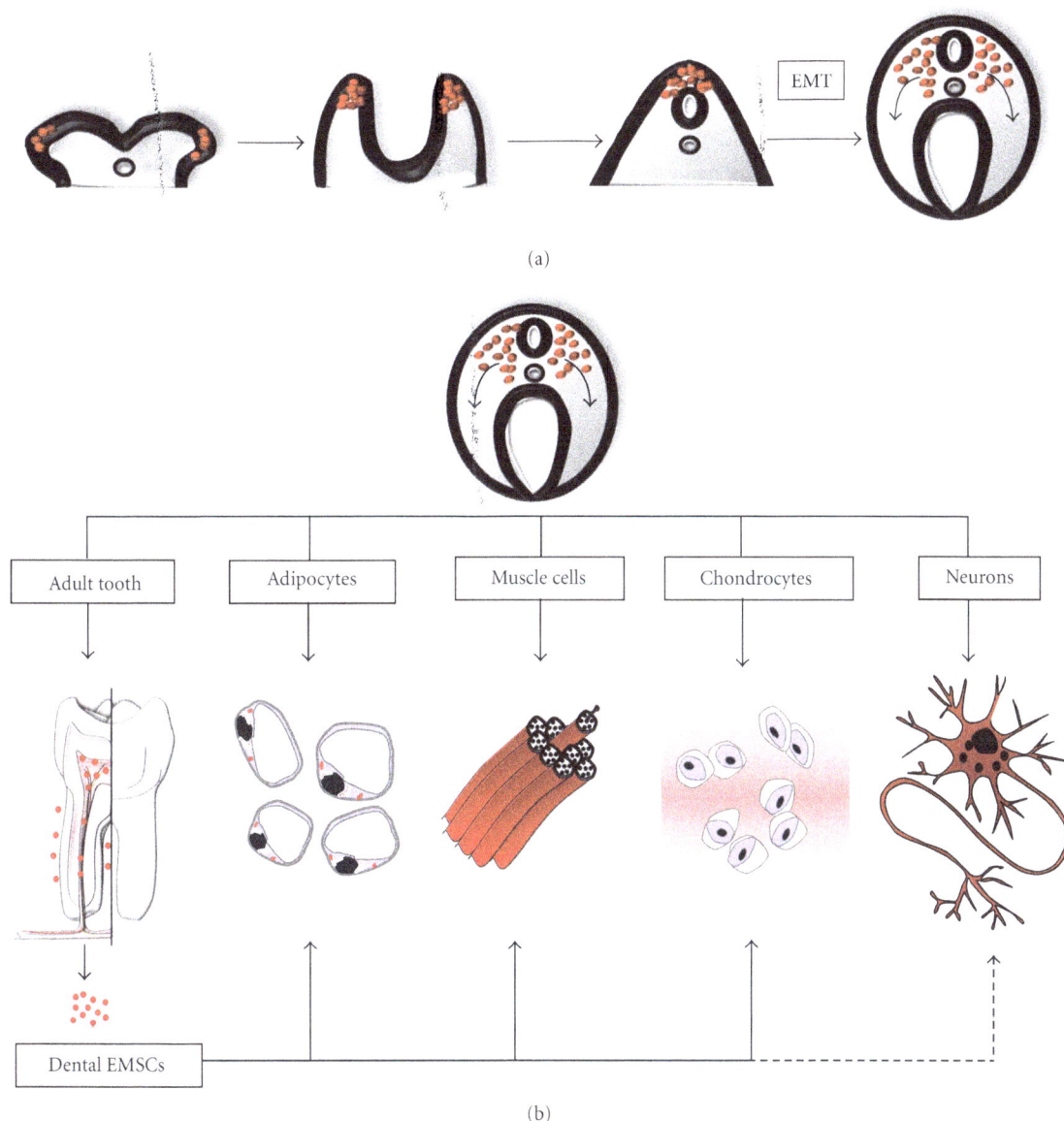

FIGURE 1: Origin and differentiation potential of dental ectomesenchymal stem cells (EMSCs). (a) Origin of neural crest stem cells (NCSCs). The neural crest arises as a cell population belonging to the fusing edges of the neuroectoderm. After neural tube fusion, neural crest cells undergo an epithelial-mesenchymal transition (EMT), where they transform into EMSCs. EMSCs migrate to generate the majority of craniofacial tissues, including tooth tissues fat, muscle, bone, and cartilage tissues, as well as cranial peripheral ganglia and nerves, among others. (b) EMSCs are retained in the adult dental pulp and periodontal tissues. These cells keep the potential to differentiate to various cell lineages and thus regenerate different dental and connective tissues. Dental EMSCs appear to hold a particularly high neurogenic potential and may also be used to regenerate nerve tissue.

Dental and periodontal stem cells present a substantial advantage for their use in nerve tissue restoration, in that they present a neural crest phenotype. Contrary to mesoderm-derived MSCs, EMSCs from dental tissues constitutively express neural-progenitor protein markers, even in basal culture conditions [41, 44–46]. This suggests that EMSCs may retain the intrinsic ability to redifferentiate to nerve cells. Due to their common embryonic origin with the peripheral nervous system, it seems reasonable to say that dental EMSCs are one step closer to nerve cells than other stem cells, such as mesodermal MSCs, and thus EMSCs

may be more amenable than other stem cells to genuine neural and glial cell differentiation, under the appropriate conditions [41, 47]. This propensity to differentiate to neural lineages is not exclusive to dental EMSCs, and other NCSC types, such as those present in the skin and hair follicles, show similar neural differentiation ability [48, 49].

The amount of cells that can be obtained from a healthy human molar tooth pulp ranges between 500.000 and 2 million, which may seem quite modest. However, it is estimated that between 0.2% and 0.7% of the cells plated after pulp dissociation represent true colony-forming dental

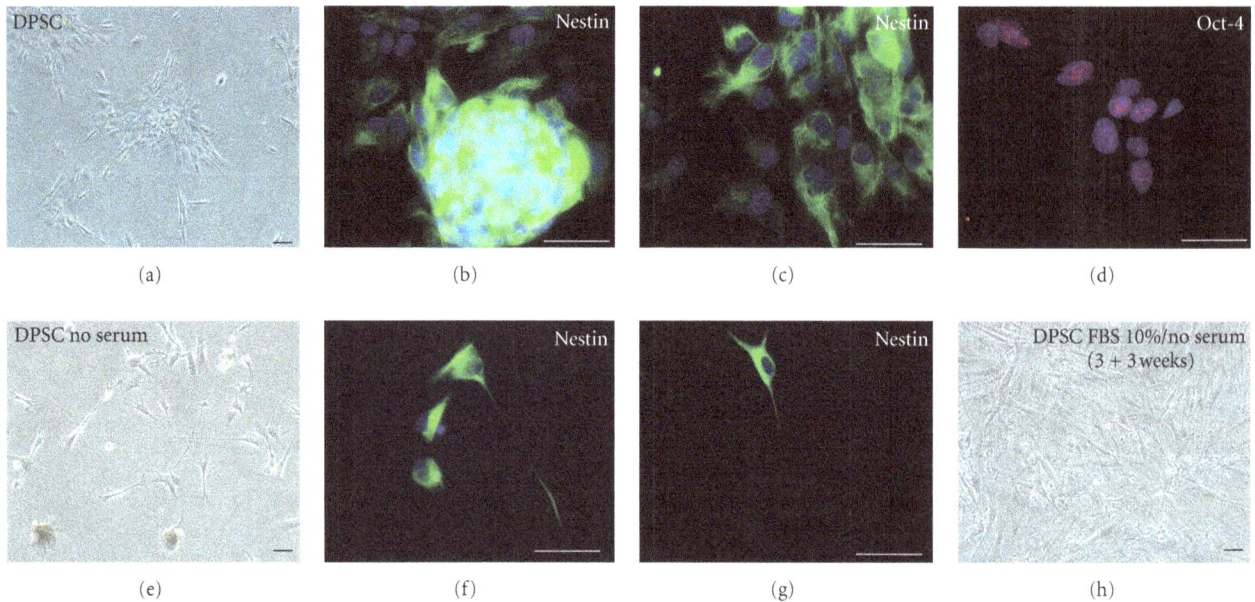

FIGURE 2: Dental EMSCs express neural differentiation and pluripotency markers and can acquire a prominent neural-like morphology *in vitro*. Dental EMSCs isolated from dental pulp (DPSCs) form clonogenic adherent colonies (a), which present Nestin+ immunoreactivity (b) and from which equally Nestin+ migrating cells spread to eventually bring the culture plate to full confluency (c). Dental EMSCs also express pluripotency markers such as Oct-4, in the absence of any genetic or pharmacological manipulation (d). The cellular morphology and proliferation rates of dental EMSCs vary depending on the presence of FBS in the culture medium. DPSCs proliferate slowly in the absence of serum. Cells cultured without serum are equally Nestin+ but display very variable morphologies, including the appearance of cells with striking neuron-like shape, that show very thin and long cytoplasmic processes, resembling dendrites and axons (f, g). When DPSC are expanded for 3 weeks with 10% FBS, following another 3 weeks of serum deprivation, a sheet of nerve-like tissue is formed (h). Times after seeding: (a) 1 week; (e) 3 weeks; (h) 6 weeks (3 + 3); (b–d; f–g) double merged images of Nestin (green) and Oct-4 (red) immunolabeled cells, with DAPI (blue) introduced as a nuclear counterstain. Scale bars: 50 μm.

EMSCs, also referred to as dental pulp stem cells (DPSC) [39]. In our experience with these dental pulp cultures, when placed in a culture medium specific for MSC, nonstem cells deadhere and only adherent dental EMSCs remain. These EMSCs rapidly generate Oct-4+/Vimentin+/Nestin+ clonogenic colonies. After 5 days in culture, each of the colonies may show around 40–50 cells on average, and some peripheral cells with fibroblastic migratory shape, showing big lamellipodia, begin to spread apart of the colony cell mass (Figures 2(a)-2(b)). Then, a significant change is observed, notably depending on the absence or presence of fetal bovine serum (FBS) in the culture medium. Cells placed in 10% FBS continue to proliferate at high rate and can be maintained in this condition for very long periods, over 4–6 months, while preserving Oct-4+/Vimentin+/Nestin+ immunoreactivity (Figures 2(c)-2(d)). We estimate that, in the presence of FBS, about 1000 plated EMSCs are capable of bringing a 6-well culture plate area to full confluence (roughly 1 million cells) in the course of merely 2 weeks. Thus, it seems reasonable to say that, although the number of EMSCs that can be obtained from a single tooth piece is indeed small, their high proliferative capacity *in vitro* makes dental tissues very promising alternatives to provide sufficient amounts of EMSCs, even for clinical purposes.

Interestingly, dental EMSCs can also be cultured *in vitro* in the absence of serum for long periods, comparable to those with serum. However, important differences are observed in no-serum conditions. In the absence of FBS, once after the initial steps of colony formation, dental EMSCs cease to proliferate. At this point, some specific cells with a shape surprisingly similar to neuronal cells begin to emerge, displaying long and thin cytoplasmic processes resembling dendrites and axons (Figures 2(e)–2(g)), whereas other cells maintain a fibroblast-like morphology. Overall, in the absence of serum, cell extension throughout the culture plate is limited, restricted to the initially formed stable colonies and a few migrating cells. 6-well culture plates are not brought to confluency even after several months after seeding. To what concerns neural marker expression, the neural progenitor marker Nestin as well as the mature neuron marker β-3tubulin is increased under serum-absence conditions, and some cells out of the colonies present a very striking neural-like elongated morphology (Figures 2(f)–2(d)). Therefore, the absence of serum might favor the acquisition of a neural-like phenotype by dental EMSCs, as opposed to a fibroblast-like one. To this date, there is a need to evaluate if these dental EMSCs cultured *in vitro* could represent genuine neuron-like cells. They present strong Nestin+ immunoreactivity, β-3tubulin+ immunoreactivity, and surprisingly similar neural-like morphology in the absence of any kind of genetic or pharmacological stimulation of neural differentiation, but further research, including a more detailed information of their transcriptome and electrophysiological assessment of their electrical activity, will be necessary to clarify this. Another important point is to determine if fibroblast-like cells expanded on FBS can be effectively reverted to a neuron-like phenotype after subsequent serum deprivation. Our preliminary results suggest a positive answer to this (Figure 2(h)). This is an important matter, since the presence of xenoproteins on the culture medium might be inappropriate for the use of these cells in human cell therapy [50].

3. EMSCs Derived from Human Adult Teeth

Different EMSC types can be isolated from dental and periodontal tissues. In this section, we proceed to discuss the main characteristics of the different dental and periodontal stem cell types. Overall, EMSCs derived from adult teeth or those derived from developing teeth can be distinguished.

EMSCs derived from adult teeth would be the most interesting from the clinical viewpoint, because it permits their extraction on demand, whenever they are required, precluding the need of long periods of cryopreservation and storage in cell banks, and therefore saving considerable economic and human resources. Very often, tooth pieces are extracted for other reasons than to obtain stem cells. The most clear example of this constitutes the third molars (or wisdom teeth) of young individuals, which are daily extracted by orthodontic reasons and discarded by thousands as chirurgical waste, in dental clinics worldwide. Therefore, dental tissues may well provide a steady supply of stem cells to be employed in autologous and/or allogeneic transplants in human patients. Finally, third molars have a significant advantage over fully adult erupted teeth, in that they are not completely developed and thus present a more immature phenotype at the time of extraction, which seems to favor the presence of pluripotent-like EMSCs [51].

3.1. Dental Pulp Stem Cells (DPSCs). The human adult tooth pulp contains a population of neural crest-derived EMSCs that can be isolated by enzymatic digestion and which forms adherent clonogenic colonies of fibroblast-like cells when cultured *in vitro* ([39, 41]; Figure 1(a)). These EMSCs from dental pulp, termed DPSCs, display a great variability in growth rate and may exhibit a wide range of cell morphologies and tissue marker expression, which appears to reflect their high multilineage differentiation potential to both mesenchymal and nonmesenchymal lineages, characteristic of neural crest stem cells [41, 52]. Notably, DPSCs *in vivo* appear to reside at the perivascular and periodontoblastic compartments within the adult tooth pulp [41, 53], and their cellular phenotype corresponds to pericyte-like smooth-muscle-actin- (SMA-) expressing cells [54]. DPSCs proliferate faster than bone marrow MSCs (BMMSCs) [39, 42]. Finally, and similarly to other MSC types, protocols have been devised that permit long-term cryopreservation of DPSCs without affecting their stemness potential [55].

DPSCs have been reported to *in vitro* differentiate to multiple cell lineages, including odontoblasts, chondroblasts, adipocytes, muscle cells, and neurons [44, 56]. Differentiation of DPSC to dentinogenic cell lineages specifically seems to be favored after serial *in vitro* culture passaging [57]. When DPSCs are xenotypically transplanted in immunocompromised mice, combined with mineralized biocompatible hydroxyapatite/tricalcium phosphate (HA/TCP) scaffolding materials, they can generate a complete dentin-pulp complex containing odontoblastic cells. Conversely, BMMSCs in the same conditions give rise to highly vascularized bone-like tissue, containing adipocytes and lamellar bone trabeculae [39, 58]. These different outcomes after *in vivo* transplantation seem to be at least partly related with a differential secretion of paracrine signals by the grafted stem cells, which act upon surrounding host cells to generate specific tissue phenotypes [59, 60].

3.2. Dental Pulp Pluripotent Stem Cells (DPPSCs). Very recently, a new stem population from the human dental pulp of third molars has been isolated and characterized [51, 61]. These cells, termed dental pulp pluripotent stem cells (DPPSCs), may correspond to the aforementioned population of tooth pulp NCSCs [41]. DPPSCs express pluripotency markers such as Oct-4, Lin-28, Sox-2, and Nanog, which are four factors whose induced expression alone is sufficient to revert human-differentiated cells to a pluripotential phenotype [62]. DPPSCs have been shown to differentiate to cells from the three embryonic layers: endoderm, mesoderm, and ectoderm, thus displaying a potency that was widely thought to be exclusive from embryonic stem (ES) cells and induced pluripotent stem (IPS) cells [41, 51]. Similar stem cells with basal pluripotency marker expression have been isolated from the periodontal ligament [63], and our own studies confirm that stem cells derived from the dental pulp of third molars express pluripotency markers, such as Oct-4, which were traditionally associated with pluripotent ES and IPS cells (Figure 2(d)).

3.3. Stem Cells from Human Exfoliated Teeth (SHED). Like adult permanent teeth, pulp tissue of primary exfoliated human teeth (children's milk teeth) also contains an EMSC population. SEHD possess remarkable proliferative capacity, even higher than DPSC [46]. SHED basally express neural markers and can be readily induced to differentiate to neuron-like cells, and transplanted SHED have been shown to survive for a long term and integrate in recipient brain tissues [46]. A basal expression of pluripotency markers has been documented for SHED as well [64]. Therefore, it is quite likely that a population of pluripotent cells, similar to the DPPSCs found in the adult dental pulp, may also be isolated from exfoliated milk teeth. However, the clinical use of SHED in clinical therapy might be hampered by their limited temporary availability and the fact that milk teeth undergo intense root resorption during exfoliation, which may reduce the amount of collected material.

3.4. Periodontal Ligament Stem Cells (PDLSCs). Enzyme-mediated digestion of the PDL also yields a MSC population with clonogenic potential, and similar proliferation rates to adult DPSCs [43], and PDLSCs also display a multilineage differentiation potential [65] and a basal expression of pluripotency markers [63]. When transplanted *in vivo* in the presence of HA/TCP scaffolds, these PDLSCs are able to generate properly arranged cementum and PDL-like structures, including Sharpey's fiber bundles providing cementum attachment [43]. These properties make PDLSCs a good choice for their use in periodontal tissue engineering therapies, possibly in combination with other adjuvant factors such as platelet-derived plasma rich in growth factors, or PRGFs [66]. Moreover, PDLSCs also maintain their stem cell properties after cryopreservation [67].

4. EMSCs Derived from Developing Teeth

The formation of the dental pulp and periodontium during tooth development requires the coordinated action of different neural crest stem cells [68]. These stem cells, given their embryonic nature, may not be considered for isolation with clinical purposes, for obvious ethic reasons. They represent nonetheless interesting alternative animal NCSC sources for experimental research in tissue engineering. No pluripotency features have been described yet for EMSCs from developing teeth, although because of their common origin with EMSCs from adult teeth and other nondental NCSC types, it is conceivable that they might share this property as well.

4.1. Stem Cells from Apical Papilla (SCAP). The apical papilla is the tissue which surrounds the apices of developing teeth near Hertwig's epithelial root sheath and which takes part in tooth root formation. An EMSC population presenting a high proliferative capacity can be isolated from there [69, 70]. The apical papilla may also be present in some preerupting little developed wisdom teeth. SCAP can be induced to differentiate to multiple cell lineages and possess a large potential for dental and periodontal repair therapies [71]. SCAP can also be cryopreserved without losing stem cell activity [72].

4.2. Stem Cells from Dental Follicle (SCDF). The dental sac or follicle is the ectomesenchymal embryonic tissue surrounding the tooth germ. This tissue is still present in preerupting impacted wisdom teeth [73]. SCDF can be differentiated *in vitro* to various cell lineages, particularly those involved in the formation of periodontal tissues [74–76].

5. Neural Crest Stem Cells and Pluripotency

One outstanding feature reported for dental EMSCs is their apparent pluripotency. As already mentioned, some recents studies suggest that EMSCs from dental and periodontal tissues may possess a superior multilineage differentiation potential, even comparable to that of ES and IPS cells [41, 61]. This may not be so surprising, if we consider the nature of the NCSC phenotype [77]. Already during early embryo development, neural crest cells must undergo a major phenotype switch, to become connective tissue-like migrating cells (i.e. ectomesenchymal cells), out of cells primitively belonging to the epithelial neuroectoderm. This transformation from neuroectoderm to ectomesenchyme, also termed epithelial-mesenchymal transition (EMT), is a clear example of how classic embryonic layer boundaries

can be naturally crossed by neural crest cells, and gives evidence of their high multidifferentiation potential [78]. The ability to undergo EMT appears to be important for the emergence of the stem cell phenotype [79], and this is a particularly remarkable and intrinsic feature of adult NCSCs. Consistently, dental EMSCs present upregulated bone morphogenetic protein (BMP) signaling, compared to other mesoderm-derived and phenotypically related stem cells, like BMMSCs [59]. Since transforming growth factor (TGF)/BMP signaling is a major inductor of EMT [80], this may reflect important differences between neural crest-derived stem cells and other adult stem cells, with regard to their multilineage differentiation potential.

Consistent with the finding of DPPSCs in adult teeth, other NCSCs with similar pluripotency characteristics have been found in additional locations within the adult human body, notably in the skin, and typically associated with hair follicles [81–83]. These skin-derived pluripotent NCSC appear to arise from different locations and correspond to cells that have intense migratory activity [84, 85]. Similarly to DPPSCs, skin-derived NCSCs can be maintained for long periods (months or years) *in vitro*, and they also express neural and pluripotency markers, while retaining the ability to differentiate to different cell lineages, including nerve and glial cells [48, 85]. Notably, skin-derived NCSCs have been successfully used to contribute to functional recovery in animal models of peripheral nerve and spinal cord injury as well as demyelinating disease [86–89]. It remains to be determined whether NCSCs derived from skin and tooth share fully similar characteristics and which might be the conditions that favor the use of one or another type in cell-based regenerative strategies. A substantial advantage of these adult tissue-derived NCSCs for their use in cell therapy is that, contrary to pluripotent ES and IPS cells, they do not appear to form tumors *in vivo* [49, 83, 90].

6. Dental and Periodontal Stem Cells in Regenerative Dentistry

Dental EMSCs present an obvious interest for dental tissue bioengineering, because these cells have shown to be able to regenerate various dental and periodontal tissues, after transplantation to immunocompromised animals [91–93]. Affections like dental caries or periodontal disease are very common worldwide, and current procedures to replace missing or degraded dental tissues often rely on synthetic materials, which may not adapt to the patient in the same way as a fully biological graft. In the future, regenerative procedures employing autologous or allogeneic stem cells might become a common dental practice, due to the significant advantages these bioengineered structures would offer, with regard to their better dynamic integration in the oral tissue environment.

Tooth enamel and dentin are degraded in dental caries, whose extreme complication is infection of dental pulp. Nowadays, the most common treatment for such deep caries relies on endodontics, which involves replacement of infected pulp tissue with inert materials. This leaves a devitalized (dead) pulp chamber that results in a much more fragile tooth piece, and may often require placement of a synthetic crown to avoid tooth breakage. Therefore, it is of considerable interest to find bioactive substitutes of pulp refilling materials and in this scenario, dental EMSCs may constitute a very good alternative. Recently, it has been reported that DPSsC, transplanted together with synthetic scaffolds to emptied mice pulp, are able to regenerate pulp chamber tissue and create new layers of dentin *de novo* [94, 95].

Periodontitis is an infective disease that destroys tissues providing tooth anchorage, such as the PDL and surrounding alveolar bone. Severe periodontitis results in a chronic inflammatory condition where risk of tooth loss by detachment is elevated, hence the importance of devising periodontal repair therapies. From the clinical point of view, periodontal repair is a challenging issue, since different tissues (cementum, Sharpey's fibers, PDL, and alveolar bone) need to be restored in a spatially organized way. Notably, positive results of functional periodontal regeneration have been obtained in experimental animals, using stem cell-based strategies [43, 71]. Stem cell therapy thus promises to warrant further research in the field of dental and periodontal repair.

Another research direction of dental and periodontal EMSC biology seeks to exploit the ability of these cells to generate bone [96]. In a dental clinic, boosting alveolar bone generation is of great importance for artificial tooth replacement, given that implants are directly anchored to a predrilled hole in the jaw or maxilla, and these bone areas need to be sufficiently solid to withstand implant screwing and subsequent mastication forces. Regarding this, MSC-based strategies have been proven successful, both experimentally and clinically, to increase bone mass and allow better implant placement and performance [97]. Traditional synthetic implants present a nonnegligible risk of defective integration in the alveolar bone. Another important reason why to switch to autologous cell-based therapies in this context would be to prevent peri-implant disease, which is a far more frequent complication, with prevalence rates estimated of about 8%–14% [98–100]. Experimental evidence reports a significantly better implant tolerance, better bone formation, and higher bone-to-implant contact, when biomaterial-designed implants are placed in combination with PDLSCs or BMMSCs, in animal models of peri-implant defect [101].

The ultimate achievement in regenerative dentistry would be to generate a whole functional replacement tooth, out of cultured and dissociated dental stem cells. Once considered to be chimeric, this has already been successfully accomplished in animal models. Complete and functional mouse teeth can be generated from dissociated dental epithelial and mesenchymal stem cells, properly recombined *in vitro* to reconstitute fully functional bioengineered tooth germs. These tooth germs develop normally to form a well-calcified tooth piece, which integrates well into surrounding tissues, supports masticatory forces, and gets normally innervated [102, 103]. Nevertheless, in spite of these encouraging results, there are several issues to be addressed before this kind of approaches can be translated to dental practice. One of them, not trivial, is patterning of the engineered biotooth

germ to achieve optimal dental shape and occlusion [104]. However, the main issue to be solved is the lack of consistent sources of epithelial stem cells with odontogenic potential in the adult human individual to be recombined with mesenchymal stem cells. Despite the inherent difficulty to obtain epithelial odontogenic stem cells (which mostly disappear after tooth eruption), new alternatives are emerging to solve this issue. Recently, positive results have been described using PDL-derived epithelial rests of Mallassez, and oral mucosal epithelial cells [105, 106]. Another interesting alternative to obtain epithelial odontogenic cells would be to derive them from autologous IPS cells [107].

7. Dental and Periodontal Stem Cells in Neural Regeneration

Interest in dental stem cell research goes far beyond applications for dentistry. Because of their shared common origin with the nervous system, dental EMSCs may be ideal candidates to generate large pools of neural cells for cellular therapy, in conditions such as ischemic stroke, spinal cord trauma, and neurodegenerative diseases. As already commented before, the properties of dental EMSCs are largely shared by other NCSC types found in other adult human tissues, like the skin and hair follicles. Because of their high accessibility and apparent safety, these adult NCSC types may be regarded as very convenient sources of autologous stem cells for neural regeneration. In this last section, we outline some important aspects with regard to nerve tissue regeneration by cell therapy and discuss the evidence that supports a beneficial effect of dental and periodontal EMSC transplantation for the treatment of neural lesions.

First of all, when it comes to consider the choice of new stem cell sources like dental tissues, size matters. Millions of transplanted cells may be required to repair specific damages, the amount of course depending on the actual lesion volume. Small localized lesions may require fewer transplanted cells, but any suitable stem cell therapy should take the magnitude factor into account. Dental tissues have been partly neglected so far because they constitute a relatively little amount of biological material for the isolation of stem cells, especially when comparing it with large available fat, umbilical cord, or bone marrow tissue sources. However, despite being less abundantly available, dental EMSCs present higher proliferation rates than bone marrow MSCs [39, 46], and their populations can be readily expanded in a few weeks *in vitro*, thus making them a real alternative to classic MSCs. A similar conclusion may be drawn when it comes to evaluate the potential of other related NCSC types, such as those derived from the skin. Large pools of cells can be generated, within 3 months, out of relatively small (2–16 square cm) human skin biopsies [82, 85].

Stem cells derived from adult individuals are particularly interesting with a view to cell therapy of neural disorders, because this would permit to obtain a population of autologous stem cells that would elicit no eventual long-term immune rejection after transplantation. Inflammation is a particularly harmful phenomenon when it refers to nerve tissue. Liquid accummulation characteristic of inflammation increases hydrostatic pressure. Within the central nervous system (CNS), this constitutes a dangerous event which would lead to a rapid collapse of neural function. The CNS has a sophisticated mechanism to avoid liquid filtration across its irrigating blood vessel walls (the blood-brain barrier) and thus prevents a potentially mortal brain edema [108]. The resident macrophages of the central nervous system (the microglia) have evolved to adapt to the specific immune requirements of the CNS as well [109].

For all these reasons, it is very advisable that any eventual clinical trial of cell transplantation to the human CNS attempts to minimize any chance, however little, of immune rejection. Some nonneural crest stem cell types, like MSCs, have been reported to improve neural function in a variety of animal models, which was attributed to an immunosuppressant role, by secretion of a large number of anti-inflammatory cytokines, even when these cells were allogenically transplanted [25]. However, when devising a cell therapy protocol for CNS repair, owing to its extraordinary immune sensitivity, it is highly convenient that the cells of use are autologous, or "patient specific." Therefore, research on stem cell transplantation to nerve tissue should not only rely on allogeneic cells from compatible human donors, but also and possibly mainly on autologous cells isolated from the own patient. With regard to autologous cell neurotherapy, NCSCs from skin and dental tissues constitute very interesting alternatives, since these can be easily extracted, even in aged patients that may not support well the complicated surgery that is required for the extraction of fat or bone marrow tissue [110]. Moreover, NCSCs from dental and skin tissues may be a far better choice than other stem cell types for neural regeneration [47, 49, 86, 90, 111]. Finally, the immune-regulation benefits described when MSCs are transplanted to the CNS may be comparable, if not better, using autologous dental EMSCs [112, 113].

Dental pulp EMSCs are characterized by a strong expression of neural and glial cell markers, even in basal conditions and in the absence of any pharmacological or genetic manipulation. Moreover, under specific culture conditions, dental EMSCs can be induced to acquire a neural-like morphology, which includes the appearance of very long cytoplasmic processes resembling dendrites and axons (Figure 2). Some studies have already shown that cultured dental EMSCs also show neuron-like electrical activity, characterized by the expression of functional neurotransmitter receptors and the generation of action potentials [47, 114]. Therefore, if properly stimulated, dental EMSCs could constitute a privileged source to obtain neural cells. Furthermore, transplantation of dental EMSCs in experimental animals has shown that these exogenous cells can integrate and survive in the host neural tissue, adopting a neural phenotype according to their specific CNS or PNS location, and even promoting de novo neurogenesis [46, 115, 116].

Importantly, the healing potential of stem cell transplantation is known to be based on mechanisms far more complex than a mere engraftment and replacement of damaged cells. Indeed, dental EMSCs have been shown to secrete a wide variety of paracrine factors such as neurotrophins and chemokines [117], which can play critical roles in the survival of neighboring cells, immunomodulation [112, 113], and even axonal guidance [118]. Remarkably, and similar to other MSCs types, dental EMSC have been shown to present strong immunosuppressive properties [112, 113, 119], which constitutes a fundamental factor to understand the achieved therapeutic success of stem cell therapies for nerve injury [120].

The possibility to obtain autologous NCSCs from dental and/or skin tissue and transplant them in the brain or spinal cord of human patients affected by neural damage could yield considerable expectation, since these lesions are usually quite hopeless with regard to spontaneous tissue regeneration and functional recovery. There is a high social demand to devise innovative neural regeneration boosting strategies for these patients, but dramatically at the same time, endogenous sources of human neural stem cells, which could perfectly fit into that picture, are very scarce and nonaccessible. Experimental evidence of dental and skin-derived NCSC engraftment shows damage recovery in animal models of both central and peripheral nervous system injury [49, 86–89, 121, 122]. This clearly opens new doors for hope on the treatment of largely invalidating human neural disorders, like brain and spinal cord trauma, stroke, and neurodegenerative diseases. However, a comprehensive understanding of the healing processes triggered by stem-cell transplant is yet to be achieved. The repair mechanisms are likely to be more complex and diverse than a differentiation to neurons/glia and replacement of damaged cells, and immunomodulatory effects may play an important role. It is becoming clear that dental EMSCs may hold a broad application potential, not only regarding regeneration of oral, dental, and neural tissues, but even for more general conditions requiring a dynamic immune system regulation, like autoimmune diseases.

8. Concluding Remarks

Human adult teeth and periodontium retain populations of NCSCs that show characteristics of pluripotency. These stem cells, similar to other NCSCs types in the human body, are highly accessible and offer substantial additional advantages that make them good alternatives for their manipulation and clinical use: they present a high multilineage differentiation potential, high proliferative capacity, they are not oncogenic, and its obtention does not raise ethical concerns. Since the isolation of these cells does not require to make a large tissue biopsy, dental NCSCs are particularly suited for autologous cell therapies. Dental and periodontal stem cells are currently being experimentally tested in various tooth and oral tissue regeneration scenarios. Another great application ground for dental NCSCs is nervous system repair. Both dental and nondental NCSCs express immature neural/glial cell markers and are particularly amenable to neural/glial differentiation. Remarkable positive results of neural regeneration and functional improvement have been obtained in experimental models of brain, spinal cord, and nerve injury therapy, using transplanted dental and nondental NCSCs. Time and future experiments will tell whether NCSCs from dental tissues become a privileged source of the very much needed neural cells for clinical cell therapy in human patients.

Acknowledgments

This work was supported by research projects from the University of the Basque Country (UPV/EHU): GIU09/70 and Unidades de Formación e Investigación (UFI11/44), projects from Jesús Gangoiti Barrera Foundation, and projects from the Basque Government: Saiotek (SPEDTC; S-PE11UN051).

References

[1] P. Rama, S. Matuska, G. Paganoni, A. Spinelli, M. De Luca, and G. Pellegrini, "Limbal stem-cell therapy and long-term corneal regeneration," *The New England Journal of Medicine*, vol. 363, no. 2, pp. 147–155, 2010.

[2] A. Hayani, E. Lampeter, D. Viswanatha, D. Morgan, and S. N. Salvi, "First report of autologous cord blood transplantation in the treatment of a child with leukemia," *Pediatrics*, vol. 119, no. 1, pp. e296–e300, 2007.

[3] K. Greenow and A. R. Clarke, "Controlling the stem cell compartment and regeneration in vivo: the role of pluripotency pathways," *Physiological Reviews*, vol. 92, no. 1, pp. 75–99, 2012.

[4] L. Teri, "Behavior and caregiver burden: behavioral problems in patients with Alzheimer disease and its association with caregiver distress," *Alzheimer Disease and Associated Disorders*, vol. 11, no. 4, pp. S35–S38, 1997.

[5] O. L. Lopez, "The growing burden of Alzheimer's disease," *The American Journal of Managed Care*, vol. 17, supplement 13, pp. S339–S345, 2011.

[6] M. V. Sofroniew, "Molecular dissection of reactive astrogliosis and glial scar formation," *Trends in Neurosciences*, vol. 32, no. 12, pp. 638–647, 2009.

[7] A. Ramón-Cueto, M. I. Cordero, F. F. Santos-Benito, and J. Avila, "Functional recovery of paraplegic rats and motor axon regeneration in their spinal cords by olfactory ensheathing glia," *Neuron*, vol. 25, no. 2, pp. 425–435, 2000.

[8] A. Ramón-Cueto and C. Muñoz-Quiles, "Clinical application of adult olfactory bulb ensheathing glia for nervous system repair," *Experimental Neurology*, vol. 229, no. 1, pp. 181–194, 2011.

[9] G. L. Ming and H. Song, "Adult neurogenesis in the mammalian brain: significant answers and significant questions," *Neuron*, vol. 70, no. 4, pp. 687–702, 2011.

[10] T. D. Palmer, P. H. Schwartz, P. Taupin, B. Kaspar, S. A. Stein, and F. H. Gage, "Progenitor cells from human brain after death," *Nature*, vol. 411, no. 6833, pp. 42–43, 2001.

[11] H. K. Väänänen, "Mesenchymal stem cells," *Annals of Medicine*, vol. 37, no. 7, pp. 469–479, 2005.

[12] D. Woodbury, E. J. Schwarz, D. J. Prockop, and I. B. Black, "Adult rat and human bone marrow stromal cells differentiate into neurons," *Journal of Neuroscience Research*, vol. 61, no. 4, pp. 364–370, 2000.

[13] G. C. Kopen, D. J. Prockop, and D. G. Phinney, "Marrow stromal cells migrate throughout forebrain and cerebellum, and they differentiate into astrocytes after injection into neonatal mouse brains," *Proceedings of the National Academy of Sciences of the United States of America*, vol. 96, no. 19, pp. 10711–10716, 1999.

[14] G. Muñoz-Elias, A. J. Marcus, T. M. Coyne, D. Woodbury, and I. B. Black, "Adult bone marrow stromal cells in the embryonic brain: engraftment, migration, differentiation, and long-term survival," *Journal of Neuroscience*, vol. 24, no. 19, pp. 4585–4595, 2004.

[15] S. Wislet-Gendebien, G. Hans, P. Leprince, J. M. Rigo, G. Moonen, and B. Rogister, "Plasticity of cultured mesenchymal stem cells: switch from nestin-positive to excitable neuron-like phenotype," *Stem Cells*, vol. 23, no. 3, pp. 392–402, 2005.

[16] K. J. Cho, K. A. Trzaska, S. J. Greco et al., "Neurons derived from human mesenchymal stem cells show synaptic transmission and can be induced to produce the neurotransmitter substance P by interleukin-1α," *Stem Cells*, vol. 23, no. 3, pp. 383–391, 2005.

[17] C. B. Choi, Y. K. Cho, K. V. Prakash et al., "Analysis of neuron-like differentiation of human bone marrow mesenchymal stem cells," *Biochemical and Biophysical Research Communications*, vol. 350, no. 1, pp. 138–146, 2006.

[18] P. Lu, A. Blesch, and M. H. Tuszynski, "Induction of bone marrow stromal cells to neurons: differentiation, transdifferentiation, or artifact?" *Journal of Neuroscience Research*, vol. 77, no. 2, pp. 174–191, 2004.

[19] N. Bertani, P. Malatesta, G. Volpi, P. Sonego, and R. Perris, "Neurogenic potential of human mesenchymal stem cells revisited: analysis by immunostaining, time-lapse video and microarray," *Journal of Cell Science*, vol. 118, part 17, pp. 3925–3936, 2005.

[20] M. Dezawa, H. Kanno, M. Hoshino et al., "Specific induction of neuronal cells from bone marrow stromal cells and application for autologous transplantation," *The Journal of Clinical Investigation*, vol. 113, no. 12, pp. 1701–1710, 2004.

[21] B. Neuhuber, G. Gallo, L. Howard, L. Kostura, A. Mackay, and I. Fischer, "Reevaluation of in vitro differentiation protocols for bone marrow stromal cells: disruption of actin cytoskeleton induces rapid morphological changes and mimics neuronal phenotype," *Journal of Neuroscience Research*, vol. 77, no. 2, pp. 192–204, 2004.

[22] D. J. Maltman, S. A. Hardy, and S. A. Przyborski, "Role of mesenchymal stem cells in neurogenesis and nervous system repair," *Neurochemistry International*, vol. 59, no. 3, pp. 347–356, 2011.

[23] D. G. Phinney and D. J. Prockop, "Concise review: Mesenchymal stem/multipotent stromal cells: the state of transdifferentiation and modes of tissue repair - Current views," *Stem Cells*, vol. 25, no. 11, pp. 2896–2902, 2007.

[24] A. Gebler, O. Zabel, and B. Seliger, "The immunomodulatory capacity of mesenchymal stem cells," *Trends in Molecular Medicine*, vol. 18, no. 2, pp. 128–134, 2012.

[25] D. J. Prockop and J. Y. Oh, "Mesenchymal stem/stromal cells (MSCs): role as guardians of inflammation," *Molecular Therapy*, vol. 20, no. 1, pp. 14–20, 2012.

[26] L. Crigler, R. C. Robey, A. Asawachaicharn, D. Gaupp, and D. G. Phinney, "Human mesenchymal stem cell subpopulations express a variety of neuro-regulatory molecules and promote neuronal cell survival and neuritogenesis," *Experimental Neurology*, vol. 198, no. 1, pp. 54–64, 2006.

[27] D. G. Phinney, K. Hill, C. Michelson et al., "Biological activities encoded by the murine mesenchymal stem cell transcriptome provide a basis for their developmental potential and broad therapeutic efficacy," *Stem Cells*, vol. 24, no. 1, pp. 186–198, 2006.

[28] T. Kamada, M. Koda, M. Dezawa et al., "Transplantation of human bone marrow stromal cell-derived Schwann cells

reduces cystic cavity and promotes functional recovery after contusion injury of adult rat spinal cord," *Neuropathology*, vol. 31, no. 1, pp. 48–58, 2011.

[29] P. Dharmasaroja, "Bone marrow-derived mesenchymal stem cells for the treatment of ischemic stroke," *Journal of Clinical Neuroscience*, vol. 16, no. 1, pp. 12–20, 2009.

[30] A. Uccelli, L. Moretta, and V. Pistoia, "Mesenchymal stem cells in health and disease," *Nature Reviews Immunology*, vol. 8, no. 9, pp. 726–736, 2008.

[31] E. Ben-Ami, S. Berrih-Aknin, and A. Miller, "Mesenchymal stem cells as an immunomodulatory therapeutic strategy for autoimmune diseases," *Autoimmunity Reviews*, vol. 10, no. 7, pp. 410–415, 2011.

[32] D. J. Prockop and J. Y. Oh, "Medical therapies with adult stem/progenitor cells (MSCs): a backward journey from dramatic results in vivo to the cellular and molecular explanations," *Journal of Cellular Biochemistry*, vol. 113, no. 5, pp. 1460–1469, 2012.

[33] A. Chen, B. Siow, A. M. Blamire, M. Lako, and G. J. Clowry, "Transplantation of magnetically labeled mesenchymal stem cells in a model of perinatal brain injury," *Stem Cell Research*, vol. 5, no. 3, pp. 255–266, 2010.

[34] X. Wang, H. Willenbring, Y. Akkari et al., "Cell fusion is the principal source of bone-marrow-derived hepatocytes," *Nature*, vol. 422, no. 6934, pp. 897–901, 2003.

[35] A. Acquistapace, T. Bru, P. F. Lesault et al., "Human mesenchymal stem cells reprogram adult cardiomyocytes toward a progenitor-like state through partial cell fusion and mitochondria transfer," *Stem Cells*, vol. 29, no. 5, pp. 812–824, 2011.

[36] Y. H. Song, K. Pinkernell, and E. Alt, "Stem cell-induced cardiac regeneration: fusion/mitochondrial exchange and/or transdifferentiation?" *Cell Cycle*, vol. 10, no. 14, pp. 2281–2286, 2011.

[37] J. L. Spees, S. D. Olson, M. J. Whitney, and D. J. Prockop, "Mitochondrial transfer between cells can rescue aerobic respiration," *Proceedings of the National Academy of Sciences of USA*, vol. 103, no. 5, pp. 1283–1288, 2006.

[38] Y. Zhuge, Z. J. Liu, and O. C. Velazquez, "Adult stem cel diferentiation and trafficking and their implications in disease," *Advances in Experimental Medicine and Biology*, vol. 695, pp. 169–183, 2010.

[39] S. Gronthos, M. Mankani, J. Brahim, P. G. Robey, and S. Shi, "Postnatal human dental pulp stem cells (DPSCs) in vitro and in vivo," *Proceedings of the National Academy of Sciences of the United States of America*, vol. 97, no. 25, pp. 13625–13630, 2000.

[40] Y. Chai, X. Jiang, Y. Ito et al., "Fate of the mammalian cranial neural crest during tooth and mandibular morphogenesis," *Development*, vol. 127, no. 8, pp. 1671–1679, 2000.

[41] K. Janebodin, O. V. Horst, N. Ieronimakis et al., "Isolation and characterization of neural crest-derived stem cells from dental pulp of neonatal mice," *PLoS One*, vol. 6, no. 11, article e27526, 2011.

[42] G. T. Huang, S. Gronthos, and S. Shi, "Mesenchymal stem cells derived from dental tissues vs. those from other sources: their biology and role in regenerative medicine," *Journal of Dental Research*, vol. 88, no. 9, pp. 792–806, 2009.

[43] B. M. Seo, M. Miura, S. Gronthos et al., "Investigation of multipotent postnatal stem cells from human periodontal ligament," *Lancet*, vol. 364, no. 9429, pp. 149–155, 2004.

[44] S. Gronthos, J. Brahim, W. Li et al., "Stem cell properties of human dental pulp stem cells," *Journal of Dental Research*, vol. 81, no. 8, pp. 531–535, 2002.

[45] R. M. Davidson, "Neural form of voltage-dependent sodium current in human cultured dental pulp cells," *Archives of Oral Biology*, vol. 39, no. 7, pp. 613–620, 1994.

[46] M. Miura, S. Gronthos, M. Zhao, B. Lu, L. W. Fisher, P. G. Robey et al., "SHED: stem cells from human exfoliated deciduous teeth," *Proceedings of the National Academy of Sciences of USA*, vol. 100, no. 10, pp. 5807–5812, 2003.

[47] A. Arthur, G. Rychkov, S. Shi, S. A. Koblar, and S. Gronthose, "Adult human dental pulp stem cells differentiate toward functionally active neurons under appropriate environmental cues," *Stem Cells*, vol. 26, no. 7, pp. 1787–1795, 2008.

[48] K. J. L. Fernandes, N. R. Kobayashi, C. J. Gallagher et al., "Analysis of the neurogenic potential of multipotent skin-derived precursors," *Experimental Neurology*, vol. 201, no. 1, pp. 32–48, 2006.

[49] Y. Amoh, K. Katsuoka, and R. M. Hoffman, "The advantages of hair follicle pluripotent stem cells over embryonic stem cells and induced pluripotent stem cells for regenerative medicine," *Journal of Dermatological Science*, vol. 60, no. 3, pp. 131–137, 2010.

[50] G. A. Tonti and F. Mannello, "From bone marrow to therapeutic applications: different behaviour and genetic/epigenetic stability during mesenchymal stem cell expansion in autologous and foetal bovine sera?" *International Journal of Developmental Biology*, vol. 52, no. 8, pp. 1023–1032, 2008.

[51] M. Atari, M. Barajas, F. Hernández-Alfaro et al., "Isolation of pluripotent stem cells from human third molar dental pulp," *Histology and Histopathology*, vol. 26, no. 8, pp. 1057–1070, 2011.

[52] A. Abzhanov, E. Tzahor, A. B. Lassar, and C. J. Tabin, "Dissimilar regulation of cell differentiation in mesencephalic (cranial) and sacral (trunk) neural crest cells in vitro," *Development*, vol. 130, no. 19, pp. 4567–4579, 2003.

[53] S. Shi and S. Gronthos, "Perivascular niche of postnatal mesenchymal stem cells in human bone marrow and dental pulp," *Journal of Bone and Mineral Research*, vol. 18, no. 4, pp. 696–704, 2003.

[54] X. Zhao, P. Gong, Y. Lin, J. Wang, X. Yang, and X. Cai, "Characterization of α-smooth muscle actin positive cells during multilineage differentiation of dental pulp stem cells," *Cell Proliferation*, vol. 45, no. 3, pp. 259–265, 2012.

[55] E. J. Woods, B. C. Perry, J. J. Hockema, L. Larson, D. Zhou, and W. S. Goebel, "Optimized cryopreservation method for human dental pulp-derived stem cells and their tissues of origin for banking and clinical use," *Cryobiology*, vol. 59, no. 2, pp. 150–157, 2009.

[56] X. Yang, W. Zhang, J. van den Dolder et al., "Multilineage potential of STRO-1+ rat dental pulp cells in vitro," *Journal of Tissue Engineering and Regenerative Medicine*, vol. 1, no. 2, pp. 128–135, 2007.

[57] J. Yu, H. He, C. Tang et al., "Differentiation potential of STRO-1+ dental pulp stem cells changes during cell passaging," *BMC Cell Biology*, vol. 11, article 32, 2010.

[58] S. Batouli, M. Miura, J. Brahim et al., "Comparison of stem-cell-mediated osteogenesis and dentinogenesis," *Journal of Dental Research*, vol. 82, no. 12, pp. 976–981, 2003.

[59] K. Hara, Y. Yamada, S. Nakamura, E. Umemura, K. Ito, and M. Ueda, "Potential characteristics of stem cells from human exfoliated deciduous teeth compared with bone marrow-derived mesenchymal stem cells for mineralized tissue-forming cell biology," *Journal of Endodontics*, vol. 37, no. 12, pp. 1647–1652, 2011.

[60] J. Yu, Y. Wang, Z. Deng et al., "Odontogenic capability: bone marrow stromal stem cells versus dental pulp stem cells," *Biology of the Cell*, vol. 99, no. 8, pp. 465–474, 2007.

[61] M. Atari, C. Gil-Recio, M. Fabregat et al., "Dental pulp of the third molar: a new source of pluripotent-like stem cells," *Journal of Cell Science*, vol. 125, part 14, pp. 3343–3356, 2012.

[62] J. Yu, M. A. Vodyanik, K. Smuga-Otto et al., "Induced pluripotent stem cell lines derived from human somatic cells," *Science*, vol. 318, no. 5858, pp. 1917–1920, 2007.

[63] O. Trubiani, S. F. Zalzal, R. Paganelli et al., "Expression profile of the embryonic markers nanog, OCT-4, SSEA-1, SSEA-4, and Frizzled-9 receptor in human periodontal ligament mesenchymal stem cells," *Journal of Cellular Physiology*, vol. 225, no. 1, pp. 123–131, 2010.

[64] I. Kerkis, A. Kerkis, D. Dozortsev et al., "Isolation and characterization of a population of immature dental pulp stem cells expressing OCT-4 and other embryonic stem cell markers," *Cells Tissues Organs*, vol. 184, no. 3-4, pp. 105–116, 2007.

[65] J. Xu, W. Wang, Y. Kapila, J. Lotz, and S. Kapila, "Multiple differentiation capacity of STRO-1+/CD146+ PDL Mesenchymal Progenitor Cells," *Stem Cells and Development*, vol. 18, no. 3, pp. 487–496, 2009.

[66] E. Anitua, M. Sánchez, A. T. Nurden, P. Nurden, G. Orive, and I. Andía, "New insights into and novel applications for platelet-rich fibrin therapies," *Trends in Biotechnology*, vol. 24, no. 5, pp. 227–234, 2006.

[67] B. M. Seo, M. Miura, W. Sonoyama, C. Coppe, R. Stanyon, and S. Shi, "Recovery of stem cells from cryopreserved periodontal ligament," *Journal of Dental Research*, vol. 84, no. 10, pp. 907–912, 2005.

[68] M. Rothová, R. Peterková, and A. S. Tucker, "Fate map of the dental mesenchyme: dynamic development of the dental papilla and follicle," *Developmental Biology*, vol. 366, no. 2, pp. 244–254, 2012.

[69] W. Sonoyama, Y. Liu, D. Fang et al., "Mesenchymal stem cell-mediated functional tooth regeneration in swine," *PLoS One*, vol. 1, article e79, 2006.

[70] A. Bakopoulou, G. Leyhausen, J. Volk et al., "Comparative analysis of in vitro osteo/odontogenic differentiation potential of human dental pulp stem cells (DPSCs) and stem cells from the apical papilla (SCAP)," *Archives of Oral Biology*, vol. 56, no. 7, pp. 709–721, 2011.

[71] G. T. J. Huang, W. Sonoyama, Y. Liu, H. Liu, S. Wang, and S. Shi, "The hidden treasure in apical papilla: the potential role in pulp/dentin regeneration and bioroot engineering," *Journal of Endodontics*, vol. 34, no. 6, pp. 645–651, 2008.

[72] G. Ding, W. Wang, Y. Liu et al., "Effect of cryopreservation on biological and immunological properties of stem cells from apical papilla," *Journal of Cellular Physiology*, vol. 223, no. 2, pp. 415–422, 2010.

[73] C. Morsczeck, W. Götz, J. Schierholz et al., "Isolation of precursor cells (PCs) from human dental follicle of wisdom teeth," *Matrix Biology*, vol. 24, no. 2, pp. 155–165, 2005.

[74] S. Yao, F. Pan, V. Prpic, and G. E. Wise, "Differentiation of stem cells in the dental follicle," *Journal of Dental Research*, vol. 87, no. 8, pp. 767–771, 2008.

[75] M. J. Honda, M. Imaizumi, S. Tsuchiya, and C. Morsczeck, "Dental follicle stem cells and tissue engineering," *Journal of Oral Sciences*, vol. 52, no. 4, pp. 541–552, 2010.

[76] K. Handa, M. Saito, A. Tsunoda et al., "Progenitor cells from dental follicle are able to form cementum matrix in vivo," *Connective Tissue Research*, vol. 43, no. 2-3, pp. 406–408, 2002.

[77] M. S. Prasad, T. Sauka-Spengler, and C. Labonne, "Induction of the neural crest state: control of stem cell attributes by gene regulatory, post-transcriptional and epigenetic interactions," *Developmental Biology*, vol. 366, no. 1, pp. 10–21, 2012.

[78] J. P. Thiery, H. Acloque, R. Y. J. Huang, and M. A. Nieto, "Epithelial-mesenchymal transitions in development and disease," *Cell*, vol. 139, no. 5, pp. 871–890, 2009.

[79] D. Medici and R. Kalluri, "Endothelial-mesenchymal transition and its contribution to the emergence of stem cell phenotype," *Seminars in Cancer Biology*, vol. 22, pp. 5379–5684, 2012.

[80] L. A. van Meeteren and P. ten Dijke, "Regulation of endothelial cell plasticity by TGF-β," *Cell and Tissue Research*, vol. 347, no. 1, pp. 177–186, 2012.

[81] Y. Amoh, L. Li, K. Katsuoka, and R. M. Hoffman, "Embryonic development of hair follicle pluripotent stem (hfPS) cells," *Medical Molecular Morphology*, vol. 43, no. 2, pp. 123–127, 2010.

[82] J. G. Toma, I. A. McKenzie, D. Bagli, and F. D. Miller, "Isolation and characterization of multipotent skin-derived precursors from human skin," *Stem Cells*, vol. 23, no. 6, pp. 727–737, 2005.

[83] M. Sieber-Blum and Y. Hu, "Epidermal neural crest stem cells (EPI-NCSC) and pluripotency," *Stem Cell Reviews*, vol. 4, no. 4, pp. 256–260, 2008.

[84] A. Uchugonova, J. Duong, N. Zhang, K. König, and R. M. Hoffman, "The bulge area is the origin of nestin-expressing pluripotent stem cells of the hair follicle," *Journal of Cellular Biochemistry*, vol. 112, no. 8, pp. 2046–2050, 2011.

[85] C. E. Wong, C. Paratore, M. T. Dours-Zimmermann et al., "Neural crest-derived cells with stem cell features can be traced back to multiple lineages in the adult skin," *Journal of Cell Biology*, vol. 175, no. 6, pp. 1005–1015, 2006.

[86] I. A. McKenzie, J. Biernaskie, J. G. Toma, R. Midha, and F. D. Miller, "Skin-derived precursors generate myelinating Schwann cells for the injured and dysmyelinated nervous system," *Journal of Neuroscience*, vol. 26, no. 24, pp. 6651–6660, 2006.

[87] Y. Amoh, L. Li, R. Campillo et al., "Implanted hair follicle stem cells form Schwann cells that support repair of severed peripheral nerves," *Proceedings of the National Academy of Sciences of the United States of America*, vol. 102, no. 49, pp. 17734–17738, 2005.

[88] Y. F. Hu, K. Gourab, C. Wells, O. Clewes, B. D. Schmit, and M. Sieber-Blum, "Epidermal neural crest stem cell (EPI-NCSC)-mediated recovery of sensory function in a mouse model of spinal cord injury," *Stem Cell Reviews and Reports*, vol. 6, no. 2, pp. 186–198, 2010.

[89] F. Liu, A. Uchugonova, H. Kimura et al., "The bulge area is the major hair follicle source of nestin-expressing pluripotent stem cells which can repair the spinal cord compared to the dermal papilla," *Cell Cycle*, vol. 10, no. 5, pp. 830–839, 2011.

[90] Y. Amoh, M. Kanoh, S. Niiyama et al., "Human hair follicle pluripotent stem (hfPS) cells promote regeneration of peripheral-nerve injury: an advantageous alternative to ES and iPS cells," *Journal of Cellular Biochemistry*, vol. 107, no. 5, pp. 1016–1020, 2009.

[91] A. H. Yen and P. T. Sharpe, "Stem cells and tooth tissue engineering," *Cell and Tissue Research*, vol. 331, no. 1, pp. 359–372, 2008.

[92] G. Bluteau, H. U. Luder, C. De Bari, and T. A. Mitsiadis, "Stem cells for tooth engineering," *European Cells and Materials*, vol. 16, pp. 1–9, 2008.

[93] A. A. Volponi, Y. Pang, and P. T. Sharpe, "Stem cell-based biological tooth repair and regeneration," *Trends in Cell Biology*, vol. 20, no. 12, pp. 715–722, 2010.

[94] T. Srisuwan, D. J. Tilkorn, S. Al-Benna, K. Abberton, H. H. Messer, and E. W. Thompson, "Revascularization and tissue regeneration of an empty root canal space is enhanced by a direct blood supply and stem cells," *Dental Traumatology*. In press.

[95] G. T. J. Huang, T. Yamaza, L. D. Shea et al., "Stem/Progenitor cell-mediated de novo regeneration of dental pulp with newly deposited continuous layer of dentin in an in vivo model," *Tissue Engineering A*, vol. 16, no. 2, pp. 605–615, 2010.

[96] G. Laino, F. Carinci, A. Graziano et al., "In vitro bone production using stem cells derived from human dental pulp," *Journal of Craniofacial Surgery*, vol. 17, no. 3, pp. 511–515, 2006.

[97] J. B. Park, "Use of cell-based approaches in maxillary sinus augmentation procedures," *Journal of Craniofacial Surgery*, vol. 21, no. 2, pp. 557–560, 2010.

[98] L. J. Heitz-Mayfield, "Diagnosis and management of peri-implant diseases," *The Australian Dental Journal*, vol. 53, supplement 1, pp. S43–S48, 2008.

[99] B. E. Pjetursson, U. Brägger, N. P. Lang, and M. Zwahlen, "Comparison of survival and complication rates of tooth-supported fixed dental prostheses (FDPs) and implant-supported FDPs and single crowns (SCs)," *Clinical Oral Implants Research*, vol. 18, no. 3, pp. 97–113, 2007.

[100] C. Fransson, U. Lekholm, T. Jemt, and T. Berglundh, "Prevalence of subjects with progressive bone loss at implants," *Clinical Oral Implants Research*, vol. 16, no. 4, pp. 440–446, 2005.

[101] S. H. Kim, K. H. Kim, B. M. Seo et al., "Alveolar bone regeneration by transplantation of periodontal ligament stem cells and bone marrow stem cells in a canine peri-implant defect model: a pilot study," *Journal of Periodontology*, vol. 80, no. 11, pp. 1815–1823, 2009.

[102] E. Ikeda, R. Morita, K. Nakao et al., "Fully functional bioengineered tooth replacement as an organ replacement therapy," *Proceedings of the National Academy of Sciences of USA*, vol. 106, no. 32, pp. 13475–13480, 2009.

[103] M. Oshima, M. Mizuno, A. Imamura et al., "Functional tooth regeneration using a bioengineered tooth unit as a mature organ replacement regenerative therapy," *PLoS One*, vol. 6, no. 7, article e21531, 2011.

[104] B. Hu, A. Nadiri, S. Kuchler-Bopp, F. Perrin-Schmitt, H. Peters, and H. Lesot, "Tissue engineering of tooth crown, root, and periodontium," *Tissue Engineering*, vol. 12, no. 8, pp. 2069–2075, 2006.

[105] Y. Shinmura, S. Tsuchiya, K. I. Hata, and M. J. Honda, "Quiescent epithelial cell rests of malassez can differentiate into ameloblast-like cells," *Journal of Cellular Physiology*, vol. 217, no. 3, pp. 728–738, 2008.

[106] E. Nakagawa, T. Itoh, H. Yoshie, and I. Satokata, "Odontogenic potential of post-natal oral mucosal epithelium," *Journal of Dental Research*, vol. 88, no. 3, pp. 219–223, 2009.

[107] G. Ibarretxe, M. Alvarez, M. Cañavate -L, E. Hilario, A. Maitane, and U. Fernando, "Cell reprogramming, IPS limitations and overcoming strategies in dental bioengineering," *Stem Cells International*, vol. 2012, Article ID 365932, 2012.

[108] N. J. Abbott, "Astrocyte-endothelial interactions and blood-brain barrier permeability," *Journal of Anatomy*, vol. 200, no. 6, pp. 629–638, 2002.

[109] M. Tremblay, B. Stevens, A. Sierra, H. Wake, A. Bessis, and A. Nimmerjahn, "The role of microglia in the healthy brain," *The Journal of Neuroscience*, vol. 31, no. 45, pp. 16064–16069, 2011.

[110] M. Lehnhardt, H. H. Homann, A. Daigeler, J. Hauser, P. Palka, and H. U. Steinau, "Major and lethal complications of liposuction: a review of 72 cases in germany between 1998 and 2002," *Plastic and Reconstructive Surgery*, vol. 121, no. 6, pp. 396e–403e, 2008.

[111] K. Kadar, M. Kiraly, B. Porcsalmy et al., "Differentiation potential of stem cells from human dental origin—promise for tissue engineering.," *Journal of Physiology and Pharmacology*, vol. 60, pp. 167–175, 2009.

[112] L. Pierdomenico, L. Bonsi, M. Calvitti et al., "Multipotent mesenchymal stem cells with immunosuppressive activity can be easily isolated from dental pulp," *Transplantation*, vol. 80, no. 6, pp. 836–842, 2005.

[113] T. Yamaza, A. Kentaro, C. Chen et al., "Immunomodulatory properties of stem cells from human exfoliated deciduous teeth," *Stem Cell Research & Therapy*, vol. 1, no. 1, article 5, 2010.

[114] M. Király, B. Porcsalmy, Á. Pataki et al., "Simultaneous PKC and cAMP activation induces differentiation of human dental pulp stem cells into functionally active neurons," *Neurochemistry International*, vol. 55, no. 5, pp. 323–332, 2009.

[115] A. H. C. Huang, B. R. Snyder, P. H. Cheng, and A. W. S. Chan, "Putative dental pulp-derived stem/stromal cells promote proliferation and differentiation of endogenous neural cells in the hippocampus of mice," *Stem Cells*, vol. 26, no. 10, pp. 2654–2663, 2008.

[116] M. Király, K. Kádár, D. B. Horváthy et al., "Integration of neuronally predifferentiated human dental pulp stem cells into rat brain in vivo," *Neurochemistry International*, vol. 59, no. 3, pp. 371–381, 2011.

[117] I. V. Nosrat, C. A. Smith, P. Mullally, L. Olson, and C. A. Nosrat, "Dental pulp cells provide neurotrophic support for dopaminergic neurons and differentiate into neurons in vitro; implications for tissue engineering and repair in the nervous system," *European Journal of Neuroscience*, vol. 19, no. 9, pp. 2388–2398, 2004.

[118] A. Arthur, S. Shi, A. C. W. Zannettino, N. Fujii, S. Gronthos, and S. A. Koblar, "Implanted adult human dental pulp stem cells induce endogenous axon guidance," *Stem Cells*, vol. 27, no. 9, pp. 2229–2237, 2009.

[119] G. Ding, Y. Liu, Y. An et al., "Suppression of T cell proliferation by root apical papilla stem cells in vitro," *Cells Tissues Organs*, vol. 191, no. 5, pp. 357–364, 2010.

[120] Y. Ziv, H. Avidan, S. Pluchino, G. Martino, and M. Schwartz, "Synergy between immune cells and adult neural stem/progenitor cells promotes functional recovery from spinal cord injury," *Proceedings of the National Academy of Sciences of the United States of America*, vol. 103, no. 35, pp. 13174–13179, 2006.

[121] I. V. Nosrat, J. Widenfalk, L. Olson, and C. A. Nosrat, "Dental pulp cells produce neurotrophic factors, interact with trigeminal neurons in vitro, and rescue motoneurons after spinal cord injury," *Developmental Biology*, vol. 238, no. 1, pp. 120–132, 2001.

[122] F. M. Almeida, S. A. Marques, B. D. Ramalho et al., "Human dental pulp cells: a new source of cell therapy in a mouse model of compressive spinal cord injury," *Journal of Neurotrauma*, vol. 28, no. 9, pp. 1939–1949, 2011.

2

Retinal Pigment Epithelium and Müller Progenitor Cell Interaction Increase Müller Progenitor Cell Expression of PDGFRα and Ability to Induce Proliferative Vitreoretinopathy in a Rabbit Model

Gisela Velez,[1,2,3] **Alexa R. Weingarden,**[3] **Budd A. Tucker,**[2,3] **Hetian Lei,**[2,3] **Andrius Kazlauskas,**[2,3] **and Michael J. Young**[2,3]

[1] *Department of Ophthalmology, University of Massachusetts Medical School, Worcester, MA 01605, USA*
[2] *Department of Ophthalmology, Harvard Medical School, Boston, MA 02115, USA*
[3] *The Schepens Eye Research Institute, Massachusetts Eye and Ear, Boston, MA 02114, USA*

Correspondence should be addressed to Gisela Velez, gisela.velez@umassmed.edu

Academic Editor: B. Bunnell

Purpose. Proliferative vitreoretinopathy (PVR) is a complication of retinal detachment characterized by redetachment of the retina as a result of membrane formation and contraction. A variety of retinal cells, including retinal pigment epithelial (RPE) and Müller glia, and growth factors may be responsible. Platelet-derived growth factor receptor alpha (PDGFRα) is found in large quantities in PVR membranes, and is intrinsic to the development of PVR in rabbit models. This study explores the expression of PDGFR in cocultures of RPE and Müller cells over time to examine how these two cell types may collaborate in the development of PVR. We also examine how changes in PDGFRα expression alter Müller cell pathogenicity. *Methods.* Human MIO-M1 Müller progenitor (MPC) and ARPE19 cells were studied in a transmembrane coculture system. Immunocytochemistry and Western blot were used to look at PDGFRα, PDGFRβ, and GFAP expression. A transfected MPC line cell line expressing the PDGFRα (MIO-M1α) was generated, and tested in a rabbit model for its ability to induce PVR. *Results.* The expression of PDGFRα and PDGFRβ was upregulated in MIO-M1 MPCs cocultured with ARPE19 cells; GFAP was slightly decreased. Increased expression of PDGFRα in the MIO-M1 cell line resulted in increased pathogenicity and enhanced ability to induce PVR in a rabbit model. *Conclusions.* Müller and RPE cell interaction can lead to upregulation of PDGFRα and increased Müller cell pathogenicity. Müller cells may play a more active role than previously thought in the development of PVR membranes, particularly when stimulated by an RPE-cell-rich environment. Additional studies of human samples and in animal models are warranted.

1. Introduction

Proliferative vitreoretinopathy (PVR) occurs in 5–10% of rhegmatogenous retinal detachments [1]. It is a complex cellular process characterized by preretinal and subretinal membrane formation, intraretinal degeneration, gliosis, and contraction. The disease is characterized by (1) migration and proliferation of retinal pigment epithelial cells (RPE) and glial cells along with synthesis of extracellular matrix (ECM) proteins, such as collagen or fibronectin, which organize into retinal and vitreous membranes; (2) intraretinal glial cell proliferation, photoreceptor degeneration, and disorganization of retinal cell layers [2, 3]. In a way, PVR can be viewed as maladaptive and/or aberrant wound healing [4], the severity of which is often determined by the circumstances in which it occurs.

Certain clinical characteristics are associated with an increased risk of PVR development [5, 6]. These can be classified into two categories. In the first group are risk factors which increase RPE cell dispersion into the subretinal and preretinal space, and cellular proliferation. These include large retinal tears and detachments, cryotherapy and sclera indentation, and retinal detachments of long duration. In the second group are characteristics which increase the presence of growth factors and inflammatory cytokines in the environment, with or without breakdown of the blood-ocular barrier [7]. This includes vitreous hemorrhage, choroidal hemorrhage, and cryotherapy. These risk factors for PVR are additive—the more characteristics, the higher the risk of PVR development. Patients with traits in both categories are faced with a perfect storm, in which cell migration and proliferation occur in an environment primed for cellular misbehavior.

There has been controversy in the literature regarding the extent of involvement of cells other than RPE, such as Müller glia, in the pathogenesis of PVR. It is a fact that Müller cells are active participants. Recent work demonstrating the reactivity of Müller glia during retinal detachment and other forms of retinal injury suggests that these cells play a significant role in diseases involving retinal injury and degeneration, such as PVR. Although RPE cells have long been considered the principal mediators of this disease, Müller cell activation, migration, proliferation and transformation in retinal detachment, and retinal injury have all been documented [8–10]. Increased expression of GFAP and vimentin, indicative of increased reactivity, has been demonstrated in Müller glia in detached human retinas and experimental models of retinal detachment [11, 12]. Experimental detachment models have also shown Müller cell proliferation which peaks at 3-4 days retinal detachment and continues at a slower rate for weeks to months [13], as well as migration of Müller cell processes and nuclei throughout the retinal layers and into the subretinal space [8]. Certainly, the data supports the need to explore more closely how these cells participate in PVR pathogenesis, and what drives them to do so.

The question then arises of whether the behavior of Müller cells, already primed and activated in the context of retinal detachment, can be altered by the presence of RPE cells and growth factors in the vitreous environment. Our experiments were designed to help us understand how RPE and Müller cells might affect each other when forced to interact in the context of retinal detachment, and how Müller glia altered by this environment participate in PVR. Because our goal is to better understand this process in human disease, we have chosen to work with the ARPE19 and MIO-M1 Müller progenitor cell lines.

2. Methods

2.1. Major Reagents.
Antibodies against PDGFRα and PDGFRβ were purchased from Cell Signaling Technology (Beverly, MA, USA), anti-GFAP from Zymed (San Francisco, CA, USA), and β-actin from Abcam (Cambridge, MA, USA). Secondary antibodies (antirabbit IgG) were purchased from Jackson ImmunoResearch Laboratories, Inc (West Grove, PA, USA). ARPE19 cells were purchased from American Type Culture Collection; MIO-M1 Müller progenitor cells (MIIO-M1 MPCs) were obtained by material transfer agreement from the Institute of Ophthalmology, University College London, from Drs. GA Limb and Professor PT Khaw

(patent application PCT/GB2004/005101). Primary rabbit conjunctival fibroblasts (RCFs) were obtained as previously described [14].

2.2. Cell Cultures.
Transmembrane cell cultures were set up using MIO-M1 and ARPE19 cells in DMEM/F12 media with 10%FBS (Gibco). MIO-M1 cells were plated in six-well plates and allowed to reach confluency. ARPE19 cells were plated on transwell inserts with 0.4 μm pores and allowed to grow to confluency. Upon reaching confluency, the inserts containing ARPE19 cells were placed in MIIO-M1 containing six-well plates and cultured in a total volume of 3 mL of media. Control groups of each single-cell type were grown concurrently. Cells were fed with 1.5 mL of media on day 2 and 6, with complete media changes at day 4.

2.3. Western Blotting.
MIO-M1 and ARPE19 cells were harvested at days 1, 3, 5, and 7. Lysates were made for Western blot analysis. Media was removed and cells were collected from experimental and control plates and inserts using sterile cell scrapers in PBS. Lysates of these cells were created by incubation for 30 min at 4°C in Ripa buffer 50 mM Tris HCl [pH 8.0], 0.1% SDS, 0.5% sodium deoxycholate, 1% NP-40, 150 mM NaCl, 2% protease inhibitor cocktail, 2% phosphatase inhibitor cocktail 1, and 2% phosphatase inhibitor cocktail 2 (Sigma), followed by 15 seconds of sonication and removal of cellular debris by centrifugation at 12,000 rpm for 12 min at 4°C. The protein content of the lysates was determined with the BCA protein assay (Thermo Scientific). Expression of PDGFRα and PDGFRβ in the control and experimental samples was compared by Western blotting. 50 μg of protein was resolved by 10% sodium dodecyl sulfate-polyacrylamide gel electrophoresis (SDS-PAGE). The protein bands were transferred onto nitrocellulose membranes (Bio-Rad Laboratories), and the membrane was subjected to Western blot analysis using anti-PDGFRα or anti-PDGFRβ primary antibodies. Band density was quantified using Image J and normalized to β-actin expression.

2.4. Immunocytochemistry.
MIO-M1 and ARPE19 cells were cocultured as described above on 16-well glass slides with ARPE19 cells in 8-well strips of 0.2 μm membrane inserts. Inserts were removed after 5 days and the plated cells were fixed for 20 minutes with 4% paraformaldehyde and permeabilized for one hour at room temperature with 10% goat serum and 0.1% Triton X-100 in PBS. MIO-M1 cells were stained with primary antibodies directed against PDGFRα, PDGFRβ, and incubated at 4°C overnight. Primary and secondary antibodies were prepared in 10% GS in PBS solutions at a concentration of 1 : 100 for PDGFRα and β. The slides were then washed with PBS. Secondary antibodies were added to the slides for 1 hour. Slides were then washed with PBS, coated with mounting media containing DAPI, and covered. The cells were examined by fluorescent microscopy with Cy2 filter.

2.5. Preparation of MIO-M1α Cell Line and Rabbit Model for PVR.
The pLHDCX^2-PDGFRα retrovirus was used to

Retinal Pigment Epithelium and Müller Progenitor Cell Interaction Increase Müller Progenitor Cell Expression of PDGFRα and Ability to Induce Proliferative Vitreoretinopathy in a Rabbit Model

15

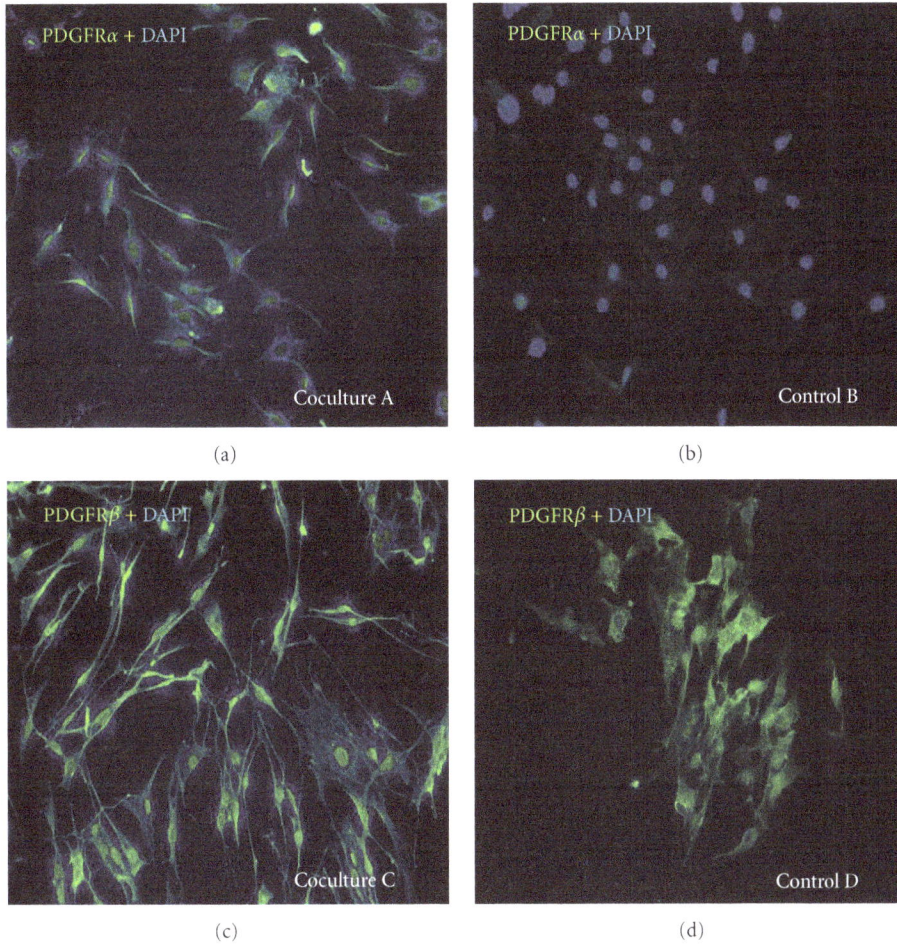

FIGURE 1: Immunocytochemical staining for PDGFRα and β (green) in MIO-M1 MPCs. Expression of PDGFRα after 5 days when cocultured with ARPE19 cells (A) and expression of PDGFRα in control culture (B). Expression of PDGFRβ after 5 days when cocultured with ARPE19 cells (C) and expression of PDGFRβ in control culture (D). PDGFRβ expression appears relatively stable, while PDGFRα expression increases more significantly.

stably express the PDGFRα in immortalized MIO-M1 Müller progenitor cells (MIO-M1 MPCs). Transfected cells with increased PDGFRα expression were selected for resistance to histidinol toxicity and designated as MIO-M1α.

PVR was induced in the right eyes of pigmented rabbits purchased from Covance (Denver, PA, USA). Briefly, a gas vitrectomy was performed by injecting 0.1 mL of perfluoropropane (C_3F_8) (Alcon, Fort Worth, TX, USA) into the vitreous cavity 4 mm posterior to the corneal limbus. One week later, all rabbits received two injections: (1) 0.1 mL of PRP (platelet-rich plasma) and (2) 0.1 mL DMEM containing 2×10^5 of rabbit conjunctival fibroblasts (RCFs), MIO-M1, and MIO-M1α cells. The extent of retinal detachment was evaluated by indirect ophthalmoscopy with a handheld +30 D fundus lens at days 2, 4, 7, and weekly thereafter for a total of 4 weeks. Extent of PVR was graded according to the Fastenberg classification from grade 0 through 5 [15]. On day 28 the animals were sacrificed and the eyes were enucleated. All surgeries were performed under aseptic conditions and pursuant to the ARVO Statement for the Use of Animals in Ophthalmic and Vision Research. The protocol for the use

of animals was approved by the Schepens Animal Care and Use Committee. Mann-Whitney test for nonparametric data ($P < 0.05$) was used for statistical analysis.

3. Results

As previously discussed, the goal of these experiments is to determine if RPE cells induce a change in Muller cells that would result in a PVR-inducing cell.

Immunocytochemical staining of MIO-M1 MPCs after 5 days of coculture with ARPE19 cells confirms MIO-M1 MPCs upregulate their expression of PDGFRα (Figures 1(a)-1(b)), with a moderate increase in expression of PDGFRβ (Figures 1(c)-1(d)). Consistent with these results, Western blot analysis showed upregulation of PDGFRα expression in experimental MIO-M1 MPCs by day 5 after-plating (Figure 2). In contrast, expression of PDGFRβ remained low in MIO-M1 and ARPE 19 cells across the same time, with a measurable increase in MIO-M1 cells by day 7 only (Figure 2). A small but detectable decrease in GFAP

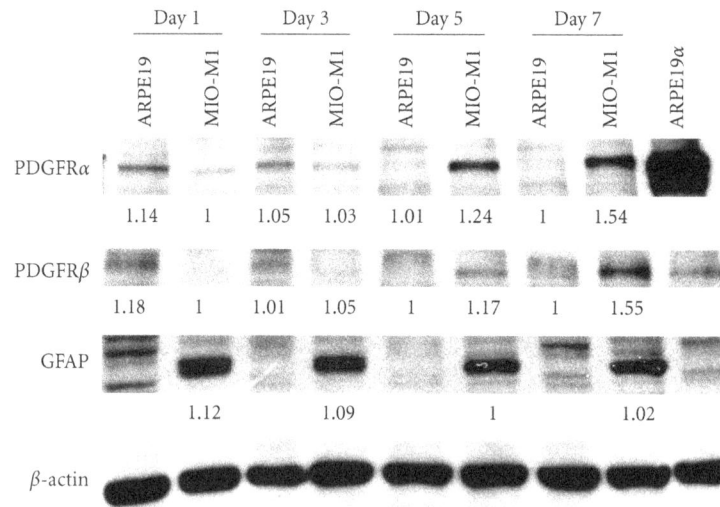

FIGURE 2: Western blot analysis of coculture samples at days 1, 3, 5, and 7 shows noticeable increases in PDGFRα expression in MIO-M1 MPCs. Transfected ARPE19 cells with increased expression of PDGFRα (RPEα) are used as control for comparison. PDGFRβ levels remain relatively low in both cell types throughout the course of the experiment, with a small increase in MIO-M1 MPCs on day 5 and a more significant increase by day 7. MIO-M1 cells show a small but measurable and consistent decrease in expression of GFAP between days 1 and 7 of the experiment. RPEα cells are included for control. Protein concentrations were standardized by Bradford assay. Band intensity was standardized by β-Actin expression (shown). Relative expression ratios are shown.

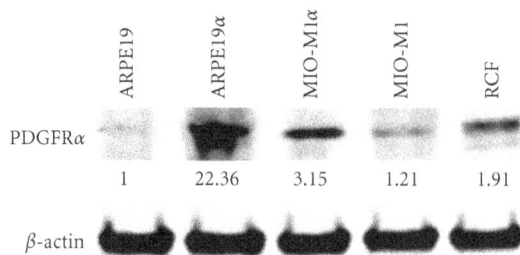

FIGURE 3: Western blot of ARPE19, ARPE19α, MIO-M1 MPCs, MIO-M1α-transfected MPCs, and rabbit conjunctival fibroblast (RCF) lysates shows comparable expression of PDGFRα in transfected MPCs (MIO-M1α) and RCFs, with levels comparable to those developed in cocultured cells. MIO-M1α MPCs have an approximate 2.56X increase in PGFRα expression when compared to untransfected MIO-M1 MPCs, and a 1.65X increase in expression when compared to RCFs. Relative expression ratios are shown.

expression was observed in MIIO-M1 MPCs as early as day 3 after coculture (Figure 2).

The above data suggests that upregulation of PDGFRα could lead to stimulation of fibroblastic behavior consistent with PVR in Müller cells. Given our knowledge of the importance of PDGFRα and not PDGFRβ (see discussion below), we overexpressed PDGFRα in MIO-M1 MPCs to test our hypothesis that Müller cells alone can induce PVR. As confirmed by Western blot analysis, transfection of MIO-M1 cells with pLHDCX²-PDGFRα resulted in increased expression of PDGFRα (Figure 3) in MIO-M1 cells comparable to that observed in cells cocultured with ARPE19 and with the expression of rabbit conjunctival fibroblasts

(RCFs). Comparison of MIO-M1, MIIO-M1α, and RCF behavior in a rabbit model showed a dramatic increase in PVR pathogenicity of the MIIO-M1α cell line comparable to that of RCF's. MIIO-M1α cells were equally effective as RCFs in inducing PVR after-transplantation (Figure 4).

4. Discussion

PDGFRα has long been implicated in the pathogenesis of PVR. It is found extensively in preretinal membranes from PVR patients [16, 17]. Experimental models using mouse embryonic fibroblasts as well as rabbit conjunctival fibroblasts have demonstrated the intrinsic role that PDGFRα, and not PDGFRβ, plays in the pathogenesis of the disease [14, 18]. In fact, inhibition of the PDGFRα, either through inhibition of its tyrosine kinase or the ROS pathway, has been shown to be sufficient in these models to attenuate and/or inhibit the development of PVR [19, 20].

Studies show that Müller cells are present in PVR membranes [21]. However, RPE rather than Müller cells, have dominated the literature and have been the focus of most studies and theories of PVR [22, 23]. This is partly due to the fact that RPE cell markers are more abundant in PVR membranes. The assumption has been made that Müller cells play a less important role, yet this may not be the case.

Our in-vitro study observations and correlating rabbit model results suggest that one of the mechanisms by which Müller cells may play a role in PVR is by upregulating the expression of PDGFRα. When comparing with previous studies in the literature, this change has a bigger impact on Müller cell behavior than RPE cell behavior [24]. These experiments also suggest that Müller cell up-regulation of PDGFR might be the result of the changes in the RPE cell

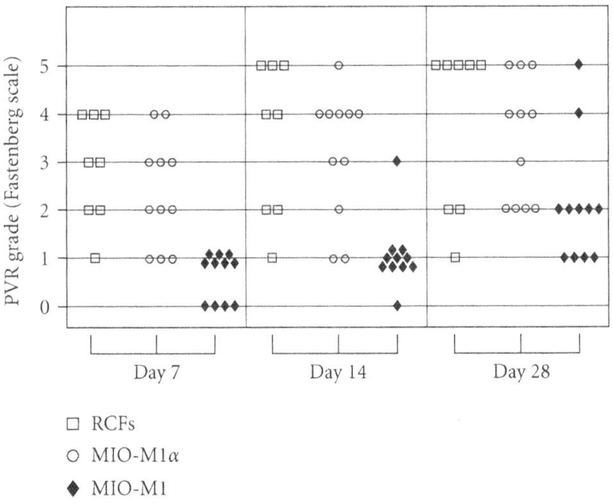

FIGURE 4: Overexpression of PDGFRα in MIO-M1 MPCs induces a phenotypic switch to fibroblast-like cells that effectively induce PVR postintravitreal injection in rabbit. Classification is as follows: stage 0—no PVR; stage 1—presence of fibrous bands; stage 2—fibrous bands with traction; stage 3—retinal detachment involving less than 2 quadrants; stage 4—retinal detachment involving more than 2 quadrants; stage 5—total retinal detachment. For statistical purposes, stage 3 or higher is considered severe PVR. Mann-Whitney statistical analysis for nonparametric data showed a statistically significant difference ($P < 0.05$) at all three time points between RCFs versus MIO-M1 MPCs, and MIO-M1 MPCs versus MIO-M1α MPCs. No statistically significant difference was observed between RFCs versus MIO-M1α MPCs.

rich environment which exists in retinal detachments with high-risk characteristics. High-risk retinal detachments for the development of PVR are more commonly characterized by increased RPE cell migration and presence in the vitreous cavity. In the presence of RPE cells in our study, Müller progenitor cells do two very important things—they change their expression of traditional Müller cell markers such as GFAP, and they increase their expression of PDGFR. Though these changes do not appear to be significant at first glance, studies in the rabbit model suggest that only a small increase in PDGFRα expression is necessary to dramatically alter the behavior of these cells to resemble that of fibroblasts. This is in stark contrast to studies performed using RPE cells, in which a more than 80-fold increase in receptor expression was necessary to significantly alter their behavior, with invivo results which were still inferior when compared to those using fibroblasts [24].

Müller cell plasticity and their capacity to transform their phenotype have already been demonstrated [25, 26]. The ability of this cell type to alter its expression of GFAP in different environments helps to support our observations [9]. Dedifferentiation in particular is thought to play an important role in how Müller cells participate in PVR. Müller cells in the peripheral retina, where PVR most often occurs, have been shown to express stem cell markers, indicative of active proliferation, and dedifferentiation [27]. In-vitro, human-derived Müller cells, including the MIO-M1 Müller

progenitor cell line, have been shown to exhibit neural stem cell traits [28, 29].

We therefore propose the following theory to PVR development invivo. During retinal detachment, depending on the size and longevity of the detachment as well as the size and location of the retinal tear, there is an opportunity for RPE cells to abandon their natural monolayer and migrate onto the subretinal and preretinal space. The vitreous often acts as a scaffold onto which these cells can attach. Once allowed to migrate, RPE cells begin to produce cytokines and cofactors (yet to be fully identified) which can alter Müller cell phenotype and growth factor surface protein expression, leading to an increase in fibroblastic behavior and pathogenicity. Whether there is complete transformation of Müller cells invivo remains a question. It is possible that the abundance of RPE cells in PVR membranes is a "red-herring", and that RPE cells play more of an effector role, with Müller cells doing most of the membrane formation and contraction.

The drawback of our study is that it is based on observations in an in-vitro setup and a limited rabbit animal model. These observations would be more difficult to make invivo, given the progressive and dynamic nature of the disease and the plasticity of Müller cells. Despite its limitations, our in-vitro model allows us to capture specific changes, and our rabbit model allows us to confirm their importance.

Certainly more work needs to be performed invivo. The next step would be a series of experiments in retinal detachment models looking at intraretinal GFAP and PDGFRα expression. Another set of experiments would be aimed at identifying those molecules which trigger Müller cell transformation and growth factor receptor expression. Once identified, therapeutic interventions can be designed to interfere with and redirect this process.

Acknowledgment

This work is supported by NEI 5K08EY17383 and presented in part at the Association for Research in Vision and Ophthalmology 2009 (abstract 2707) and 2011 (abstract 2065), available at http://www.arvo.org/.

References

[1] R. Machemer, T. M. Aaberg, H. M. Freeman, A. R. Irvine, J. S. Lean, and R. M. Michels, "An updated classification of retinal detachment with proliferative vitreoretinopathy," *American Journal of Ophthalmology*, vol. 112, no. 2, pp. 159–165, 1991.

[2] S. K. Fisher, P. A. Erickson, G. P. Lewis, and D. H. Anderson, "Intraretinal proliferation induced by retinal detachment," *Investigative Ophthalmology and Visual Science*, vol. 32, no. 6, pp. 1739–1748, 1991.

[3] G. P. Lewis, D. G. Charteris, C. S. Sethi, and S. K. Fisher, "Animal models of retinal detachment and reattachment: identifying cellular events that may affect visual recovery," *Eye*, vol. 16, no. 4, pp. 375–387, 2002.

[4] M. Weller, P. Wiedemann, and K. Heimann, "Proliferative vitreoretinopathy—is it anything more than wound healing at the wrong place?" *International Ophthalmology*, vol. 14, no. 2, pp. 105–117, 1990.

[5] P. A. Campochiaro, I. H. Kaden, J. Vidaurri-Leal, and B. M. Glaser, "Cryotherapy enhances intravitreal dispersion of viable retinal pigment epithelial cells," *Archives of Ophthalmology*, vol. 103, no. 3, pp. 434–436, 1985.

[6] R. H. Y. Asaria and D. G. Charteris, "Proliferative vitreo-retinopathy: developments in pathogenesis and treatment," *Comprehensive Ophthalmology Update*, vol. 7, no. 4, pp. 179–185, 2006.

[7] E. H. Jaccoma, B. P. Conway, and P. A. Campochiaro, "Cryotherapy causes extensive breakdown of the blood-retinal barrier. A comparison with argon laser photocoagulation," *Archives of Ophthalmology*, vol. 103, no. 11, pp. 1728–2730, 1985.

[8] G. Luna, G. P. Lewis, C. D. Banna, O. Skalli, and S. K. Fisher, "Expression profiles of nestin and synemin in reactive astrocytes and Müller cells following retinal injury: a comparison with glial fibrillar acidic protein and vimentin," *Molecular Vision*, vol. 16, pp. 2511–2523, 2010.

[9] C. Guidry, J. L. King, and J. O. Mason, "Fibrocontractive müller cell phenotypes in proliferative diabetic retinopathy," *Investigative Ophthalmology and Visual Science*, vol. 50, no. 4, pp. 1929–1939, 2009.

[10] M. A. Tackenberg, B. A. Tucker, J. S. Swift et al., "Müller cell activation, proliferation and migration following laser injury," *Molecular Vision*, vol. 15, pp. 1886–1896, 2009.

[11] M. Okada, M. Matsumura, N. Ogino, and Y. Honda, "Muller cells in detached human retina express glial fibrillary acidic protein and vimentin," *Graefe's Archive for Clinical and Experimental Ophthalmology*, vol. 228, no. 5, pp. 467–474, 1990.

[12] G. P. Lewis, C. J. Guerin, D. H. Anderson, B. Matsumoto, and S. K. Fisher, "Rapid changes in the expression of glial cell proteins caused by experimental retinal detachment," *American Journal of Ophthalmology*, vol. 118, no. 3, pp. 368–376, 1994.

[13] S. F. Geller, G. P. Lewis, D. H. Anderson, and S. K. Fisher, "Use of the MIB-1 antibody for detecting proliferating cells in the retina," *Investigative Ophthalmology and Visual Science*, vol. 36, no. 3, pp. 737–744, 1995.

[14] A. Andrews, E. Balciunaite, F. L. Leong et al., "Platelet-derived growth factor plays a key role in proliferative vitreoretinopathy," *Investigative Ophthalmology and Visual Science*, vol. 40, no. 11, pp. 2683–2689, 1999.

[15] D. M. Fastenberg, K. R. Diddie, J. M. Delmage, and K. Dorey, "Intraocular injection of silicone oil for experimental proliferative vitreoretinopathy," *American Journal of Ophthalmology*, vol. 95, no. 5, pp. 663–667, 1983.

[16] S. G. Robbins, R. N. Mixon, and D. J. Wilson, "Platelet-derived growth factor ligands and receptors immunolocalized in proliferative retinal diseases," *Investigative Ophthalmology and Visual Science*, vol. 35, no. 10, pp. 3649–3663, 1995.

[17] J. Cui, H. Lei, A. Samad et al., "PDGF receptors are activated in human epiretinal membranes," *Experimental Eye Research*, vol. 88, no. 3, pp. 438–444, 2009.

[18] Y. Ikuno and A. Kazlauskas, "An in vivo gene therapy approach for experimental proliferative vitreoretinopathy using the truncated platelet-derived growth factor α receptor," *Investigative Ophthalmology and Visual Science*, vol. 43, no. 7, pp. 2406–2411, 2002.

[19] Y. Zheng, Y. Ikuno, M. Ohj et al., "Platelet-derived growth factor receptor kinase inhibitor AG1295 and inhibition of experimental proliferative vitreoretinopathy," *Japanese Journal of Ophthalmology*, vol. 47, no. 2, pp. 158–165, 2003.

[20] H. Lei, G. Velez, J. Cui et al., "N-acetylcysteine suppresses retinal detachment in an experimental model of proliferative vitreoretinopathy," *American Journal of Pathology*, vol. 177, no. 1, pp. 132–140, 2010.

[21] D. G. Charteris, J. Downie, G. W. Aylward, C. Sethi, and P. Luthert, "Intraretinal and periretinal pathology in anterior proliferative vitreoretinopathy," *Graefe's Archive for Clinical and Experimental Ophthalmology*, vol. 245, no. 1, pp. 93–100, 2007.

[22] M. A. Peters, J. M. Burke, M. Clowry, G. W. Abrams, and G. A. Williams, "Development of traction retinal detachments following intravitreal injections of retinal Muller and pigment epithelial cells," *Graefe's Archive for Clinical and Experimental Ophthalmology*, vol. 224, no. 6, pp. 554–563, 1986.

[23] B. Kirchhof and N. Sorgente, "Pathogenesis of proliferative vitreoretinopathy. Modulation of retinal pigment epithelial cell functions by vitreous and macrophages," *Developments in Ophthalmology*, vol. 16, pp. 1–53, 1989.

[24] H. Lei, M.-A. Rhéaume, G. Velez, S. Mukai, and A. Kazlauskas, "Expression of PDGFRα is a determinant of the PVR potential of ARPE19 cells," *Investigative Ophthalmology and Visual Science*, vol. 52, no. 9, pp. 5016–5021, 2011.

[25] S. G. Giannelli, G. C. Demontis, G. Pertile, P. Rama, and V. Broccoli, "Adult human Müller glia cells are a highly efficient source of rod photoreceptors," *Stem Cells*, vol. 29, no. 2, pp. 344–356, 2011.

[26] C. Tian, T. Zhao, Y. Zeng, and Z. Q. Yin, "Increased Müller cell de-differentiation after grafting of retinal stem cell in the sub-retinal space of royal college of surgeons rats," *Tissue Engineering Part A*, vol. 17, no. 19-20, pp. 2523–2532, 2011.

[27] E. O. Johnsen, R. C. Frøen, R. Albert et al., "Activation of neural progenitor cells in human eyes with proliferative vitreoretinopathy," *Experimental Eye Research*, vol. 98, no. 1, pp. 28–36, 2012.

[28] B. Bhatia, H. Jayaram, S. Singhal, M. F. Jones, and G. A. Limb, "Differences between the neurogenic and proliferative abilities of Müller glia with stem cell characteristics and the ciliary epithelium from the adult human eye," *Experimental Eye Research*, vol. 93, no. 6, pp. 852–861, 2011.

[29] J. M. Lawrence, S. Singhal, B. Bhatia et al., "MIO-M1 cells and similar Müller glial cell lines derived from adult human retina exhibit neural stem cell characteristics," *Stem Cells*, vol. 25, no. 8, pp. 2033–2043, 2007.

3

Amniotic Fluid and Amniotic Membrane Stem Cells: Marker Discovery

Maria G. Roubelakis,[1, 2] Ourania Trohatou,[1, 2] and Nicholas P. Anagnou[1, 2]

[1] *Laboratory of Biology, University of Athens School of Medicine, 115 27 Athens, Greece*
[2] *Cell and Gene Therapy Laboratory, Centre of Basic Research II, Biomedical Research Foundation of the Academy of Athens (BRFAA), 115 27 Athens, Greece*

Correspondence should be addressed to Maria G. Roubelakis, mroubelaki@bioacademy.gr

Academic Editor: Mahmud Bani

Amniotic fluid (AF) and amniotic membrane (AM) have been recently characterized as promising sources of stem or progenitor cells. Both not only contain subpopulations with stem cell characteristics resembling to adult stem cells, such as mesenchymal stem cells, but also exhibit some embryonic stem cell properties like (i) expression of pluripotency markers, (ii) high expansion in vitro, or (iii) multilineage differentiation capacity. Recent efforts have been focused on the isolation and the detailed characterization of these stem cell types. However, variations in their phenotype, their heterogeneity described by different groups, and the absence of a single marker expressed only in these cells may prevent the isolation of a pure homogeneous stem cell population from these sources and their potential use of these cells in therapeutic applications. In this paper, we aim to summarize the recent progress in marker discovery for stem cells derived from fetal sources such as AF and AM, using novel methodologies based on transcriptomics, proteomics, or secretome analyses.

1. Introduction

Both amniotic fluid (AF) and amniotic membrane (AM) represent rich sources of stem cells that can be used in the future for clinical therapeutic applications. Ethical concerns regarding the isolation of stem cells from these sources are minimized [1–3], in contrary to the issues emerging from human embryonic stem cell (ESC) research [4–6]. AF is collected during scheduled amniocenteses between 15th and 19th week of gestation for prenatal diagnosis and the excess of sample can be used for cell sourcing [2, 4–9], whereas AM is usually collected during the caesarean sections of term pregnancies [10, 11]. Given the heterogeneity of the stem cell populations derived from these sources, the isolation of specific cell types is difficult and requires a detailed phenotypic and molecular characterization of the respective cells. Studies that include *omics* approaches are fundamental in better understanding the mechanisms of molecular expression of these cells and defining the correct methodologies for their isolation, prior to their use in therapeutic approaches.

This paper aims to present the main biological and molecular characteristics of AF- and AM-derived stem cells and also to highlight the recent advances in marker discovery using global methodologies, such as transcriptomics, proteomics, or secretome analyses.

1.1. Amniotic Fluid. AF serves as a protective liquid for the developing embryo, providing mechanical support and the required nutrients during embryogenesis [1, 3]. Amniocentesis has been used for many decades as a routine procedure for fetal karyotyping and prenatal diagnosis, allowing the detection of a variety of genetic diseases [1, 3, 12].

The major component of AF is water; however its overall composition varies throughout pregnancy. At the beginning of pregnancy, the amniotic osmolarity is similar to the fetal plasma. After keratinization of the fetal skin amniotic osmolarity decreases relatively to maternal or fetal plasma, mainly due to the inflow of fetal urine [1]. More interestingly, AF also represents a rich source of a stem cell population deriving from either the fetus or the surrounding amniotic membrane [1, 12]. Additional investigations by several groups have been recently focused on the cellular properties of amniotic derived cells and their potential use in preclinical models [13–18] and in transplantation therapies [7, 17, 19–24].

1.1.1. Amniotic Fluid Stem Cells (AFSCs). The amniotic fluid cells (AFCs) represent a heterogeneous population derived from the three germ layers. These cells share an epithelial origin and are derived from either the developing embryo or the inner surface of the amniotic membrane, which are characterized as amniotic membrane stem cells [12]. The AFCs are mainly composed of three groups of adherent cells, categorized based on their morphological, growth, and biochemical characteristics [12]. Epithelioid (E-type) cell are cuboidal to columnar cells derived from the fetal skin and urine, amniotic fluid (AF-type) cells are originating from fetal membranes, and fibroblastic (F-type) cells are generated mainly from fibrous connective tissue. Both AF- and F-type cells share a fibroblastoid morphology and the dominant cell type appears to be the AF-type, coexpressing keratins and vimentins [1–3, 8, 9, 25–27]. Several studies have documented that human amniotic fluid stem cells (AFSCs) can be easily obtained from a small amount of second trimester AF, collected during routine amniocenteses [2, 4–9], a procedure with spontaneous abortion rate ranging from 0.06 to 0.5% [2, 28, 29]. Up to date, a number of different cultivation protocols have been reported, leading to enriched stem cell populations. The isolation of AFSC and the respective culture protocols were summarized in a recent review by Klemmt et al. [3] and can be categorized as follows: (i) a single step cultivation protocol, where the primary culture was left undisturbed for 7 days or more until the first colonies appear [2, 3, 30–32], (ii) a two-step cultivation protocol, where amniocytes, not attached after 5 days in culture, were collected and further expanded [3, 5, 33], (iii) cell surface marker selection for CD117 (c-kit receptor) [3, 7, 34, 35], (iv) mechanical isolation of the initial mesenchymal progenitor cell colonies formed in the initial cultures [9], and (v) short-term cultures to isolate fibroblastoid colonies [36]. The majority of the AFSCs, isolated following these methodologies, shared a multipotent mesenchymal phenotype and exhibited higher proliferation potential and a wider differentiation potential compared to adult MSCs [2, 4–7, 9, 24, 37].

1.2. Amniotic Membrane (AM). The amniotic membrane, lacking any vascular tissue, forms most of the inner layer of the fetal membrane [12, 38] and is composed of 3 layers: (i) an epithelial monolayer consisting of epithelial cells, (ii) an acellular intermediate basement layer, and (iii) an outer mesenchymal cell layer, rich in mesenchymal stem cells and placed in close proximity to the chorion [12, 38]. AM was used in clinic for many decades for wound healing in burns, promoting epithelium formation and protecting against infection [39, 40]. Recently, the use of AM has been evaluated as a wound dressing material for surgical defects of the oral

mucosa [41], ocular surface reconstruction [40, 42], corneal perforations [43, 44], and bladder augmentation [45].

1.2.1. Amniotic Membrane Stem Cells (AMSCs). Amniotic membrane stem cells (AMSCs) include two types, the amniotic epithelial cells (AECs) and the amniotic membrane mesenchymal stem cells (AM-MSCs) derived from the amniotic epithelial and the amniotic mesenchymal layers, respectively [12, 46]. Both cell types are originated during the pregastrulation stages of the developing embryo, before the delineation of the three primary germ layers and are mostly of epithelial nature [38, 47]. A variety of protocols have been established for AECs and AM-MSCs isolation, primarily based on the mechanical separation of the AM from the chorionic membrane and the subsequent enzymatic digestion [47–50]. AM-MSCs exhibited plastic adherence and fibroblastoid morphology, while AECs displayed a cobblestone epithelial phenotype. AM-MSCs shared similar phenotypic characteristics with the ones derived from adult sources. More interestingly, AM-MSCs, similarly to AF-MSCs, exhibited a higher proliferation rate compared to MSCs derived from adult sources [12, 51] and a multilineage differentiation potential into cells derived from the three germ layers [27].

2. Immunophenotype

2.1. Amniotic Fluid Stem Cells. The AF has recently emerged as an alternative fetal source of a variety of cells of stem cell origin [1, 3]. Herein, we aim to summarize the key markers that characterize AFSCs. To date, MSCs represent the best characterized subpopulation of AFSCs. The AF-MSCs exhibited typical mesenchymal marker expression, such as CD90, CD73, CD105, CD29, CD166, CD49e, CD58, and CD44, determined by flow cytometry analyses [2, 5–8, 10, 12, 21, 32, 33, 52, 53]. Additionally, these cells expressed the HLA-ABC antigens, whereas the expression of the hematopoietic markers CD34 and CD45, the endothelial marker CD31, and the HLA-DR antigen was undetected [2, 5, 6, 32]. More importantly, the majority of cultured AF-MSCs expressed pluripotency markers such as the octamer binding protein 3/4 (Oct-3/4), the homebox transcription factor Nanog (Nanog), and the stage-specific embryonic antigen 4 (SSEA-4) [2, 5–7, 9, 21, 32, 33, 52].

It was also reported that amniocyte cultures contain a small population of CD117 (a tyrosine kinase specific for stem cell factor present primarily in ESCs and primordial germ cells) positive cells that can be clonally expanded in culture [7]. The differentiation properties of CD117$^+$ AFS were tested for the first time in vivo, proving in this way their stem cell identity [7]. Experimental evidence suggested that AFSCs are derived from spindle-shaped fibroblastoid cells [10].

In an attempt to analyze the AFSCs subpopulations, our group recently identified two morphologically distinct populations of AFSCs of mesenchymal origin, with different proliferation and differentiation properties, termed as spindle shaped (SS) and round shaped (RS) [9]. Both subpopulations were expressing mesenchymal stem cell markers at similar levels. However, it was identified that SS colonies expressed higher levels of CD90 and CD44 antigens compared to RS colonies [9].

2.2. Amniotic Membrane Stem Cells (AMSCs). A detailed immunophenotype analysis of AMSCs revealed the expression of antigens, such as CD13, CD29, CD44, CD49e, CD54, CD73, CD90, CD105, CD117^{low}, CD166, CD27^{low}, stromal stem cell marker 1 (Stro-1), SSEA-3, SSEA-4, collagen I and III (Col1/Col3), alpha-smooth muscle actin (α-SMA), CD44, vimentin (Vim), fibroblast surface protein (FSP), and HLA-ABC antigen [10, 12, 27]. However, intercellular adhesion molecule 1 (ICAM-1) was expressed in very low levels and proteins TRA-1-60, vascular cell adhesion protein 1 (VCAM-1), von Willebrand factor (vWF), platelet endothelial cell adhesion molecule (PECAM-1), CD3, and HLA-DR were not detected [10, 27]. One of the most abundant proteins found in AM derived cells is laminin, which plays a key role in differentiation, cell shape and migration, and tissue regeneration [54, 55]. RT-PCR analysis further showed that AMSCs expressed genes, such as Oct-3/4, zinc finger protein 42 (zfp42 or Rex-1), stem cell factor protein (SCF), neural cell adhesion molecule (NCAM), nestin (NES), bone morphogenetic protein 4 (BMP-4), GATA binding protein 4 (GATA-4), and hepatocyte nuclear factor 4α (HNF-4α) even in high passages. Brachyury, fibroblast growth factor 5 (FGF5), paired box protein (Pax-6), and bone morphogenetic protein 2 (BMP2) transcripts were not detected [10, 12]. Similarly, AECs were positive for CD10, CD13, CD29, CD44, CD49e, CD73, CD90, CD105, CD117, CD166, Stro-1, HLA-ABC, and HLA-DQ^{low} and negative for CD14, CD34, CD45, CD49d, and HLA-DR expressions, as determined by FACS analyses [27, 47–50]. Further investigation showed that AECs were expressing stem cell markers such as SSEA-1, SSEA-3, SSEA-4, Nanog, sex determining region Y-box 2 (Sox2), Tra1-60 and Tra1-80, fibroblast growth factor 4 (FGF4), Rex-1, cryptic protein (CFC-1), and prominin 1 (PROM-1) [38, 50].

3. Transcriptomics

3.1. Amniotic Fluid Stem Cells. A functional analysis of the gene expression signature of AF-MSCs compared to bone-marrow- (BM-), cord-blood- (CB-), and AM-MSCs was initially performed by Tsai et al. [11]. Genes expressed in MSCs from all three sources could be categorized in groups related to (i) extracellular matrix remodeling (CD44, collagen II (COL2), insulin-like growth factor 2 (IGF2), and tissue inhibitor of metalloproteinase 1 (TIMP1)), (ii) cytoskeletal regulation (urokinase-type plasminogen activator (PLAU) and receptor (PLAUR)), (iii) chemokine regulation and adhesion (alpha actinin 1 (ACTN1), actin-related protein complex subunit 1B (ARPC1B) and thrombospondin 1 (THBS1)), (iv) plasmin activation (tissue factor pathway inhibitor 2 (TFPI2)), (v) transforming growth factor β (TGFβ) receptor signaling (caveolin 1 (Cav1), caveolin 2 (Cav2), cyclin-dependent kinase inhibitor 1A (CDKN1A)), and (vi) genes encoding E3 ubiquitin ligases (SMURF) [11]. The upregulated genes in AF-MSCs compared to BM-, CB-,

and AM-MSCs included molecules involved in uterine maturation and contraction, such as oxytocin receptor (OXTR) and regulation of prostaglandin synthesis, such as phospholipase A2 (PLA2G10). Other upregulated genes in this group were involved in signal transduction related to (i) thrombin triggered response ((F2R and F2RL)), (ii) hedgehog signaling ((hedgehog acyltransferase (HHAT)), and (iii) G-protein-related pathways (rho-related GTP-binding protein (RHOF), regulator of G protein signaling 5 and 7 (RGS5, RGS7), and phospholipase C beta 4 (PLCB4)) [11].

In recent studies on AFSCs, Kim et al. described for the first time the gene expression changes in total AFSC population during different passages by illumina microarray analysis. 1970 differentially expressed genes were detected and categorized according to their expression profiles into 9 distinct clusters [56]. Genes with gradually increasing expression levels included chemokine (C-X-C motif) ligand 12 (CXCL12), cadherin 6 (CDH6), and folate receptor 3 (FOLR3). Downregulated genes were among others, cyclin D2 (CCND2), keratin 8 (K8), IGF2, natriuretic peptide precursor (BNP) B, and cellular retinoic acid binding protein 2 (CRABPII) [56]. To obtain further information, chip data analysis on aging genes was performed and revealed upregulation of gene transcripts, such as nerve growth factor beta (NGFβ), insulin receptor substrate 2 (IRS-2), insulin-like growth factor binding protein 3 (IGFBP-3), and apolipoprotein E (APOE). Expression of genes, such as PLAU, E2F transcription factor 1 (E2F1), IGF2, breast cancer type 1 susceptibility gene (BRCA1), DNA topoisomerase 2-alpha (TOP2A), proliferating cell nuclear antigen (PCNA), forkhead box M1 (FOXM1), cyclin-A2 gene (CCNA2), budding uninhibited by benzimidazoles 1 homolog beta (BUB1B), and cyclin dependent kinase 1 (CDC2), was gradually downregulated during culture [56].

Wolfrum et al. performed a global gene expression analysis of AFSCs compared to iPSCs derived from AF (AFiPSC) and ESCs [57]. Among these, genes related to self renewal and pluripotency (1299 genes e.g., POU class 5 homeobox 1 (POU5F1), Sox2, Nanog, microRNA-binding protein LIN28) and AFSCs-specificity (665 genes, e.g., OXTR, HHAT, RGS5, neurofibromatosis type 2 (NF2), protectin (CD59), tumor necrosis factor superfamily member 10 (TNFSF10), 5′-nucleotidase (NT5E)) were detected in AFSCs [57]. Furthermore, the authors examined the expression of senescence and telomere associated genes in AFSCs of early and later passage, in order to study the effect of reprogramming on bypassing senescence observed in AFSC cultures. Sixty-four genes were identified as differentially expressed in AFSCs compared to AFiPSC lines. Of these, telomere-associated genes and genes involved in regulating cell cycle, such as the mitotic arrest deficient-like 2 (MAD2L2), the poly ADP-ribose polymerase 1 (PARP1), replication protein A3 (RPA3), the dyskeratosis congenita 1 (DKC1), the mutS homolog 6 (MSH6), the CHK1 checkpoint homolog (CHEK1), the polo-like kinase 1 (PLK1), the POU class 2 homeobox 1 (POU2F1), the CDC2, the Bloom syndrome gene RecQ helicase-like (BLM), the Werner syndrome RecQ helicase-like (WRN), the DNA methyltransferase 1 (DNMT1), the DNA methyltransferase 3 beta (DNMT3B), the lamin B1 (LMNB1), and the DNA replication factor 1

(CDT1), were downregulated in AFSCs compared to AFiPSCs and ESCs. In contrast, peptidylprolyl cis/trans isomerase (PIN1), lamin A/C (LMNA), growth arrest and DNA damage inducible alpha (GADD45A), chromobox homolog 6 (CBX6), NADPH oxidase 4 (NOX4), endoglin (ENG), histone H2B type 2-E (HIST2H2BE), CDKN1A, CDKN2A growth differentiation factor 15 (GDF15), and serine protease inhibitor 1 (SERPINE1), among others, were upregulated in AFSCs compared to AFiPSCs and ESCs [57].

3.2. Amniotic Membrane Stem Cells. Transcriptomic analysis using DNA microarrays has been reported for AM-MSCs [11]. These experimental data provided information on the AM-MSC gene expression pattern compared to gene expression profiles of AF, CB, and BM-MSCs. Several upregulated genes in AM-MSCs involved in immune adaptation regulation between the maternoplacental interface were identified. Among others, spondin 2 (SPON2), interferon, alpha inducible protein 27 (IFI27), bradykinin receptor B1 (BDKRB1), small inducible cytokine subfamily B member 5 and 6 (SCYB5, SCYB6), and Yamaguchi sarcoma viral-related oncogene homolog (LYN) were found to be upregulated [11]. In addition, other genes with increased expression in AM-MSCs compared to AF, CB, and BM-MSCs included (i) transcription factors, such as forkhead box F1 (FOXF1), heart and neural crest derivatives expressed 2 (HAND2), and transcription factor 21 (TCF21) and (ii) metabolic enzymes, such as dipeptidyl-peptidase 6 (DPP6), tryptophan 2,3-dioxygenase (TDO2), and sialyltransferases (STs) [11].

4. Proteomics

4.1. Amniotic Fluid Stem Cells. Proteomic studies on the total AFSC population, including epithelioid (E-type), amniotic fluid specific (AF-type), and fibroblastic (F-type) cells, revealed 2400 spots that resulted in the identification of 432 different gene products. The majority of the proteins was localized in cytoplasm (33%), mitochondria (16%), and nucleus (15%) and represented mainly enzymes (174 proteins) and structural proteins (75 proteins). A relatively high percentage of membrane and membrane-associated proteins were also present (7%) [58]. Among the detected proteins, 9 were corresponding to epithelial cells, such as ATP synthase D chain (ATP5H), NADH-ubiquinone oxidoreductase 30 kDa subunit (NUIM), annexin II (Anx2), annexin IV (Anx4), 40S ribosomal protein SA (Rpsa), glutathione S-transferase P (GSTP), major vault protein, and cytokeratins 19 and 7 (CK-19, CK-7), whereas 12 proteins were reported to be expressed in fibroblasts, including fibronectins, tropomyosins, transgelin (TAGLN), arp2/3 complex 34 kDa subunit (P34-arp), gelsolin (Gsn), elongation factor 1-β (EF-1β), and others. Eight proteins were found to be expressed in keratinocytes, including keratins, ribonucleoproteins, Anx2, aetyl-CoA acetyl-transferase (ACAT1), and others, three to be expressed in epidermis, including tropomyosins and keratins and one in mesenchymal cell type (vimentin 1 (Vim 1)) [58].

Recent studies provided evidence that a diversity of metabolic enzyme expression in the amnion cells is involved

in metabolic and genetic syndromes, and thus, their detection might be important for prenatal diagnosis. A more detailed analysis for determining specific metabolic enzymes present in AFSCs was reported by Oh et al. [59]. Ninety-nine proteins had been identified, such as carbohydrate handing enzymes, amino acid handling enzymes, proteins of purine metabolism, and enzymes of intermediary metabolism [59, 60].

A proteomic analysis was also performed on different culture passages of CD117$^+$ AFSCs, exhibiting variations in protein expression that mainly occurred in early passages [35]. Twenty-three proteins were differentially expressed between early and late passages with the most sticking downregulated proteins, the Col1, the Col2, the vinculin (Vcl), the CRABP II, the stathmin (STMN1), and the cofilin-1 (CFL1). In contrast, TAGLN and Col3 are increased during passages [35]. Proteins that showed dysregulated levels along the passages were the 26S protease regulatory subunit 7 (PSMD7), the ubiquitin carboxyl terminal hydrolase isoenzyme L1 (UCH-L1), the heterogeneous nuclear ribonuclear protein H (hnRNP H), and the TAR DNA-binding protein 43 (TDP-43) [35].

In 2007, the proteomic map of human AF-MSCs was constructed and directly compared to the one derived from BM-MSCs [2]. 261 different proteins were identified in AF-MSCs with the majority of the proteins localized in the cytoplasm (41%), whereas others were found in the endoplasmic reticulum (8%), nucleus (13%), mitochondria (12%), ribosomes (1%), cytoskeleton (6%), cytoplasm and the nucleus (5%), and secreted (2%) proteins [2]. AF-MSCs expressed a number of proteins related to proliferation and cell maintenance, such as ubiquilin-1 (UBQLN1), which is known to control cell cycle progression and cell growth, the proliferation associated protein 2G4 (PA2G4), a nucleolar growth-regulating protein, the secreted protein acidic and rich in cysteine (SPARC), which is regulated during embryogenesis and is involved in the control of the cell cycle and cell adhesion, and the enhancer of rudimentary homolog (ERH) that also regulates cell cycle [2]. TAGLN and galectin 1 (Gal 1), both present in stem cells and related to differentiation, were also abundantly expressed in AF-MSCs. Other proteins expressed in high levels in AF-MSCs were related to (i) development, such as Deltex-3-like (DTX3L), and (ii) cytoskeletal organization and movement, such as CFL1, the coactosin-like protein (CLP), and the enabled protein homolog (Enah). As expected, Vim was also expressed in high amounts in AF-MSCs. In this study, a detailed comparison of the common identified proteins in AF cells [58] and AF-MSCs was also described [2].

In our later study [9], we established the proteomic map of the two morphologically distinct AF mesenchymal progenitor cell types (SS and RS) by 2-DE. Twenty-five proteins were differentially expressed in the two subpopulations. Proteins upregulated in SS-AF-MSCs compared to RS-AF-MSCs included reticulocalbin-3 precursor (RCN3), collagen α1 (I) (COL1α1), FK506-binding protein 9 precursor (FKBP9), Rho GDP-dissociation inhibitor 1 (RhoGDI), chloride intracellular channel protein 4 (CLIC4), tryptophanyl-tRNA synthetase (TrpRS), and 70 kD heat shock protein (HSP70). Peroxiredoxin 2 (Prdx2), 60 kD heat shock protein (HSP60), GSTP, and Anx4 were upregulated in RS-AFMPCs. However, proteins identified in RS-AF-MSCs only included cytokeratin-8, -18, and -19 (CK-8, -18, and CK-19), cathepsin B (CTSB), CLP, and integrin αV protein (CD51). Mesenchymal-related proteins, such as Vim, Gal, Gsn, and prohibitin (PHB), were expressed at the same levels in both populations [9].

4.2. Amniotic Membrane Stem Cells. A detailed approach for studying human AM proteins was described by Hopkinson et al. [61]. In this study, the authors performed a proteomic analysis of AM samples that were prepared for human transplantation, by using 2-DE gels. The wash media from the AM samples were also examined and the secreted proteins were identified. Proteins detected in both AM and the wash media suggested that partial protein release had occurred. These proteins were mostly soluble cytoplasmic proteins and were categorized according to their subcellular localization and function [61]. One example of the most abundant and consistent proteins in AM is THBS1 which is reported to play role in wound repair, inflammatory response, and angiogenesis [62, 63]. Mimecan (also named osteoglycin/OGN) is another protein detected in AM that represents a small leucine-rich proteoglycan, found in the ECM of connective tissue. Mimecan is reported to maintain the tensile strength and hydration of the tissue [61, 64–66]. In addition, the larger form of mimecan was expressed in AM cells and was susceptible to proteolytic cleavage [65]. TGF-β-induced protein ig-h3 (βIG-H3), an ECM adhesive molecule acting as a membrane-associated growth factor during cell differentiation and wound healing, and intergrin α6 (CD49f), a component of α6β4 integrin, were also present in significant amounts in AM cells [61, 67, 68]. It is well known that α6β4-βIG-H3 interaction plays an important role in mediating cell adhesion and wound repair signaling pathways [69].

Another important study by Baharvand et al. [70] was focused on the analysis of epithelium-denuded human AM showing both quantitative and qualitative differences compared to nontreated AM [61]. They investigated the proteome of the human AM epithelium, which was used as a limbal stem cell niche for treating ocular surface reconstruction [71, 72]. 515 spots were detected in all the 2-DE gels and 43 proteins were identified using MALDI TOF/TOF MS in AM. The most abundant proteins were different isoforms of lumican (LUM) and OGN, both members of the proteoglycan (PG) family. In particular, OGN might play role in many biological processes including cell growth, angiogenesis, and inflammation [66]. Other proteins detected included collagen VI α-1/α-2 (Col6a1/Col6a2), fibrinogen beta chain (FGB), transglutaminase 2 isoform A (TGM2A), b-actin variant (ACTB), 70 kD heat shock protein 5 (HSPA5), nidogen 2 (NID2), CD49f, βIG-H3, and tubulointerstitial nephritis (TIN) [70]. Some of the proteins identified in this study were also related to extracellular matrix (ECM). Among the detected ones, fibronectin (FN), laminins, and collagen IV (Col4) and VII were reported to promote epithelial adhesion and migration [73, 74].

5. Secretome

Recently, significant progress has been made regarding the analysis of the secreted proteins from AFSCs. It has been documented that AFSC secretome was responsible for enhancing vasculogenesis and was capable of evoking a strong angiogenic response in murine recipients [75]. According to this study, a detailed analysis of the AFSC-conditioned media revealed the presence of known proangiogenic and antiangiogenic factors using Luminex's MAP Technology. Vascular endothelial growth factor (VEGF), stromal cell-derived factor 1 (SDF-1), interleukin 8 (IL-8), monocyte chemotactic protein 1 (MCP-1), and two angiogenesis inhibitors, interferon-gamma (IFNγ) and interferon gamma-induced protein 10 (IP-10), were identified as secreted proteins [75–77]. It was also demonstrated that a relative small number of AFSC was enough to secrete a detectable amount of proangiogenic growth factors and cytokines. The secretion of these can be regulated in a dose-dependent manner according to the initial cell number of the cells used [24, 75].

A systematic study on AFSC-secreted proteins led to the conclusion that proangiogenic soluble factors from AFSCs can mediate the recruitment of endothelial progenitors in an ischemic rat model [78]. In particular, conditioned medium derived from AFSCs could topically deliver angiogenic growth factors and cytokines into the skin flap of the ischemic rat model and was responsible for triggering the endogenous repair by recruiting endothelial progenitor cells [78].

In our recent studies, we examined the therapeutic potential of an AF-MSCs and their secreted molecules in mice with acute hepatic failure [24]. A variety of cytokines and growth factor were detected in AF-MSC conditioned medium. Cytokines such as interleukin 10 (IL-10), interleukin 27 (IL-27), interleukin 17 family (IL-17E), interleukin 12p70 (IL-12p70), interleukin-1 beta (IL-1β), and interleukin-1 receptor antagonist (IL-1ra), responsible for inducing local and systemic downregulation of pro-inflammatory mediators, were detected. SERPINE1, MCP-1, and SDF-1, responsible for promoting tissue repair, were also secreted [24, 79, 80]. Interestingly, among the highly expressed growth factors were platelet-derived endothelial cell growth factor (PD-ECGF), endostatin/collagen XVII (EN/Col17), urinary plasminogen activator (uPA), TIMP1, TIMP2, heparin-binding EGF-like growth factor (HB-EGF), fibroblast growth factor 7 (FGF7), and epidermal growth factor (EGF), responsible for liver regeneration and tissue repair [24, 81].

6. Summary

The current data so far suggest that amniotic fluid and amniotic membrane may represent promising sources for stem cells of mesenchymal origin. Indeed, MSCs are more abundant and a wide range of protocols has been described for their isolation. However, it is reported that different culture conditions of the same type of cells may affect their differential gene expression pattern, which represents a limitation for their isolation and expansion in vitro. Studies

Transcriptomics

AFSCs:
IGF2, PLAU, OXTR, HHAT, RCS5 [11, 57], CDC2 [56, 57], CD44, COL2, TIMP1, ACT1, ARPC1B, TSP1, TFRI2, TGFβ, Cav1, Cav2, CDKN1A, SMURF, F2R, F2RL, IL7R, RHOF, RGS7 [11], CXCL12, CDH6, FOLR3, CCND2, K8, CRABPII, NGFB, IRS2, APOE, IGFBP3, E2F1, TOP2A, FOXM1, BUBB1 [56], Nanog, Sox2, POU5F1, NF2, CD59, NTSE, MAD2L2, PARP1, RPA3, DKC1, MSH6, PLK1, CHEK1, BLM, WRN, CDT1, PIN1, DNMT1, DNMT3B, LMNB1, LMNA, CDKN2A, GADD45A, GDF15, SERPINE 1 [57]
- - - - - - - - - - - - - - -
AMSCs:
SPON2, IFI27, BDBKRB1, SCYB5, SCYB6, FOXF1, HAND2, TCF21, DPP6, TDO2, STs [11]

Proteomics

AFSCs:
TAGLN [2, 34, 58], Gsn, Anx4, GSTP, CK-19 [9, 58], Vim [2, 9, 53], CFL1 [2, 34], Col1 [9, 34], Gal, CLP [2, 9], Anx2, Rpsa , ATP5H, CK-7, EF-1β, ACAT1, P34-arp, NUIM [58],
Col2, Col3, VCL, CRABPII, STMN1, PSMD7, UCH-L1, hnRNPH, TDP43 [34], UBQLN1, PA2GA, SPARC, ERH, DTXEL, Enah [2], RCN3, FKBP9, CLIC4, HSP60, HSP70, Prdx2, RhoGDI, CTSB, CD51, CK-8, CK-18 [9]
- - - - - - - - - - - - - - -
AMSCs:
OGN, βIG-H3, CD49F [61, 70], THBS1 [61], LUM, COL, TGM2A, ACTB, FGB, NID2, HSPA5 [70]

Secretome

AFSCs:
SDF-1, MCP-1 [75, 23], VEGF, IFNγ, IP-10, IL-8 [70], SERPINE 1, PD-ECGF, FGF7, HB-EGF, EGF, TIMP1, TIMP2, uPA, EN, Col17, IL-10, IL-27, IL-1β, IL-1ra, IL-12p70, IL-17E [23]

Immunophenotype

AFSCs:
CD90, CD73, CD105, CD29, CD166, CD49e, CD58, CD44, HLA-ABC, SSEA-4 [2, 58, 10, 12, 24, 31, 32, 52, 53], CD117 [7]
- - - - - - - - - - - - - - -
AMSCs:
CD13, CD29, CD44, CD49e, CD73, CD90, CD105, CD117, CD166, Stro-1, HLA-ABC, SSEA-3, SSEA-4, Rex-1 [10,12, 37, 46–50], Nanog , Sox2, Tra1-60, Tra1-80, FGF-4, CFC-1, PROM1 [37, 49], CD10, HLA-DQ [46–50] CD27, Col1, Col3, α-SMA, Vim, FSP, Oct-3/4, SCF, NCAM, NES, BMP-4, GATA-4, HNF-4 α [10, 12, 50]

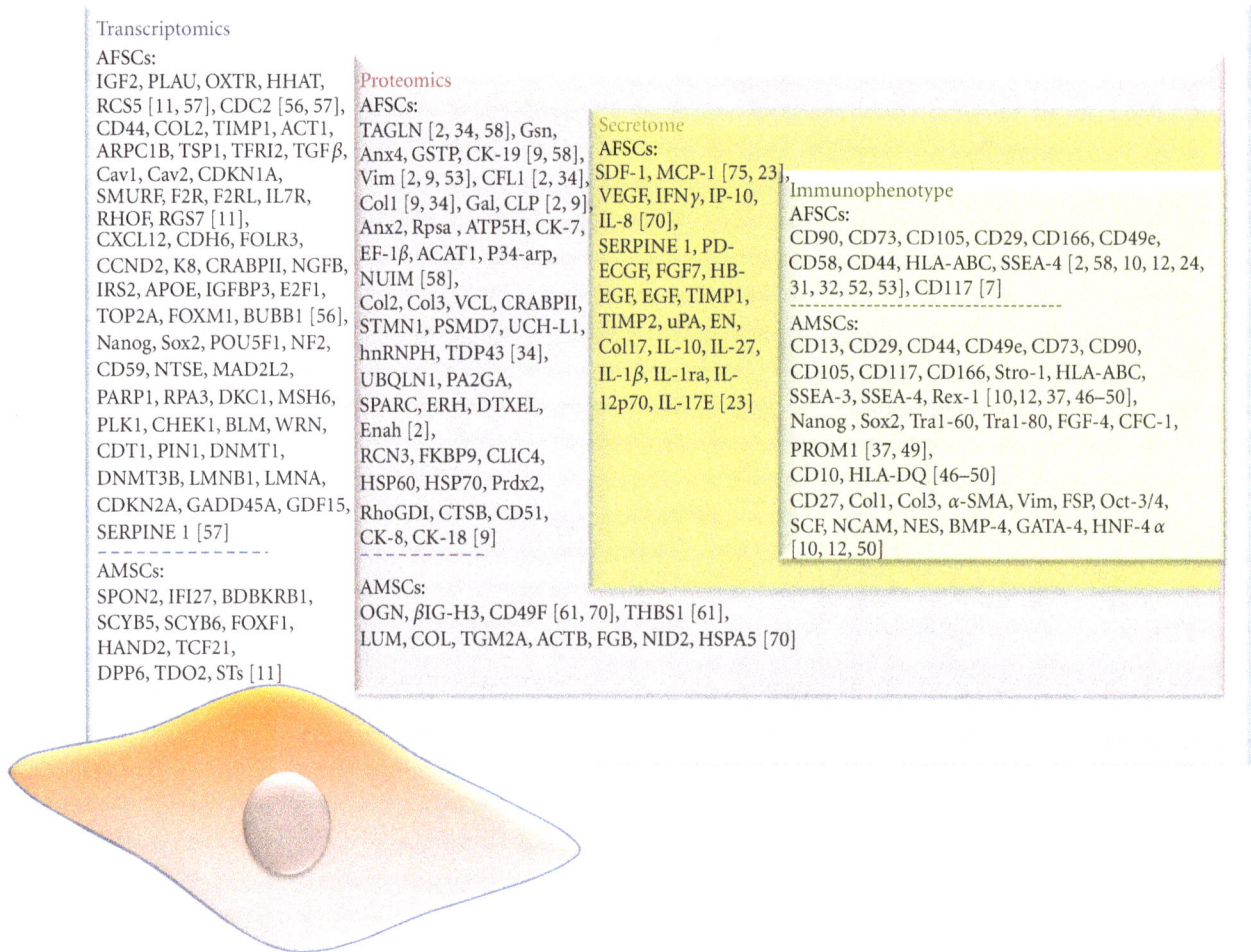

FIGURE 1: Summary of the most important markers identified in AFCs and AMCs by the use of transcriptomics, proteomics, secretome, and immunophenotypic analyses. Proteins identified in more than one study are marked in bold.

including phenotypic analysis, using methodologies such as flow cytometry and immunohistochemistry, as well as transcriptomics, proteomics, and secretome analyses approaches, aim to determine the protein profile of these cells (Figure 1). Data generated by such studies are expected to clarify their differential repertoire and validate the molecular profile of these stem cells. However, the main issue urged to be addressed is the isolation of a homogenous population that may facilitate systematic studies for the elucidation of the function of these multipotent cells.

Such approaches may lead to the identification of key antigens that mirror the phenotype of these cells and explain their distinct features properties. This type of studies will open the way for a systematic and efficient isolation of these cells prior to their use at the clinical setting.

Appendix

Questions for Further Investigation

Which are the appropriate isolation methods and culture conditions of AFSCs or AMSCs that will allow the identification of a consistent phenotype?

Is there a single marker that can be used for AFSCs or AMSCs isolation?

The AFSC and AMSC populations are heterogeneous and differ in their phenotypic and molecular properties. Methods of isolation can result in a homogeneous cell population.

AFSCs or AMSCs can be used as tools in regenerative medicine: establishment of culture conditions with minimal or no animal substances.

Marker Discovery. The AFSCs and the AMSCs initial characterization can be performed by immunophenotype analysis by using well-characterized cell surface markers such as AFSCs: CD90, CD73, CD105, CD29, CD166, CD49e, CD58, CD44, HLA-ABC, SSEA-4; AMSCs: CD13, CD29, CD44, CD49e, CD73, CD90, CD105, CD117, CD166, Stro-1, HLA-ABC, SSEA-3, SSEA-4, Nanog, Sox2, Tra1-60, Tra1-80, FGF-4, CFC-1, and PROM1.

Transcriptomics and Proteomics Revealed the Identification of Key Markers Expressed such as. AFSCs: Nanog, Sox2, POU5F1, NF2, IGF2, PLAU, OXTR, HHAT, RCS5, CDC2, COL2, TAGLN, Gsn, Anx4, GSTP, CK-19, Vim, Col1, and Gal; AMSCs: OGN, βIG-H3, and CD49F.

Since there is no common marker available for AFSC and AMSC, a wider panel of markers needs to be employed. This also urges the conduction of further detailed array and functional analyses in order to define the most appropriate markers for AFSC and AMSC characterization.

Conflict of Interests

The authors declare that they have no conflict of interests.

References

[1] D. Fauza, "Amniotic fluid and placental stem cells," *Best Practice and Research*, vol. 18, no. 6, pp. 877–891, 2004.

[2] M. G. Roubelakis, K. I. Pappa, V. Bitsika et al., "Molecular and proteomic characterization of human mesenchymal stem cells derived from amniotic fluid: comparison to bone marrow mesenchymal stem cells," *Stem Cells and Development*, vol. 16, no. 6, pp. 931–951, 2007.

[3] P. A. Klemmt, V. Vafaizadeh, and B. Groner, "The potential of amniotic fluid stem cells for cellular therapy and tissue engineering," *Expert Opinion on Biological Therapy*, vol. 11, no. 10, pp. 1297–1314, 2011.

[4] P. S. In't Anker, S. A. Scherjon, C. Kleijburg-van der Keur et al., "Amniotic fluid as a novel source of mesenchymal stem cells for therapeutic transplantation [1]," *Blood*, vol. 102, no. 4, pp. 1548–1549, 2003.

[5] M. S. Tsai, J. L. Lee, Y. J. Chang, and S. M. Hwang, "Isolation of human multipotent mesenchymal stem cells from second-trimester amniotic fluid using a novel two-stage culture protocol," *Human Reproduction*, vol. 19, no. 6, pp. 1450–1456, 2004.

[6] M. S. Tsai, S. M. Hwang, Y. L. Tsai, F. C. Cheng, J. L. Lee, and Y. J. Chang, "Clonal amniotic fluid-derived stem cells express characteristics of both mesenchymal and neural stem cells," *Biology of Reproduction*, vol. 74, no. 3, pp. 545–551, 2006.

[7] P. De Coppi, G. Bartsch, M. M. Siddiqui et al., "Isolation of amniotic stem cell lines with potential for therapy," *Nature Biotechnology*, vol. 25, no. 1, pp. 100–106, 2007.

[8] A. R. Prusa and M. Hengstschläger, "Amniotic fluid cells and human stem cell research - A new connection," *Medical Science Monitor*, vol. 8, no. 11, pp. RA253–RA257, 2002.

[9] M. G. Roubelakis, V. Bitsika, D. Zagoura et al., "In vitro and in vivo properties of distinct populations of amniotic fluid mesenchymal progenitor cells," *Journal of Cellular and Molecular Medicine*, vol. 15, no. 9, pp. 1896–1913, 2011.

[10] J. Kim, H. M. Kang, H. Kim et al., "Ex vivo characteristics of human amniotic membrane-derived stem cells," *Cloning and Stem Cells*, vol. 9, no. 4, pp. 581–594, 2007.

[11] M. S. Tsai, S. M. Hwang, K. D. Chen et al., "Functional network analysis of the transcriptomes of mesenchymal stem cells derived from amniotic fluid, amniotic membrane, cord blood, and bone marrow," *Stem Cells*, vol. 25, no. 10, pp. 2511–2523, 2007.

[12] K. I. Pappa and N. P. Anagnou, "Novel sources of fetal stem cells: where do they fit on the developmental continuum?" *Regenerative Medicine*, vol. 4, no. 3, pp. 423–433, 2009.

[13] S. Bollini, K. K. Cheung, J. Riegler et al., "Amniotic fluid stem cells are cardioprotective following acute myocardial infarction," *Stem Cells and Development*, vol. 20, no. 11, pp. 1985–1994, 2011.

[14] P. V. Hauser, R. De Fazio, S. Bruno et al., "Stem cells derived from human amniotic fluid contribute to acute kidney injury recovery," *American Journal of Pathology*, vol. 177, no. 4, pp. 2011–2021, 2010.

[15] W. Y. Lee, H. J. Wei, W. W. Lin et al., "Enhancement of cell retention and functional benefits in myocardial infarction using human amniotic-fluid stem-cell bodies enriched with endogenous ECM," *Biomaterials*, vol. 32, no. 24, pp. 5558–5567, 2011.

[16] T. Maraldi, M. Riccio, E. Resca, A. Pisciotta, G. B. La Sala et al., "Human amniotic fluid stem cells seeded in fibroin scaffold produce in vivo mineralized matrix," *Tissue Engineering Part A*, vol. 17, no. 21-22, pp. 2833–2843, 2011.

[17] S. W. S. Shaw, A. L. David, and P. De Coppi, "Clinical applications of prenatal and postnatal therapy using stem cells retrieved from amniotic fluid," *Current Opinion in Obstetrics and Gynecology*, vol. 23, no. 2, pp. 109–116, 2011.

[18] C. G. Turner, J. D. Klein, S. A. Steigman et al., "Preclinical regulatory validation of an engineered diaphragmatic tendon made with amniotic mesenchymal stem cells," *Journal of Pediatric Surgery*, vol. 46, no. 1, pp. 57–61, 2011.

[19] A. Angelini, C. Castellani, B. Ravara et al., "Stem-cell therapy in an experimental model of pulmonary hypertension and right heart failure: role of paracrine and neurohormonal milieu in the remodeling process," *Journal of Heart and Lung Transplantation*, vol. 30, no. 11, pp. 1281–1293, 2011.

[20] V. Bitsika, M. G. Roubelakis, D. Zagoura, O. Trohatou, and M. Makridakis, "Human amniotic fluid-derived mesenchymal stem cells as therapeutic vehicles: a novel approach for the treatment of bladder cancer," *Stem Cells and Development*. In press.

[21] L. Perin, S. Sedrakyan, S. Giuliani et al., "Protective effect of human amniotic fluid stem cells in an immunodeficient mouse model of acute tubular necrosis," *PLoS ONE*, vol. 5, no. 2, Article ID e9357, 2010.

[22] M. Rosner, K. Schipany, C. Gundacker, B. Shanmugasundaram, K. Li et al., "Renal differentiation of amniotic fluid stem cells: perspectives for clinical application and for studies on specific human genetic diseases," *European Journal of Clinical Investigation*. In press.

[23] C. Rota, B. Imberti, M. Pozzobon, M. Piccoli, P. De Coppi et al., "human amniotic fluid stem cell preconditioning improves their regenerative potential," *Stem Cells and Development*. In press.

[24] D. S. Zagoura, M. G. Roubelakis, V. Bitsika, O. Trohatou, K. I. Pappa et al., "Therapeutic potential of a distinct population of human amniotic fluid mesenchymal stem cells and their secreted molecules in mice with acute hepatic failure," *Gut*. In press.

[25] C. M. Gosden, "Amniotic fluid cell types and culture," *British Medical Bulletin*, vol. 39, no. 4, pp. 348–354, 1983.

[26] H. Hoehn and D. Salk, "Morphological and biochemical heterogeneity of amniotic fluid cells in culture," *Methods in Cell Biology*, vol. 26, pp. 12–34, 1982.

[27] U. Manuelpillai, Y. Moodley, C. V. Borlongan, and O. Parolini, "Amniotic membrane and amniotic cells: potential therapeutic tools to combat tissue inflammation and fibrosis?" *Placenta*, vol. 32, supplement 4, pp. S320–S325, 2011.

[28] N. J. Leschot, M. Verjaal, and P. E. Treffers, "Risks of midtrimester amniocentesis; assessment in 3000 pregnancies," *British Journal of Obstetrics and Gynaecology*, vol. 92, no. 8, pp. 804–807, 1985.

[29] K. A. Eddleman, F. D. Malone, L. Sullivan et al., "Pregnancy loss rates after midtrimester amniocentesis," *Obstetrics and Gynecology*, vol. 108, no. 5, pp. 1067–1072, 2006.

[30] P. S. In't Anker, S. A. Scherjon, C. Kleijburg-Van Der Keur et al., "Isolation of mesenchymal stem cells of fetal or maternal origin from human placenta," *Stem Cells*, vol. 22, no. 7, pp. 1338–1345, 2004.

[31] S. Cipriani, D. Bonini, E. Marchina et al., "Mesenchymal cells from human amniotic fluid survive and migrate after transplantation into adult rat brain," *Cell Biology International*, vol. 31, no. 8, pp. 845–850, 2007.

[32] J. Kim, Y. Lee, H. Kim et al., "Human amniotic fluid-derived stem cells have characteristics of multipotent stem cells," *Cell Proliferation*, vol. 40, no. 1, pp. 75–90, 2007.

[33] P. Bossolasco, T. Montemurro, L. Cova et al., "Molecular and phenotypic characterization of human amniotic fluid cells and their differentiation potential," *Cell Research*, vol. 16, no. 4, pp. 329–336, 2006.

[34] A. Ditadi, P. De Coppi, O. Picone et al., "Human and murine amniotic fluid c-Kit+Lin- cells display hematopoietic activity," *Blood*, vol. 113, no. 17, pp. 3953–3960, 2009.

[35] W. Q. Chen, N. Siegel, L. Li, A. Pollak, M. Hengstschläger, and G. Lubec, "Variations of protein levels in human amniotic fluid stem cells CD117/2 over passages 5-25," *Journal of Proteome Research*, vol. 8, no. 11, pp. 5285–5295, 2009.

[36] N. Sessarego, A. Parodi, M. Podestà et al., "Multipotent mesenchymal stromal cells from amniotic fluid: solid perspectives for clinical application," *Haematologica*, vol. 93, no. 3, pp. 339–346, 2008.

[37] D. M. Delo, P. De Coppi, G. Bartsch, and A. Atala, "Amniotic fluid and placental stem cells," *Methods in Enzymology*, vol. 419, pp. 426–438, 2006.

[38] S. Ilancheran, A. Michalska, G. Peh, E. M. Wallace, M. Pera, and U. Manuelpillai, "Stem cells derived from human fetal membranes display multilineage differentiation potential," *Biology of Reproduction*, vol. 77, no. 3, pp. 577–588, 2007.

[39] B. Bose, "Burn wound dressing with human amniotic membrane," *Annals of the Royal College of Surgeons of England*, vol. 61, no. 6, pp. 444–447, 1979.

[40] Y. Hao, D. H. K. Ma, D. G. Hwang, W. S. Kim, and F. Zhang, "Identification of antiangiogenic and antiinflammatory proteins in human amniotic membrane," *Cornea*, vol. 19, no. 3, pp. 348–352, 2000.

[41] N. Arai, H. Tsuno, M. Okabe, T. Yoshida, C. Koike et al., "clinical application of a hyperdry amniotic membrane on surgical defects of the oral mucosa," *Journal of Oral and Maxillofacial Surgery*. In press.

[42] J. C. Kim and S. C. G. Tseng, "Transplantation of preserved human amniotic membrane for surface reconstruction in severely damaged rabbit corneas," *Cornea*, vol. 14, no. 5, pp. 473–484, 1995.

[43] K. Kitagawa, M. Okabe, S. Yanagisawa, X. Y. Zhang, T. Nikaido, and A. Hayashi, "Use of a hyperdried cross-linked amniotic membrane as initial therapy for corneal perforations," *Japanese Journal of Ophthalmology*, vol. 55, no. 1, pp. 16–21, 2011.

[44] K. Kitagawa, S. Yanagisawa, K. Watanabe et al., "A hyperdry amniotic membrane patch using a tissue adhesive for corneal perforations and bleb leaks," *American Journal of Ophthalmology*, vol. 148, no. 3, pp. 383–389, 2009.

[45] K. Iijima, Y. Igawa, T. Imamura et al., "Transplantation of preserved human amniotic membrane for bladder augmentation in rats," *Tissue Engineering*, vol. 13, no. 3, pp. 513–524, 2007.

[46] J. Cai, W. Li, H. Su et al., "Generation of human induced pluripotent stem cells from umbilical cord matrix and amniotic membrane mesenchymal cells," *Journal of Biological Chemistry*, vol. 285, no. 15, pp. 11227–11234, 2010.

[47] O. Parolini, F. Alviano, G. P. Bagnara et al., "Concise review: isolation and characterization of cells from human term placenta: outcome of the First International Workshop on Placenta Derived Stem Cells," *Stem Cells*, vol. 26, no. 2, pp. 300–311, 2008.

[48] T. Miki, F. Marongiu, K. Dorko, E. C. S. Ellis, and S. C. Strom, "Isolation of amniotic epithelial stem cells," *Current Protocols in Stem Cell Biology*, no. 12, pp. 1E.3.1–1E.3.10, 2010.

[49] M. Soncini, E. Vertua, L. Gibelli et al., "Isolation and characterization of mesenchymal cells from human fetal membranes," *Journal of Tissue Engineering and Regenerative Medicine*, vol. 1, no. 4, pp. 296–305, 2007.

[50] F. Marongiu, R. Gramignoli, Q. Sun et al., "Isolation of amniotic mesenchymal stem cells," *Current Protocols in Stem Cell Biology*, vol. 1, unit 1E.5, 2010.

[51] T. Miki, K. Mitamura, M. A. Ross, D. B. Stolz, and S. C. Strom, "Identification of stem cell marker-positive cells by immunofluorescence in term human amnion," *Journal of Reproductive Immunology*, vol. 75, no. 2, pp. 91–96, 2007.

[52] A. R. Prusa, E. Marton, M. Rosner, G. Bernaschek, and M. Hengstschläger, "Oct-4-expressing cells in human amniotic fluid: a new source for stem cell research?" *Human Reproduction*, vol. 18, no. 7, pp. 1489–1493, 2003.

[53] P. Zhao, H. Ise, M. Hongo, M. Ota, I. Konishi, and T. Nikaido, "Human amniotic mesenchymal cells have some characteristics of cardiomyocytes," *Transplantation*, vol. 79, no. 5, pp. 528–535, 2005.

[54] A. Toda, M. Okabe, T. Yoshida, and T. Nikaido, "The potential of amniotic membrane/amnion-derived cells for regeneration of various tissues," *Journal of Pharmacological Sciences*, vol. 105, no. 3, pp. 215–228, 2007.

[55] S. Takashima, M. Yasuo, N. Sanzen et al., "Characterization of laminin isoforms in human amnion," *Tissue and Cell*, vol. 40, no. 2, pp. 75–81, 2008.

[56] Y. W. Kim, H. J. Kim, S. M. Bae, Y. J. Kim, J. C. Shin et al., "Time-course transcriptional profiling of human amniotic fluid-derived stem cells using microarray," *Cancer Research and Treatment*, vol. 42, no. 2, pp. 82–94, 2010.

[57] K. Wolfrum, Y. Wang, A. Prigione, K. Sperling, H. Lehrach, and J. Adjaye, "The LARGE principle of cellular reprogramming: lost, acquired and retained gene expression in foreskin and amniotic fluid-derived human iPS cells," *PLoS ONE*, vol. 5, no. 10, Article ID e13703, 2010.

[58] G. Tsangaris, R. Weitzdörfer, D. Pollak, G. Lubec, and M. Fountoulakis, "The amniotic fluid cell proteome," *Electrophoresis*, vol. 26, no. 6, pp. 1168–1173, 2005.

[59] J. E. Oh, M. Fountoulakis, J. F. Juranville, M. Rosner, M. Hengstschlaeger, and G. Lubec, "Proteomic determination of metabolic enzymes of the amnion cell: basis for a possible diagnostic tool?" *Proteomics*, vol. 4, no. 4, pp. 1145–1158, 2004.

[60] S. H. Kim, R. Vlkolinsky, N. Cairns, and G. Lubec, "Decreased levels of complex III core protein 1 and complex V β chain in brains from patients with Alzheimer's disease and down syndrome," *Cellular and Molecular Life Sciences*, vol. 57, no. 12, pp. 1810–1816, 2000.

[61] A. Hopkinson, R. S. McIntosh, V. Shanmuganathan, P. J. Tighe, and H. S. Dua, "Proteomic analysis of amniotic membrane prepared for human transplantation: characterization of proteins and clinical implications," *Journal of Proteome Research*, vol. 5, no. 9, pp. 2226–2235, 2006.

[62] J. C. Adams and J. Lawler, "The thrombospondins," *International Journal of Biochemistry and Cell Biology*, vol. 36, no. 6, pp. 961–968, 2004.

[63] A. Zaslavsky, K. H. Baek, R. C. Lynch et al., "Platelet-derived thrombospondin-1 is a critical negative regulator and potential biomarker of angiogenesis," *Blood*, vol. 115, no. 22, pp. 4605–4613, 2010.

[64] J. L. Funderburgh, L. M. Corpuz, M. R. Roth, M. L. Funderburgh, E. S. Tasheva, and G. W. Conrad, "Mimecan, the 25-kDa corneal keratan sulfate proteoglycan, is a product of the gene producing osteoglycin," *Journal of Biological Chemistry*, vol. 272, no. 44, pp. 28089–28095, 1997.

[65] E. S. Tasheva, A. Koester, A. Q. Paulsen et al., "Mimecan/osteoglycin-deficient mice have collagen fibril abnormalities," *Molecular Vision*, vol. 8, pp. 407–415, 2002.

[66] A. Kampmann, B. Fernández, E. Deindl et al., "The proteoglycan osteoglycin/mimecan is correlated with arteriogenesis," *Molecular and Cellular Biochemistry*, vol. 322, no. 1-2, pp. 15–23, 2009.

[67] M. O. Kim, S. J. Yun, I. S. Kim, S. Sohn, and E. H. Lee, "Transforming growth factor-β-inducible gene-h3 (βig-h3) promotes cell adhesion of human astrocytoma cells in vitro: implication of $\alpha6\beta4$ integrin," *Neuroscience Letters*, vol. 336, no. 2, pp. 93–96, 2003.

[68] N. S. Corsini and A. Martin-Villalba, "Integrin alpha 6: anchors away for glioma stem cells," *Cell Stem Cell*, vol. 6, no. 5, pp. 403–404, 2010.

[69] K. I. Endo, T. Nakamura, S. Kawasaki, and S. Kinoshita, "Human amniotic membrane, like corneal epithelial basement membrane, manifests the $\alpha5$ chain of type IV collagen," *Investigative Ophthalmology and Visual Science*, vol. 45, no. 6, pp. 1771–1774, 2004.

[70] H. Baharvand, M. Heidari, M. Ebrahimi, T. Valadbeigi, and G. H. Salekdeh, "Proteomic analysis of epithelium-denuded human amniotic membrane as a limbal stem cell niche," *Molecular Vision*, vol. 13, pp. 1711–1721, 2007.

[71] M. Grueterich, E. M. Espana, and S. C. G. Tseng, "Ex vivo expansion of limbal epithelial stem cells: amniotic membrane serving as a stem cell niche," *Survey of Ophthalmology*, vol. 48, no. 6, pp. 631–646, 2003.

[72] W. Li, H. He, C. L. Kuo, Y. Gao, T. Kawakita, and S. C. G. Tseng, "Basement membrane dissolution and reassembly by limbal corneal epithelial cells expanded on amniotic membrane," *Investigative Ophthalmology and Visual Science*, vol. 47, no. 6, pp. 2381–2389, 2006.

[73] K. Fukuda, T. I. Chikama, M. Nakamura, and T. Nishida, "Differential distribution of subchains of the basement membrane components type IV collagen and laminin among the amniotic membrane, cornea, and conjunctiva," *Cornea*, vol. 18, no. 1, pp. 73–79, 1999.

[74] V. H. Lobert, A. Brech, N. M. Pedersen et al., "Ubiquitination of $\alpha5\beta1$ integrin controls fibroblast migration through lysosomal degradation of fibronectin-integrin complexes," *Developmental Cell*, vol. 19, no. 1, pp. 148–159, 2010.

[75] M. Teodelinda, C. Michele, C. Sebastiano, C. Ranieri, and G. Chiara, "Amniotic liquid derived stem cells as reservoir of secreted angiogenic factors capable of stimulating neo-arteriogenesis in an ischemic model," *Biomaterials*, vol. 32, no. 15, pp. 3689–3699, 2011.

[76] I. F. Charo and M. B. Taubman, "Chemokines in the pathogenesis of vascular disease," *Circulation Research*, vol. 95, no. 9, pp. 858–866, 2004.

[77] M. Heil and W. Schaper, "Arteriogenic growth factors, chemokines and proteases as a prerequisite for arteriogenesis," *Drug News and Perspectives*, vol. 18, no. 5, pp. 317–322, 2005.

[78] T. Mirabella, J. Hartinger, C. Lorandi, C. Gentili, M. van Griensven et al., "Pro-angiogenic soluble factors from amniotic fluid stem cells mediate the recruitment of endothelial progenitors in a model of ischemic fasciocutaneous flap," *Stem Cells and Development*. In press.

[79] A. Maroof and P. M. Kaye, "Temporal regulation of interleukin-12p70 (IL-12p70) and IL-12-related cytokines in splenic dendritic cell subsets during Leishmania donovani infection," *Infection and Immunity*, vol. 76, no. 1, pp. 239–249, 2008.

[80] H. Yoshidome, A. Kato, M. Miyazaki, M. J. Edwards, and A. B. Lentsch, "IL-13 activates STAT6 and inhibits liver injury induced by ischemia/reperfusion," *American Journal of Pathology*, vol. 155, no. 4, pp. 1059–1064, 1999.

[81] D. van Poll, B. Parekkadan, I. H. M. Borel Rinkes, A. W. Tilles, and M. L. Yarmush, "Mesenchymal stem cell therapy for protection and repair of injured vital organs," *Cell and Molecular Biology*, vol. 1, no. 1, pp. 42–50, 2008.

4

Feline Neural Progenitor Cells I: Long-Term Expansion under Defined Culture Conditions

Jing Yang,[1] Jinmei Wang,[1] Ping Gu,[1,2] X. Joann You,[1] and Henry Klassen[1]

[1] Department of Ophthalmology, Ophthalmology Research Laboratories, The Gavin Herbert Eye Institute, University of California, Irvine, CA 92697, USA
[2] Department of Ophthalmology, Shanghai Ninth People's Hospital, School of Medicine, Shanghai Jiaotong University, Shanghai 200011, China

Correspondence should be addressed to Henry Klassen, hklassen@uci.edu

Academic Editor: Heuy-Ching Hetty Wang

Neural progenitor cells (NPCs) of feline origin (cNPCs) have demonstrated utility in transplantation experiments, yet are difficult to grow in culture beyond the 1 month time frame. Here we use an enriched, serum-free base medium (Ultraculture) and report the successful long-term propagation of these cells. Primary cultures were derived from fetal brain tissue and passaged in DMEM/F12-based or Ultraculture-based proliferation media, both in the presence of EGF + bFGF. Cells in standard DMEM/F12-based medium ceased to proliferate by 1-month, whereas the cells in the Ultraculture-based medium continued to grow for at least 5 months (end of study) with no evidence of senescence. The Ultraculture-based cultures expressed lower levels of progenitor and lineage-associated markers under proliferation conditions but retained multipotency as evidenced by the ability to differentiate into neurons and glia following growth factor removal in the presence of FBS. Importantly, later passage cNPCs did not develop chromosomal aberrations.

1. Introduction

The mammalian central nervous system (CNS) has a restricted capacity for self-repair and regeneration and, as a consequence, the extent of clinical recovery from CNS injury or disease is generally limited. Because of this unmet clinical need, much work has been devoted to exploring potential ways of enhancing clinical outcomes in the setting of debilitating neurological conditions. One particularly interesting approach is the transplantation of allogeneic neural progenitor cells (NPCs). These multipotent cells are derived from the developing nervous system and, under defined serum-free conditions, are capable of at least limited expansion in culture, followed by differentiation into mature neurons and glia, either following cessation of mitogenic stimulation in vitro or transplantation to the diseased CNS [1, 2].

There are a number of characteristics of NPCs that recommend them for application to neural repair strategies. From a practical standpoint, the proliferative capability of the cells mentioned above allows for the generation of cell banks [3], thereby decreasing the need for continued derivation from donor tissue. From a biological standpoint, the ability of NPCs to exhibit directed migration to areas of disease and integrate into the local cytoarchitecture represents a major breakthrough compared to previous work, for example, with fetal tissue transplantation [4, 5]. From a clinical standpoint, the immune tolerance-afforded allogeneic NPCs in animal studies [6–8] would appear to obviate the need for mandatory immune suppression in many cases, hopefully including allografts in humans. If this is the case, it would substantially decrease the therapeutic risk to patients. In addition, it would appear that progenitor cells of this type convey a substantially decreased risk of tumor formation, particularly when compared to analogous cells derived from pluripotent cell types [9].

In addition to their potential role in cell replacement, NPCs also represent an attractive method for gene delivery, particularly with respect to neuroprotective cytokines. These molecules are gene products that are rapidly degraded in vivo by endogenous proteases and notably include trophic factors such as glial cell line-derived neurotrophic factor (GDNF). It has been demonstrated that NPCs can be genetically modified to express these types of factors ex vivo, expanded in number, and subsequently transplanted for study [10, 11]. Given that these cells are typically well tolerated immunologically, genetically modified NPCs could provide a method of sustained drug delivery to local sites within the brain, retina, and spinal cord. This option is of interest in species, where NPCs can be successfully isolated, and where models of CNS disease are available.

Progenitor or precursor cells have now been isolated and grown from viable brain tissue in a broad range of mammalian species, including mouse, rat, cat, pig, sheep, dog, monkey, and human [12]. The cat represents a model of interest for neural repair strategies because of the potential for detailed electrophysiological and behavioral studies. In previous work, we and another group have reported the isolation of feline neural progenitor-like cells, combined with successful transplantation to the dystrophic retina [13] and the normal brain [14] of allorecipients. Nevertheless, it has proven difficult to grow these cells for extended periods in culture using conventional protocols. This lack of in vitro expansion hampers further research by restricting the number of studies that can be performed from a given isolation. Here, we identify a modified culture method that allows for sustained, abundant growth of feline neural progenitor cells sufficient for banking. We provide additional characterization of these cells, including examination of karyotype and analysis of gene expression at multiple time points in culture.

2. Materials and Methods

2.1. Isolation and Culture of NPCs from the Cat (cNPCs).
The isolation of cNPCs followed a protocol similar to that described previously [13], but in this case the donor was a 47-day timed-pregnant domestic cat (E47). Fetuses were removed under terminal anesthesia at an academic veterinary facility and shipped on ice to the site of cell isolation and culture. Upon arrival, brains were removed by dissection and the forebrain separated from the cerebellum and brainstem. Forebrain tissue was relocated to a petridish containing cold DMEM (Invitrogen, Carlsbad, CA, USA). The tissue was minced using 2 scalpels and then enzymatically digested using 0.05% TrypLE Express (Invitrogen). The resulting cell suspension was washed repeatedly and dissociated by repeated, gentle aspiration using a flame-polished glass pipette. The resulting cells were then divided and seeded into 1 of 2 different complete culture media, namely, standard medium (SM) or Ultraculture-based medium (UM). SM consisted of Advanced DMEM/F12 (Invitrogen), 1% by volume N2 neural supplement (Invitrogen), 1% GlutaMax (Invitrogen), 50 U/mL penicillin-streptomycin (Invitrogen), 20 ng/mL epidermal growth factor (recombinant human EGF, Invitrogen) and 20 ng/mL basic fibroblast growth factor (recombinant human bFGF; Invitrogen). To promote adherence, 5% FBS (Sigma) was also included at the time of initial plating. The following day all medium in cultures was completely replaced with serum-free SM. The remaining half of the primary cells were seeded in an alternate proliferation medium, henceforth designated UltraCulture-based medium (UM), containing Ultraculture (Lonza), 1% GlutaMax, 50 U/mL penicillin-streptomycin, 20 ng/mL epidermal growth factor, and 20 ng/mL basic fibroblast growth factor. The plating density was 0.5×10^6 cells/mL for both conditions. Subsequently, cells were fed by medium exchange every 2 to 3 days and passaged at confluence using TrypLE Express and gentle trituration through a flame-polished glass pipette. At each passage, cell number was counted using a hemocytometer.

2.2. Cytogenetic Analysis (Chromosome Counting and Karyotyping).
Confluent cNPCs generated in UM were harvested at culture passages 8 and 14 and prepared for analysis, as follows. Cells were plated onto a T-25 flask, and the media were changed 24 hours before harvesting the culture to stimulate cell division and maximize the mitotic index. The cells were then mitotically arrested with colcemid (KaryoMax Colcemid solution, Invitrogen) at a final working concentration of 0.12 μg/mL at 37°C for 20 minutes. Isolated cNPCs were harvested for hypotonic treatment in 0.075 M KCl solution at room temperature for 25 minutes. The cells were pelleted by centrifugation at 1000 rpm for 8 minutes and fixed in ice-cold fixative (3:1 methanol: glacial acetic acid) for 10 min. After a second wash in fixative, the cells were resuspended in 2 mL fixative. Slides were prepared by dropping the cell suspension onto dry microscope slides prewashed with fixative. G-banded karyotyping was performed by Cell Line Genetics LLC (Madison, WI, USA).

2.3. RNA Isolation and cDNA Synthesis.
Total RNA was extracted from passage 8 cNPCs using the RNeasy Mini Kit (Qiagen, Valencia, CA, USA) according to the manufacturer's protocol. DNase I was used to digest and eliminate any contaminating genomic DNA. Two micrograms of total RNA in a 20 μL reaction were reverse-transcribed using an Omniscript cDNA Synthesis Kit (Qiagen, Valencia, CA, USA).

2.4. Quantitative PCR (qPCR).
qPCR was performed on an Applied Biosystems 7500 Fast Real-Time PCR Detection System (Applied Biosystems, Foster, CA, USA) following protocols previously described [15]. Briefly, 20 μL total reaction was made up of 10 μL 2x Power SYBR Green PCR Master Mix (Applied Biosystems, Foster, CA, USA), 100 ng cDNA, and gene specific primers (Table 1) at a concentration of 300 μM. Samples were initially denatured at 95°C for 10 min, followed by 40 cycles of PCR amplification (15 seconds at 95°C and 1 minute at 60°C). To normalize template input, β-actin (endogenous control) transcript level was measured for each sample. Melting curves were determined to confirm amplification of the expected fragment. Fold change and heat map were generated using JMP 4.1 and DataAssist 2.0 software.

2.5. Induction of cNPC Differentiation.
The cNPCs were cultured in UM or UM-FBS that contained 10% FBS but no added growth factors with the same cell density, 0.3×10^6 cells/mL. Culture media was exchanged every 2 days.

TABLE 1: Cat-specific primers for real-time PCR.

Genes	Description	Forward (5′–3′)	Reverse (5′–3′)	Annealing temperature (°C)	Product size (base pairs)
Nestin	Intermediate filament, Progenitor	CTGGAGCAGGAGAAGGAGAG	GAAGCTGAGGGAAGCCTTG	60	180
Sox-2	Transcription factor, progenitor	ACCAGCTCGCAGACCTACAT	TGGAGTGGGAGGAAGAGGTA	60	154
Vimentin	Intermediate filament, progenitor	ATCCAGGAGCTACAGGCTCA	GGACCTGTCTCCGGTACTCA	60	247
Pax 6	Transcription factor, progenitor	AGGAGGGGGAGAGAATACCA	CTTTCTCGGGCAAACACATC	60	183
Notch1	Surface receptor, progenitor	CAGTGTCTGCAGGGCTACAC	CTCGCACAGAAACTCGTTGA	60	231
CD133	Progenitor	AGGAAGTGCTTTGCGGTCT	TGCCAGTTTCCGAGTCTTTT	60	120
Cyclin D2	Cell cycle protein	CAAGATCACCAACACGGATG	ATATCCCGCACGTCTGTAGG	60	162
Ki-67	Cell cycle protein, proliferation	TCGTCTGAAGCCGGAGTTAT	TCTTCTTTTCCCGATGGTTG	60	150
CD81	Tetraspaniin	CCACAGACCACCAACCTTCT	CAGGCACTGGGACTCCTG	60	156
EGFR	EGF receptor, surface marker	AACTGTGAGGTGGTCCTTGG	CGCAGTCCGGTTTTATTTGT	60	231
FABP7	fatty acid binding protein	TGGAGGCTTTCTGTGCTACC	TGCTTTGTGTCCTGATCACC	60	165
β3-tubulin	Microtubule protein, neural precursor	CATTCTCGTGGACCTTGAGC	GCAGTCGCAATTCTCACATT	60	199
Map2	Microtubule-associated, neuron	ACCTAAGCCATGTGACATCCA	CTCCAGGTACATGGTGAGCA	60	152
GFAP	Intermediate filament, glia	CGGTTTTTGAGGAAGATCCA	TTGGACCGATACCACTCCTC	60	188
AQP4	water channel protein	TACACTGGTGCCAGCATGA	CACCAGCGAGGACAGCTC	60	118
SDF 1	stromal-cell-derived factor-1	ACAGATGTCCTTGCCGATTC	CCACTTCAATTTCGGGTCAA	60	152
CXCR4	fusin	TCTGTGGCAGACCTCCTCTT	TTTCAGCCAACAGCTTCCTT	60	220
Dcx	Doublecortin, neuroblast marker	GGCTGACCTGACTCGATCTC	GCTTTCATATTGGCGGATGT	60	222
Lhx2	Homeobox transcription factor	GATCTGGCGGCCTACAAC	AGGACCCGTTTGGTGAGG	60	224
NCAM (CD56)	Adhesion molecule, surface marker	AGAACAAGGCTGGAGAGCAG	TTTCGGGTAGAAGTCCTCCA	60	172
NogoA	Reticulon 4, surface protein	TTTGCAGTGTTGATGTGGGTA	TAACAGGAACGCTGAAGAGTGA	60	100
nucleostemin	Nucleolar protein	CAGTGGTGTTCAGAGCCTCA	CCGAATGGCTTTGCTGTAA	60	165
Pbx 1	Transcription factor	CTCCGATTACAGAGCCAAGC	GCTGACCATACGCTCGATCT	60	166
β-actin	Housekeeping gene	GCCGTCTTCCCTTCCATC	CTTCTCCATGTCGTCCCAGT	60	168

The morphology of cells was monitored every day, and the cells were photographed on days 1, 3, 5, and 7.

2.6. Immunocytochemistry. After 4 months in culture, cNPCs were plated on four-well chamber slides in either UM or UM-FBS medium and fed every two days. On day 5, cells were fixed with freshly prepared 4% paraformaldehyde (Invitrogen) in 0.1 M phosphate-buffered saline (PBS) for 20 minutes at room temperature. Fixed cells were washed with PBS,

then they were incubated for 1 hour at room temperature in antibody blocking buffer containing the following: PBS containing 10% (v/v) normal donkey serum (Sigma), 0.3% Triton X-100, and 0.1% NaN3 (Sigma-Aldrich, Saint Louis, MO, USA). Slides were then incubated in primary antibodies (Table 2) at 4°C overnight. After washing, slides were incubated for 1 hour at room temperature in fluorescent-conjugated secondary antibody, 1 : 400 Alexa Fluor[546] goat antimouse, followed by washings. Cell nuclei were counterstained with 1.5 μg/mL 4′,6-diamidino-2-phenylindole (DAPI;

TABLE 2: Primary antibodies for immunocytochemistry.

Antigen	Host species and reactivity in retina	Dilution	Source
Nestin	Mouse monoclonal; progenitors, reactive glia	1 : 200	BD, 611658
Vimentin	Mouse monoclonal; progenitors, reactive glia	1 : 200	Sigma, V6630
βIII-tubulin	Mouse monoclonal; immature neurons	1 : 200	Chemicon, MAB1637
Ki-67	Mouse monoclonal; proliferating cells	1 : 200	BD, 556003
GFAP	Mouse monoclonal; Astrocyte, reactive glia	1 : 200	Chemicon, MAB3402

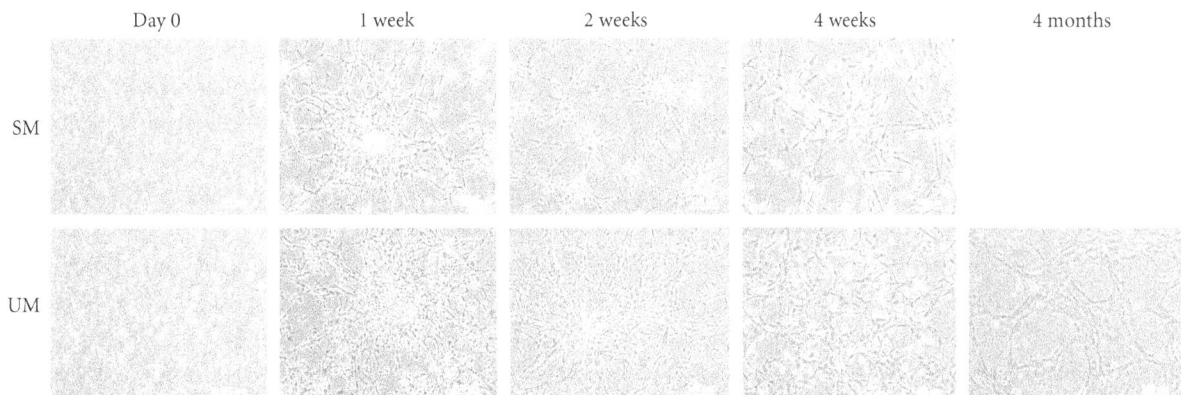

FIGURE 1: Morphology of cNPCs in different proliferation media at serial time points. Upper panel shows cNPCs cultured in SM and the lower panel cells of the same age in UM. Cultures are shown on day 0, after 1, 2, and 4 weeks as well as 4 months (UM only). In both media the cells exhibited morphologic features consistent with primitive neural cells throughout the period examined. In both cases, the adherent cells extended processes and expanded greatly during the initial week. The cells in SM ceased expanding during the first month and were not evaluated beyond the 3-month time point, whereas those in UM continued to expand throughout the course of the study. Scale bar: 100 μm.

Invitrogen, Molecular Probes, Eugene, OR, USA) in Vectashield Hard Set Mounting Medium (Vector Laboratories, Burlingame, CA, USA) for 15 min at room temperature. Negative controls for immunolabeling were performed in parallel using the same protocol but with omission of the primary antibody. Fluorescent labeling was judged as positive only with reference to the negative controls. Immunoreactive cells were visualized and images recorded using a Nikon fluorescent microscope (Eclipse E600; Nikon, Melville, NY, USA).

3. Results

3.1. Comparison of cNPCs Grown in Different Proliferation Media.
Proliferative cultures were obtained from forebrain-derived feline NPCs seeded and maintained in both types of media (SM and UM); however, only those seeded in UM continued to expand throughout the duration of the study (5 months). The cells in both types of media exhibited morphologic features consistent with primitive neuroectodermal cells throughout their growth period (Figure 1). In both cultures, the majority of cells were adherent to the surface of the flask and continued to proliferate, forming a pattern of random networks and nodal clusters as is typical of mammalian neural progenitors when not grown as suspended neurospheres.

The morphology of cNPCs cultured in the two different growth media was also examined. In both conditions, the initially dissociated cells divided and formed small clusters over the first week in culture. During this period, cellular processes had started to form by day 3 and were greatly elaborated by the end of the first week. Cells cultured in SM showed little evidence of proliferation beyond week 3, but continued to survive up to 3 months. In contrast, cells cultured in UM established stably expanding populations. The cNPCs continued to expand vigorously, while maintaining progenitor morphology, although a tendency of the cells to enlarge and flatten was observed (Figure 1).

3.2. Long-Term Expansion of cNPC Cells Is Possible in UM.
The growth characteristics of cNPCs are plotted in Figure 2. Initial growth of cells was observed in either medium, but sustained expansion was only achieved using UM. The number of cells in SM medium increased initially and peaked shortly after day 20. After that, the total cell count began to drop, and no further passaging or counting was performed although the cells continued to survive up to at least 3 months. In contrast, the cNPCs in UM continued to increase steadily, without indications of senescence, throughout the 5-month duration of this study.

3.3. Cytogenetics of cNPCs during Extended Culture.
Because increased rates of cellular proliferation can be the result of chromosomal abnormalities arising during extended periods of cell culture, the karyotypic stability of cNPCs cultures in UM was evaluated by chromosome counting and G-banded karyotyping. Cytogenetic analysis was performed on twenty

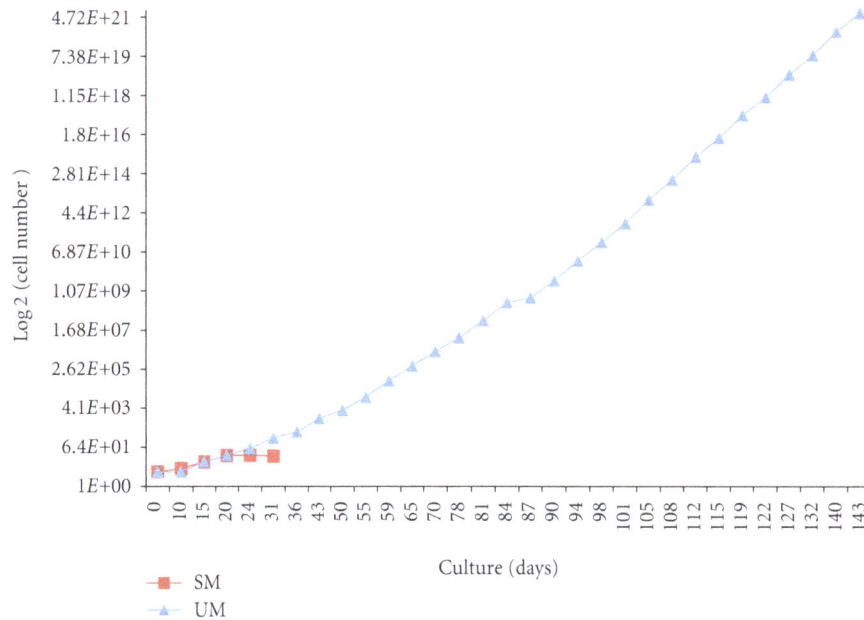

FIGURE 2: Expansion capacity of cNPC cells in long-term culture. Cells were cultured in 1 of 2 proliferation media of differing composition and counted at each passage using a hemocytometer. The number of cells in SM medium (red) increased initially, then began to drop shortly after day 20, with no measurable proliferation beyond 1 month. In contrast, cultures grown in UM (blue) exhibited sustained growth throughout the course of the study (143 days), with no evidence of senescence. The rate of expansion did not diminish with passage number. Numbers on x-axis represent days in culture at each passage, the y-axis shows cell number as total estimated yield.

G-banded metaphase cells from passage 8 (day 50) and from passage 14 (day 87) time points that roughly corresponded to possible upward inflections in the growth curve. The results showed that the cells from both time points possessed normal feline 38XX karyotypes (Figure 3), indicating that the increased proliferation rate seen was not the result of a culture-induced chromosomal abnormality.

3.4. Quantitative Evaluation of the Effect of Different Culture Media on cNPC Gene Expression.

Having determined that UM effectively sustains the proliferation of NPCs of feline origin, whereas the conventional media formation did not, it was of interest to compare the phenotype of the cells grown using these methods. In order to look for differences related to the alternate proliferation conditions used, we compared gene expression profiles for cNPCs grown in SM versus UM at the 1 month time point using quantitative RT-PCR (Figures 4(a) and 4(b)).

Both sampled populations expressed the neural progenitor-associated genes nestin, sox-2, vimentin, and notch1 as well as the proliferation markers cyclinD2 and Ki-67 (Figure 4(a)). Expression of the markers CD81 and FABP7, which are also known to be expressed by NPCs [16–18], was detected as well. Low expression of the early neuronal marker β-III tubulin was seen, as reported previously [13]. The mature neuronal and astroglial markers Map2 and GFAP were detectable, the latter more prominently than the former. Overall, these results were consistent with the maintenance of markers associated with neural progenitor populations by cNPCs when grown in UM, including the modest but detectable tendency for ongoing, spontaneous differentiation along the neuronal lineage, as previously reported in analogous cells from various mammalian species.

Looked at more closely, there were similarities and differences in the level of expression for particular markers (Figure 4(b)). Less than 2 fold variance between conditions was observed for expression of the majority of markers including AQP4, β3-tubulin, CD9, CD81, CyclinD2, EGFR, GFAP, Lhx2, NCAM, nestin, nogoA, notch1, Pax6, Sox2, and vimentin. Growth in UM was associated with greater than 2 fold increased expression in the neuroblast marker DCX, the neuronal marker Map2, the transcription factor Pbx1, and the migration-associated marker SDF1. Markers that were greater than 2 fold lower in UM were CXCR4, FABP7 and Ki-67. Of note, the most upregulated marker (SDF1) is a receptor for the migration factor CXCR4, which was downregulated.

3.5. Sequential Analysis of cNPC Gene Profile with Time in Culture.

To examine the phenotypic stability of cRPCs during extended culture in UM, we employed qPCR, in this case to compare the expression profile obtained at 2 weeks to that present at 1, 2, 3, and 5 months (Figure 5). A preponderance of the markers examined showed a tendency to decrease with time in culture. This trend included progenitor-associated and neurodevelopmental markers as well as some markers associated with further lineage restriction. Both heat map and cluster analysis indicated an overall drop in marker expression between the 1- and 2-month time points (Figure 5(a)). Interestingly, this is the same time frame in

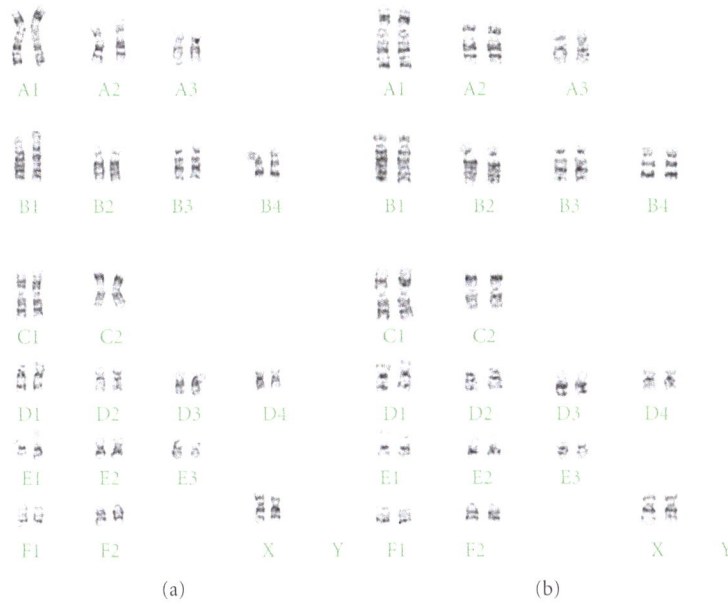

(a) (b)

FIGURE 3: G-banded karyotyping of cNPCs at early and later passage. Cytogenetic G-banded karyotyping results based on analysis of 20 metaphase cNPCs. (a) passage 8 (day 50); (b) passage 14 (day 87). The cells from both time points exhibited a normal 38XX feline karyotype.

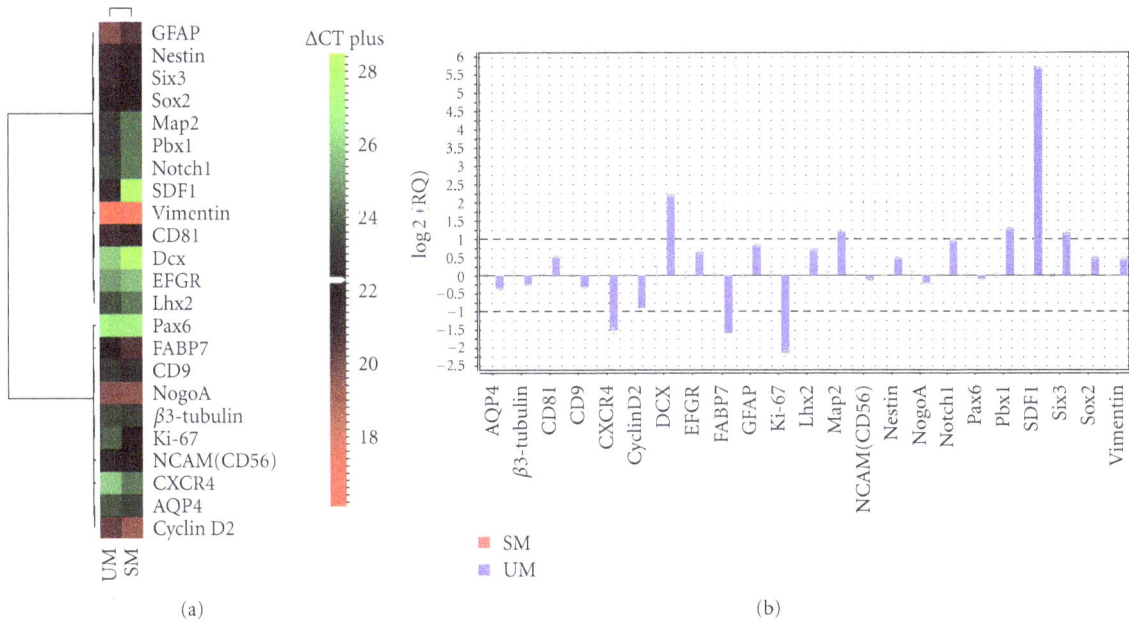

(a) (b)

FIGURE 4: Comparison by qPCR of gene expression profile for cNPCs in different culture media. The cNPCs were cultured in either SM or UM for 1 month prior to testing. (a) heat map display showing relative expression levels of 23 genes expressed by NPCs or related progeny of neural lineage. The scale to the right shows that moderate expression level (as determined by CT value) is shown as black, while lower expression appears increasingly green, and higher expression increasingly red. Viewed in this way, the general similarity of the 2 conditions is evident in that the color of a particular gene tends to be conserved across conditions, even if the intensity often varies. (b) fold change, with SM used as calibrator. Note that expression is represented on a log2 scale, such that 1.00 corresponds to a 2 fold change. Viewed in this way, differences in expression are highlighted. The majority of genes showed less than 2 fold change (between 1.00 to −1.00, on log2 scale), again confirming the general similarity between conditions; however, a number of individual genes fell outside this range. The error bars-show standard deviation.

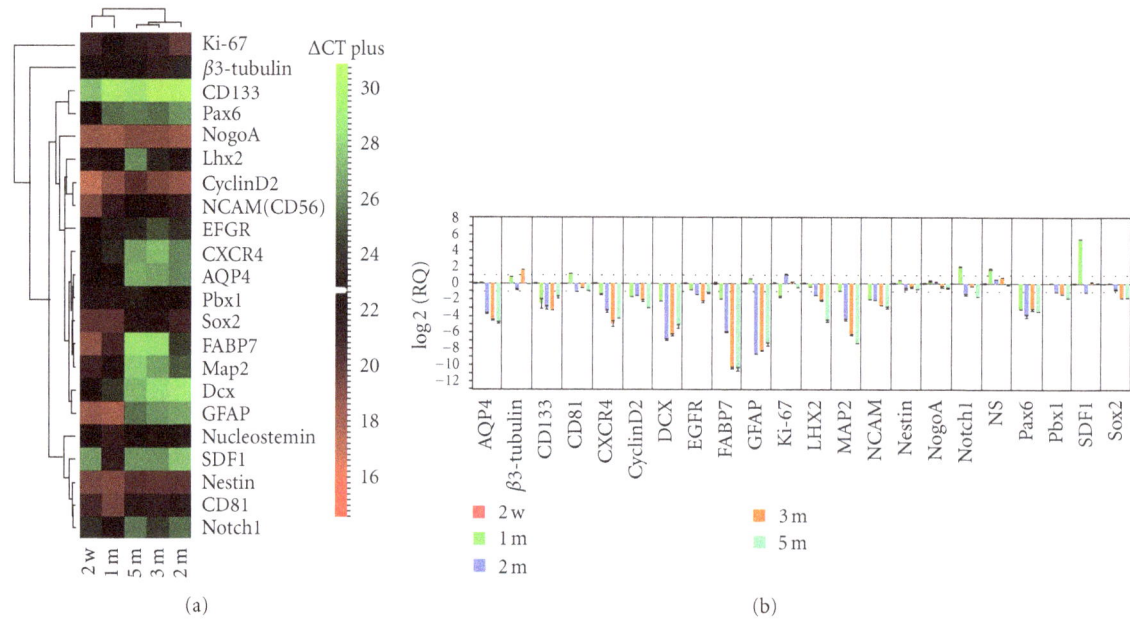

FIGURE 5: Comparison of gene expression from cNPCs at different time points in UM via qPCR. A 22-gene profile was assayed at each time point. The initial time point for comparison was 2 weeks (calibrator), followed by 1, 2, 3 and 5 months. (a) viewed as a heat map, there was an apparent overall drop in marker expression (shift from red towards green end of spectrum), and this was most evident between the 1- and 2-month time points, both visually and by cluster analysis (dendrogram at top). (b) data viewed as RQ (fold change) confirms the prevalent downward trend with time as well as highlighting the quantitative differences in fold change between markers. Error bars show standard deviation.

which the cells in UM diverged in growth characteristics from those in SM, as seen above in Figure 2. Viewed as a histogram, the qPCR data showed a sequential downward trend, although expression levels appeared to be leveling off at the latter time points (Figure 5(b)). Again, this is concomitant to the robust proliferation seen beyond 1 month in the UM condition.

3.6. Differentiation. Having determined that cNPCs can be grown beyond the 1-month time point using UM, it was important to confirm whether cNPCS grown in this medium retain the potential to differentiate into both neuronal and glial cell types. As a first step, cNPCs (4 months, P26) were dissociated into single cells and induced to differentiate by culture in UM without growth factors, but containing 10% serum (UM-FBS), for 7 days. The cells cultured in UM-FBS appeared similar but exhibited a more flattened morphology than undifferentiated controls (Figure 6). Interestingly, the cultures in UM-FBS reached confluence more rapidly than those in UM. The next step was to examine the expression of relevant markers.

3.7. Effect of UM-FBS on Marker Expression of cNPCs, Evaluated by Immunocytochemistry. Immunocytochemical analysis (Figure 7) at the same time point (4 months, P26) confirmed that feline cells cultured in UM expressed a numbers of markers associated with neural precursor cells. These included strong expression of the intermediate filaments nestin and vimentin as well as the proliferation marker Ki-67. There was also trace labeling for the lineage markers β3-tubulin and

GFAP, both of which are cytoskeletal proteins. β3-tubulin is a marker of neurons, and GFAP is strongly expressed by astrocytes. These data are suggestive of a small but detectable level of spontaneous differentiation in the cultures under proliferation conditions, as is expected with cells of this type.

At 5 days after induction of differentiation in UM-FBS, very few cells remained nestin positive, the signal for vimentin persisted at a diminished level, and expression of Ki-67 had decreased notably. In contrast, many more cells were positive for β3-tubulin and a subset of cells GFAP was strongly positive for GFAP, consistent with differentiation along neuronal as well as glial lineages (Table 3).

4. Discussion

Since their initial isolation, neural progenitor cells have been viewed as a powerful research tool for experimental investigation of novel approaches to cell replacement throughout the central nervous system (CNS). The recognized potential of NPC transplantation-based regenerative therapy for CNS diseases has generated considerable enthusiasm among many investigators and resulted in rapid growth of the field. The scientific understanding of NPCs has increased accordingly, although transplantation of these cells has yet to achieve accepted clinical use. One challenge has been growing sufficient quantities of the cells, and this is, therefore, a fundamental area deserving of additional attention. Refinement and the optimization of culture conditions is an obvious initial approach to further sustaining the proliferation of NPCs *in vitro*. It is also important to consider that the culture

TABLE 3: Estimated percentage and intensity of labeling of cultured cNPCs for specific markers after 5-day exposure to differentiation conditions (UM-FBS). +: weak expression; ++: moderate expression; +++: strong expression.

	Nestin	Vimentin	β3-tubulin	Ki-67	GFAP
UM	100/++	100/+++	60/+	85/++	5/+
UM-FBS	2/+	100/++	85/++	60/+	35/+++

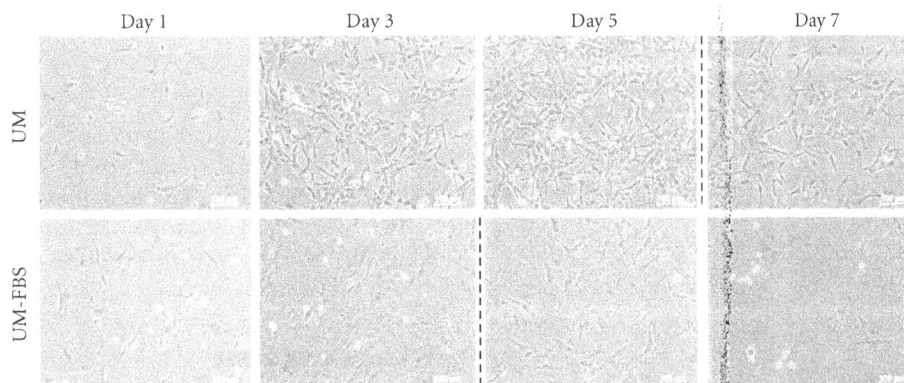

FIGURE 6: Morphology of cNPCs grown under proliferation versus differentiation conditions. Cultured cNPCs grown under proliferation conditions (UM), beginning at P26 (4 months), maintained the appearance of neural progenitors, while those grown under differentiation conditions (UM-FBS) appeared similar but exhibited a more flattened morphology. Dotted vertical lines represent passaging/reseeding, thereby accounting for the decreased cell density in images to the right of those points. Cells in the UM-FBS condition reached confluence more quickly.

requirements of progenitor cells may differ between species. Research has shown that extended culture of neural progenitors is often associated with loss of multipotency, particularly a reduced potential to generate neurons, together with loss of self-renewal, as reflected in a marked propensity towards early senescence [19, 20]. A pertinent issue is the extent to which changes in culture conditions might enhance the expansion of functionally multipotent NPCs.

Feline NPCs can be difficult to propagate using conventional serum-free conditions. Here, we directly compared two variations on serum-free proliferation media, SM and UM, which differed in base medium but contained the same growth factors. Both formulations were used to examine their ability to sustain the proliferation and development of cNPCs derived from E47 brain tissue. In the more conventional SM medium, cNPCs stopped dividing and began to senesce by 1-month in culture. In UM, the cells continued to exhibit vigorous growth for up to 5 months, the latest time point examined, thereby allowing the banking of considerable numbers of mitotically active cNPCs. Although cNPCs grown in SM and UM appear similar in terms of certain key genes expressed, quantitative analysis of expression level did reveal differences between the conditions at the 1 month point. Interestingly, the expression level of the majority of genes, including progenitor and lineage markers, was down-regulated in UM versus SM. Furthermore, this tendency toward downregulation in UM was even more pronounced beyond the 1-month time point, although the possible trend toward a new, lower set point in expression was noted. The reason for this is not clear, but might relate to a state of continuous, rapid cell division. What is clear is that UM is strongly permissive of feline NPCs survival and proliferation *in vitro*, whereas use of conventional SM medium rapidly leads to a failure to propagate.

One possible explanation for the facile growth exhibited by cNPCs in UM could be spontaneous immortalization. The cells in UM displayed repeated upward inflections in growth rate with time in culture that might reflect dysregulation of the cell cycle. It is known that immortalization of NPCs can occur with extended time in culture, and that such events are frequently associated with abnormalities in karyotype. To examine this, we evaluated whether karyotypic alterations were present in our cells, and the results showed that despite 14 passages in UM, the karyotype remained stable. Therefore, the improved growth seen in UM cannot be attributed to changes in karyotype.

Because altered gene expression might be associated with a loss of multipotency, it was important to confirm whether NPCs grown in UM maintain their ability to differentiate into cells of neural lineage. Comparing various progenitor markers and differentiation markers in UM versus UM-FBS conditions, we found that expression levels of progenitor markers decreased while neuronal and glial markers increased. These data indicate that cNPCs cultured in UM retain multipotency and the capacity to differentiate.

The source of the improvement in growth of cBPCs seen in UM thus appears to reside in the beneficial effects of the media constituents rather than aberrations of cellular proliferation. There is no question that Ultraculture is a much richer base medium, containing approximately 6 fold greater total protein than SM. While it is tempting to speculate that certain serum proteins or peptides may be critical to

UM   UM-FBS

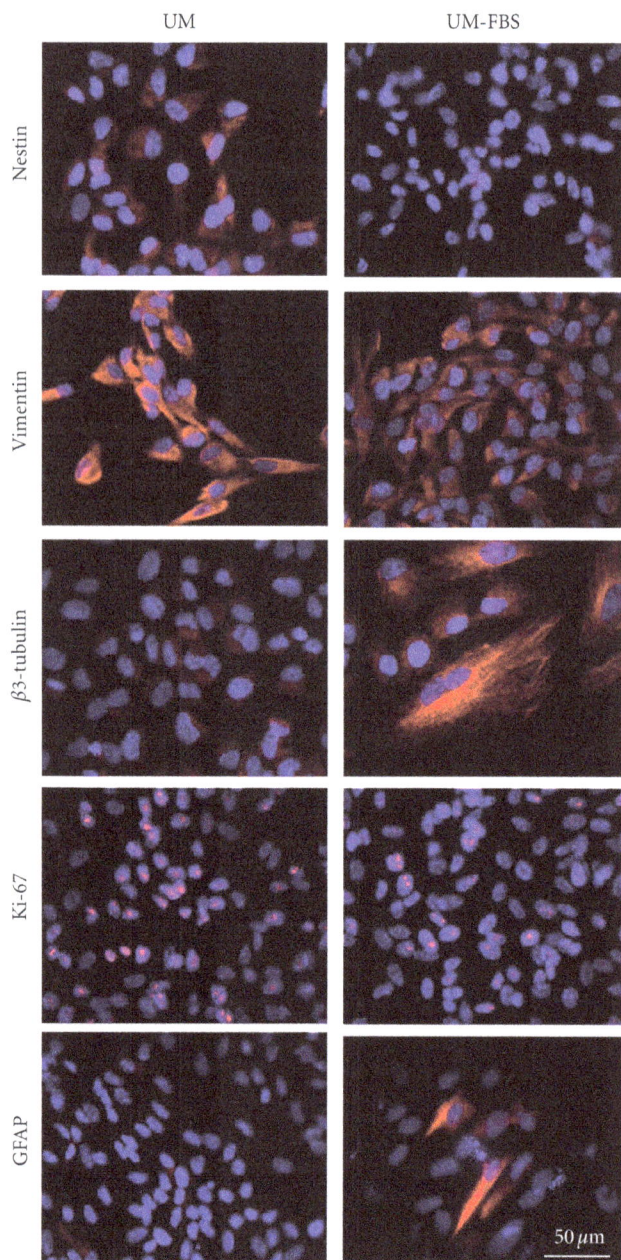

FIGURE 7: Effect of differentiation conditions on expression of markers by immunocytochemistry. To examine the lineage potential of cNPCs, P26 (4 month) cultures were grown in UM or UM-FBS for 5 days and immunolabeled with antibodies (red) against nestin, vimentin, β3-tubulin, Ki-67, and GFAP. Cell nuclei were labeled with DAPI (blue). Scale bars represent 50 μm.

the growth of feline progenitors, further work is needed to define which particular components are responsible for the dramatic improvements seen in the current study.

In summary, we have shown that the use of a highly enriched, serum-free medium allows the long-term propagation of feline neural progenitor cells, something that standard serum-free conditions does poorly, if at all. The resulting cells retain multipotency and the ability to differentiate, as well as a normal karyotype. This does not rule out the possibility

that the cells may have taken a significant, but less obvious, step towards spontaneous immortalization, and that the growth-promoting influence of UM might be causative. Fortunately, the resulting ability to generate and bank large numbers of cNPCs should greatly facilitate additional examination of these cells, including both safety concerns and the potential for therapeutic benefits following transplantation.

Abbreviations

AQP4:   Aquaporin 4
FABP7:   Fatty acid binding protein 7
GFAP: Glial fibrillary acidic protein
NCAM: Neural cell adhesion molecule
SDF1:   Stromal cell-derived factor 1
RT-PCR: Reverse transcriptase-polymerase chain
          reaction.

Acknowledgments

The authors are grateful to Victor David for providing the cat-specific primer sequences used in this study and to Kristina Narfstrom for her longstanding involvement in cat models of retinal dystrophy as well as the provenance of fetal feline tissue used for our original derivation of feline neural progenitor cells. In addition, the authors thank the Lincy Foundation, the Discovery Eye Foundation, the Andrei Olenicoff Memorial Foundation, and the Polly and Michael Smith Foundation for their generous financial support of this paper.

References

[1] F. H. Gage, "Mammalian neural stem cells," Science, vol. 287, no. 5457, pp. 1433–1438, 2000.

[2] D. van der Kooy and S. Weiss, "Why stem cells?" Science, vol. 287, no. 5457, pp. 1439–1441, 2000.

[3] R. J. Thomas, A. D. Hope, P. Hourd et al., "Automated, serum-free production of ctx0e03: a therapeutic clinical grade human neural stem cell line," Biotechnology Letters, vol. 31, no. 8, pp. 1167–1172, 2009.

[4] C. Lundberg, A. Martínez-Serrano, E. Cattaneo, R. D. G. McKay, and A. Björklund, "Survival, integration, and differentiation of neural stem cell lines after transplantation to the adult rat striatum," Experimental Neurology, vol. 145, no. 2, pp. 342–360, 1997.

[5] M. Olsson, "Incorporation of mouse neural progenitors transplanted into the rat embryonic forebrain is developmentally regulated and dependent on regional and adhesive properties," European Journal of Neuroscience, vol. 10, no. 1, pp. 71–85, 1998.

[6] J. Hori, T. F. Ng, M. Shatos, H. Klassen, J. W. Streilein, and M. J. Young, "Neural progenitor cells lack immunogenicity and resist destruction as allografts," Stem Cells, vol. 21, no. 4, pp. 405–416, 2003.

[7] H. Klassen, K. Warfvinge, P. H. Schwartz et al., "Isolation of progenitor cells from gfp-transgenic pigs and transplantation to the retina of allorecipients," Cloning and Stem Cells, vol. 10, no. 3, pp. 391–402, 2008.

[8] S. J. Van Hoffelen, M. J. Young, M. A. Shatos, and D. S. Sakaguchi, "Incorporation of murine brain progenitor cells

into the developing mammalian retina," *Investigative Ophthalmology and Visual Science*, vol. 44, no. 1, pp. 426–434, 2003.

[9] P. G. Hess, "Risk of tumorigenesis in first-in-human trials of embryonic stem cell neural derivatives: ethics in the face of long-term uncertainty," *Accountability in Research*, vol. 16, no. 4, pp. 175–198, 2009.

[10] S. Behrstock, A. D. Ebert, S. Klein, M. Schmitt, J. M. Moore, and C. N. Svendsen, "Lesion-induced increase in survival and migration of human neural progenitor cells releasing gdnf," *Cell Transplantation*, vol. 17, no. 7, pp. 753–762, 2008.

[11] A. D. Ebert, E. L. McMillan, and C. N. Svendsen, "Isolating, expanding, and infecting human and rodent fetal neural progenitor cells," *Current Protocols in Stem Cell Biology*, no. 6, pp. 2D.2.1–2D.2.16, 2008.

[12] H. Klassen, "Transplantation of cultured progenitor cells to the mammalian retina," *Expert Opinion on Biological Therapy*, vol. 6, no. 5, pp. 443–451, 2006.

[13] H. Klassen, P. H. Schwartz, B. Ziaeian et al., "Neural precursors isolated from the developing cat brain show retinal integration following transplantation to the retina of the dystrophic cat," *Veterinary Ophthalmology*, vol. 10, no. 4, pp. 245–253, 2007.

[14] L. Wang, D. R. Martin, H. J. Baker et al., "Neural progenitor cell transplantation and imaging in a large animal model," *Neuroscience Research*, vol. 59, no. 3, pp. 327–340, 2007.

[15] M. W. Pfaffl, "A new mathematical model for relative quantification in real-time rt-pcr," *Nucleic Acids Research*, vol. 29, no. 9, article e45, 2001.

[16] H. Klassen, M. R. Schwartz, A. H. Bailey, and M. J. Young, "Surface markers expressed by multipotent human and mouse neural progenitor cells include tetraspanins and non-protein epitopes," *Neuroscience Letters*, vol. 312, no. 3, pp. 180–182, 2001.

[17] P. H. Schwartz, P. J. Bryant, T. J. Fuja, H. Su, D. K. O'Dowd, and H. Klassen, "Isolation and characterization of neural progenitor cells from post-mortem human cortex," *Journal of Neuroscience Research*, vol. 74, no. 6, pp. 838–851, 2003.

[18] P. H. Schwartz, H. Nethercott, I. I. Kirov, B. Ziaeian, M. J. Young, and H. Klassen, "Expression of neurodevelopmental markers by cultured porcine neural precursor cells," *Stem Cells*, vol. 23, no. 9, pp. 1286–1294, 2005.

[19] L. Anderson, R. M. Burnstein, X. He et al., "Gene expression changes in long term expanded human neural progenitor cells passaged by chopping lead to loss of neurogenic potential *in vivo*," *Experimental Neurology*, vol. 204, no. 2, pp. 512–524, 2007.

[20] L. S. Wright, K. R. Prowse, K. Wallace, M. H. K. Linskens, and C. N. Svendsen, "Human progenitor cells isolated from the developing cortex undergo decreased neurogenesis and eventual senescence following expansion in vitro," *Experimental Cell Research*, vol. 312, no. 11, pp. 2107–2120, 2006.

5

Ex Vivo Expansion of Human Mesenchymal Stem Cells in Defined Serum-Free Media

Sunghoon Jung,[1] Krishna M. Panchalingam,[1] Lawrence Rosenberg,[2] and Leo A. Behie[1]

[1] *Pharmaceutical Production Research Facility (PPRF), Schulich School of Engineering, University of Calgary, Calgary, AB, Canada T2N 1N4*
[2] *Department of Surgery, McGill University, Montreal, QC, Canada H3G 1A4*

Correspondence should be addressed to Leo A. Behie, behie@ucalgary.ca

Academic Editor: Selim Kuçi

Human mesenchymal stem cells (hMSCs) are presently being evaluated for their therapeutic potential in clinical studies to treat various diseases, disorders, and injuries. To date, early-phase studies have indicated that the use of both autologous and allogeneic hMSCs appear to be safe; however, efficacy has not been demonstrated in recent late-stage clinical trials. Optimized cell bioprocessing protocols may enhance the efficacy as well as safety of hMSC therapeutics. Classical media used for generating hMSCs are typically supplemented with ill-defined supplements such as fetal bovine serum (FBS) or human-sourced alternatives. Ideally, culture media are desired to have well-defined serum-free formulations that support the efficient production of hMSCs while maintaining their therapeutic and differentiation capacity. Towards this objective, we review here current cell culture media for hMSCs and discuss medium development strategies.

1. Introduction

Human mesenchymal stem cells (hMSCs), also referred to as mesenchymal stromal cells [1], demonstrate regenerative properties and multipotentiality, and thus have been proposed as a potential candidate for cell therapies and tissue engineering. Clinical studies employing hMSCs derived from different sources have been initiated for the treatment of several diseases and injuries such as myocardial infarction, osteogenesis imperfecta, graft-versus-host disease (GVHD), and Crohn's disease, spinal cord injury, multiple sclerosis, and diabetes (http://www.clinicaltrials.gov/). Early-phase studies with thousands of patients have indicated that the use of both autologous and allogeneic hMSCs appears to be safe; however, efficacy has not been demonstrated in recent late-stage clinical trials [2]. In general, clinical protocols employ cell culture technologies by which a small fraction of primary hMSCs are isolated from a selected tissue source and expanded for multiple passages in order to generate a clinically relevant number of cells. Consequently, once the tissue source of hMSCs is determined for an intended clinical application, the safety and efficacy of cell therapeutics produced may be significantly influenced by cell bioprocessing protocols [3]. As a consequence, developing robust production processes by optimizing culture variables is critical to efficiently and consistently generate hMSCs that retain desired regenerative and differentiation properties while minimizing any potential risks.

Cell culture variables include medium formulation (basal media and supplements), culture surface substrate, cell seeding density, physiochemical environment (dissolved oxygen and carbon dioxide concentrations, temperature, pH, osmolality, and buffer system), along with subculture protocols. In particular, the development of well-formulated culture media for both the isolation and expansion of hMSCs is imperative, but has been recognized as an extremely difficult process due to the high complexity of media formulations. Herein, we review various types of media that are currently used for clinical studies or under evaluation, along with the biological characteristics and *ex vivo* expansion procedures for hMSCs. It is clear that defined media optimized for hMSC isolation and expansion would greatly facilitate the development of robust, clinically acceptable bioprocesses for reproducibly generating quality-assured cells. Although several serum-free formulations have recently been developed, the performance of most media seems to be suboptimal. Identifying critical factors and their concentrations towards designing an ideally formulated, chemically defined serum-free medium should be carried out using rational and systematic approaches. Hence, in the second part of this paper, we discuss crucial strategies and important decisions needed for serum-free medium development.

2. Mesenchymal Stem Cells

2.1. What Is an MSC? Friedenstein and colleagues first reported a small fraction of cells in bone marrow (BM) attached to and proliferated on tissue culture substrates and that these cells were able to differentiate into multiple cell types such as adipocytes, osteoblasts, and chondrocytes both *in vitro* and *in vivo* [reviewed in [4]]. These cells were fibroblastic spindle-shaped and readily generated single-cell-derived colonies and were originally referred to as colony-forming unit-fibroblasts (CFU-F). Later, these cells were demonstrated by many investigators to be heterogeneous populations of nonhematopoietic adult stem/progenitor cell-like cells residing in marrow stroma and, thus, were called marrow stromal cells, mesenchymal stem cells, or multipotent mesenchymal stromal cells [1, 4]. In addition to BM, similar MSC-like cells have also been shown to be present in most tissues, including adipose tissue (AT), synovial membranes, bone, skin, pancreas, blood, fetal liver, lung, and umbilical cord blood (UCB) [4, 5].

2.2. Characteristics of hMSCs. BM has been the traditional source of hMSCs for basic research and therapeutic use because BM harvest is a routine and safe procedure. Therefore, the characteristics of *ex vivo* expanded hMSCs described below mostly represent BM-derived hMSCs unless otherwise stated.

2.2.1. Morphology. Typically, hMSCs isolated and expanded in classical FBS-containing media are mostly spindle-shaped (or fusiform) and cuboidal fibroblast-like cells. More specifically, Prockop and colleagues demonstrated that hMSCs undergo a time-dependent morphological transition from thin (small), spindle-shaped cells (considered stem cells or early progenitors) to wider (larger), spindle-shaped cells (looked like more mature cells) when cells are plated at 1 to $1,000 \, cells/cm^2$ [6]. They further showed that the small, spindle-shaped cells proliferate more rapidly and have a higher level of multipotentiality, compared to the slowly replicating large cells, which have lost most of their multipotentiality but can still differentiate into a lineage (e.g., osteogenic) as a default pathway. The morphology (and size) of hMSCs may also be dependent upon culture conditions (e.g., growth media, culture surface). For example, hMSCs expanded in bFGF-supplemented media were smaller and

proliferated more rapidly, compared to those in bFGF-lacking control conditions [7]. Culture surfaces (e.g., treated with Matrigel) might also affect the morphology [8].

2.2.2. Growth and Adherence Characteristics. hMSCs are anchorage-dependent cells, which attach to a plastic surface, spread out, and grow, when maintained in standard culture conditions (e.g., DMEM supplemented with 10% FBS). The initial growth of hMSCs in primary BM cell culture on a plastic surface is characterized by the formation of single-cell-derived colonies, when the cells are plated at appropriate numbers. The cells in colonies generated in the primary culture can typically be subcultured through multiple passages at various plating densities. In general, hMSCs have great propensity for expansion in culture, although their proliferation potential is highly variable, depending on many aspects such as donor age, tissue source, and culture conditions. For example, Sekiya et al. demonstrated that hMSCs proliferate more rapidly when passaged by plating the cells at low densities (e.g., 10–$100 \, cells/cm^2$, compared to $1,000$–$10,000 \, cells/cm^2$) [6]. hMSC proliferation is also highly variable depending on growth media [9].

2.2.3. Immunophenotype. Currently, no prospective markers exclusively defining hMSCs are available. In general, hMSCs are negative for hematopoietic surface markers including Cluster of Differentiation (CD) 34, CD45, CD14, CD11b, CD19, CD79α, CD31, CD133 and positive for CD63, CD105, CD166, CD54, CD55, CD13, CD44, CD73, and CD90 [10, 11]. However, differences exist among the studies reporting the surface marker characteristics, which may be explained by variations in culture methods and/or differentiation stage of the cells [11].

2.2.4. Multilineage Differentiation Potential. hMSCs have at least trilineage differentiation potential *in vitro* (i.e., the ability to differentiate into bone, cartilage and fat upon proper induction conditions). This is the most well-established characteristic of hMSCs and thus is considered the hallmark of these cells [12]. It has also been observed that hMSCs could give rise to other mesodermal cells and nonmesodermal cell types, such as neuron-like and endoderm-like cells [11].

2.2.5. Minimal Criteria for Defining hMSCs. Standard culture protocols for the isolation and expansion of hMSCs have not been well established, in particular for growth medium. Therefore, different laboratories often use various methods of isolation/expansion and also different approaches to characterize the cells. This makes it difficult to compare and contrast the outcomes from various investigators. To minimize the variations, the Mesenchymal and Tissue Stem Cell Committee of the International Society for Cellular Therapy has proposed minimal criteria to define hMSC populations. These include the following: (i) hMSCs must be plastic-adherent when maintained in classical culture conditions; (ii) hMSCs must express high levels ($\geq$95% positive) of CD105, CD73, and CD90 and lack expression

($\leq$2% positive) of CD45, CD34, CD14, or CD11b, CD79α or CD19, and HLA-DR (unless stimulated by interferon-γ) surface molecules; (iii) hMSCs must differentiate into osteoblasts, adipocytes, and chondroblasts under specific *in vitro* differentiation conditions [10].

2.3. Potential Therapeutic Properties of hMSCs. hMSCs show various properties that could be important in therapeutic applications. Indeed, some of these functions are currently being exploited in clinical trials with great promise.

2.3.1. Multipotentiality. As described earlier, hMSCs can differentiate into distinctive mesenchymal phenotypes, and thus they have been used to reconstruct damaged tissues upon transplantation in association with scaffolds. In addition, due to their differentiation potential into nonmesodermal cell types, hMSCs cells have also been proposed for replacement therapies to treat various diseases and disorders such as neuronal diseases and diabetes [13, 14].

2.3.2. Tropism for Sites of Disease. hMSCs appear to be capable of homing to sites of disease or damage. It has been reported that hMSCs systematically infused into diabetic mice migrated to damaged sites (i.e., pancreatic islets and renal glomeruli) and contributed to the repair of tissue [15] by certain mechanism(s) yet unidentified.

2.3.3. Secretion of Bioactive Factors. hMSCs inherently synthesize and secrete a broad range of bioactive agents such as cytokines and growth factors [16]. This intrinsic secretory activity of hMSCs may significantly contribute to tissue repair or regeneration, presumably by establishing a regenerative microenvironment at sites of tissue injury or damage [16]. Originally, therapeutic effects observed with the use of hMSCs were thought to be due to their transdifferentiation (i.e., differentiation into nonmesodermal cell types) potential. However, these beneficial effects were often demonstrated without evidence for the engraftment and transdifferentiation of transplanted hMSCs in animal model studies. Therefore, these indirect, secretory functions of hMSCs have been proposed as an alternative mechanism explaining the therapeutic effects, and importantly, these characteristics have generated clinical interest to use undifferentiated hMSCs for various applications such as repair or regeneration of damaged tissues [16].

2.3.4. Immunomodulation. hMSCs also display immune regulatory properties that might represent a critical role in the therapeutic application of these cells [17]. *In vitro* studies using hMSCs demonstrated that these cells suppress the proliferation of T cells. Further, it was also revealed that hMSCs inhibit the differentiation and maturation of dendritic cells (DCs) and decrease the production of inflammatory cytokines by various immune cell populations [18]. DCs are the most potent antigen-presenting cells, which specialize in antigen uptake, transport, and presentation and have the unique capacity to stimulate naïve and memory T cells [17]. In addition to the *in vitro* effects, it has

been seen in animal model studies that hMSCs may also display immunosuppressive capacities *in vivo*. For example, hMSCs facilitated engraftment of hematopoietic stem cells and prolonged skin allograft survival [19]. Further, it has been demonstrated that the use of hMSCs reversed severe acute GVHD [19]. However, while *in vitro* results consistently show the immunosuppressive capacity of hMSCs, studies in animals and humans suggest that hMSCs are less effective in producing systemic immunosuppression *in vivo* [20]. Therefore, further studies using standardized hMSC populations are urgently needed to verify their *in vivo* immunosuppressive potential and to define the optimal conditions for the use of hMSCs as immunotherapy.

2.3.5. Immune Privileged or Hypoimmunogenic Property. When undifferentiated hMSCs were transplanted into recipients in preclinical and clinical trials, these cells produced various cytokines and growth factors and had an ability to modify the response of immune cells. Another important observation is that hMSCs escape immune recognition or at least possess a hypoimmunogenic character upon allogeneic transplantation [21]. Indeed, clinical studies showed that hMSCs evoke little or no immune reactivity in allogeneic recipients [5]. This indicates that, in addition to the transplantation of autologous cells to patients to minimize the risk of immune response, allogeneic hMSCs could also be safely used. If this is the case, the use of allogeneic hMSCs has an important advantage in that the culture-expanded cells could be considered as an "off the shelf" therapeutic product. Indeed, clinical studies using allogeneic, as well as autologous, hMSCs from BM have been initiated for the treatment of several diseases and injuries such as osteogenesis imperfecta, GVHD, leukemia, myocardial infarcts, Crohn's Disease, cartilage and meniscus injury, stroke, and spinal cord injury [5, 16].

2.4. Safety of Using hMSCs. A large body of safety data has been gained from the use of hMSCs in various clinical applications including the treatment of GVHD and the facilitation of BM engraftment [14]. That is, until present, only few adverse effects attributed to hMSC transplantation have been reported [22]. This has facilitated the rapid translation of basic research into clinical trials. However, there are some obvious issues that need to be addressed before the wide implementation of clinical trials using hMSCs.

2.4.1. Tumor Formation. In general, it is considered that hMSCs can be safely cultured *in vitro* with no risk of malignant spontaneous transformation [23]. Stenderup and colleagues cultured several strains of hMSCs from BM at various ages (i.e., aged 18–81 years) until the cells reached their maximal life span without any evidence of transformation [24]. Further, there have been no reports with human trials demonstrating the formation of tumors by culture-expanded hMSCs [22]. Nonetheless, a potential risk for spontaneous transformation associated with hMSC proliferation *in vitro*, in particular after long-term culture, cannot be ruled out.

The transplantation of primitive stem/progenitor cells with considerable proliferative potential can raise the possibility of tumor formation, and any *ex vivo* manipulation will increase the chances of transformation [14]. It has been recommended by the Food and Drug Administration (FDA) that "minimally manipulated" cells be used for human clinical trials. In this regard, attempts are being made to develop an efficient production system to produce clinically relevant numbers of hMSCs at relative shorter periods of time with lower passage numbers [25].

2.4.2. Promotion of Tumor Growth and Development. A potential risk of treatment with hMSCs can paradoxically arise from the fact that these cells are capable of suppressing various immune cells, which may promote tumor growth and metastasis. The role of hMSCs in tumors is controversial: some studies have demonstrated enhancement of tumor growth and metastasis, while others have shown no apparent effect or inhibition of tumor growth with the use of hMSCs [26].

2.4.3. Immune Response. Although hMSCs themselves appear to escape immune recognition, those "cultured in medium containing FBS" can produce immune reactions in patients receiving repeated administrations of these cells [27]. Conventionally, the optimal conditions for hMSC expansion require media supplemented with FBS at a concentration of 10–20%, which corresponds to approximately 5–10 mg FBS proteins/mL of medium. Spees et al. demonstrated that, when hMSCs were cultured in medium containing 20% FBS and harvested, 7–30 mg of FBS proteins were still associated with a standard preparation of 100 million hMSCs, a dosage that probably will be needed for clinical therapies [28]. Thus, immunological reactions caused by medium-derived FBS proteins will be a concern, in particular for certain types of cell therapy involving multiple administrations of hMSCs. The safety issue associated with the use of FBS in culture media will be avoided by developing an alternative culture protocol to produce hMSCs *in vitro* in the absence of FBS.

2.5. Sources of hMSCs. Although the traditional source of hMSCs is BM, it has been demonstrated that cells displaying similar characteristics with BM-hMSCs can also be derived from other sources including AT, UCB, umbilical cord tissue, placenta, amniotic fluid, liver, lung, pancreas, and muscle [29–34]. The ideal source of hMSCs for therapeutic use would be one that is readily available and can be expanded in culture rapidly to yield large numbers of cells. In this regard, hMSCs from readily obtainable tissue otherwise discarded, such as AT, may offer a preferable alternative to BM, because the collection of BM is an invasive procedure. Moreover, AT is a source of abundant hMSCs, and the AT-derived hMSCs have shown various potential therapeutic properties both *in vitro* and *in vivo* [29]. UCB, umbilical cord tissue, and placenta also represent attractive sources of hMSCs because these tissues are readily available and the derived cells may contain less genetic abnormalities and greater proliferative capacity than adult tissue-derived hMSCs [30–32].

It is important to note that there is much evidence demonstrating that hMSCs (or similar populations) derived from various sources showed different characteristics in gene expression profile, proliferation and differentiation potential, and functional properties although most of these satisfied the minimal criteria for defining MSCs and, thus, were considered as hMSCs as a whole [35–38]. For example, studies have shown that AT-hMSCs exhibited *in vitro* immunomodulatory properties at higher efficiencies, compared to BM-derived counterparts [35]. Another example can be found from a study comparing the differentiation potential of hMSCs from BM and pancreas into insulin-producing endocrine cells [36]. This study revealed that hMSCs derived from the pancreas are committed to an endocrine fate and thus have a greater propensity to generate insulin-producing cells compared to BM-hMSCs. Therefore, to select an ideal source of hMSCs for therapeutic use, their functional properties (e.g., differentiation potential, immunomodulation, secretion of bioactive factors) should be critically evaluated in comparison with those from other potential sources, in addition to the availability of tissue and cell proliferation capacity as mentioned earlier.

3. Generation of Mesenchymal Stem Cells

3.1. hMSC Number. The frequency of hMSCs in BM is very low. The CFU-F assay is widely used to estimate the number of MSCs in primary BM cells as well as passaged cell populations in culture [39, 40]. Using this assay, it has been reported that MSCs represent 0.01% to 0.001% of human BM mononuclear cells (MNCs) [39]. It was also demonstrated that hMSCs comprise approximately 1 in 10,000, 100,000, and 250,000 BM-hMNCs of newborns, teens, and 30 year-olds, respectively, indicating that the hMSC frequency is highly variable with age [16].

There is a significant difference in the frequency of hMSCs present in other tissues/organs, heavily depending on the source. Kern et al. reported different frequencies of hMSCs in BM, AT, and UCB. In their study, with culture-initiating populations (i.e., MNCs of BM and UCB, and stromal vascular fraction of AT), it was demonstrated that the number of CFU-Fs (i.e., corresponding to hMSCs) calculated at the basis of 1×10^6 initially plated cells was highest for AT (557), followed by BM (83) [37]. In contrast, the frequency of CFU-Fs in UCB was considerably lower. Similar observations were reported by others [41, 42].

Although the dosage of hMSCs for their optimal use in therapeutic applications is still unclear and should be dependent upon the type of cell therapy, at least 1 to 2×10^6 hMSCs per kg body weight of the adult patient is generally suggested [43]. Consequently, the number of primary hMSCs, regardless of the sources, is insufficient for research as well as clinical use. Hence, it is necessary to isolate hMSCs and then subsequently expand them for multiple passages on tissue culture substrates in order to generate clinically relevant numbers of cells.

3.2. Isolation and Expansion of hMSCs

3.2.1. Isolation of hMSCs (Primary Culture).
As there are no universal surface markers available for exclusively defining hMSCs, these cells have traditionally been isolated from initial primary cell fractions (e.g., BM MNCs), based on their selective adherence, compared to hematopoietic cells, to plastic surfaces. Therefore, the hMSCs obtained are intrinsically heterogeneous. Importantly, it has been demonstrated that the characteristics of isolated cells are highly dependent upon culture conditions used. For BM cells, either unfractionated whole BM, fractionated MNCs by density gradient, or separated cells by depletion of certain subpopulations are used, with the fractioned MNCs being the most popular.

3.2.2. Expansion of hMSCs.
As a large number of hMSCs is needed for their clinical use, cells obtained from the primary culture are further expanded through multiple passages. Typically, hMSCs obtained from young donors can undergo 24–40 population doublings (PD) in culture before they reach senescence, while those from older donors retain reduced proliferative potential [11]. Similar to other diploid cells, hMSCs grow at a rather constant rate during early passages (typically for the first 2 to 3 weeks) and then with a gradual increase in cell doubling times as the passage number increases until the growth ceases due to senescence [11]. It is also known that, after the initial culture, hMSCs progressively show loss of multipotentiality [44] under classical media and possibly other culture conditions.

3.3. Culture Media for hMSCs

3.3.1. Classical FBS-Based Media.
Conventional media used for isolating and expanding hMSCs include supplementation of FBS at 10–20% (v/v). FBS contains a high content of attachment and growth factors as well as nutritional and physiochemical compounds required for cell maintenance and growth. The function and characteristic of serum is further reviewed later in this paper. FBS-based media remain a common standard in generating hMSCs for basic research and clinical studies; however, the use of FBS is not desirable, raising several safety and other concerns. The inherent potential problems associated with the ill-defined FBS and other animal-derived supplements are as follows [45–47]:

(i) risk of contamination associated with harmful pathogens such as viruses, mycoplasma, prions, or unidentified zoonotic agents and transmissions of these contaminants to cells being used for cellular therapy,

(ii) high content of xenogeneic proteins that can be associated with cell therapeutics during culture, causing concerns relating to immune reaction in patients, as described earlier,

(iii) high degree of batch-to-batch variation causing inconsistency in the generation of quality-assured cells and thus making standardization of the production process difficult,

(iv) presence of growth inhibitors, cytotoxic substances, and/or differentiation agents. (Beyond its growth-promoting property, serum may also contain components that are inhibitory for the growth of certain cell types. It has been demonstrated that some cell types cannot be cultured in the presence of serum at its typical concentrations in medium due to its unidentified cytotoxic constituents. It is also well known that serum is toxic at high concentrations for most cell types [48]),

(v) requirement of a set of strict quality controls to minimize the risk of contamination and to select appropriate FBS lots supporting growth of cells while retaining their regenerative and differentiation properties,

(vi) interference of unidentified factors on the effect of hormones, growth factors, or other additives under investigation,

(vii) limited availability,

(viii) ethical issues [49].

Considered together, despite strict selection and testing for safety and growth-promoting capacity, the use of FBS represents a *major obstacle* for the wide implementation of hMSC-related therapies.

3.3.2. Humanized Media.
In order to alleviate the safety and regulatory concerns raised by the use of animal serum for generating hMSCs, autologous or allogeneic human blood-derived materials, including human serum, plasma, platelet derivatives (e.g., platelet lysate), and cord blood serum, are currently under investigation for their clinical utility as an alternative medium supplement.

Human autologous serum has been reported to support hMSC expansion [50–53]. It would be problematic, however, to acquire amounts sufficient to generate clinically relevant numbers of hMSCs. Moreover, the use of autologous serum may not be applicable for elderly patients as its capacity to support cell growth may decrease with their age. The performance of human allogeneic serum from adult donors is rather controversial because contradictory results have been reported [52, 54–58]. Allogeneic human serum from UCB [59, 60] and placenta [61] has also been proposed as potential alternatives to replace FBS because these primitive tissues are a rich source of growth factors [49].

Attempts have also been made by many investigators to examine the utility of human platelet lysate (hPL), which has been prepared by mechanical disruption or chemical lysis of the platelet membrane [49], for the cultivation of hMSCs. Most of the studies reported that the growth factor-enriched allogeneic hPLs have considerable growth-promoting properties for hMSCs while maintaining their differentiation potential and immunomodulatory properties [62–70]. However, some other studies reported data that showed a reduction of osteogenic or adipogenic differentiation potential when hMSCs were cultured in hPL-based media [67, 71]. Moreover, a recent report illustrated that, although cell proliferation was greatly enhanced, the use of hPL (supplemented into RMPI 1640 medium) altered the expression of some hMSC surface molecules and led to a decrease in their *in vitro* immunosuppressive capacity [72]. This study also showed that the production of prostaglandin E_2, which has previously been demonstrated to play a major role in the suppression of immune cells [73], was lowered under the use of hPL compared to FBS.

Although considered relatively safer than FBS for human therapeutic applications, the use of human-sourced supplements is still a matter of substantial debate, prompting some concerns [74, 75]. There is a risk that allogeneic human growth supplements may be contaminated with human pathogens that might not be detected by routine screening of blood donors. Moreover, these crude blood derivatives are poorly defined and suffer from batch-to-batch variation, and thus their ability to maintain hMSC growth and therapeutic potentials could be widely variable. In particular, the variability can be a significant hindrance for implementing the clinical-scale production of hMSCs simply because it could make it difficult to obtain cells retaining desired qualities in a consistent and predictable manner, which is crucial for minimizing treatment failures.

3.3.3. Defined Serum-Free Media.
The concerns raised from the use of ill-defined serum or human-sourced supplements demonstrate the need for the development of defined serum-free media. While reducing the problems associated with such crude materials, defined serum-free media may further provide additional advantages as follows.

(i) Defined formulations designed to support the generation of a population enriched with a desired cell type (i.e., hMSCs) while preventing overgrowth of undesired cells in primary cultures will lead to the production of more homogeneous hMSCs (i.e., more precisely, a population of adherent cells containing a high content of colony-forming multipotent mesenchymal cells). It has been shown that medium formulations greatly affect the frequency and size of colonies in the primary and passaged hMSC culture, and a systematically optimized defined medium for hMSCs led to significant increased colony-formation compared to FBS-based cultures [76].

(ii) The well-defined nature of the medium would facilitate enhancing cell bioprocessing protocols, which may be crucial for increasing clinical efficacy by producing cells with desired properties. For instance, based on the proposed mechanism that hMSCs exert therapeutic benefits via the secretion of certain soluble molecules, the medium formulations may need to be modified to enhance expression of specific genes to achieve an optimal cytokine profile [3].

(iii) When *ex vivo* differentiated cells are desirable for therapeutic use, the transition of an expansion state to a differentiation phase under defined conditions could facilitate the production of such desired cell types in a more favorable and controllable environment. Davani et al. demonstrated that, in an effort

to differentiate hMSCs (pancreas-derived) to insulin-expressing cells, the shift of a serum-based expansion condition to a serum-free differentiation condition led to considerable cell death [36]. In principle, it may be less harsh to cells to switch only key "growth-promoting factor(s)" to "differentiation-inducing factor(s)" while maintaining the base condition.

Attempts have been made to develop defined serum-free media for animal or human MSC growth; however, most of them have demonstrated only limited performance [77–80]. These media formulations were only shown to support cell expansion for single-passage cultures or at slow rates through multiple passages. Moreover, all of these studies used cells which had previously been exposed to serum during the initial isolation/expansion phases. Serum-derived contaminants are probably carried over with the cells when they are placed under serum-free conditions after exposure to serum, and thus, exposure to serum may ultimately limit their therapeutic use.

The ideal media should consist of chemically defined constituents that support the attachment and growth of hMSCs primary cultures as well as passaged cultures, while maintaining their therapeutic properties. Towards this objective, our group has recently carried out a study to identify key attachment and growth factors required for both primary and passaged cultures, and this study led to the development of a defined serum-free medium (PPRF-msc6) for hMSC isolation and expansion [76]. We demonstrated that PPRF-msc6 medium supported the generation of hMSCs from multiple BM samples in a rapid and consistent manner, maintaining their multipotency and hMSC-specific immunophenotype. Furthermore, compared to a classical serum-supplemented media (i.e., DMEM supplemented with prescreened FBS), hMSCs cultured in PPRF-msc6 exhibited numerous advantages from a production standpoint. Specifically, these hMSCs had a greater colony-forming capacity in primary as well as passaged cultures, negligible lag phase and explicit exponential growth, lower population doubling times (21–26 h versus 35–38 h; between passage levels 1 and 10), a greater number of population doublings (62 ± 4 versus 43 ± 2; over a two-month period), and a more homogeneous cell population, which was smaller in size [81]. Consequently, the sustained production of smaller hMSCs in a rapid manner requires less time and surface area to obtain clinically relevant numbers of hMSCs, while reducing risk of contamination and saving cost and labor. Moreover, from a therapeutic viewpoint, the size of cells to be transplanted into patients could be an important issue because it has been shown in animal-model studies that most of hMSCs grown in FBS-supplemented media were trapped in the lung [82]. Small hMSCs may offer a significant benefit in transplantation therapies because the small cells may travel through the lung and home to the site of injury or disease at high efficiencies [83]. Similar to the performance with BM cells, PPRF-msc6 also allowed for the isolation and extended expansion of hMSCs from other sources, including AT and pancreatic tissue samples, more rapidly and efficiently compared to control

FBS-supplemented media [our unpublished data]. In view of the "defined" status, PPRF-msc6 contains some serum components, such as insulin, transferrin, serum albumin, and fetuin, which are often associated with traces of other serum constituents, and thus further investigations need to be conducted to refine this medium to a true chemically defined medium by replacing these components with synthetic alternatives. Recently, for instance, we have successfully replaced native insulin with a recombinant insulin without any decrease in the performance of PPRF-msc6 for hMSC culture. The replacement of native transferrin, albumin, and fetuin in this medium with recombinant alternatives or other supplements is currently underway. Nonetheless, PPRF-msc6 represents the most well-defined serum-free formulation to support both the isolation and expansion of hMSCs in the literature to date and a significant step forward for producing hMSC therapeutics. The protocol for PPRF-msc6 preparation has been described in detail [76] so that the disclosed formulation or its modifications can be further developed by any interested party.

Efforts have also been made to test or modify existing defined medium formulations designed for other stem cell types in order to cultivate hMSCs. Rajala et al. illustrated that a defined, xeno-free medium for human embryonic stem cells (hESCs) allowed, during a single-passage culture, the expansion of hMSCs previously isolated from AT samples in the presence of allogeneic human serum [84]. This study did not report whether this medium supported the growth of hMSCs in primary culture as well as through multiple passages. Also, Mimura et al. modified a defined hESC medium to promote the expansion of an immortalized genetically modified hMSC line [85]. The cells grown in their disclosed medium formulation demonstrated differentiation capacity towards osteogenic and adipogenic lineages while displaying a rather different gene expression profile compared to those cultured in FBS-based medium.

3.3.4. Commercially Available Media for Expanding hMSCs. Several commercially available serum-free media have recently been introduced for the expansion of hMSCs [reviewed in [86]]. StemPro MSC SFM from Invitrogen represents the first commercial serum-free medium that allows the isolation and expansion of hMSCs from BM and has recently been cleared by the FDA as a medical device for clinical trials in the United States (http://www.invitrogen.com/). Agata et al. demonstrated that this medium supported hMSC growth more rapidly at early passages while reaching senescence earlier (at passage 5) with gradually reduced proliferation rate, compared to a control FBS medium [87]. In addition, although most of the hMSC-specific surface antigens were expressed on both cell populations expanded in the serum-free medium and an FBS-based reference medium, some molecules were expressed in different levels (i.e., CD105 and CD146). Moreover, it appears that both cell populations displayed different levels of stemness as well as different differentiation potential (i.e., cells expanded in serum-free medium exhibited lower ALP activity in noninduced state, but a greater response to osteogenic

induction compared to serum-based controls). In summary, this commercial serum-free medium seems to generate hMSCs with different characteristics in comparison with those derived in classical FBS media.

Aiming towards the widespread implementation of hMSC-related therapy in later stage of clinical trials, serum-free, xeno-free media for hMSC culture have also been commercialized. However, the formulations of these commercial media are not disclosed, which may restrict their wide utility in hMSC research and clinical studies. The identification of specific medium components allowing for the serum-free isolation and expansion of hMSCs would contribute significantly to the research and therapeutic applications of these cells. Moreover, as medium formulations determine cell characteristics (i.e., growth pattern, gene expression, phenotype, and functional properties), it is important to evaluate carefully each of these commercial media for intended therapeutic applications, preferably in parallel to select the best choice for each specific target.

We have recently initiated a study to compare these commercial media along with other existing media. The media under investigation include Mesencult-XF (STEMCELL Technologies), StemPro MSC SFM Xeno-Free (Invitrogen), MSCGM-CD (Lonza), PPRF-msc6, and DMEM +10% FBS (Lonza). Our initial data show that the performance of the commercial hMSC media on the attachment and growth of primary BM-hMSCs is questionable and thus should be open to discussion. Specifically, in a preliminary experiment, the commercial media were evaluated in parallel with PPRF-msc6 and 10% FBS DMEM by plating human BM MNCs into human fibronectin-coated T-25 flasks containing each of the media. Cells were inoculated at 150,000 cells/cm^2, and nonadherent cells in each medium were removed after 60 hours with 100% medium change. Thereafter, the adherent cells were allowed to grow with 50% medium replacement every other day, and then stained on day 12. In this experiment, none of the commercial media demonstrated cell growth (Figures 1(a)–1(c)). In contrast, a significant number of well-developed colonies were found in the culture with PPRF-msc6 (Figure 1(d)). The serum-based control culture with 10% FBS DMEM also resulted in the formation of colonies although most of them were still premature. Lindroos et al. reported that StemPro MSC SFM Xeno-Free medium provided significantly higher proliferation rates of AT MSCs when compared with serum-containing media [88]. In their study, however, the authors tested the commercial serum-free medium using cells that were previously isolated and expanded in a serum-containing medium (10% human serum), and the ability of StemPro MSC SFM Xeno-Free medium to allow the growth of primary hMSCs was not addressed. Moreover, Hartmann et al. stated that they were not able to culture hMSCs derived from the UC tissue using StemPro MSC SFM Xeno-Free medium without serum [73]. In contrast, the authors demonstrated that Mesencult-XF medium supported the isolation and expansion of UC-hMSCs without the use of serum. In an attempt to culture hMSCs from BM using a xeno-free protocol (i.e., proprietary Mesencult-XF Attachment Substrate as well as medium), Miwa et al. also showed that the use of

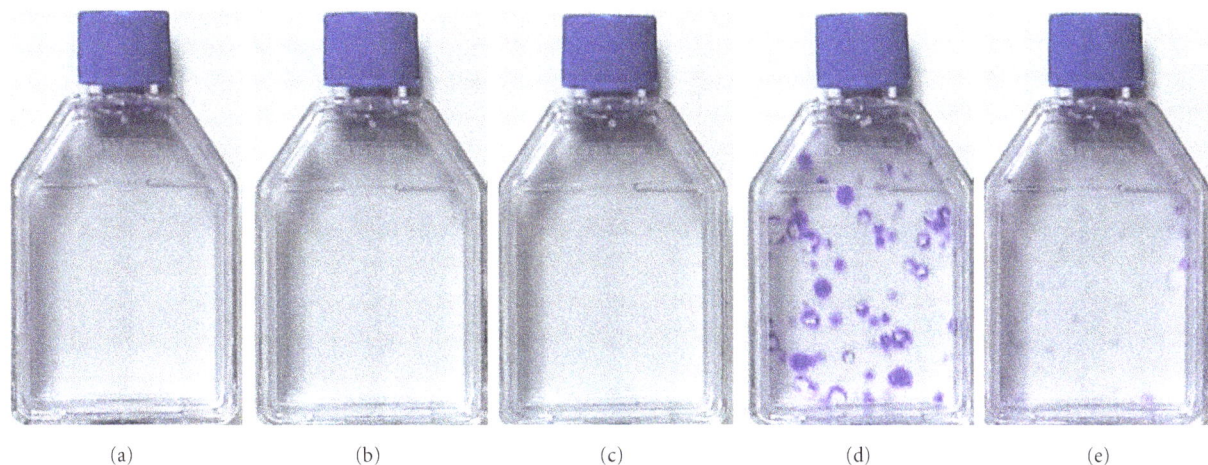

| (a) | (b) | (c) | (d) | (e) |

FIGURE 1: Cultivation of primary human BM MNCs using different media including three commercial media. Cells were inoculated at 150,000 BM MNCs/cm^2 into fibronectin-coated T-25 flasks, each containing 8 mL of Mesencult-XF (a), StemPro MSC SFM Xeno-Free (b), MSCGM-CD (c), and PPRF-msc6 (d), and a classical FBS medium (10% FBS DMEM) (e). After 60 h, nonadherent cells in each medium were removed, and fresh medium was added to the adherent cells (100% medium change). The adherent cells were allowed to grow for additional 10 days with 50% medium change every other day, and then stained with crystal violet to visualize colonies generated.

Mesencult-XF medium resulted in the growth of primary BM-hMSCs more rapidly than a serum-containing medium [89].

The contradictory data between our work and the literature [73, 89] regarding Mesencult-XF medium may be due, at least in part, to the use of different substrate materials. Specifically, we used human fibronectin-coated flasks, while Miwa et al. used a proprietary substrate-coating product. In this regard, we plated the nonadherent cells, which were removed from the first medium change during the primary culture with each medium described earlier, into new flasks containing the same medium to allow them to attach to the new substrate and grow. For convenience, here we call these as "secondary" cultures as opposed to their original cultures described in the previous paragraph and Figure 1. The "secondary" flasks were coated with gelatin (bovine), which is widely used to facilitate the attachment of many types of anchorage-dependent cells to the substrate. In these secondary cultures, we observed that a number of colonies were formed in the culture with Mesencult-XF medium (Figure 2(a)). Together with the data obtained from the original culture (Figure 1(a)), this demonstrates the ability of Mesencult-XF medium to allow the growth of primary hMSCs, but implying that the performance of the medium could be improved by manipulating the substrate-coating materials. In contrast, StemPro MSC SFM Xeno-Free medium and MSCGM-CD medium did not allow for colony formation (Figures 2(b) and 2(c), resp.). These data suggest that factors required for the isolation of hMSCs from primary cultures seem to be missed in both media. Similar with the study by Hartmann et al. [73], we also observed that the addition of low serum (i.e., 2% prescreened FBS) into StemPro MSC SFM Xeno-Free medium (and MSCGM-CD medium) supported the growth of primary BM-hMSCs (data not shown). Based on these observations, therefore, we would argue that it should be desirable to further optimize

all the commercial media described here for the serum-free, xeno-free isolation of hMSCs. Regarding PPRF-msc6, beyond the high number of large colonies generated in the original culture (Figure 1(d)), a number of colonies also appeared in the secondary cultures (Figure 2(d)), which were initiated with the nonadherent cells that had been normally discarded in our previous work [81]. In contrast, the FBS-based culture led to the appearance of only a few colonies in its secondary culture (Figure 2(e)), indicating that the majority of hMSCs obtainable from the use of 10% FBS DMEM attached to the surface of original culture in the presence of known and unknown attachment factors included in serum. Considered together, these data imply that the yield of hMSCs obtained from the primary culture of BM cells with PPRF-msc6 could further be increased by modifying the culture protocols, particularly by identifying optimal attachment factors and/or substrate-coating materials to enhance initial cell attachment efficiencies.

A commercial medium (mTeSR) with disclosed composition, which was originally developed for the expansion of hESCs, has also been tested for hMSC culture [90]. Although this defined medium together with human fibronectin-treated substrate allowed the expansion of BM-hMSCs previously isolated using FBS-based medium, it did not support cell growth in primary BM cultures. In addition, when hMSCs were plated into the mTeSR at a very low density for a CFU-F assay, the colonies derived were significantly smaller at lower frequency, compared to a control case with FBS-based medium. Moreover, mTeSR-derived cells demonstrated significantly decreased adipogenic potential. Therefore, further studies should be carried out with this medium to identify factors affecting multipotency as well as growth of hMSCs to make the disclosed formulation viable for research and clinical applications.

In summary, although numerous defined hMSC media are commercially available or have been introduced in

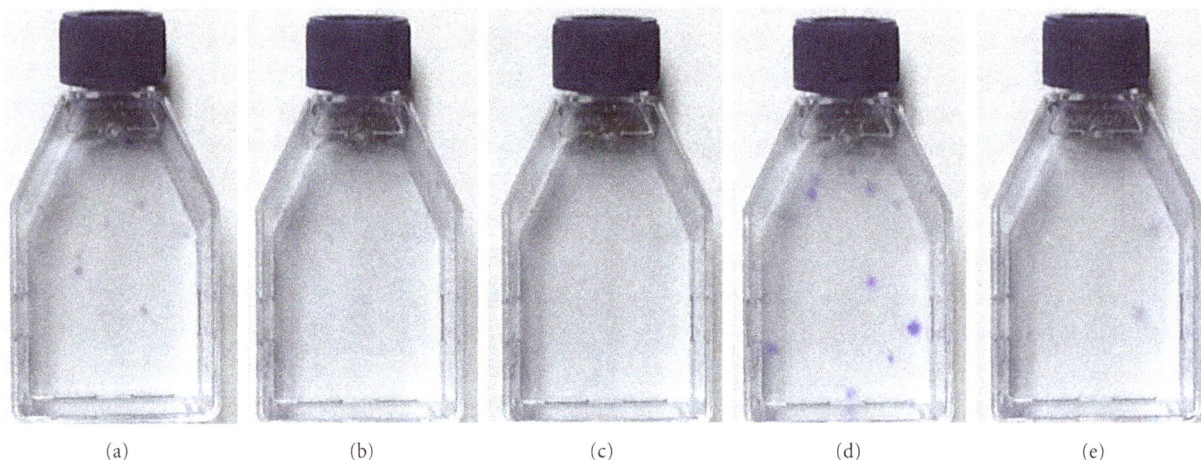

(a)   (b)   (c)   (d)   (e)

FIGURE 2: Cultivation of nonadherent cell fractions removed from the culture of primary BM MNCs in different media. Nonadherent cells and spent medium removed from each of the flasks, demonstrated in Figure 1, were replated into a new T-25 flask coated with gelatin containing 4 mL of the fresh medium—that is, Mesencult-XF (a), StemPro MSC SFM Xeno-Free (b), MSCGM-CD (c), PPRF-msc6 (d), and 10% FBS DMEM (e). After 60 h, nonadherent cells and medium in each flask were discarded, and fresh medium was added to the adherent cells (8 mL per flask). The adherent cells were allowed to grow for additional 8 days with 50% medium change every other day and then stained with crystal violet to visualize colonies generated.

the literature to support the growth of hMSCs, one must realize that the therapeutically relevant properties of culture-expanded hMSCs could be significantly affected by medium components. Considering the safety and efficacy required to produce hMSC therapeutics for intended clinical applications, it is crucial to compare different media (and their formulations if the recipe is disclosed) and probably further optimize the formulations in a systematic manner. In this regard, the disclosed medium formulations for hMSCs (e.g., those reported in [76, 80, 85, 90]) are best positioned to be further developed by the many investigators interested in therapeutic applications of hMSCs.

4. Development of Defined Serum-Free Media

Defined serum-free medium development or optimization for a specific cell type is a very complicated process because multiple variables that affect the maintenance, growth, and characteristics of cells are interrelated. Moreover, designing a new serum-free formulation for anchorage-dependent cells such as hMSCs tends to be more fastidious compared to those grown in suspension culture, as the interaction of cells with the substrate on which they attach and spread prior to growth needs to be understood. Medium development studies should involve rational approaches: (i) to select appropriate factors (e.g., basal medium formulations and growth/attachment proteins) and (ii) to screen them in a stepwise, systematic manner for their effect on cell properties and growth.

4.1. Cell Culture Requirements. An understanding of the requirements for successful cell culture is a prerequisite for designing a rational strategy towards the efficient development/optimization of a new serum-free medium. In addition, since anchorage-dependent hMSCs normally require

serum, namely, some serum components yet unidentified but responsible for their attachment, spread, and growth, it is particularly crucial to understand the functions that serum serve in cell culture in order to identify such components. Hence, specific requirements of nutrients and nonnutrient elements for cell culture are briefly reviewed below with a special emphasis on the constituents and functions of serum.

4.1.1. Nutrients. Nutrients refer to chemical substances that are taken into cells and utilized as substrates in energy metabolism or biosynthesis, as catalysts in those processes, or as structural components of cellular organelles. The nutrients are divided into organic nutrients, inorganic salts, and trace elements, and the organic nutrients are further subdivided into amino acids, carbohydrates, lipids, vitamins, and others [91]. Generally, the nutrients are considered as the "defined" portion of culture media. In addition to the "nutrient" roles, the nutrients also have regulatory functions. It has been demonstrated that these nutrients could represent the only requirements for *in vitro* growth of certain transformed cell lines [92]; however, more fastidious nontransformed normal cells typically require additional growth-promoting supplements for their growth in culture.

Organic Nutrients. Amino acids represent essential elements of media as building blocks for protein synthesis. In addition, certain amino acids have other key roles in multiplication of cells in culture, especially under serum-free conditions. In particular, glutamine appears to play major roles in many metabolic pathways, and thus an adequate extracellular concentration of glutamine is typically needed in cell culture media. It is common to add 2–4 mM of glutamine to hMSC media. It is important to note that glutamine is labile under cell culture conditions, and thus the amount of glutamine for hMSC culture should be determined considering both the requirement for cell growth and its breakdown during the culture. Moreover, nonessential amino acids have been added into a defined medium developed for hMSC growth [80].

A carbohydrate source is essential for the growth of cells in culture, since neither amino acids nor fats can readily be used either as the sole energy source or as substrates to build up a sufficient pool of intracellular carbohydrate intermediates. Glucose is the commonly provided source of energy for cells in culture, and together with amino acids it is included in most defined basal medium formulations. It is known that glucose at high concentrations has harmful effects on some cell types in culture. For this reason, low concentrations of glucose (~ 5 mM) are commonly used for hMSC culture. However, recent evidence reveals that high glucose concentrations (~ 25 mM) led to comparable or higher growth of animal and human MSCs [93–95].

It is known that certain lipids, such as cholesterol, free linoleic acid and its metabolites, free oleic acid, and phospholipids containing linoleic acid, stimulate growth of mammalian cells. Lipids are frequently not included in the defined portions of cell culture media. Large amounts of bound lipids are contained in serum; therefore, normally serum-containing media do not need the supplementation of additional lipids. In contrast, externally supplied lipids are generally required in serum-free culture [91]. Lipid supplements have been added to serum-free media for hMSCs [76, 80].

In general, mammals require 12 vitamins, including the 4 fat-soluble vitamins (A, D, E, and K) and the 8 members of the B complex (thiamine, riboflavin, niacin, pyridoxine, pantothenic acid, folacin, vitamin B_{12}, and biotin). In addition, primates, guinea pigs and flying mammals require vitamin C (ascorbic acid). In contrast, normal diploid cells in culture exhibit requirements for the B vitamins, while some cells have shown growth responses to ascorbic acid. For this reason, most cell culture media include all the B vitamins but variably contain vitamin C [91]. Other vitamins are not included in media. The B vitamins function as cofactors for specific enzymes, and their deficiency can result in death of the animal. Ascorbic acid functions as an oxygen acceptor in several mixed-function oxidase systems. Rowe et al. reported that ascorbic acid had an effect on collagen synthesis by human diploid fibroblasts and played a role as a growth-promoting factor for many cell types [96]. The use of ascorbic acid for hMSC culture seems to be a matter of debate. Gronthos and Simmons demonstrated that ascorbic acid was a critical component under serum-free conditions for supporting the formation of CFU-F colonies in primary cultures of human BM cells [97]. We and others also demonstrated that ascorbic acid promoted hMSC growth [76, 98]. Moreover, it was observed that the lack of ascorbic acid in medium significantly reduced osteogenic potential of hMSCs [76]. On the other hand, ascorbic acid has typically been used as a supplement in some MSC differentiation media. Mimura et al. reported that ascorbic acid increased osteoblastic marker expression in hMSCs grown in a serum-free condition, and thus the authors removed this component from their defined medium

formulation [85]. It should be noted that ascorbic acid is very labile under cell culture conditions [99]; therefore, care should be taken when this substance is used in cell culture.

Inorganic Salts. The salts that are included in most media are those of Na^+, K^+, Mg^{2+}, Ca^{2+}, Cl^-, SO_4^{2-}, PO_4^{3-}, and HCO_3^-, and they play several functions. The salts primarily contribute to retaining the osmotic balance of the cells. The osmolality of most cell culture media is approximately 300 mOsm/kg, and this represents an optimal value for most cell lines. It has been shown that many cell lines tolerate variation of approximately 10% of this optimal value, and thus care should be taken when extra salts are added into a medium [45]. Divalent cations, particularly Ca^{2+}, are required by some cell adhesion molecules, such as the cadherins. Ca^{2+} also acts as an intermediary in signal transduction, and the concentration of Ca^{2+} in the medium can have an influence on cell proliferation or differentiation. Na^+, K^+, and Cl^- regulate membrane potential, while SO_4^{2-}, PO_4^{3-}, and HCO_3^- have roles as anions required by the matrix and nutritional precursors for macromolecules, as well as regulators of intracellular charge. HCO_3^- also plays a role as a buffer and its concentration is determined by the concentration of CO_2 in the gas phase [100].

Trace Elements. In addition to the inorganic salts, other inorganic elements, such as Mn^{2+}, Cu^{2+}, Zn^{2+}, Mo^{6+}, Va^{5+}, Se^{8+}, Fe^{2+}, Ca^{2+}, Mg^{2+}, Si^{4+}, Ni^{2+} are present in serum in trace amounts. These substances are referred to as trace elements and are included in most medium formulations. Although the role of these trace elements has been only partially elucidated, it has been demonstrated that many of these elements act as enzyme cofactors and are essential to the survival and growth of most cells [45, 101]. For instance, selenium is well recognized as an activator of glutathione peroxidase, a key enzyme essential for detoxifying cytotoxic oxygen radicals, and has been considered as an essential trace element for many cell types in culture [92, 102, 103]. It was also observed that selenium increased the proliferation of hMSCs from AT [104]. In contrast, numerous reports demonstrated that selenium suppressed cell proliferation in culture and induced cytotoxicity [105]. In our study, the addition of selenium into a serum-based medium reduced the colony-forming ability of hMSCs [76]. Considered together, the effect of selenium on hMSC expansion seems to depend on culture conditions or cell sources.

4.1.2. Nonnutrient Factors. Beyond the nutrients, the growth of mammalian cells requires additional substances (provided from serum or other sources). These nonnutrient factors, including growth and attachment factors and hormones, generally function in regulatory roles on cellular differentiation as well as growth and proliferation. These regulatory factors are not included in most basal media and are frequently supplemented to serum-free media. Often, the requirements of nutrients for the growth of cells of interest could be satisfied by selecting appropriate defined basal media; therefore, identifying growth-stimulating regulatory factors has typically been the key subject in the development of serum-free media. Much effort has been made to investigate the effect of cytokines and growth factors on hMSC growth. Many reports showed that bFGF promotes the proliferation of hMSCs [76, 106–109]. TGF-β1 is also known to support hMSC proliferation in combination with other growth factors [85, 106]. It is important to note that TGF-β1 alone showed a growth-inhibitory effect on hMSCs, while demonstrating a significant degree of synergistic effect with bFGF [76]. The impact of PDGF on hMSCs is controversial. Several studies reported that PDGF enhanced the proliferation of MSCs from human and animal BM [77, 97, 106]. Moreover, PDGF-enriched plasma or platelet lysate has been shown to support the isolation and expansion of hMSCs. In contrast, our group observed that PDGF reduced considerably the colony-forming property of hMSCs [76]. It is presumed that the contradictory data are due, at least in part, to different modes of interactions with different factors present in different culture conditions. Other growth factors, such as EGF, Activin A, aFGF, and FGF4, have also been shown to promote hMSC proliferation (e.g., [76, 110, 111]); however, their effects could be masked in the presence of more potent factors (e.g., bFGF) [76].

Binding proteins such as albumin and transferrin are commonly added to serum-free media. Parker et al. reported that the absence of albumin in their serum-free formulation reduced hMSC growth [80]. Supplementation of key hormone components into serum-free media is also crucial. We observed no stimulatory effects of insulin and progesterone under FBS-based conditions in our study [76]. Nonetheless, these components showed growth-promoting effects for many cell types in serum-free condition [112]. Hydrocortisone has been shown to increase the proliferation of adherent human BM cells [113]. It has also been demonstrated that dexamethasone, a synthetic reagent of fluoridated hydrocortisone, is an essential component in serum-free medium for the growth of CFU-F colonies in primary cultures of human BM cells [97]. Interestingly, our experiments showed that the supplementation of hydrocortisone into an FBS-containing medium significantly inhibited cell proliferation and caused a change in cell morphology from spindle-shaped to cuboidal (data not shown); however, this hormone was found to be a key component in our serum-free media for hMSC growth, displaying a considerable combined effect with fetuin, particularly in primary culture [76]. This indicates that the effect of hydrocortisone is highly dependent upon culture conditions. Fetuin, a major plasma glycoprotein, has been used as a requirement for serum-free primary cultures of hMSCs and other cell types such as mouse fibroblast and epithelial cells [76, 114]. Heparin, a glycosaminoglycan that typically acts as an anticoagulant factor, has been shown to have proliferative or antiproliferative effects on various cell types [115, 116]. Addition of heparin into culture media led to a reduced growth of hMSCs from AT and BM [66, 76]. In contrast, Mimura et al. reported the growth-enhancing effect of heparin on a genetically modified hMSC line [85].

4.1.3. Other Variables. For successful cell cultures, it is also important to control other key variables, particularly when serum-free media are used. Beyond the nutrients and nonnutrient factors, medium pH, osmolality, and partial pressure of dissolved gases in culture are important for cell growth. In addition, environmental conditions, including temperature and the nature of culture surface, have significant impacts. Finally, culture techniques, such as trypsinization and passaging protocol, are also important factors. Review of these variables on hMSCs in serum-free conditions is out of the scope of this paper.

4.2. Serum Components and Functions. Media for the culture of stem cells must provide all the essential requirements for cell survival and growth while maintaining their undifferentiated characteristics. These requirements (both defined and undefined) are normally provided by using serum in hMSC cultures. Serum is an extremely complex fluid, which is prepared by defibrination of plasma. It contains a broad spectrum of biological factors (Table 1) having physiologically balanced growth-promoting, growth-inhibiting, and/or differentiation-inducing activities [101, 112]. The important components of serum and their main functions are as follows [45, 48, 101, 112]:

(i) growth factors (e.g., PDGF, EGF, FGF, IGF-1, IGF-2) promoting cell proliferation: some of these factors may be cytostatic and induce differentiation;

(ii) components of base membrane (e.g., fibronectin) and other adhesion factors (e.g., fetuin and hydrocortisone, particularly present in fetal serum) supporting cell attachment and spreading;

(iii) trace elements (e.g., selenium), minerals, vitamins (e.g., ascorbic acid), lipids, and hormones (e.g., insulin, hydrocortisone): many of these are bound to carrier proteins, stimulating cell growth, and are involved in many other biological activities;

(iv) other nutrients (e.g., amino acids, nucleosides): some of these are present in solution and the others are bound to proteins. These nutrient components are largely included in basal media, but serum also provides necessary nutrients that may not be present in basal media or may not be present in sufficient amounts to promote growth;

(v) binding proteins (e.g., albumin, transferrin) carrying minerals, vitamins, lipids, hormones, and other nutrients: these proteins play a role to stabilize and modulate the activity of the components which they bind;

(vi) buffer (e.g., albumin and others) modulating pH: the role of serum for increasing the buffering capacity is particularly important where the seeding density is low (e.g., cell cloning experiments);

(vii) protease inhibitors (e.g., α2-macroglobulin) neutralizing proteases: these antiproteases protect cells from damage caused by their exposure to proteases such as trypsin used in the passaging procedure or proteases

TABLE 1: Constituents of serum [Adapted from [112]].

Constituent	Range of concentration	Constituent	Range of concentration[a]
Proteins and polypeptides	40–80 mg/mL	Polyamines:	0.1–1.0 μM
Albumin	20–50 mg/mL	Putrescine, Spermidine	
Fetuin[b]	10–20 mg/mL		
Fibronectin	1.0–10 μg/mL	Urea	170–300 μg/mL
Globulins	1.0–15 mg/mL		
Protease inhibitors:	0.5–2.5 mg/mL	Inorganics	0.14–0.16 M
α1-antitrypsin,		Calcium	4.0–7.0 mM
α2-macroglobulin		Chlorides	100 μM
Transferrin	2.0–4.0 mg/mL	Iron	10–50 μM
		Potassium	5.0–15 mM
Growth factors:		Phosphate	2.0–5.0 mM
EGF, PDGF, IGF1 and 2,	1.0–100 ng/mL	Selenium	0.01 μM
FGF, IL-1, IL-6		Sodium	135–155 mM
		Zinc	0.1–1.0 μM
Amino acids	0.01–1.0 μM		
		Hormones	0.1–200 nM
Lipids	2.0–10 mg/mL	Hydrocortisone	10–200 nM
Cholesterol	10 μM	Insulin	1.0–100 ng/mL
Fatty acids	0.1–1.0 μM	Triiodothyronine	20 nM
Linoleic acid	0.01–0.1 μM	Thyroxine	100 nM
Phospholipids	0.7–3.0 mg/mL	⋮	
		Vitamins	0.01–10 μg/mL
Carbohydrates	1.0-2.0 mg/mL	Vitamin A	10–100 ng/mL
Glucose	0.6–1.2 mg/mL	Folate	5.0–20 ng/mL
Hexosamine	0.6–1.2 mg/mL		
Lactic acid	0.5–2.0 mg/mL		
Pyruvic acid	2.0–10 μg/mL		

[a] The range of concentrations is approximate and is intended to convey only the order of magnitude.
[b] In fetal serum only.

released by the cells during culture. They may also promote cell attachment;

(viii) protection factors (e.g., albumin and others) contributing to viscosity and thus protecting circulating cells from mechanical damage (e.g., shear stress induced by pipetting or agitation in suspension culture): these elements are considered less important in monolayer culture, but they may be important in protecting trypsinized cells from the pipetting;

(ix) antitoxins: these factors bind and neutralize toxins.

When serum is omitted from culture media, it is important to find substitutes (i.e., alternative medium supplements together with appropriate culture protocols) that can replace the serum functions essentially required for cell survival and proliferation. In most cases, the requirements are multiple, and thus it is necessary to investigate the effects of both nutritional factors and regulatory factors. Typically, native proteins purified from serum (e.g., albumin, insulin, transferrin, fetuin) and synthetic substances (e.g., recombinant growth factors) are added into serum-free formulations. The requirements of these and other supplements vary greatly, depending on the cell type being studied and the basal medium selected. Moreover, it is very important to employ appropriate culture protocols (e.g., culture surface, trypsinization) to properly examine the effects of the supplements.

4.3. Proposed Approaches for Defined Serum-Free Medium Development. Typically, to select basal media, growth factors and other medium supplements in a logical way (i.e., understanding serum factors and their functions, and finding related information from the literature) and then to perform trial and error experiments may be the only method to identify the best candidates. The most well-known fundamental strategies for the development of a new serum-free medium were proposed in the 1960s and 1970s by separate groups. Together with these classical methods, some practical approaches are summarized below.

4.3.1. Ham's Approach. Ham developed a method for substantially reducing (or eliminating in certain cases) the amount of serum in a medium. This approach is based on the careful manipulation of media components and culture conditions (i.e., by modifying the defined constituents of an existing medium formulation and a culture protocol previously developed for a related cell type without adding growth factors) in order to provide cells with an optimal nutrient balance [92]. In other words, the adjustment of concentrations of the nutrients to optimum values and the manipulation of culture protocols enables significant reduction of the concentration of serum proteins, although it is unknown what functions of serum are exactly replaced. It has been demonstrated that variables whose modification has contributed to reducing the requirement for serum proteins include (i) the nature of the culture surface, (ii) the type of trypsinization procedure, (iii) buffering, (iv) pH, (v) osmolarity, (vi) the availability of all nutrients, and (vii) quantitative adjustment of their concentrations. The basic concept of Ham's approach to reduce serum in the medium is (i) to reduce the amount of serum to a level that restricts growth and then (ii) to look for changes in the medium or culture conditions that will improve growth. During their work, Ham and colleagues found it important to reexamine, at lower serum concentrations, those factors that had no effect on growth at higher amounts of serum.

Procedure of Ham's Approach. In the attempt to replace the functions of serum with the quantitative adjustment of the nutrient concentrations and culture conditions, Ham and colleagues used the following approach.

(1) The amount of serum is reduced to a level that yields suboptimal growth in a medium. The medium is selected, based on its performance for the growth of a related cell type.

(2) To identify those components whose quantitative adjustment is the most limiting to growth with the low concentration of serum, the effect of increasing and decreasing the concentration of each individual component of the medium by 5 or 10 times is tested.

(3) The component that has the greatest effect in this preliminary survey is then tested over a wide range of concentrations. In this step, a typical growth-response curve is generated and divided into three parts as follows:

   (i) The first is a direct growth response, in which growth improves as the nutrient concentration is increased until a saturation value is reached.

   (ii) The second is a plateau where further increases in the nutrient concentration have no effect on growth.

   (iii) The third is a toxic response in which increasing the nutrient concentration has a detrimental effect on growth.

Figure 3 shows a schematic growth-response curve typical for most components, although the growth stimulation to certain factors is biphasic in rare cases [92]. At the upper end of the curve in Figure 3, serum proteins have the ability

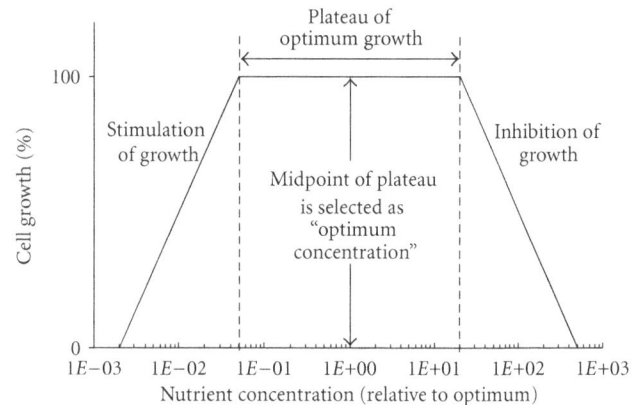

FIGURE 3: Idealized growth response curve versus nutrient concentration illustrating the procedure for determining the "optimum" concentration of a nutrient. The range of concentrations that support optimum growth (referred to as a "plateau") is determined, and its midpoint on the plot is selected as the concentration to be used in future media (Adapted from [92]).

to protect cells from the inhibitory effect of excess amounts of nutrients. At the lower end of the curve, a large amount of serum proteins permit cells to grow at concentrations of essential nutrients that would be inadequate with lesser amounts of serum protein. Each time that such a titration is performed, the midpoint of the plateau region on the growth response curve is selected as the optimum concentration for use in future media. This process is useful to keep the selected nutrient concentration as far separated as possible both from nutritional inadequacy and from toxicity (i.e., the lower end and upper end, respectively, of the growth-response curve in Figure 3).

(4) Once the quantitative adjustment improves growth, the concentration of serum is reduced until it again becomes limiting.

(5) At the readjusted lower concentration of serum, the next most critical component whose concentration needs to be adjusted is determined repeating the steps 2 and 3.

(6) These steps above are repeated until serum is reduced to the minimum level or is completely eliminated in certain cases of transformed cells.

Based on the results obtained using this approach, Ham and colleagues classified the growth-promoting functions of serum into two operational categories, "replaceable" and "nonreplaceable". The replaceable category consists of those functions of serum that could be replaced by making changes in the defined portion of the medium or in the culture conditions. In contrast, the nonreplaceable functions are those that could not be replaced using this approach. Ham's group reported that serum was completely eliminated by using their method for the growth of some cell lines including certain normal cells; however, it was later found that these cell lines underwent subtle transformations, which enabled their growth in the absence of serum proteins [117].

Using this approach, Ham's group was able to formulate a variety of basal media, such as Ham's F12 and MCDB series, providing optimal nutrient balances to certain cell types. These medium formulations supported the clonal growth of many specific cell lines in the presence of a minimized amount of serum. However, this approach is extremely labor intensive and time consuming. Further, as the "nonreplaceable functions" of serum could not be replaced for the growth of normal cells using this approach, externally supplied growth-promoting substances, in the form of dialyzed serum, purified fractions from serum, or synthetic materials, should still be provided to the cells to obtain satisfactory growth even with the optimized media and culture conditions.

4.3.2. Sato's Approach.

In contrast to Ham's approach, which is analytical in nature, Sato and colleagues developed a synthetic method for the replacement of serum in culture media. This approach was based on attempts (i) to understand what roles serum play for the maintenance and growth of cells in culture and then (ii) to supplement an existing basal medium formulation with a combination of key hormones and growth factors mimicking the growth-stimulatory function of whole serum while restricting the manipulation of the basal media components [48]. For example, one of the main functions of serum is to provide a mixture of hormones, which is stimulatory for cell growth. In order to identify the active additives, an array of factors is tested under suboptimal conditions—for example, at lowered serum concentrations, as described below.

Procedure of Sato's Approach

(1) The growth promoting capacity of serum is first lowered to a level that yields suboptimal growth by reducing the concentration of serum, in order to see a stimulation of growth when various factors under investigation are added to the medium.

(2) Upon understanding what functions serum serve for cells in culture and the specific requirements of nutrients and nonnutrient growth factors, a large array of factors is selected and tested under the suboptimal conditions.

(3) As active factors are identified, the serum concentration is further lowered and the search continued.

Through their extensive work on many cell types, Sato's group identified various key essential supplements, hormones, binding proteins, lipids, trace elements, and attachment factors, required for addition to basal medium. In particular, they demonstrated that insulin, transferrin, and selenium were essential for the growth of most cells while hydrocortisone and EGF were additionally needed for certain cell types. Using their approach, Sato and colleagues were able, for a number of different types of cells, to replace serum with hormones and growth factors while leaving the basal medium essentially unchanged.

However, Sato's approach is still labor intensive and time consuming.

4.3.3. Top-Down and Bottom-Up Approaches.

Considered as more practical approaches, top-down and bottom-up approaches can be used effectively for the development of a new serum-free medium formulation for the growth of a cell population of interest [45].

Top-Down Approach. This approach involves employing an existing medium formulation for a similar cell type, and identifying stimulatory components in the presence of serum for the growth of the target cells. This process proceeds as the concentration of serum is gradually reduced. This concept evolved from the premise that a cell type, which belongs to a group of cells with similar characteristics, often requires the same combination of growth factors for growth. When this approach is used, care should be taken to identify the existence of any cytotoxic or growth-inhibitory components in the medium for the cells being studied.

Bottom-Up Approach. This approach involves first selecting an appropriate basal medium (e.g., a medium used for the growth of a related cell type) and then screening various selected exogenous factors for their growth-stimulatory effects. Since only the active components required for the growth of cells of interest are added into the medium, the final formulation will represent an efficient and easily amendable medium. However, this approach is likely to be labor-intensive and time-consuming. Further, since the screening of factors being examined is performed in the absence of serum, the critical functions of serum required to see their effects should be carefully considered and satisfied by alternative means (e.g., well-controlled physiochemical parameters, treatment of culture surface, trypsinization and passage protocols), because normally the serum-free basal medium does not provide such functions.

We would like to point out that there is no universal guideline for screening selected medium additives towards the development of a new medium, and thus it is important for investigators to understand the advantages and disadvantages of all the approaches previously proposed and then to exploit beneficial features of each approach for designing their own strategies in a rational, effective manner. As an example, in our study for hMSC serum-free medium development [76], we selected various medium ingredients (basal media, extra nutrients, binding proteins, buffering agents, hormones, vitamins, and growth and attachment factors) based on the understanding of cell culture requirement including the role of serum constituents. And then the selected factors were examined in a sequential manner, employing some useful suggestions of each approach described earlier, in order to determine chronologically their impact on proliferation, attachment, and isolation of hMSCs (Figure 4). In addition, an effective serum-free medium development can be achieved by considering other important issues as discussed below.

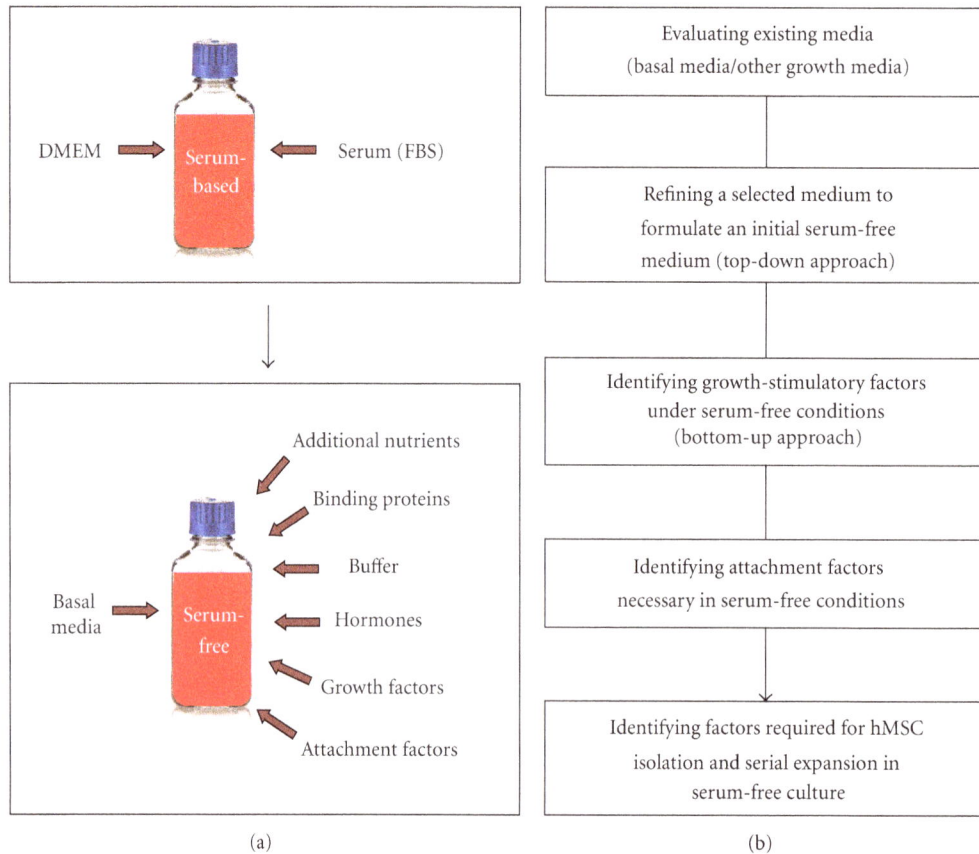

FIGURE 4: An overview demonstrating a process for the development of a defined serum-free medium for hMSCs. (a) To replace ill-defined serum with defined supplements, a variety of medium constituents, including basal media, additional nutrients (e.g., lipids and vitamins), binding proteins, physiochemical reagents (e.g., buffer), hormones, growth factors, and attachment factors were selected. (b) A sequential strategy was designed for screening effectively the selected basal media and medium additives to develop a defined serum-free condition that supports the isolation and expansion of hMSCs [76].

4.4. Considerations for the Development of a New Serum-Free Medium

4.4.1. Selection of Materials and Testing Methods

Selection of Basal Media. hMSCs are typically cultured in Dulbecco's Modified of Eagle's Medium (DMEM) or Minimum Essential Medium Alpha (αMEM) with the supplementation of FBS. However, whether these basal media are appropriate for serum-free culture should be critically considered for the cell type being investigated, because each basal medium has been developed or optimized for a specific application. For example, Ham's F12, which was developed for the clonal growth of Chinese Hamster Ovary cells in low serum, contains a wide range of ingredients at low concentrations, while DMEM, which was optimized at higher cell densities for viral propagation, contains fewer constituents but at high concentrations [45]. For this reason, a 1:1 mixture of DMEM and Ham's F12 has been used for the culture of many cell types with serum or as a basis for serum-free media, since this combination provides a reasonable compromise between high concentrations and a wide range of ingredients. The DMEM/F-12 mixture has been employed as a basal medium for the development of serum-free media for hMSCs [76, 80].

Selection of Factors to Be Tested. Recent trends towards the development of serum-free media for the growth of a cell type often exclusively focus on the effect of "regulatory growth factors" such as peptide growth factors and hormones. When an established serum-free medium exists for those cells or a closely related cell type, this approach represents a reasonable method, because this type of study is more likely to be characterized as a medium optimization or modification process, rather than a "significant" development. When such a medium is not available, the medium development process will be more extensive and complicated. In this case, together with the wide-ranging investigation on growth-promoting growth factors and other medium supplements, considerations should also be placed on other properties of cells (e.g., attachment, in particular in primary culture). In this regard, an understanding of serum functions and related constituents is important to select candidates to be examined.

Culture Protocol for Screening Factors. In the development of serum-free media for anchorage-dependent cells, as described earlier, conventional approaches for screening growth factors include the use of serum with gradual reduction of its content in media to (a) provide unidentified adherent proteins for facilitating cell attachment to the substrate and (b) support sufficient growth levels to observe meaningfully the impact of the additives [48, 92]. However, this procedure is very labor intensive and time consuming. As a more practical approach, it has been suggested to plate the cells initially in serum-containing medium, remove the medium after the cells attach, and screen the factors in serum-free medium [48]. It was further recommended that this protocol would work best in the presence of insulin and transferrin because these two components are required for most cell types and their presence is necessary for the appearance of a stimulatory effect of other factors [48]. This screening protocol has also been effectively employed for a serum-free medium development for hMSCs [76].

Necessity of Reexamination of Factors. Through their extensive work on medium development, both Ham and Sato demonstrated that the composition of a medium formulation could mask effects of certain factors under screening that could reveal their impact at different medium compositions or their concentrations [48, 92]. For example, it was shown that some factors, such as transferrin, were not stimulatory until the serum concentration was substantially reduced [48]. This is because some serum components at high concentrations covered the effect of transferrin, which became unmasked at the decrease of their concentrations to certain levels. Conversely, effects of certain factors under screening could also be unrevealed in the absence of some medium components. Therefore, both Ham and Sato proposed that the examination of selected factors and the adjustment of their concentrations to optimum values be done in a stepwise manner at progressively defined compositions and concentrations of the medium formulation and that certain factors having no effects at a condition be reevaluated under a revised screening condition.

Synergistic Effects. Growth factors often act synergistically or additively with each other or with other hormones. In this regard, statistical approaches have been widely used to investigate specific interactions between growth factors under screening. This method will be powerful when a good screening medium, which includes requirements for cell maintenance and at least "minimal" growth as well as attachment, is available to examine effectively the individual and synergistic effects of the selected growth factors.

Contamination with Other Trace Elements. It is known that purified serum proteins, such as albumin, insulin, transferrin, and fetuin, often carry other trace components, which may affect cell growth. Therefore, it is desirable to use highly purified substances or completely defined synthetic materials, if available, to determine conclusively the effect of such proteins.

4.4.2. Cell Culture Aspects in Serum-Free Conditions

Cell Handling. Cells grown in serum-free conditions are more delicate than those grown in the presence of serum and thus should be handled very gently to minimize cell damage during the harvesting and passaging procedures.

Buffer System of Media. Since the buffering function of serum to modulate pH is omitted in serum-free cultures, it may be beneficial to further supplement the medium with a chemical buffer such as HEPES, in addition to the bicarbonate-CO_2 system, in order to improve the buffering capacity of the medium. The HEPES concentration could be increased above 15 mM without toxicity for some cell lines, but it may be necessary to adjust the osmolality of the medium accordingly [48].

Lack of Detoxifying Substances. As serum proteins that could bind and neutralize toxic contaminants are not present in serum-free conditions, its protective, detoxifying activity is also omitted. Thus, care should be taken in selecting water, reagents, as well as culture techniques. The *level of purity of water and reagents and the degree of cleanliness of all apparatus must be very high* [45, 48, 112]. In general, basal media are recommended to be kept at 4°C no longer than 2 weeks because their constituents are more likely to be decomposed in the absence of those detoxifying serum components. Growth factors and other medium supplements, in particular labile components such as transferrin, hormones, and ascorbic acid, should be reconstituted, stored and used strictly according to the manufacturer's instruction.

Lack of Protease Inhibitors. The addition of serum to cells exposed to trypsin during trypsinization neutralizes any residual proteolytic activity. Protease inhibitors such as aprotinin and soybean trypsin inhibitor could be used to replace this function. However, the level of their antiproteolytic action and their potential impact on cell growth should be examined by testing these materials in a dose-dependent manner in comparison with a control case using serum. In addition, as an alternative trypsinization protocol, the use of native trypsin could be replaced by a less detrimental protease (e.g., recombinant trypsin) for cell harvesting. Moreover, recombinant trypsin has effectively been used for hMSC culture in serum-free conditions [84, 87–90]. When recombinant trypsin is used to detach cells from the substrate, the use of FBS or other trypsin inhibitors may not be necessary for serum-free culture. In contrast, Hudson et al. used serum albumin (1%) in PBS to wash cells after trypsinization with recombinant trypsin [90].

5. Conclusions

Clinical efficacy for the use of hMSCs has been variable and probably still insufficient for widespread implementation of hMSC therapies. Enhancing culture protocols may be a critical issue to meet efficacy endpoints in upcoming clinical studies. Well-formulated chemically defined serum-free media for hMSC isolation and expansion would greatly contribute to the achievement of this goal. Towards this objective, significant progress has been made to generate various medium formulations for hMSC culture in the absence of ill-defined FBS and human-sourced supplements. These defined media should be critically evaluated through *in vitro* and *in vivo* analyses and most likely further refined for optimal performance. In this regard, fully disclosed formulations should represent important platforms for enhancing the therapeutic potential of hMSCs. We also emphasize that the identification of key elements towards the development and optimization of serum-free media should follow rational, systematic approaches in order to maximize the possibility of finding their true effects on hMSCs. All the issues reviewed herein should thus be considered seriously when medium development and optimization studies are carried out.

Acknowledgments

The authors acknowledge appreciatively the financial support of the Canadian Institutes of Health Research (CIHR), the Natural Sciences and Engineering Research Council of Canada (NSERC), and the Canada Research Chairs (CRC) program.

References

[1] E. M. Horwitz, K. Le Blanc, M. Dominici et al., "Clarification of the nomenclature for MSC: the international society for cellular therapy position statement," *Cytotherapy*, vol. 7, no. 5, pp. 393–395, 2005.

[2] J. Ankrum and J. M. Karp, "Mesenchymal stem cell therapy: two steps forward, one step back," *Trends in Molecular Medicine*, vol. 16, no. 5, pp. 203–209, 2010.

[3] E. M. Horwitz, R. T. Maziarz, and P. Kebriaei, "MSCs in Hematopoietic Cell Transplantation," *Biology of Blood and Marrow Transplantation*, vol. 17, no. 1, pp. S21–S29, 2011.

[4] D. J. Prockop, ""Stemness" does not explain the repair of many tissues by mesenchymal stem/multipotent stromal cells (MSCs)," *Clinical Pharmacology and Therapeutics*, vol. 82, no. 3, pp. 241–243, 2007.

[5] K. Le Blanc and O. Ringdén, "Immunomodulation by mesenchymal stem cells and clinical experience," *Journal of Internal Medicine*, vol. 262, no. 5, pp. 509–525, 2007.

[6] I. Sekiya, B. L. Larson, J. R. Smith, R. Pochampally, J. G. Cui, and D. J. Prockop, "Expansion of human adult stem cells from bone marrow stroma: conditions that maximize the yields of early progenitors and evaluate their quality," *Stem Cells*, vol. 20, no. 6, pp. 530–541, 2002.

[7] L. A. Solchaga, K. Penick, J. D. Porter, V. M. Goldberg, A. I. Caplan, and J. F. Welter, "FGF-2 enhances the mitotic and chondrogenic potentials of human adult bone marrow-derived mesenchymal stem cells," *Journal of Cellular Physiology*, vol. 203, no. 2, pp. 398–409, 2005.

[8] L. Qian and W. M. Saltzman, "Improving the expansion and neuronal differentiation of mesenchymal stem cells through culture surface modification," *Biomaterials*, vol. 25, no. 7-8, pp. 1331–1337, 2004.

[9] A. Apel, A. Groth, S. Schlesinger et al., "Suitability of human mesenchymal stem cells for gene therapy depends on the expansion medium," *Experimental Cell Research*, vol. 315, no. 3, pp. 498–507, 2009.

[10] M. Dominici, K. Le Blanc, I. Mueller et al., "Minimal criteria for defining multipotent mesenchymal stromal cells. The International Society for Cellular Therapy position statement," *Cytotherapy*, vol. 8, no. 4, pp. 315–317, 2006.

[11] M. Kassem, "Stem cells: potential therapy for age-related diseases," *Annals of the New York Academy of Sciences*, vol. 1067, no. 1, pp. 436–442, 2006.

[12] M. F. Pittenger, A. M. Mackay, S. C. Beck et al., "Multilineage potential of adult human mesenchymal stem cells," *Science*, vol. 284, no. 5411, pp. 143–147, 1999.

[13] O. Karnieli, Y. Izhar-Prato, S. Bulvik, and S. Efrat, "Generation of insulin-producing cells from human bone marrow mesenchymal stem cells by genetic manipulation," *Stem Cells*, vol. 25, no. 11, pp. 2837–2844, 2007.

[14] C. M. Rice and N. J. Scolding, "Autologous bone marrow stem cells-properties and advantages," *Journal of the Neurological Sciences*, vol. 265, no. 1-2, pp. 59–62, 2008.

[15] R. H. Lee, M. J. Seo, R. L. Reger et al., "Multipotent stromal cells from human marrow home to and promote repair of pancreatic islets and renal glomeruli in diabetic NOD/scid mice," *Proceedings of the National Academy of Sciences of the United States of America*, vol. 103, no. 46, pp. 17438–17443, 2006.

[16] A. I. Caplan, "Adult mesenchymal stem cells for tissue engineering versus regenerative medicine," *Journal of Cellular Physiology*, vol. 213, no. 2, pp. 341–347, 2007.

[17] W. E. Fibbe, A. J. Nauta, and H. Roelofs, "Modulation of immune responses by mesenchymal stem cells," *Annals of the New York Academy of Sciences*, vol. 1106, pp. 272–278, 2007.

[18] S. Aggarwal and M. F. Pittenger, "Human mesenchymal stem cells modulate allogeneic immune cell responses," *Blood*, vol. 105, no. 4, pp. 1815–1822, 2005.

[19] K. Le Blanc and O. Ringdén, "Mesenchymal stem cells: properties and role in clinical bone marrow transplantation," *Current Opinion in Immunology*, vol. 18, no. 5, pp. 586–591, 2006.

[20] B. J. Jones and S. J. McTaggart, "Immunosuppression by mesenchymal stromal cells: from culture to clinic," *Experimental Hematology*, vol. 36, no. 6, pp. 733–741, 2008.

[21] I. Rasmusson, "Immune modulation by mesenchymal stem cells," *Experimental Cell Research*, vol. 312, no. 12, pp. 2169–2179, 2006.

[22] A. Uccelli, L. Moretta, and V. Pistoia, "Mesenchymal stem cells in health and disease," *Nature Reviews Immunology*, vol. 8, no. 9, pp. 726–736, 2008.

[23] M. E. Bernardo, N. Zaffaroni, F. Novara et al., "Human bone marrow-derived mesenchymal stem cells do not undergo transformation after long-term in vitro culture and do not exhibit telomere maintenance mechanisms," *Cancer Research*, vol. 67, no. 19, pp. 9142–9149, 2007.

[24] K. Stenderup, J. Justesen, C. Clausen, and M. Kassem, "Aging is associated with decreased maximal life span and accelerated senescence of bone marrow stromal cells," *Bone*, vol. 33, no. 6, pp. 919–926, 2003.

[25] C. Bartmann, E. Rohde, K. Schallmoser et al., "Two steps to functional mesenchymal stromal cells for clinical application," *Transfusion*, vol. 47, no. 8, pp. 1426–1435, 2007.

[26] S. Kidd, E. Spaeth, A. Klopp, M. Andreeff, B. Hall, and F. C. Marini, "The (in) auspicious role of mesenchymal stromal cells in cancer: be it friend or foe," *Cytotherapy*, vol. 10, no. 7, pp. 657–667, 2008.

[27] E. M. Horwitz, P. L. Gordon, W. K. K. Koo et al., "Isolated allogeneic bone marrow-derived mesenchymal cells engraft and stimulate growth in children with osteogenesis imperfecta: implications for cell therapy of bone," *Proceedings of the National Academy of Sciences of the United States of America*, vol. 99, no. 13, pp. 8932–8937, 2002.

[28] J. L. Spees, C. A. Gregory, H. Singh et al., "Internalized antigens must be removed to prepare hypoimmunogenic mesenchymal stem cells for cell and gene therapy," *Molecular Therapy*, vol. 9, no. 5, pp. 747–756, 2004.

[29] A. Schaffler and C. Buchler, "Concise review: adipose tissue-derived stromal cells—Basic and clinical implications for novel cell-based therapies," *Stem Cells*, vol. 25, no. 4, pp. 818–827, 2007.

[30] A. Flynn, F. Barry, and T. O'Brien, "UC blood-derived mesenchymal stromal cells: an overview," *Cytotherapy*, vol. 9, no. 8, pp. 717–726, 2007.

[31] D. L. Troyer and M. L. Weiss, "Concise review: wharton's Jelly-derived cells are a primitive stromal cell population," *Stem Cells*, vol. 26, no. 3, pp. 591–599, 2008.

[32] S. Barlow, G. Brooke, K. Chatterjee et al., "Comparison of human placenta- and bone marrow-derived multipotent mesenchymal stem cells," *Stem Cells and Development*, vol. 17, no. 6, pp. 1095–1107, 2008.

[33] M. G. Roubelakis, K. I. Pappa, V. Bitsika et al., "Molecular and proteomic characterization of human mesenchymal stem cells derived from amniotic fluid: comparison to bone marrow mesenchymal stem cells," *Stem Cells and Development*, vol. 16, no. 6, pp. 931–951, 2007.

[34] L. D. S. Meirelles, P. C. Chagastelles, and N. B. Nardi, "Mesenchymal stem cells reside in virtually all post-natal organs and tissues," *Journal of Cell Science*, vol. 119, no. 11, pp. 2204–2213, 2006.

[35] I. Bochev, G. Elmadjian, D. Kyurkchiev et al., "Mesenchymal stem cells from human bone marrow or adipose tissue differently modulate mitogen-stimulated B-cell immunoglobulin production in vitro," *Cell Biology International*, vol. 32, no. 4, pp. 384–393, 2008.

[36] B. Davani, L. Ikonomou, B. M. Raaka et al., "Human islet-derived precursor cells are mesenchymal stromal cells that differentiate and mature to hormone-expressing cells in vivo," *Stem Cells*, vol. 25, no. 12, pp. 3215–3222, 2007.

[37] S. Kern, H. Eichler, J. Stoeve, H. Klüter, and K. Bieback, "Comparative analysis of mesenchymal stem cells from bone marrow, umbilical cord blood, or adipose tissue," *Stem Cells*, vol. 24, no. 5, pp. 1294–1301, 2006.

[38] W. Wagner, F. Wein, A. Seckinger et al., "Comparative characteristics of mesenchymal stem cells from human bone marrow, adipose tissue, and umbilical cord blood," *Experimental Hematology*, vol. 33, no. 11, pp. 1402–1416, 2005.

[39] H. Castro-Malaspina, R. E. Gay, and G. Resnick, "Characterization of human bone marrow fibroblast colony-forming cells (CFU-F) and their progeny," *Blood*, vol. 56, no. 2, pp. 289–301, 1980.

[40] C. M. Digirolamo, D. Stokes, D. Colter, D. G. Phinney, R. Class, and D. J. Prockop, "Propagation and senescence of

human marrow stromal cells in culture: a simple colony-forming assay identifies samples with the greatest potential to propagate and differentiate," *British Journal of Haematology*, vol. 107, no. 2, pp. 275–281, 1999.

[41] M. M. Bonab, K. Alimoghaddam, F. Talebian, S. H. Ghaffari, A. Ghavamzadeh, and B. Nikbin, "Aging of mesenchymal stem cell in vitro," *BMC Cell Biology*, vol. 7, p. 14, 2006.

[42] S. A. Wexler, C. Donaldson, P. Denning-Kendall, C. Rice, B. Bradley, and J. M. Hows, "Adult bone marrow is a rich source of human mesenchymal 'stem' cells but umbilical cord and mobilized adult blood are not," *British Journal of Haematology*, vol. 121, no. 2, pp. 368–374, 2003.

[43] K. Schallmoser, E. Rohde, A. Reinisch et al., "Rapid large-scale expansion of functional mesenchymal stem cells from unmanipulated bone marrow without animal serum," *Tissue Engineering*, vol. 14, no. 3, pp. 185–196, 2008.

[44] L. Sensebe, "Clinical grade production of mesenchymal stem cells," *Bio-Medical Materials and Engineering*, vol. 18, no. 1, pp. S3–S10, 2008.

[45] A. Burgener and M. Butler, "Medium development," in *Cell Culture Technology for Pharmaceutical and Cell-Based Therapies*, S. Ozturk and W. S. Hu, Eds., pp. 41–79, CRC Press, Boca Raton, Fla, USA, 2006.

[46] I. Dimarakis and N. Levicar, "Cell culture medium composition and translational adult bone marrow-derived stem cell research," *Stem Cells*, vol. 24, no. 5, pp. 1407–1408, 2006.

[47] F. Mannello and G. A. Tonti, "Concise review: no breakthroughs for human mesenchymal and embryonic stem cell culture: Conditioned medium, feeder layer, or feeder-free; medium with fetal calf serum, human serum, or enriched plasma; serum-free, serum replacement nonconditioned medium, or ad hoc formula? All that glitters is not gold!," *Stem Cells*, vol. 25, no. 7, pp. 1603–1609, 2007.

[48] D. Barnes and G. Sato, "Methods for growth of cultured cells in serum-free medium," *Analytical Biochemistry*, vol. 102, no. 2, pp. 255–270, 1980.

[49] C. Tekkatte, G. P. Gunasingh, K. M. Cherian, and K. Sankaranarayanan, "'Humanized' stem cell culture techniques: the animal serum controversy," *Stem Cells International*, vol. 2011, Article ID 504723, 14 pages, 2011.

[50] J. A. Dahl, S. Duggal, N. Coulston et al., "Genetic and epigenetic instability of human bone marrow mesenchymal stem cells expanded in autologous seum or fatal bovine serum," *International Journal of Developmental Biology*, vol. 52, no. 8, pp. 1033–1042, 2008.

[51] N. Mizuno, H. Shiba, Y. Ozeki et al., "Human autologous serum obtained using a completely closed bag system as a substitute for foetal calf serum in human mesenchymal stem cell cultures," *Cell Biology International*, vol. 30, no. 6, pp. 521–524, 2006.

[52] A. Shahdadfar, K. Frønsdal, T. Haug, F. P. Reinholt, and J. E. Brinchmann, "In vitro expansion of human mesenchymal stem cells: choice of serum is a determinant of cell proliferation, differentiation, gene expression, and transcriptome stability," *Stem Cells*, vol. 23, no. 9, pp. 1357–1366, 2005.

[53] N. Stute, K. Holtz, M. Bubenheim, C. Lange, F. Blake, and A. R. Zander, "Autologous serum for isolation and expansion of human mesenchymal stem cells for clinical use," *Experimental Hematology*, vol. 32, no. 12, pp. 1212–1225, 2004.

[54] S. A. Kuznetsov, M. H. Mankani, and P. G. Robey, "Effect of serum on human bone marrow stromal cells: *ex vivo*

expansion and in vivo bone formation," *Transplantation*, vol. 70, no. 12, pp. 1780–1787, 2000.

[55] K. Le Blanc, H. Samuelsson, L. Lönnies, M. Sundin, and O. Ringdén, "Generation of immunosuppressive mesenchymal stem cells in allogeneic human serum," *Transplantation*, vol. 84, no. 8, pp. 1055–1059, 2007.

[56] A. Poloni, G. Maurizi, V. Rosini et al., "Selection of CD271+ cells and human AB serum allows a large expansion of mesenchymal stromal cells from human bone marrow," *Cytotherapy*, vol. 11, no. 2, pp. 153–162, 2009.

[57] K. Tateishi, W. Ando, C. Higuchi et al., "Comparison of human serum with fetal bovine serum for expansion and differentiation of human synovial MSC: potential feasibility for clinical applications," *Cell Transplantation*, vol. 17, no. 5, pp. 549–557, 2008.

[58] K. Turnovcova, K. Ruzickova, V. Vanecek, E. Sykova, and P. Jendelova, "Properties and growth of human bone marrow mesenchymal stromal cells cultivated in different media Expansion of MSC in different media," *Cytotherapy*, vol. 11, no. 7, pp. 874–885, 2009.

[59] J. Jung, N. Moon, J. Y. Ahn et al., "Mesenchymal stromal cells expanded in human allogenic cord blood serum display higher self-renewal and enhanced osteogenic potential," *Stem Cells and Development*, vol. 18, no. 4, pp. 559–571, 2009.

[60] S. M. Phadnis, M. V. Joglekar, V. Venkateshan, S. M. Ghaskadbi, A. A. Hardikar, and R. R. Bhonde, "Human umbilical cord blood serum promotes growth, proliferation, as well as differentiation of human bone marrow-derived progenitor cells," *In Vitro Cellular and Developmental Biology*, vol. 42, no. 10, pp. 283–286, 2006.

[61] H. Shafaei, A. Esmaeili, M. Mardani et al., "Effects of human placental serum on proliferation and morphology of human adipose tissue-derived stem cells," *Bone Marrow Transplantation*, 2011.

[62] K. Bieback, A. Hecker, A. Kocaömer et al., "Human alternatives to fetal bovine serum for the expansion of mesenchymal stromal cells from bone marrow," *Stem Cells*, vol. 27, no. 9, pp. 2331–2341, 2009.

[63] C. Capelli, M. Domenghini, G. Borleri et al., "Human platelet lysate allows expansion and clinical grade production of mesenchymal stromal cells from small samples of bone marrow aspirates or marrow filter washouts," *Bone Marrow Transplantation*, vol. 40, no. 8, pp. 785–791, 2007.

[64] C. Doucet, I. Ernou, Y. Zhang et al., "Platelet lysates promote mesenchymal stem cell expansion: a safety substitute for animal serum in cell-based therapy applications," *Journal of Cellular Physiology*, vol. 205, no. 2, pp. 228–236, 2005.

[65] A. Flemming, K. Schallmoser, D. Strunk, M. Stolk, H. -D. Volk, and M. Seifert, "Immunomodulative efficacy of bone marrow-derived mesenchymal stem cells cultured in human platelet lysate," *Journal of Clinical Immunology*, vol. 31, no. 6, pp. 1143–1156, 2011.

[66] A. Kocaoemer, S. Kern, H. Klüter, and K. Bieback, "Human AB serum and thrombin-activated platelet-rich plasma are suitable alternatives to fetal calf serum for the expansion of mesenchymal stem cells from adipose tissue," *Stem Cells*, vol. 25, no. 5, pp. 1270–1278, 2007.

[67] C. Lange, F. Cakiroglu, A. N. Spiess, H. Cappallo-Obermann, J. Dierlamm, and A. R. Zander, "Accelerated and safe expansion of human mesenchymal stromal cells in animal serum-free medium for transplantation and regenerative medicine," *Journal of Cellular Physiology*, vol. 213, no. 1, pp. 18–26, 2007.

[68] I. Müller, S. Kordowich, C. Holzwarth et al., "Animal serum-free culture conditions for isolation and expansion of multipotent mesenchymal stromal cells from human BM," *Cytotherapy*, vol. 8, no. 5, pp. 437–444, 2006.

[69] A. Reinisch, C. Bartmann, E. Rohde et al., "Humanized system to propagate cord blood-derived multipotent mesenchymal stromal cells for clinical application," *Regenerative Medicine*, vol. 2, no. 4, pp. 371–382, 2007.

[70] K. Schallmoser, C. Bartmann, E. Rohde et al., "Human platelet lysate can replace fetal bovine serum for clinical-scale expansion of functional mesenchymal stromal cells," *Transfusion*, vol. 47, no. 8, pp. 1436–1446, 2007.

[71] R. Gruber, F. Karreth, B. Kandler et al., "Platelet-released supernatants increase migration and proliferation, and decrease osteogenic differentiation of bone marrow-derived mesenchymal progenitor cells under in vitro conditions," *Platelets*, vol. 15, no. 1, pp. 29–35, 2004.

[72] H. Abdelrazik, G. M. Spaggiari, L. Chiossone, and L. Moretta, "Mesenchymal stem cells expanded in human platelet lysate display a decreased inhibitory capacity on T- and NK-cell proliferation and function," *European Journal of Immunology*, vol. 41, no. 11, pp. 3281–3290, 2011.

[73] I. Hartmann, T. Hollweck, S. Haffner et al., "Umbilical cord tissue-derived mesenchymal stem cells grow best under GMP-compliant culture conditions and maintain their phenotypic and functional properties," *Journal of Immunological Methods*, vol. 363, no. 1, pp. 80–89, 2010.

[74] J. Reinhardt, A. Stuhler, and J. Blümel, "Safety of bovine sera for production of mesenchymal stem cells for therapeutic use," *Human Gene Therapy*, vol. 22, no. 6, pp. 775–756, 2011.

[75] L. Sensebé, P. Bourin, and K. Tarte, "Response to reinhardt et al.," *Human Gene Therapy*, vol. 22, no. 6, pp. 776–777, 2011.

[76] S. Jung, A. Sen, L. Rosenberg, and L. A. Behie, "Identification of growth and attachment factors for the serum-free isolation and expansion of human mesenchymal stromal cells," *Cytotherapy*, vol. 12, no. 5, pp. 637–657, 2010.

[77] D. P. Lennon, S. E. Haynesworth, R. G. Young, J. E. Dennis, and A. I. Caplan, "A chemically defined medium supports in vitro proliferation and maintains the osteochondral potential of rat marrow-derived mesenchymal stem cells," *Experimental Cell Research*, vol. 219, no. 1, pp. 211–222, 1995.

[78] C. H. Liu, M. L. Wu, and S. M. Hwang, "Optimization of serum free medium for cord blood mesenchymal stem cells," *Biochemical Engineering Journal*, vol. 33, no. 1, pp. 1–9, 2007.

[79] D. R. Marshak and J. J. Holecek, "Chemically defined medium for human mesenchymal stem cells," United States Patent 5,908,782, 1999.

[80] A. M. Parker, H. Shang, M. Khurgel, and A. J. Katz, "Low serum and serum-free culture of multipotential human adipose stem cells," *Cytotherapy*, vol. 9, no. 7, pp. 637–646, 2007.

[81] S. Jung, A. Sen, L. Rosenberg, and L. A. Behie, "Human mesenchymal stem cell culture: rapid and efficient isolation and expansion in a defined serum-free medium," *Journal of Tissue Engineering and Regenerative Medicine*, vol. 6, no. 5, pp. 391–403, 2012.

[82] R. H. Lee, A. A. Pulin, M. J. Seo et al., "Intravenous hMSCs Improve Myocardial Infarction in Mice because Cells Embolized in Lung Are Activated to Secrete the Anti-inflammatory Protein TSG-6," *Cell Stem Cell*, vol. 5, no. 1, pp. 54–63, 2009.

[83] T. J. Bartosh, J. H. Ylöstalo, A. Mohammadipoor et al., "Aggregation of human mesenchymal stromal cells (MSCs)

into 3D spheroids enhances their antiinflammatory properties," *Proceedings of the National Academy of Sciences of the United States of America*, vol. 107, no. 31, pp. 13724–13729, 2010.

[84] K. Rajala, B. Lindroos, S. M. Hussein et al., "A Defined and Xeno-Free Culture Method Enabling the Establishment of Clinical-Grade Human Embryonic, Induced Pluripotent and Adipose Stem Cells," *PLoS ONE*, vol. 5, no. 4, Article ID e10246, 2010.

[85] S. Mimura, N. Kimura, M. Hirata et al., "Growth factor-defined culture medium for human mesenchymal stem cells," *International Journal of Developmental Biology*, vol. 55, no. 2, pp. 181–187, 2011.

[86] H. Kagami, H. Agata, R. Kato, F. Matsuoka, and A. Tojo, "Fundamental technological developments required for increased availability of tissue engineering," in *Regenerative Medicine and Tissue Engineering—Cells and Biomaterials*, D. Eberli, Ed., InTech, Rijeka, Croatia, 2011.

[87] H. Agata, N. Watanabe, Y. Ishii et al., "Feasibility and efficacy of bone tissue engineering using human bone marrow stromal cells cultivated in serum-free conditions," *Biochemical and Biophysical Research Communications*, vol. 382, no. 2, pp. 353–358, 2009.

[88] B. Lindroos, S. Boucher, L. Chase et al., "Serum-free, xeno-free culture media maintain the proliferation rate and multipotentiality of adipose stem cells in vitro," *Cytotherapy*, vol. 11, no. 7, pp. 958–972, 2009.

[89] H. Miwa, Y. Hashimoto, K. Tensho, S. Wakitani, and M. Takagi, "Xeno-free proliferation of human bone marrowmesenchymal stem cells," *Cytotechnology*. In press.

[90] J. E. Hudson, R. J. Mills, J. E. Frith et al., "A defined medium and substrate for expansion of human mesenchymal stromal cell progenitors that enriches for osteo- and chondrogenic precursors," *Stem Cells and Development*, vol. 20, no. 1, pp. 77–87, 2011.

[91] W. J. Bettger and R. G. Ham, "The nutrient requirements of cultured mammalian cells," *Advances in Nutritional Research*, vol. 4, pp. 249–286, 1982.

[92] R. G. Ham and W. L. McKeehan, "Development of improved media and culture conditions for clonal growth of normal diploid cells," *In Vitro*, vol. 14, no. 1, pp. 11–22, 1978.

[93] B. Deorosan and E. A. Nauman, "The role of glucose, serum, and three-dimensional cell culture on the metabolism of bone marrow-derived mesenchymal stem cells," *Stem Cells International*, vol. 2011, Article ID 429187, 12 pages, 2011.

[94] Y. M. Li, T. Schilling, P. Benisch et al., "Effects of high glucose on mesenchymal stem cell proliferation and differentiation," *Biochemical and Biophysical Research Communications*, vol. 363, no. 1, pp. 209–215, 2007.

[95] B. R. Weil, A. M. Abarbanell, J. L. Herrmann, Y. Wang, and D. R. Meldrum, "High glucose concentration in cell culture medium does not acutely affect human mesenchymal stem cell growth factor production or proliferation," *American Journal of Physiology*, vol. 296, no. 6, pp. R1735–R1743, 2009.

[96] D. W. Rowe, B. J. Starman, W. Y. Fujimoto, and R. H. Williams, "Differences in growth response to hydrocortisone and ascorbic acid by human diploid fibroblasts," *In Vitro*, vol. 13, no. 12, pp. 824–830, 1977.

[97] S. Gronthos and P. J. Simmons, "The growth factor requirements of STRO-1-positive human bone marrow stromal precursors under serum-deprived conditions in vitro," *Blood*, vol. 85, no. 4, pp. 929–940, 1995.

[98] S. A. Kuznetsov, A. J. Friedenstein, and P. G. Robey, "Factors required for bone marrow stromal fibroblast colony formation in vitro," *British Journal of Haematology*, vol. 97, no. 3, pp. 561–570, 1997.

[99] J. Feng, A. H. Melcher, D. M. Brunette, and H. K. Moe, "Determination of L ascorbic acid levels in culture medium: concentrations in commercial media and maintenance of levels under conditions of organ culture," *In Vitro*, vol. 13, no. 2, pp. 91–99, 1977.

[100] M. Butler, *Animal Cell Culture and Technology*, BIOS Scientific Publishers, New York, NY, USA, 2004.

[101] H. Maurer, "Towards serum-free, chemically defined media for mamallian cell culture," in *Animal Cell Culture*, R. Freshney, Ed., pp. 15–46, IRL Press, New York, NY, USA, 1992.

[102] W. L. McKeehan, W. G. Hamilton, and R. G. Ham, "Selenium is an essential trace nutrient for growth of WI-38 diploid human fibroblasts," *Proceedings of the National Academy of Sciences of the United States of America*, vol. 73, no. 6, pp. 2023–2027, 1976.

[103] L. J. Guilbert and N. N. Iscove, "Partial replacement of serum by selenite, transferrin, albumin and lecithin in haemopoietic cell cultures," *Nature*, vol. 263, no. 5578, pp. 594–595, 1976.

[104] J. H. Kim, M. R. Lee, J. H. Kim, M. K. Jee, and S. K. Kang, "IFATS collection: selenium induces improvement of stem cell behaviors in human adipose-tissue stromal cells via SAPK/JNK and stemness acting signals," *Stem Cells*, vol. 26, no. 10, pp. 2724–2734, 2008.

[105] C. Ip, "Lessons from basic research in selenium and cancer prevention," *Journal of Nutrition*, vol. 128, no. 11, pp. 1845–1854, 1998.

[106] F. Ng, S. Boucher, S. Koh et al., "PDGF, tgf-2. And FGF signaling is important for differentiation and growth of mesenchymal stem cells (mscs): transcriptional profiling can identify markers and signaling pathways important in differentiation of MSCs into adipogenic, chondrogenic, and osteogenic lineages," *Blood*, vol. 112, no. 2, pp. 295 307, 2008.

[107] L. A. Solchaga, K. Penick, V. M. Goldberg, A. I. Caplan, and J. F. Welter, "Fibroblast growth factor-2 enhances proliferation and delays loss of chondrogenic potential in human adult bone-marrow-derived mesenchymal stem cells," *Tissue Engineering*, vol. 16, no. 3, pp. 1009–1019, 2010.

[108] S. Tsutsumi, A. Shimazu, K. Miyazaki et al., "Retention of multilineage differentiation potential of mesenchymal cells during proliferation in response to FGF," *Biochemical and Biophysical Research Communications*, vol. 288, no. 2, pp. 413–419, 2001.

[109] C. van den Bos, J. D. Mosca, J. Winkles, L. Kerrigan, W. H. Burgess, and D. R. Marshak, "Human mesenchymal stem cells respond to fibroblast growth factors," *Human cell*, vol. 10, no. 1, pp. 45–50, 1997.

[110] S. C. Choi, S. J. Kim, J. H. Choi, C. Y. Park, W. J. Shim, and D. S. Lim, "Fibroblast growth factor-2 and -4 promote the proliferation of bone marrow mesenchymal stem cells by the activation of the PI3K-Akt and ERK1/2 signaling pathways," *Stem Cells and Development*, vol. 17, no. 4, pp. 725–736, 2008.

[111] K. Tamama, H. Kawasaki, and A. Wells, "Epidermal growth factor (EGF) treatment on multipotential stromal cells (MSCs). Possible enhancement of therapeutic potential of MSC," *Journal of Biomedicine and Biotechnology*, vol. 2010, Article ID 795385, 10 pages, 2010.

[112] R. I. Freshney, *Culture of Animal Cells: A Manual of Basic technique*, Wiley-LISS, New York, NY, USA, 2000.

[113] T. Suda and T. M. Dexter, "Effect of hydrocortisone on long-term human marrow cultures," *British Journal of Haematology*, vol. 48, no. 4, pp. 661–664, 1981.

[114] S. Wang and S. Z. Haslam, "Serum-free primary culture of normal mouse mammary epithelial and stromal cells," *In Vitro Cellular and Developmental Biology*, vol. 30, no. 12, pp. 859–866, 1994.

[115] J. J. Castellot Jr, D. L. Cochran, and M. J. Karnovsky, "Effect of heparin on vascular smooth muscle cells. I. Cell metabolism," *Journal of Cellular Physiology*, vol. 124, no. 1, pp. 21–28, 1985.

[116] T. Imaizumi, F. Jean-Louis, M. L. Dubertret, and L. Dubertret, "Heparin induces fibroblast proliferation, cell-matrix interaction and epidermal growth inhibition," *Experimental Dermatology*, vol. 5, no. 2, pp. 89–95, 1996.

[117] P. I. Marcus, G. H. Sato, R. G. Ham, and D. Patterson, "A tribute to Dr. Theodore T. Puck (September 24, 1916-November 6, 2005)," *In vitro Cellular & Developmental Biology*, vol. 42, no. 8-9, pp. 235–241, 2006.

6

Modelling Improvements in Cell Yield of Banked Umbilical Cord Blood and the Impact on Availability of Donor Units for Transplantation into Adults

Natasha Kekre,[1] Jennifer Philippe,[2] Ranjeeta Mallick,[3] Susan Smith,[2] and David Allan[1,2,4]

[1] Blood and Marrow Transplant Program, Division of Hematology, Department of Medicine, University of Ottawa,
501 Smyth Rd., Box 704, Ottawa, ON, Canada K1H 8L6
[2] OneMatch Stem Cell and Marrow Network, Canadian Blood Services, 40 Concourse Gate, Ottawa, ON, Canada K2E 8A6
[3] Clinical Epidemiology Program, Ottawa Hospital Research Institute, 501 Smyth Rd., Ottawa, ON, Canada K1H 8L6
[4] Regenerative Medicine Program, Ottawa Hospital Research Institute, 501 Smyth Rd., Ottawa, ON, Canada K1H 8L6

Correspondence should be addressed to David Allan; daallan@ohri.ca

Academic Editor: Gesine Kogler

Umbilical cord blood (UCB) is used increasingly in allogeneic transplantation. The size of units remains limiting, especially for adult recipients. Whether modest improvements in the yield of cells surviving storage and thawing allow more patients to proceed to transplant was examined. The impact of improved cell yield on the number of available UCB units was simulated using 21 consecutive anonymous searches. The number of suitable UCB units was calculated based on hypothetical recipient weight of 50 kg, 70 kg, and 90 kg and was repeated for a 10%, 20%, and 30% increase in the fraction of cells surviving storage. Increasing the percentage of cells that survive storage by 30% lowered the threshold of cells needed to achieve similar engraftment rates and increased numbers of UCB units available for patients weighing 50 ($P = 0.011$), 70 ($P = 0.014$), and 90 kg ($P = 0.003$), controlling for differences in HLA compatibility. Moreover, if recipients were 90 kg, 12 out of 21 patients had access to at least one UCB unit that met standard criteria, which increased to 19 out of 21 patients ($P = 0.035$) when the fraction of cells surviving storage and thawing increased by 30%. Modest increases in the yield of cells in banked UCB units can significantly increase donor options for adult patients undergoing HSCT.

1. Introduction

Umbilical cord blood (UCB) is used increasingly as an alternative source of hematopoietic stem cells for allogeneic transplantation into pediatric and adult patients. The National Marrow Donor Program recently reported that 10% of adult hematopoietic stem cell transplants (HSCT) and 41% of pediatric transplants utilized UCB as the graft source [1]. There are many reasons for the increased utility of UCB. Firstly, less than 30 percent of potential HSCT recipients will have a matched related donor available [2] and the trend towards increased reliance on alternative donor sources will continue well into the future based on reduced fertility rates observed in recent decades [3]. This has led to increased

utilization of unrelated sources of stem cell grafts, including widespread public cord blood banking. UCB transplantation requires less stringent HLA matching compared with bone marrow or peripheral blood stem cell grafts [4] and thereby helps to overcome barriers to donor availability for many patients, and especially patients from ethnic minorities [5].

The size of many adult patients often limits the availability of cord blood units due to the reduced number of cells per kilogram of recipient body weight, or the effective stem cell dose. Low cell doses may preclude transplantation or contribute to delayed engraftment [6], transplant-related mortality, and survival [7, 8]. Combining more than one UCB unit for transplantation into adults has been one approach to overcome limiting cell doses [9, 10], but this approach substantially increases costs of transplantation, making it unaffordable in many jurisdictions. Measurement of post-thaw cell number, viability, and function have highlighted the significant impact of processing, cryopreservation, and thawing on cell number and function. Reports have suggested that the recovery of total nucleated cells (TNC) prior to infusion at time of transplant ranges from 50 to 80 percent [11–16]. This further limits the applicability of UCB transplantation for adult patients. Thresholds of prestorage cell numbers have been established for timely engraftment of adult recipients of UCB transplantation. Total nucleated cell dose thresholds depend on the degree of HLA disparity, with a greater TNC dose required for each additional HLA mismatch [17, 18].

Availability of donor units of sufficient size continues to be a limiting factor for many patients, especially as requests for available backup units become more common in case of graft failure [17]. Research to address improvements in cell recovery through optimization of cryopreservation conditions is ongoing [19–21]. Many studies have addressed potential cell expansion methods although this remains an area of active research and will likely be associated with significant cost [22]. In this study, we sought to quantitatively model the required improvements in TNC yield that could improve access to UCB donors for adult-sized patients undergoing HSCT. Our approach uses anonymized actual searches and simulates the impact of improved cell yield following storage and thawing on the number of available cord blood units. The goal of our study was to provide an estimate of the improvement in cell yield required to impact the pool of available donors for adult patients that could influence cord blood banking practices by blood establishments.

2. Materials and Methods

2.1. Match Selection. Twenty-one consecutive preliminary umbilical cord blood searches from the OneMatch Stem Cell Network of Canadian Blood Services were anonymized and obtained for use in the modeling analysis. In our study, we used results from the Cord Blood Match Program of the Bone Marrow Donors Worldwide (BMDW) for actual preliminary searches performed by Canadian Blood Services. The BMDW search program provides preliminary results from the inventories of 46 cord blood banks in 30 countries with a total combined inventory in excess of 500,000 units. Canadian Blood Services routinely uses the Cord Blood Match Program of BMDW to obtain preliminary search results from cord blood bank inventories. The research protocol was approved by the research ethics boards at The Ottawa Hospital Research Institute and Canadian Blood Services.

2.2. Modelling the Impact of Improved Cell Yield on Cord Blood Search Results. A model was created based on current published criteria used for selection of umbilical cord blood units for HSCT [18]. These criteria incorporate the degree of HLA-A, HLA-B, and HLA-DR compatibility with thresholds of TNC. A TNC dose of 1.5×10^7/kg was used to identify 6/6 HLA-matched units, 2.5×10^7/kg was used to identify 5/6 HLA-matched units, and 5.0×10^7/kg was used to identify 4/6

HLA-matched units. We calculated the TNC dose per kg in each search using 50 kg, 70 kg, and 90 kg to simulate the range of weights typical for adult transplant recipients. The total number of units available, including HLA-matched and HLA-mismatched units, was determined at each weight for each search. We repeated the calculation and assumed an increase of 10%, 20%, or 30% in the percentage of cells that survived storage and thawing to determine the number of available cord blood units that exceeded the minimum criteria for each of the recipient weight categories. The hypothetical increase in percentage of cells that survived the storage and thawing process allowed us to calculate a lowered effective TNC threshold that we used for identifying units that could be selected for transplantation (see Table 1). Importantly, even a 30% increase in the fraction of cells surviving over the standard level of 70% would yield an achievable 91% of cells surviving storage and thawing. As an example,

> standard TNC threshold at collection = yield after thaw/(% cells surviving).

If we assume an increase of 10% in the fraction of cells surviving storage, we can calculate a new lower threshold for identifying units associated with the same likelihood of timely engraftment (i.e., units with the same yield of cells after thawing) as follows:

(i) new TNC threshold at collection = yield after thaw/(% cells surviving × 1.1), or

(ii) new TNC threshold at collection = standard TNC threshold/1.1.

2.3. Statistical Analysis. A mixed effects model was used to determine the impact of two variables: (1) degree of HLA matching and (2) fraction of cells surviving storage and thawing, on the mean number of umbilical cord blood units available. In cases of statistical significance, multiple comparisons were performed to compare groups within the variable using Tukey's adjustment. Mean values were reported ±1 standard error unless otherwise stated. Proportions were compared using chi-squared analysis.

3. Results

An increase in the percentage of cells that survive the storage and thawing process lowered the effective threshold of TNC needed at the time of collection and demonstrated a trend towards increased mean number of available UCB units for patients weighing 50, 70, and 90 kg at all levels of HLA compatibility (see Table 2). A mixed effects model was used to assess the impact of increasing the percentage of surviving cells by 10%, 20%, and 30% and the effect of HLA-matching (6/6 versus 5/6 versus 4/6) on the mean number of umbilical cord units available per patient. Both variables were significantly associated with increased numbers of available donors ($P = 0.01$ for the increase in the fraction of cells that survive storage and thawing and $P < 0.0001$ for degree of HLA match). Multiple comparisons revealed that a 20% ($P = 0.047$) and 30% ($P = 0.0015$) improvement in the fraction

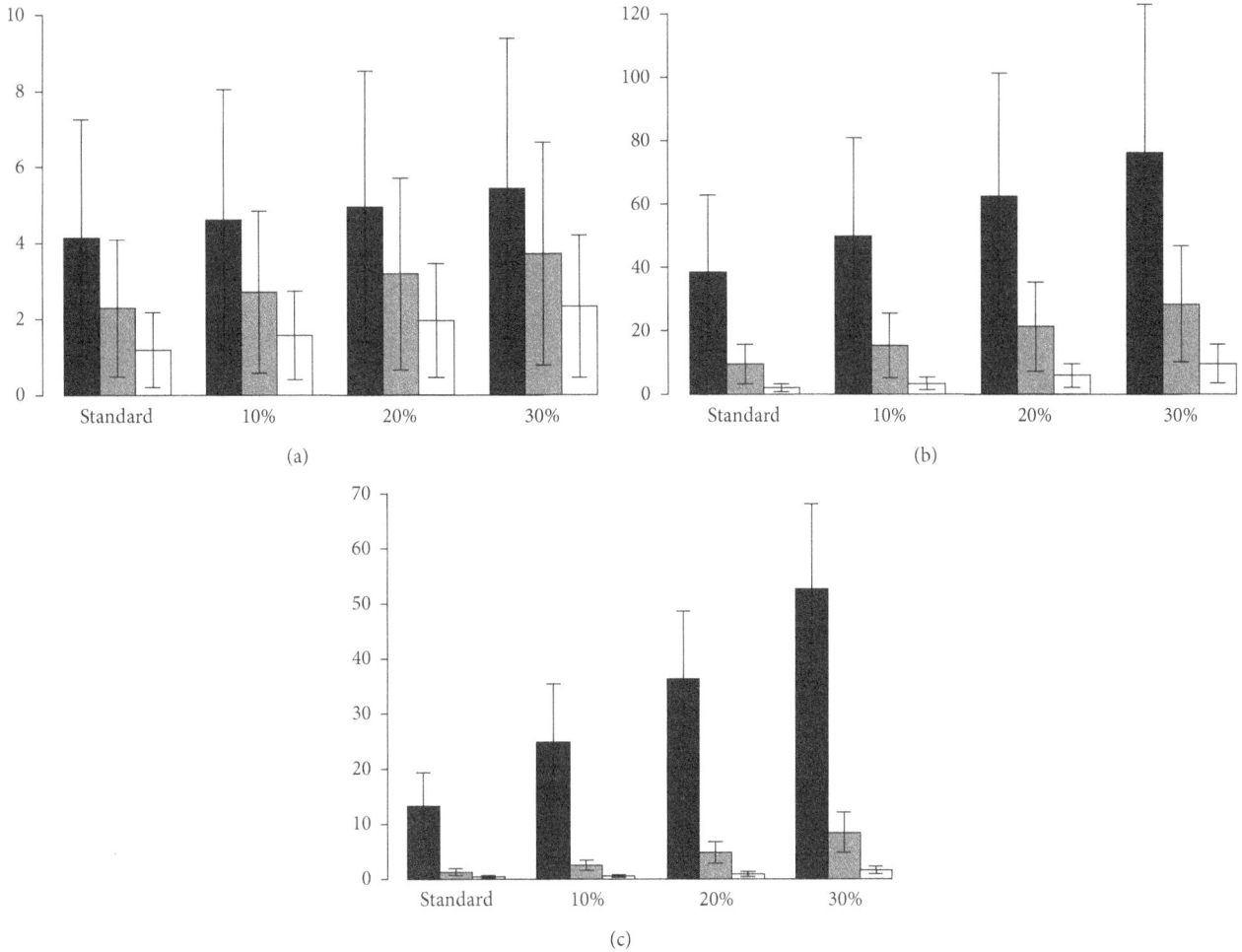

FIGURE 1: Mean number of available UCB units with increased yield of cells surviving storage and thawing. Mean number of UCB units identified if patients weighed 50 kg (black), 70 kg (grey), and 90 kg (white). Mean number of units that were 6/6 HLA matched (a), 5/6 HLA matched (b), and 4/6 HLA-matched (c) are presented using the standard threshold criteria for unit selection (standard) and if there was a 10%, 20%, or 30% increase in the fraction of cells surviving storage and thawing. Error bars represent the standard error of the mean.

of cells surviving storage and thawing for a 50 kg patient increased the mean number of UCB units available from 21.4 (standard conditions) to 37.0 (20% improvement) and 47.1 (30% improvement), respectively. For a weight of 70 kg and 90 kg, a 30% increase in the fraction of cells surviving storage and thawing ($P = 0.0021$ and $P = 0.0005$, resp.) was associated with a significant increase in the number of available units (5.1 to 14.3 (for 70 kg patients) and 1.3 to 4.7 (for 90 kg patients), resp.) (see Table 2). The number of donor units that were HLA matched or mismatched (5/6 and 4/6 matches) for patients weighing 50, 70, and 90 kg is presented in Figures 1(a)–1(c) for standard conditions and for theoretical increases of 10%, 20%, and 30% in the survival of cells surviving storage and thawing.

To better appreciate the clinical impact of improving the yield of cells that survive storage, we determined the number of patients who had at least one donor available using standard selection criteria and then determined the number of patients with available donors using the new effective TNC thresholds based on 10%, 20%, and 30% improvement in

percentage of cells that survive storage and thawing. If all patients weighed 50 kg, all patients in the study would have at least one available donor that met standard criteria. If all patients weighed 70 kg, only 19 of the 21 patients had an available unit identified using standard selection criteria; however, with a 30% increase in the fraction of cells surviving, the reduced effective TNC dose allowed all patients to have an available UCB unit. Most strikingly, if all patients weighed 90 kg, just 12 of 21 patients had an available unit and this increased to 19 of 21 patients ($P = 0.035$) when the fraction of cells surviving storage and thawing increased by 30%.

To gain insight regarding the applicability of our results on a broader scale, we modelled the number of searches needed to appreciate clinically significant changes in the number of 6/6 HLA-matched donor units that would be available for adult patients weighing 50, 70, and 90 kg in the setting of a 10% improvement in the percentage of cells that survive storage and thawing. We chose this modest level of improvement in the yield of cells to highlight the potential impact that could be realized from minimal improvement in

TABLE 1: New TNC thresholds if percentage of cells surviving storage and thawing increased by 10%, 20%, and 30%.

Thresholds $\times 10^7$/kg	6/6 HLA match	5/6 HLA match	4/6 HLA match
Standard threshold	1.5	2.5	5.0
New threshold (10%)	1.36	2.27	4.55
New threshold (20%)	1.25	2.08	4.17
New threshold (30%)	1.15	1.92	3.85

TABLE 2: Mixed effects model on the impact of increasing the fraction of cells surviving storage and thawing compared to standard yields and the impact of HLA compatibility on the number of available donor units (least square means reported).

	Available donor units for patient weight		
	50 Kg	70 kg	90 kg
Percentage of cells surviving[a]			
Standard	21.3	5.1	1.3
110% (P versus standard)	29.0 (0.33)	7.6 (0.38)	1.9 (0.50)
120% (P versus standard)	37.0 (0.047)	10.5 (0.061)	3.0 (0.068)
130% (P versus standard)	47.1 (0.002)	14.3 (0.002)	4.7 (0.0005)
Degree of HLA-match[b]			
6/6 HLA matched	4.8	3.0	1.8
5/6 (P versus 6/6)	56.6 (0.016)	18.6 (<0.0001)	5.2 (<0.0001)
4/6 (P versus 6/6)	39.4 (<0.0001)	6.5 (0.17)	1.3 (0.58)
4/6 (P versus 5/6)	39.4 (<0.0001)	6.5 (<0.0001)	1.3 (<0.0001)

[a] P values for mixed effects model considering increases in yield of cells surviving storage and thawing ($P = 0.011$ for patient weight of 50 kg, 0.014 for 70 kg, and 0.003 for 90 kg).

[b] P values for mixed effects model considering degree of HLA match ($P < 0.0001$ for patient weight of 50 kg, 70 kg, and 90 kg).

cell yield. We determined the sample size needed to achieve 90% power at 0.05 level of significance and extrapolated the results of our study using the standard deviation and mean number of HLA-matched donor units identified in the actual searches for hypothetical donors weighing 50, 70, and 90 kg. Using this approach, we determined that cord blood searches for only 37, 78, and 60 transplant recipients would be required for patients weighing 50, 70, and 90 kg, respectively, to identify a significant increase in the number of available donor units if the yield of cells that survived processing and storage increased by just 10%. That is to say, studies designed to detect a significant increase in the availability of HLA-matched cord blood units for adult patients that would be associated with a 10% increase in the yield of cells would need to enrol between 37 and 78 adult patients, depending on the weight of the patients.

4. Discussion

In this study, we have demonstrated the marked impact on the availability of banked cord blood units that would become available for transplantation into adult patients if the yield of surviving cells in banked UCB units could increase by up to 30%. Notably, our simulated modeling reveals that more patients would have at least one donor unit available if the process of storage and thawing could be improved by 30%. If the trends we observed in this small study are applied to a larger sample size, we expect that improvements of just 10% could significantly improve donor options on a

national and international scale. The results of our research are most notable for a patient weight of 90 kg which reflects an increasing proportion of the adult population. Our findings strongly support the need for improvements in storage, cryopreservation, and thawing techniques that could yield even modest benefits in the final yield of cells in thawed units.

To the best of our knowledge, our study is the first to quantify the magnitude of improvement in the yield of cells that survive storage and thawing that is needed to improve access to donors for adult patients who are candidates for cord blood transplantation. The dose of total nucleated cells remains the chief determinant that impacts on the selection of umbilical cord blood units [17, 23, 24]. Recent research suggests that a TNC count of 1.5×10^9 in collected units is associated with a marked increase in likelihood of selection by transplant centres. Many cord blood banks have increased the threshold for collection to maximize the percentage of their inventory represented by larger units that meet these criteria. This strategy, however, means that as many as 90% of collected units are not suitable for banking due to insufficient cell numbers and introduces challenges for cord blood bank viability. It is possible, however, that greater understanding of factors associated with high TNC counts could improve the efficiency associated with identifying and banking units with high cell counts. Another approach to overcoming limiting doses of cells in banked units that have been embraced by some transplant centres is a strategy of combining cord blood units to reach specific cutoffs for total nucleated cells per kg. This approach places greater strain on the resources of cord blood banking establishments as the inventory will be depleted more quickly and the high fees for retrieving banked units introduce significant financial barriers for transplant centres and health care authorities that are prohibitive in many jurisdictions. Strategies to improve the yield of cells that can survive the processing, storage, and thawing steps are less studied and could be cost-effective. Carbohydrate-based inhibitors of ice recrystallization [25], including antifreeze glycoproteins [26], are able to reduce the amount of dimethyl-sulfoxide required for safe storage of umbilical cord blood and appear promising as a means of improving the yield of viable cells. Other methods of improving the yield of cells include lyophilisation of cells [27] and novel storage methods. In addition, volume reduction techniques remain inefficient, particularly for large cellular units, and improvements in volume reduction may confer benefits on the yield of available cells [28, 29]. A final consideration for overcoming the limited cell dose in stored cord blood units is expansion of the stem and progenitor cell populations. Many groups have considered this approach using ex vivo cytokines, HOXB4, and other key regulators of hematopoietic stem cells [22, 30]. Cell expansion methods, however, will likely be resource intensive and will require specialized laboratories that will be subject to additional regulatory oversight which may limit widespread applicability.

One limitation of the current study is the sample size. Although we detected significant differences in the availability of donors using a model that increased the yield of cells by 30% when considering patients weighing 90 kg, we believe that smaller improvements in the fraction of cells that survive storage and thawing will have incremental effects on the availability for donors of patients of all weights. Extrapolation of our results suggests studies enrolling as few as 80 patients would be sufficiently powered to detect significant differences in the availability of HLA-matched cord blood units for adult patients associated with as little as a 10% increase in the fraction of cells that survive storage and thawing. The precise relationship between the degree of improvement in cell yield and impact on the availability of cord blood units for transplantation remains unproven for patients less than 50 kg. Moreover, it is important to acknowledge the evolving landscape in cell enumeration and that variable approaches to the standardization of TNC and CD34 enumeration may have impacted our results. Finally, we acknowledge that evolving practices by cord blood banks may allow one to identify particular banks that embrace practices associated with the highest quality processing and storage techniques. It would be interesting to examine the impact of improved cellular yields in the context of units derived only from banks embracing practices associated with the highest quality standards.

In conclusion, our study provides a clear demonstration that realistic and achievable improvements in the yield of cells surviving storage and thawing can have a profound impact on the availability of cord blood units for transplantation into adults recipients. Research that demonstrates modest improvements in the yield of cells in banked cord blood units could have an important effect on the field of cord blood banking and transplantation on a global scale.

Conflict of Interests

The authors declare that they have no conflict of interests.

Acknowledgments

The authors wish to acknowledge the assistance of Yiming Guo at the OneMatch Stem Cell and Marrow Network of Canadian Blood Services for her assistance with preparing the anonymized cord blood search results. They gratefully acknowledge salary support from the Department of Medicine at the University of Ottawa (DSA), a New Investigator Award from Canadian Institutes of Health Research (DSA), and a Scholar Award from the American Society of Hematology (NK).

References

[1] K. K. Ballen, R. J. King, P. Chitphakdithai et al., "The national marrow donor program 20 years of unrelated donor hematopoietic cell transplantation," *Biology of Blood and Marrow Transplantation*, vol. 14, no. 9, supplement, pp. 2–7, 2008.

[2] E. A. Copelan, "Hematopoietic stem-cell transplantation," *The New England Journal of Medicine*, vol. 354, no. 17, pp. 1813–1826, 2006.

[3] D. S. Allan, S. Takach, S. Smith, and M. Goldman, "Impact of declining fertility rates on donor options in blood and marrow transplantation," *Biology of Blood and Marrow Transplantation*, vol. 15, no. 12, pp. 1634–1637, 2009.

[4] J. Kurtzberg, M. Laughlin, M. L. Graham et al., "Placental blood as a source of hematopoietic stem cells for transplantation into unrelated recipients," *The New England Journal of Medicine*, vol. 335, no. 3, pp. 157–166, 1996.

[5] J. N. Barker, C. E. Byam, N. A. Kernan et al., "Availability of cord blood extends allogeneic hematopoietic stem cell transplant access to racial and ethnic minorities," *Biology of Blood and Marrow Transplantation*, vol. 16, no. 11, pp. 1541–1548, 2010.

[6] P. Rubinstein, C. Carrier, A. Scaradavou et al., "Outcomes among 562 recipients of placental-blood transplants from unrelated donors," *The New England Journal of Medicine*, vol. 339, no. 22, pp. 1565–1577, 1998.

[7] M. J. Laughlin, J. Barker, B. Bambach et al., "Hematopoietic engraftment and survival in adult recipients of umbilical-cord blood from unrelated donors," *The New England Journal of Medicine*, vol. 344, no. 24, pp. 1815–1822, 2001.

[8] J. E. Wagner, J. N. Barker, T. E. DeFor et al., "Transplantation of unrelated donor umbilical cord blood in 102 patients with malignant and nonmalignant diseases: Influence of CD34 cell dose and HLA disparity on treatment-related mortality and survival," *Blood*, vol. 100, no. 5, pp. 1611–1618, 2002.

[9] C. G. Brunstein, E. J. Fuchs, S. L. Carter et al., "Alternative donor transplantation after reduced intensity conditioning: results of parallel phase 2 trials using partially HLA-mismatched related bone marrow or unrelated double umbilical cord blood grafts," *Blood*, vol. 118, no. 2, pp. 282–288, 2011.

[10] K. K. Ballen, T. R. Spitzer, B. Y. Yeap et al., "Double unrelated reduced-intensity umbilical cord blood transplantation in adults," *Biology of Blood and Marrow Transplantation*, vol. 13, no. 1, pp. 82–89, 2007.

[11] Y. Kudo, M. Minegishi, O. Seki et al., "Quality assessment of umbilical cord blood units at the time of transplantation,"

International Journal of Hematology, vol. 93, no. 5, pp. 645–651, 2011.

[12] T. P. H. Meyer, B. Hofmann, J. Zaisserer et al., "Analysis and cryopreservation of hematopoietic stem and progenitor cells from umbilical cord blood," *Cytotherapy*, vol. 8, no. 3, pp. 265–276, 2006.

[13] V. Laroche, D. H. McKenna, G. Moroff, T. Schierman, D. Kadidlo, and J. McCullough, "Cell loss and recovery in umbilical cord blood processing: a comparison of postthaw and postwash samples," *Transfusion*, vol. 45, no. 12, pp. 1909–1916, 2005.

[14] D. M. Regan, J. D. Wofford, and D. A. Wall, "Comparison of cord blood thawing methods on cell recovery, potency, and infusion," *Transfusion*, vol. 50, no. 12, pp. 2670–2675, 2010.

[15] H. Yang, J. P. Acker, J. Hannon, H. Miszta-Lane, J. J. Akabutu, and L. E. McGann, "Damage and protection of UC blood cells during cryopreservation," *Cytotherapy*, vol. 3, no. 5, pp. 377–386, 2001.

[16] S. Yamamoto, H. Ikeda, D. Toyama et al., "Quality of long-term cryopreserved umbilical cord blood units for hematopoietic cell transplantation," *International Journal of Hematology*, vol. 93, no. 1, pp. 99–105, 2011.

[17] J. N. Barker, A. Scaradavou, and C. E. Stevens, "Combined effect of total nucleated cell dose and HLA match on transplantation outcome in 1061 cord blood recipients with hematologic malignancies," *Blood*, vol. 115, no. 9, pp. 1843–1849, 2010.

[18] J. N. Barker, C. Byam, and A. Scaradavou, "How I treat: the selection and acquisition of unrelated cord blood grafts," *Blood*, vol. 117, no. 8, pp. 2332–2339, 2011.

[19] L. K. Wu, J. M. Tokarew, J. L. Chaytor et al., "Carbohydrate-mediated inhibition of ice recrystallization in cryopreserved human umbilical cord blood," *Carbohydrate Research*, vol. 346, no. 1, pp. 86–93, 2011.

[20] I. B. Nicoud, D. M. Clarke, G. Taber et al., "Cryopreservation of umbilical cord blood with a novel freezing solution that mimics intracellular ionic composition," *Transfusion*, vol. 52, no. 9, pp. 2055–2062, 2012.

[21] J. Stylianou, M. Vowels, and K. Hadfield, "Novel cryoprotectant significantly improves the post-thaw recovery and quality of HSC from CB," *Cytotherapy*, vol. 8, no. 1, pp. 57–61, 2006.

[22] S. S. Tung, S. Parmar, S. N. Robinson et al., "Ex vivo expansion of umbilical cord clood for transplantation," *Best Practice & Research Clinical Haematology*, vol. 23, no. 2, pp. 245–257, 2010.

[23] J. Jaime-Pérez, R. Monreal-Robles, L. Rodríguez-Romo et al., "Evaluation of volume and total nucleated cell count as cord blood selection parameters:a receiver operating characteristic curve modeling approach," *American Journal of Clinical Pathology*, vol. 136, no. 5, pp. 721–726, 2011.

[24] D. A. Wall and K. W. Chan, "Selection of cord blood unit(s) for transplantation," *Bone Marrow Transplantation*, vol. 42, no. 1, pp. 1–7, 2008.

[25] J. Chaytor, J. Tokarew, L. Wu et al., "Inhibiting ice recrystallization and optimization of cell viability after cryopreservation," *Glycobiology*, vol. 22, no. 1, pp. 123–133, 2012.

[26] M. Leclère, B. K. Kwok, L. K. Wu et al., "Synthesis of C-linked AFGP analogues and assessment of their cryoprotective properties," *Bioconjugate Chemistry*, vol. 22, pp. 1804–1810, 2011.

[27] D. Natan, A. Nagler, and A. Arav, "Freeze-drying of mononuclear cells derived from umbilical cord blood followed by colony formation," *PLoS One*, vol. 4, no. 4, article e5240, 2009.

[28] S. Meyer-Monard, A. Tichelli, C. Troeger et al., "Initial cord blood unit volume affects mononuclear cell and CD34$^+$ cell-processing efficiency in a non-linear fashion," *Cytotherapy*, vol. 14, no. 2, pp. 215–222, 2012.

[29] P. Solves, D. Planelles, V. Mirabet, A. Blanquer, and F. Carbonell-Uberos, "Qualitative and quantitative cell recovery in umbilical cord blood processed by two automated devices in routine cord blood banking: a comparative study," *Blood Transfusion*, vol. 12, pp. 1–8, 2012.

[30] J. Antonchuk, G. Sauvageau, and R. K. Humphries, "HOXB4-induced expansion of adult hematopoietic stem cells ex vivo," *Cell*, vol. 109, no. 1, pp. 39–45, 2002.

7

Adult-Brain-Derived Neural Stem Cells Grafting into a Vein Bridge Increases Postlesional Recovery and Regeneration in a Peripheral Nerve of Adult Pig

Olivier Liard,[1] Stéphanie Segura,[2] Emmanuel Sagui,[1] André Nau,[1] Aurélie Pascual,[1] Melissa Cambon,[3] Jean-Luc Darlix,[4] Thierry Fusai,[1] and Emmanuel Moyse[2]

[1] Unité de Chirurgie et Physiologie Expérimentale (UCPE), Institut de Médecine Tropicale, 58 boulevard Charles Livon, 13007 Marseille, France
[2] Unité Physiologie de la Reproduction et des Comportements, UMR 85, Centre INRA de Tours, 37380 Nouzilly, France
[3] Laboratoire d'Ecologie fonctionnelle, Bâtiment 4R3, 118 route de Narbonne, 31062 Toulouse cedex 9, France
[4] Unité de Rétrovirologie, U421 INSERM, Ecole Normale Supérieure de Lyon, 46 Allée d'Italie, 69364 Lyon cedex 07, France

Correspondence should be addressed to Emmanuel Moyse, moyseemmanuel@yahoo.fr

Academic Editor: Henry J. Klassen

We attempted transplantation of adult neural stem cells (ANSCs) inside an autologous venous graft following surgical transsection of *nervis cruralis* with 30 mm long gap in adult pig. The transplanted cell suspension was a primary culture of neurospheres from adult pig subventricular zone (SVZ) which had been labeled *in vitro* with BrdU or lentivirally transferred fluorescent protein. Lesion-induced loss of leg extension on the thigh became definitive in controls but was reversed by 45–90 days after neurosphere-filled vein grafting. Electromyography showed stimulodetection recovery in neurosphere-transplanted pigs but not in controls. Postmortem immunohistochemistry revealed neurosphere-derived cells that survived inside the venous graft from 10 to 240 postlesion days and all displayed a neuronal phenotype. Newly formed neurons were distributed inside the venous graft along the severed nerve longitudinal axis. Moreover, ANSC transplantation increased CNPase expression, indicating activation of intrinsic Schwann cells. Thus ANSC transplantation inside an autologous venous graft provides an efficient repair strategy.

1. Introduction

Nerve injuries which are frequent in civil practice [1, 2] and catastrophe-like earthquake [3, 4] or tsunami [5] combine associative lesion with crush syndrome. War improves the risk of gap and of treatment delay with ballistic wounds [6] because these ones are less prone to emergency than vascular injuries [7]. This risk pertains after war with remanent explosive [8]. The functional pronostic is dependent on the type of wound: transsection, crush, or gap, which has been further categorized according to the length of the gap, the type of nerve (sensitive, motor or mixed), localization, association of injuries, and patient's ageing, time of surgery, and vascular environment [9–12].

Neuroguides and especially vein grafts are regularly used to bridge small nerve gaps shorter than 3 cm; for long nerve gaps, autologous nerve graft has become the gold standard

since the second war [13, 14]. But nerve repair outcome depends on fascicle concordance [15] and scar development, so expected alternatives for long nerve gaps remain a challenge to improve recovery after this type of lesion. Surgical trials to improve nerve repair have mainly targeted diversification of grafted neuroguides with resorbable materials [16]. The outcome has been improved by neuroguide preloading with extracellular matrix components [17–19], growth factors [20], or cultured regeneration-enhancing cells. The latter strategy, or cell therapy, has been attempted with primary cultures of Schwann cells [21, 22], olfactory bulb ensheating cells [23], or various types of stem cells [24]. In these studies, progenies of grafted stem cells mostly proved to be glial cells, which indirectly enhance axonal regeneration [24].

Neural stem cells from adult brain (ANSC) have been scarcely assayed to help postlesional repair of peripheral nerves, despite their strong potential of integration and development into neurons [25]. The present study is based on the hypothesis that ANSC grafting inside a venous neuroguide might be efficient to bridge a long nerve gap in adult. We tested this hypothesis in the pig, which is the non-primate animal species most closely related to human and is prone to surgery and anesthesia conditions very close to human protocols in clinic [26]. To this aim, we have characterized primary cultures of neural stem cells from adult pig brain, by optimizing the neurosphere assay on subventricular zone explants [27]. In the present study, we labeled such primary expanded ANSC *in vitro* with either BrdU or lentiviral green fluorescent protein gene transfer, and we grafted labeled neurospheres into an autologous venous bridge after a surgical 30 mm long gap in adult pig *nervi cruralis*. We compared neurosphere-grafted and control pigs for functional recovery and assessed the fate of grafted cells inside the lesioned nerve at various post-lesion intervals.

2. Material and Methods

2.1. Animals. Twenty-four adults, 4-month-old Large White Landrace pigs were used in the present study. They were housed with *ad libitum* access to water and standard food pellets, in lodges that comprised one yard and one hard infrared-heated shelter. All *in vivo* experimental protocols were approved by the local Ethics Committee on the protection of animals used for scientific activities with the protocol number 31/2006/IMTSSA/UCPE. Personal protocol number for surgery and experimentation with pigs was 2007/29/DEF/DCSSA (to O. Liard). All efforts were made to minimize the number of animals used and their suffering.

2.2. Anesthesia. Deep anesthesia was initiated by intramuscular premedication with 30 mg/kg ketamine (Imalgene 1000, Merial, Lyon, France), 0.1 mL/kg acepromazine (Vet–ranquil, Calmivet, Bayer, Puteaux, France), and 25 μg/kg atropine sulphate (Meram, Melun, France). The animal was then equipped with a peripheral intravenous perfusion delivering Ringer-lactate-5% glucose serum at 5–7 mL/kg/h, with adhesive electrocardiographic electrodes in CM5-SpO2 (ECG monitor S5, Datex Ohmeda, Madison, WI, USA), and with an artificial oxygenator. Anesthesia induction was performed by intravenous injections of 2 mg/kg propofol (Diprivan, Bayer) during 30 sec slowly, and of sufentanil (Sufenta, Bayer) three times at 1.5 μg/kg. Local glottis anesthesia was made with 5% lidocaïne spray (Xylocaine, Bayer), before orotracheal intubation with a monolight cannula (internal diameter 6.5 mm). Ventilation of lung parenchyma was checked with a stethoscope and mechanically assisted. General anesthesia was sustained with electrically driven intravenous infusion of propofol 2 mg/kg/h (Diprivan, DCI), sufentanil 1 μg/kg/h (Sufenta, DCI) and rocuronium bromide 0.15 mg/kg/h (Esmeron, DCI); curarisation was supervised by means of a S5 monitor (Entropie module) but was not released for EMG. Antibioprophylaxy was administered. All along surgery, the cardioventilatory parameters (heart and ventilation rates, electrocardiogram, blood oxygenation, ventilation pressure and volume, MAC, temperature,

hemoglucotest) as well as the sleep threshold were constantly watched with the S5 monitor.

2.3. Brain Tissue Sampling for Primary Neural Stem Cell Culture from Adult Pig. Separate animals were dedicated for primary culture and *in vitro* expansion of neural stem cells from brain subventricular zone (SVZ) as previously described [27]. On each deeply anesthetized pig, the dorsal face of the skull was cut with an electric saw and removed. A 15 mm thick coronal slice of the brain was performed with a scalpel at the commissural level of midbrain, manually explanted and transferred at 4°C on ice bed-laid sterile metal plate, beside a Bunsen flame for atmosphere sterilization. The experimental animal was thus alive until the explantation of the brain tissue slice. Each pig was sacrificed immediately after brain tissue sampling by intravenous injection of Dolethal (R) pentobarbital (DCI) at 1.5 mL/kg.

2.4. Primary Culture of SVZ Neural Stem Cells ("Neurosphere Assay"). As previously described [27], SVZ pieces were quickly microdissected from the thick midbrain slice (above) along the ventrolateral floor of lateral brain ventricles in low-calcium artificial cerebrospinal fluid (aCSF: 124 mM NaCl, 5 mM KCl, 3.2 mM MgCl$_2$, 0.1 mM CaCl$_2$, 26 mM NaHCO$_3$, 100 mM glucose, and pH 7.38). Tissue samples were rinsed twice with aCSF and digested first in 40 U cystein-EDTA-β-mercaptoethanol-preactivated papain (Sigma, L'Isle D'Abeau, France) for 10 min at 37°C, then in 250 μL undiluted TrypLE Express solution (heat-resistant, microbially produced, purified trypsinlike enzyme, Gibco # 12604-013, Invitrogen, Cergy-Pontoise, France) for 10 min at 37°C. After the addition of 750 μL of fresh aCSF and centrifugation for 8 min at 400 g at room temperature, the cell pellet was resuspended in 1 mL culture medium (DMEM (Sigma), 1x B27 (Gibco Invitrogen), 200 U/mL penicillin, and 200 μg/mL streptomycin (Gibco Invitrogen)) containing 20 ng/mL Epidermal Growth Factor (EGF, Gibco Invitrogen) and 20 ng/mL basic Fibroblast Growth Factor (bFGF, Gibco Invitrogen). The cells were dissociated gently with a 26 G steel needle on a sterile disposable 1 mL syringe, counted on a Malassez slide, and seeded at 20,000 cells per mL in 6-well plates (Falcon, BD Biosciences, Bedford, USA). Cultures were monitored daily to follow the morphological growth of the neurospheres; passage was performed when the majority of spheres were 100–120 μm in diameter. For passage, the primary spheres were collected in sterile tubes, incubated for 45–60 min at 37°C in 250 μL undiluted TrypLE Express solution (Gibco Invitrogen) per 6 mL culture-derived pellet, and dissociated gently with a 26 G steel needle on a 1 mL sterile syringe; dispersed cells were centrifuged, counted, and seeded as above. All culture media were renewed by the replacement of 2 mL of medium per 4 mL well every 2-3-days. For immunocytochemistry, coverslips bearing differentiated spheres were rinsed in PBS, fixed in 4% paraformaldehyde-containing PBS for 20 min at 4°C, and kept in PBS at 4°C until the assay.

2.5. In Vitro Labelling of Neurosphere Cells. In the first set of experiments, tertiary neurospheres were incubated with

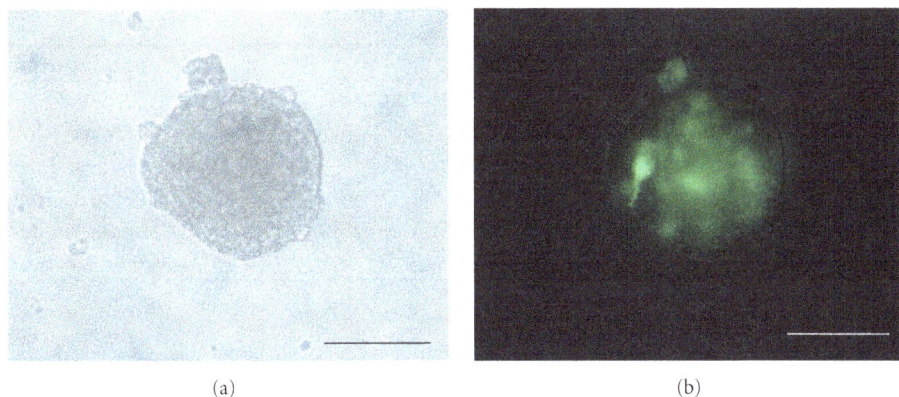

(a)   (b)

FIGURE 1: LV-GFP-labeled secondary neurosphere from adult pig SVZ, just before transplantation and 3 days after *in vitro* infection with the lentiviral vector of GFP, as observed under a photonic microscope with natural light (a) or GFP fluorescence (b). Scale bars: 50 μm.

the DNA synthesis precursor bromo-2-deoxy-uridine at 30 μM (BrdU, Sigma) from 2 DIV after passage up to 8–10 DIV, BrdU being added fresh daily from concentrated stock.

In a second set of experiments, lineage labelling was performed by infection of secondary neurospheres with a lentiviral vector of green fluorescent protein gene (LV-GFP) at 4-5 DIV after passage. LV-GFP was freshly synthetized, titrated, and tested as previously described [28], stored at −80°C and unfrozen just before use. Neurosphere cultures were preincubated 30 min in the presence of 1 mM polybrene (Sigma) and void lentiviral particles (VLP, 29) at 0.1x M.O.I., and further incubated 2 h with fresh culture medium containing 1 mM polybrene and LV-GFP at 0.3x M.O.I.; incubation medium was then replaced by fresh standard culture medium. LV-GFP-infected neurospheres were allowed 3 days culture in standard conditions for optimal lineage labelling (Figure 1); [28].

After optimal culture period (5-6 days for BrdU, 3 days for LV-GFP) and just before transplantation on the nerve lesion site (see below), neurospheres were collected, centrifuged 4 min at 800 g, and resuspended in fresh culture medium at 3×10^3 spheres per mL.

2.6. Postlesional Grafting Surgery. The surgical approach was realized on the median face of thigh to isolate *nervis cruralis*. Nerve damage was established in the right *N. cruralis* by creating a 30 mm gap, which was then bridged with an autologous vein segment sampled from *v. mammelian externalis*. This venous neuroguide was sutured at both ends over the perinevre of the sectioned nerve. In some animals, once the venous shaft was sutured at the proximal end of the lesioned nerve, 300 μL of freshly prepared neurosphere suspension (10^3 spheres) were gently infused with a micropipet into the opposite end of the neuroguide, which was then sutured onto the distal lesioned nerve end. In other animals (controls), the venous neuroguide was sutured without any additional manipulation.

In the first set of experiments, lesioned pigs were thus grafted with autologous vein shafts which were either empty (controls, $N = 2$) or filled with BrdU-prelabeled neurospheres ($N = 4$). These animals were allowed 8 or 45 days survival after lesion.

In the second set of experiments, lesioned pigs were grafted with venous neuroguides which were either empty (controls, $N = 3$) or filled with LV-GFP-labeled neurospheres ($N = 6$). These animals were allowed 8 months survival after lesion.

2.7. Functional Analysis of Lesioned Animals. Animal behaviour was evaluated by assessing muscular atrophy, deficit of leg extension over the thigh. Each animal was examined before peripheral nerve lesioning and at days 45, 90, 180, and 240 following surgical bridging.

Motor function of the crural nerve was assayed by electromyography, using pregeled surface electrodes connected to a portable electromyographic recorder (Keypoint (R) v6.01, Medtronics, MN, USA). Bipolar concentric needles (diameter 0.47 mm) were applied on muscle *quadriceps femori* for stimulodetection analyses along *N. cruralis*. Stimuli were single 100 mA shocks, ranging from 0.1 to 1 msec durations. Electromyography was performed on animals before and at 45, 90, 180, and 240 days after transection. Values were recorded in terms of voltage, amplitude and time latency of detectable electromyographic activities.

2.8. Immunohistochemistry. At the end of postlesional survival, the operated region of *N. cruralis* of each experimental pig was dissected out of the thigh under anesthesia and fixed by immersion in a 4% paraformaldehyde solution in 0.05 M, pH 7.4, NaH_2PO_4/Na_2HPO_4 buffer for 24 h at 4°C, then rinsed for 24 h at 4°C in 0.1 M, pH 7.4 phosphate-buffered saline (PBS). It was then cryoprotected for 72 h in a 30% sucrose solution, flat-embedded in OCT mounting medium and snap-frozen in liquid isopentane at −40°C for storage at −80°C. Longitudinal 20 μm-thick sections were made in a cryostat (Leica 2800), mounted on commercial precoated slides (Superfrost-Plus, Fisher-Scientific, Canada), dried overnight at ambient air, and stored at −20°C.

For immunohistofluorescent labellings, these tissue sections were brought back to room temperature and permeabilized in 0.1 M PBS with 0.5% Triton-X-100. For nuclear

TABLE 1: List of primary antibodies used.

Antigen	Antibody	Supplier	Cell-type specificity	Dilution
BrdU	Rat polyclonal	ImmunologicalDirect.com	none	1/100
CNPase	Mouse monoclonal	Sigma, L'Isle-d'Abeau, France; C-5922, clone 11-5b	Schwann cells	1/200
GFAP	Rabbit polyclonal	Dako, Trappes, France; Z0334	Astrocytes, neural stem cells	1/1000
NeuN	Mouse monoclonal	Chemicon, MAB377	Mature neurons	1/100
NF-68	Mouse monoclonal	BD-Biosciences, Heidelberg, Germany	Mature neurons	1/400
$S100\beta$	Rabbit polyclonal	Dako, Trappes, France	Astrocytes, Schwann cells	1/500

antigens, tissue sections were also treated 15 min in 10 mM sodium citrate solution (pH 5.5) at 95°C. After a PBS rinse, all preparations were incubated in blocking buffer (0.1 M PBS, 0.1% Triton, 3% bovine serum albumin, 5% normal serum) for 1 h, then overnight at 4°C with one primary antibody (Table 1). After three 5-minute-rinses in fresh 0.1 M PBS, immunohistochemical labelings were revealed by 2 h incubation at room temperature in the dark with the appropriate Alexa-594-conjugated secondary antibodies (Molecular Probes, Eugene, OR, USA; 1/400). For double-staining experiments, Alexa-594-revealed slides were rinsed three times in fresh 0.1 M PBS and further incubated overnight at 4°C with another primary antibody, which was revealed with appropriate Alexa-488-conjugated secondary antibody (Molecular Probes; 1/200). After rinsing, fluorescent staining of cell nuclei was performed by 5 min incubation in the dark with DAPI (0.5 μg/mL, Sigma). Labeled slides were coverslipped with aqueous mounting medium (Vectashield, Vector, Abcys, France) and photographed with a fluorescence microscope. CNPase immunohistochemical labeling was quantified on these photomicrographs by using the ImageJ software.

3. Results

3.1. Clinical Results. Before surgery, all experimental animals were healthy and displayed no walking deficit. After surgery, none of operated animals displayed any scar infection or host rejection response.

By clinical observation, loss of the right leg extension over the thigh was systematically observed after the surgical nerve transsection. This motor defect was maintained up to 240 days in animals which had crural nerve gap repaired by empty autologous venous bridge only. By contrast, lesioned leg extension over the thigh reappeared between 90 and 180 days in animals which had crural nerve gap repaired by the same type of autologous vein trunk filled with exogenous neurospheres.

3.2. Electromyography. Prior to surgery, electromyograms of m. quadriceps vast internal displayed amplitudes of 4.9 to 6.1 mV and poststimulus latencies of 0.89 to 3.7 ms. Immediately after surgical realization of *N. cruralis* substance loss, electromyograms of m. quadriceps were negative for all experimental animals, whatever their venous bridge had been filled or not with neurosphere suspension.

At 180 days (25 weeks) after lesion, neurosphere-transplanted pigs displayed positive electromyograms of m.

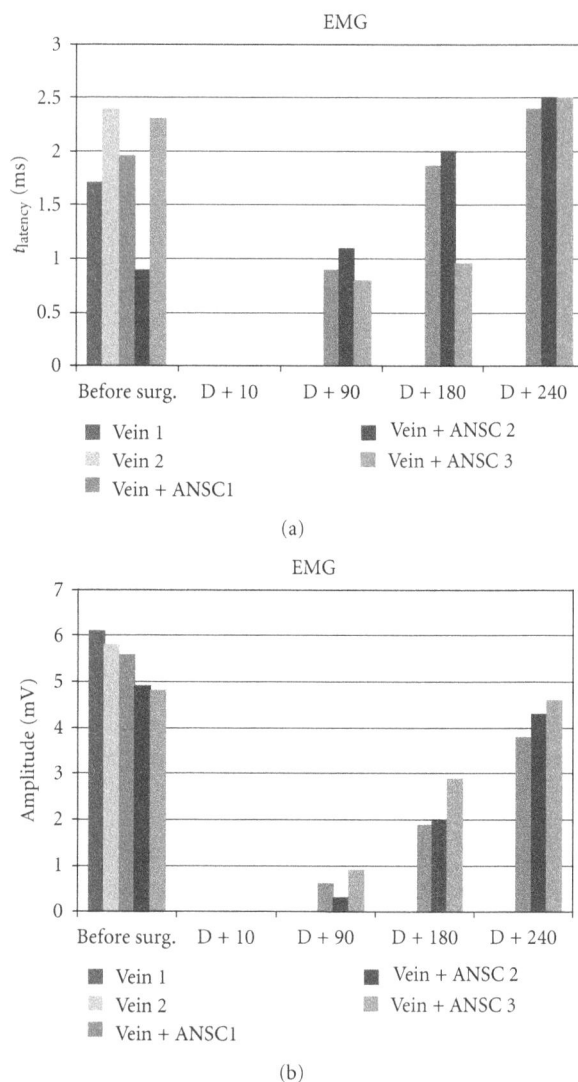

(a)

(b)

FIGURE 2: Electromyographic evaluation of muscle quadriceps femori at 90, 180, and 240 days following *N. cruralis* lesion and graft of GFP-labeled neurospheres inside a venous bridge before ("before surg.") or after ("D + 90", "D + 180", "D + 240") surgery.

quadriceps with 0.6 to 0.9 mV amplitudes and 0.96 to 2 ms latencies, whereas electromyograms of control animals remained negative (Figure 2).

At 240 days (34 weeks) after lesion, m. quadriceps electromyograms of neurosphere-transplanted pigs were improved up to 2.8–3.1 mV amplitudes with 2.4–2.5 ms

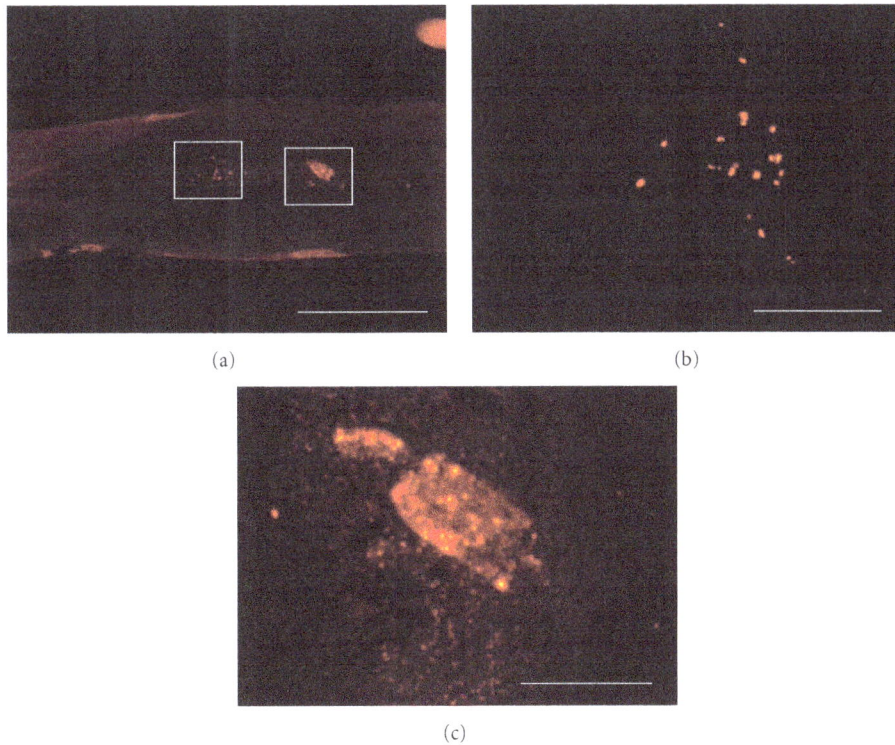

(a)

(b)

(c)

FIGURE 3: Localization of transplanted BrdU-labeled neurospheres in the bridged nerve at 8 days after lesion, by postmortem immunohistochemistry. BrdU immunoreactivity is revealed by red Alexa-594 fluorescence on longitudinal postfixed graft sections at low (a) and high (b, c) magnifications. Enlarged fields (b, c) are localized as white forms in (a). Transplanted neurosphere cells are found either sparsed (b) or clustered (c) inside the venous bridge. Scale bars: 0.5 mm (a), 100 μm (b, c).

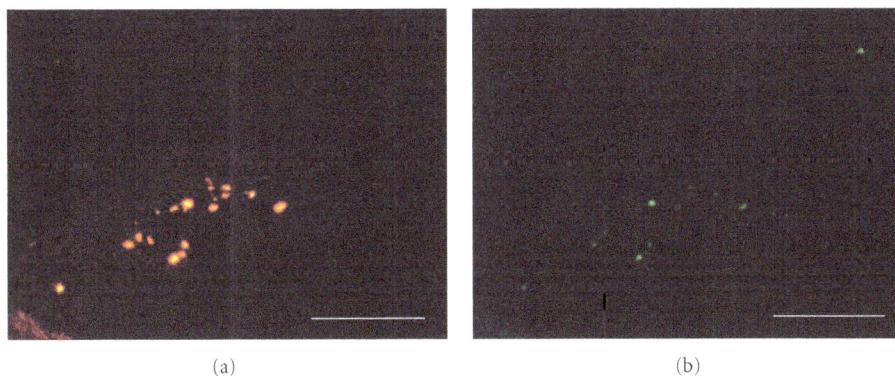

(a)

(b)

FIGURE 4: Double BrdU-DCX immunohistochemistry on a sagittal section from a neurosphere-grafted bridged nerve at 8 days after lesion. One given field was sequentially photographed with fluorescent wavelengths revealing, respectively, Alexa-594-labeled BrdU immunoreactivity (a) and Alexa-488-DCX one (b). Note the extensive nuclear colocalization of the immature neuron marker DCX with BrdU (b). Scale bars 100 mm.

latencies, while electromyograms of controls were still negative (Figure 2).

3.3. In Situ Fate of Grafted Pig Neurosphere Cells. In the first experiment, grafted neurosphere cells had been labeled by in vitro BrdU incorporation prior to graft. By immunohistochemistry on postmortem venous grafts, groups of BrdU-immunoreactive cells were detected inside the venous tube (Figure 3). In grafts sampled at 8 days after surgery, most of these BrdU+ cells were clustered in sphere-like assemblies

(Figures 3(a) and 3(c)) while some were sparsed inside the venous tube (Figure 3(b)). Most of BrdU+ cells were also immunoreactive for doublecortin (DCX) which is a specific marker of immature neurons (Figure 4). At 90 days after surgery, BrdU+ cells were still observed inside the venous tube and displayed immunoreactivity for NeuN, that is, a marker of differentiated neurons (Figure 5).

In the second experiment, expanded secondary neurospheres at 8 DIV had been stained by LV-GFP transfection just before collection and postlesional transplantation on

(a)

(b)

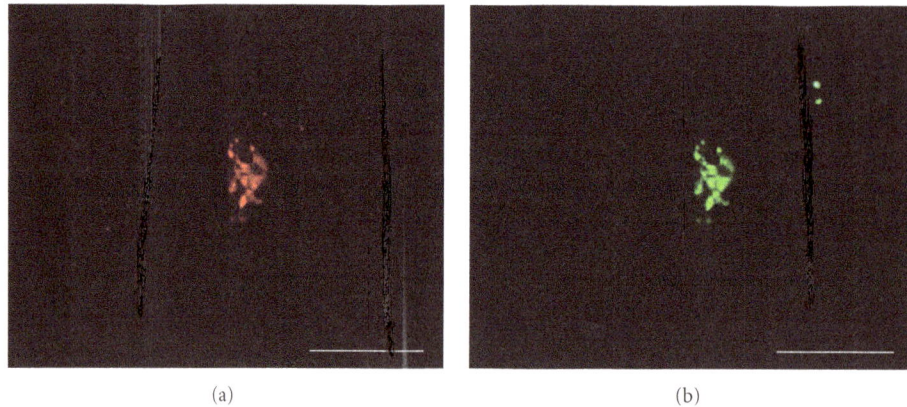

FIGURE 5: Double BrdU-NeuN immunohistochemistry on a sagittal section from a neurosphere-grafted bridged nerve at 90 days after lesion. One given field was sequentially photographed with fluorescent wavelengths revealing, respectively, Alexa-594-labeled BrdU immunoreactivity (a) and Alexa-488-NeuN one (b). Note the extensive nuclear colocalization of the mature neuron marker NeuN with BrdU (b). Scale bars 100 mm.

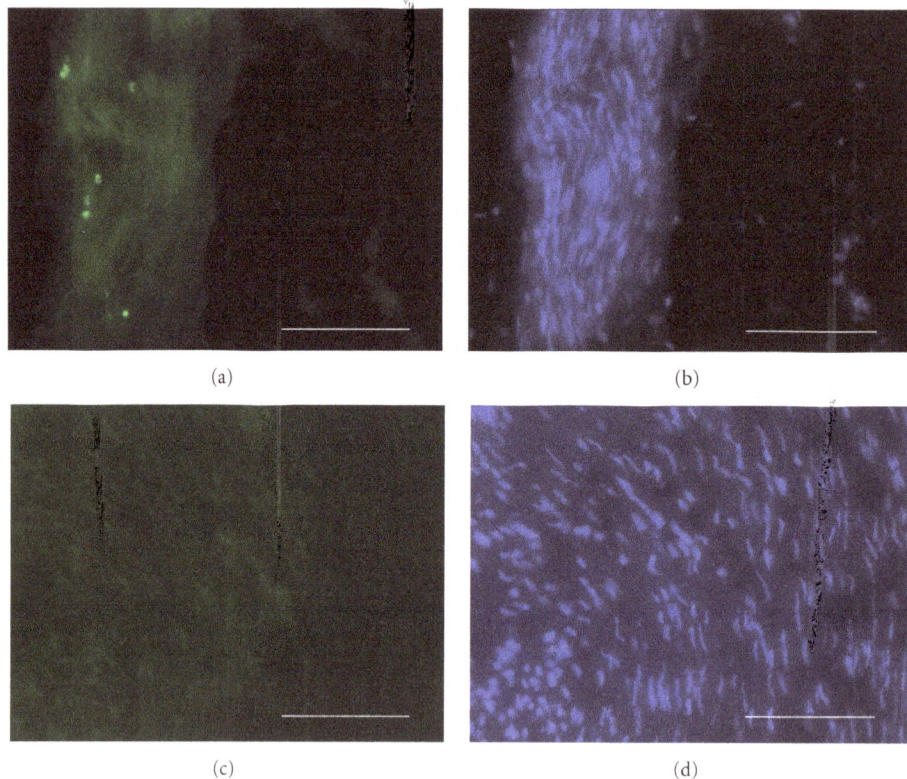

(a)

(b)

(c)

(d)

FIGURE 6: GFP lineage-labelling detection in DAPI-counterstained sagittal sections of venous bridges with (a, b) or without (c, d) transplantation of LV-GFP-labeled neurospheres, at 240 days after lesion. GFP-expressing neurosphere progeny (a, c) and DAPI-labeled tissue cell nuclei (b, d) are detected by fluorescence microscopy by using, respectively, adequate wavelengths. Scale bars: 0.5 mm (a, b), 100 μm (c, d).

the pig nerve gap. All neurospheres displayed fluorescent GFP labeling in most, but not all, cells (Figure 1). At either 45, 90, 180, or 240 days after lesion, sphere transplantation, each vein-bridged and LV-GFP sphere-transplanted nerve segment displayed a number of GFP-fluorescent cells which were exclusively localized inside the nerve fascicles (Figures 6(a) and 6(b)) and absent in nontransplanted control bridges (Figures 6(c) and 6(d)). Combined immunohistofluorescent labeling of either NeuN or neurofilament NF-68 revealed

that most of GFP fluorescence was colocalized with these neuronal markers (Figures 7(a)–7(c)). By contrast, GFP fluorescence did not colocalize with either of the glial markers assessed: S-100b (Figures 7(d)–7(f)), GFAP, CNPase.

Interestingly, at 180 and 240 days after nerve lesion and GFP-expressing neurosphere transplantation, CNPase immunohistofluorescent labeling was much higher than in vein-bridged lesioned controls which had not received neurosphere transplantation (Figure 8). Both the number of

Adult-Brain-Derived Neural Stem Cells Grafting into a Vein Bridge Increases Postlesional Recovery and Regeneration in a Peripheral Nerve of Adult Pig

71

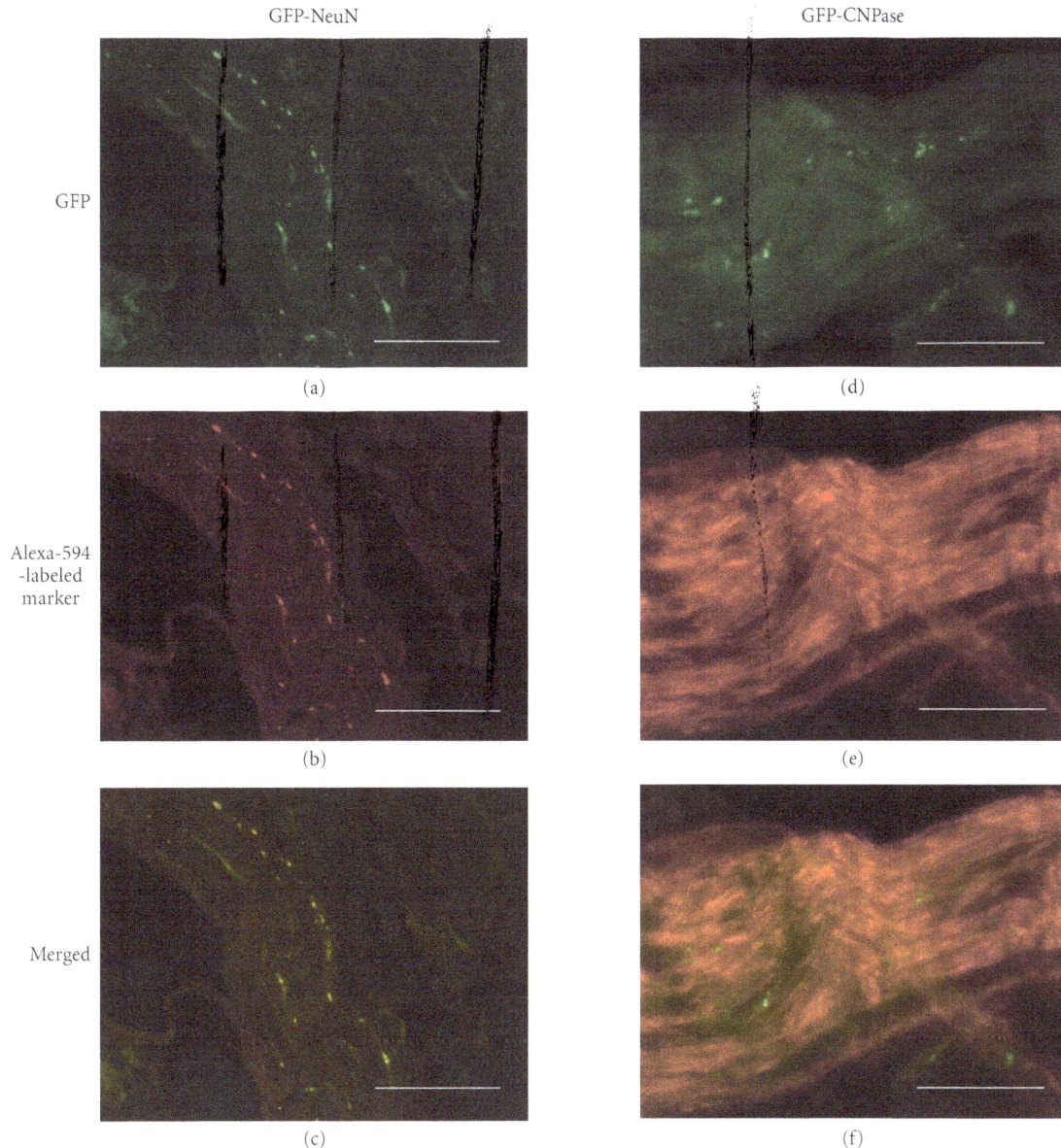

FIGURE 7: GFP detection and phenotypic marker immunohistofluorescence (NeuN on left column, Schwann cells' CNPase on right column) in sagittal sections of venous bridges which had been transplanted with LV-GFP-labeled neurospheres and were sampled at 240 days after lesion. (a, d) green endogenous fluorescence for detection of lineage-infected neurosphere progeny; (b, e) Alexa-594-revealed phenotypic marker immunoreactivities; (c, f) merged fluorescences. Note yellow-labeled colocalization of GFP-expressing neurosphere progeny with NeuN immunoreactivity (c) but not with CNPase (f). Scale bars: 0.5 mm.

CNPase-immunoreactive Schwann cell processes and their labeling intensities were higher in neurosphere-grafted nerves than in controls. By densitometric quantification with the ImageJ software, immunohistochemical CNPase labeling of neurosphere-grafted lesioned nerves, at 240 days after lesion, reached $276 \pm 2\%$ of the $100 \pm 2.9\%$ value of lesioned controls which were devoid of neurospheres; this difference being statistically significant at $P < 0.001$ by Anova.

4. Discussion

Degeneration of the distal axon segment is the consequence of axotomy and the challenge of nerve repair is to connect the proximal stump to this distal segment. For long nerve gap, it is a race between axon regeneration and distal degeneration with phenotypic change of Schwann cells [24]. Autologous nerve graft is the gold standard but results are not satisfactory [15]. Any alternative is currently believed to require a neuroguide, providing a permissive microenvironment to increase axonal regeneration and to preserve supportive cells and distal axons. Stem cells have already been studied but differentiation was mostly towards supportive cells. Neural stem cells have been reported to become integrated and provide new neurons after transplantation within central nervous system with permissive microenvironment [25]. In order to test the efficiency of this type of graft for postlesional repair

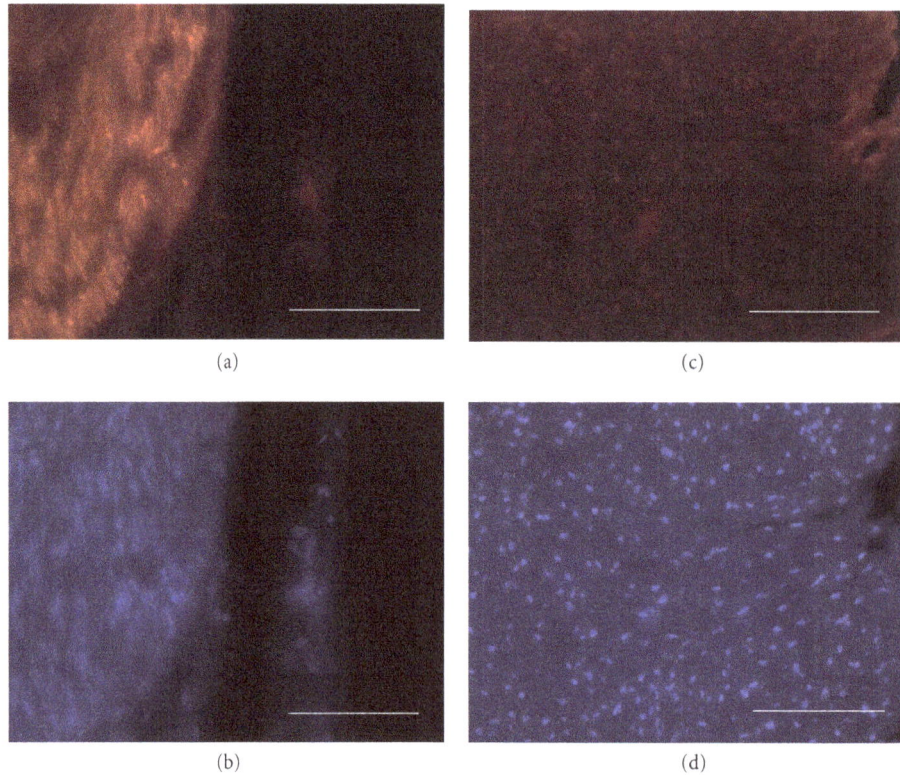

FIGURE 8: CNPase immunohistofluorescence on sagittal sections of venous bridges without (a, b) or with (c, d) transplantation of LV-GFP-labeled neurospheres, which had been sampled 240 days after lesion. Alexa-594 fluorescence-revealed CNPase immunoreactivity (a, c) is combined with histofluroescent DAPI counterstaining (b, d). Note that Schwann cell labelling density is strikingly higher in neurosphere-transplanted graft (c, d) than in void venous bridge (a, b). Σχαλεβαρσ: 100 μm.

of peripheral nerves, we have established a primary culture of adult pig neural stem cells which generate neurons *in vitro* in our previous report [27]. In the present study, we show for the first time in adult pig that transplantation of *in vitro* preexpanded adult neural stem cells into a peripheral nerve gap inside a venous bridge both leads to genesis of longitudinally aligned neurons and improves functional recovery.

4.1. Methodological Considerations.
The present experimental protocol of nerve lesion: transsection and 30 mm long nerve substance removal, has been chosen to mimic the common cases of long nerve injury in human clinics. In these cases indeed, whatever be the initial type of injury (section, tearing, crush), the surgical regularization of both nerve stumps corresponds to a model of transsection.

Autologous vein segment graft as a nerve conduit has been established as an effective treatment for the repair of nerve gaps less than 3 cm [29, 30]; it is used in hand surgery [31] and in pediatrics [32]. In a recent study [33], histomorphological examination of the sections proximal to, from, and distal to the repair zone over three months revealed less epineural scarring, a thinner epineurium, more regenerated axons and fewer inflammatory cells in groups where vein grafting was used, because the vein graft provided additional mechanical and chemical support in the size discrepancy of the nerve regeneration. A small vein graft keeps its property for end-to-side neurorrhaphy [34], but size discrepancy

between the donor and recipient nerves and length of the bypass are another problem with the risk of collapse. Vein bridging also gives excellent results in secondary repair of neglected injuries [35]. The present protocol is routinely realized in adult pig, as a convenient training system for human-operating surgeons.

The present postlesional cell therapy attempt used an *in vitro* expanded primary culture of adult pig brain neurospheres which had been extensively characterized in a previous study [27]. We had indeed shown that the present protocols of adult pig subventricular zone sampling and neurosphere assay allow to purify and maintain true neural stem cells with unlimited proliferative potential, self-renewal capacity, and ability to generate all neural cell types [27]. In particular, these neurospheres from adult pig SVZ displayed the same proportions of neurons (25%), astrocytes (70%), and oligodendrocytes (5%) as neurospheres from various adult rodent brain structures [36–38].

The procedure for fluorescent lineage labeling of grafted neurospheres used a lentiviral vector of GFP which has been validated previously [28]. Freshly prepared lentiviral particles were quantified by multiplicity of infection (MOI) determination using routine virologist assays, for optimization of the neurosphere labeling. We checked that this *in vitro* procedure allowed extensive labeling of adult pig neurospheres without alteration of their cell dynamics. It allowed subsequent identification of grafted cell progenies *in situ* merely by histofluorescence, which easily enabled to perform phenotype characterization by immunohistochemistry as revealed with different fluorophores.

4.2. Functional Recovery Enhancement by Vein-Guided Neurosphere Transplantation.

Electromyographic evaluation of the muscle which is innervated by the lesioned nerve demonstrated that our protocol of venous-graft-assisted neurosphere transplantation strongly improved functional recovery at 6 months after lesion, as compared to controls. Our subsequent histofluorescent analyses provided putative cytological substrates for such positive influence of grafted ANSC-derived cells.

In the same time, clinical evaluation was based on a simple observation. The section of the crural nerve pulled a deficient flexion of the thigh on the pond. The only recoveries of normal step were observed on the transplanted animals. The main question was to know if this recovery was bound to accelerated axonal regrowth or to the creation of a functional intermediate neuronal bypass. In fact we have a double observation of neurons and regrowth of the axons of the host.

4.3. Neuronal Outcome of Grafted Neurospheres inside the Venous Bridge.

In the present cell therapy attempt, the grafted neurospheres yielded exclusively neuronal progenies whatever be the postlesional delay. This outcome is striking since the neuronal yields from adult SVZ neural stem cells are known to reach only 25% neurons in vitro and 75% in the olfactory pathway in vivo [25, 37, 39]. The present in vivo result indicates that the venous graft provided an efficient proneurogenic environment for the transplanted neurospheres. It is in keeping with the recent demonstrations that vascular walls favor neurogenesis from adult neural stem cells [38, 40, 41], which is mediated in some rodent models by the vascular endothelium-derived growth factor (VEGF) [42]. Our results suggest that choosing a venous trunk versus an artificial neuroguide to bridge a nerve gap is an interesting solution because of intrinsic property. Furthermore, all surgeons are able to take a vein trunk on superficial vein network and this is much less expensive than neurotubes in emergency conditions. At the same time, to understand mechanism of interaction between endothelial cells and grafted neural stem cells will allow progress for the development of new artificial neurotubes. More generally, local tissue microenvironment has been formally demonstrated to be determinant on the phenotypic fate of stem-cell-derived progenies: for instance, nonneurogenic neural stem cells from the adult spinal cord generated neurons exclusively, once transplanted into the hippocampus [43].

These newly formed neurons survived at long delays after the original transplantation, which indicates they have been successfully integrated inside the severed nerve. Further, the linear distribution of these neuronal perikarya, parallel to the longitudinal axis of the lesioned nerve, suggests that the new neurons might be interconnected into multisynaptic nets bridging the lesional gap of preexisting nerve fibers. This multisynaptic nets have been described after neural stem cells graft [44, 45] This interpretation is also supported by the

evolution of transplanted cell clusters across time inside the venous graft, that is, from spherical assemblies in the first week after lesion to linear chainlike successions of sparse cells at longer delays. Such outcome arises apart of the strategies for peripheral nerve repair which have been worked out thus far and consist in stimulating either axonal regrowth into the distal nerve end or remyelination with additional Schwann cells [24].

The present results contrast with previous ones using different kinds of transplanted cells, like fœtal neural stem cells, which triggered Schwann cell like proliferation in the lesioned peripheral nerve [46], promoting in turn myelinisation and indirectly regeneration [47]. In addition, transplantation of immortalized C17.2 cells from postnatal cerebellum, which were shown to be distinct of neural stem cells [48], has been reported to trigger tumor formation in a rat model of injured sciatic nerve [49]. Adult neural stem cells are especially relevant for cell therapy from this viewpoint, because they were demonstrated to display exceptionally high resistance to tumorigenesis and senescence [50].

4.4. Possibility to Graft New Neurons into a Peripheral Nerve Gap.

There are two approaches, either to transplant neurons, or to transplant stem cells possessing neuronal differentiation potential. For primary neurons, dorsal root neurons can be prepared in vitro and their axons stretch-growth [20]. Moreover, engineered nervous tissue construct consisted of longitudinally aligned axonal tracts spanning two neuronal populations, embedded in a collagen matrix and inserted in a PGA tube [44] demonstrated neuronal survival during 112 days after surgical repair of the sciatic nerve in the rat. But only studies on the big animals allow the study of nerve gaps in good conditions.

4.5. High Survival Rate of Allogenic Transplants.

In our study, adult neural stem cells were prepared in vitro after explantation of SVZ cells from another pig, and allogenic grafted cells were integrated without immunosuppressive therapy. The same observation was noted for embryonic rat progenitors for the adult rat sciatic nerve [44] and with xenograft of embryonic rat neural stem cells into a collagen conduit for the rabbit facial nerve injury model [51]. In these attempts, grafted cells were expanded in vitro before transplantation, like in the present study.

4.6. Activation of Intrinsic Schwann Cells by Neurosphere Transplantation.

Phenotypic characterization of grafted cell progenies showed that our transplanted neurospheres generated no Schwann cell directly, but they triggered increases of the number and activity of this cell population as compared to controls. CNPase+ cells were observed along axonal regeneration but were always LV-GFP-. This result is in keeping with a previous report showing that venous graft favored Schwann cells proliferation after nerve lesion [52]. However, since in the present study controls have received a neurosphere-devoid venous graft, our results indicated that neurosphere cells emit diffusible signals that stimulate Schwann cells. Neurospheres have indeed been shown in vitro to secrete neurotrophic factors [53, 54].

5. Conclusion

The positive impact of the present cell therapy protocol can be attributed to genesis and integration of new neurons inside the lesioned nerve and/or to indirect activation of intrinsic Schwann cell population. However, Schwann cell activation was previously shown to occur after grafting a venous segment onto the lesioned nerve without neural stem cells inside. Therefore, the specific benefit of the present procedure is likely caused by the neurosphere transplantation, and hence by the genesis of new neurons inside the lesioned nerve. LV-GFP is confirmed to provide an excellent marker for grafted cells across long-time studies. Both new neuron genesis and host Schwann cell proliferation contributed to regenerate new axon fascicles in the host to bridge the long nerve gap, and the functionality of this histological repair was demonstrated in the same animals by electromyography and clinics. Large animals, and especially the pig, allow repair and study of long nerve gap with clinical conditions close to human. These results were obtained without adjunction of extracellular matrix or extrinsic growth factor. The present study thus provides a hope for improvement in human clinics.

Acknowledgments

These studies were supported by Délégation Générale pour l'Armement (DGA, France; REPAR Project, Grant 08co205). The authors express their gratitude to Professor Anne Duittoz (INRA Tours-Nouzilly) for precious advise about phenotypic marker immunohistochemistry in adult pig brain.

References

[1] J. Noble, C. A. Munro, V. S. S. V. Prasad, and R. Midha, "Analysis of upper and lower extremity peripheral nerve injuries in a population of patients with multiple injuries," *Journal of Trauma*, vol. 45, no. 1, pp. 116–122, 1998.

[2] J. A. Kouyoumdjian, "Peripheral nerve injuries: a retrospective survey of 456 cases," *Muscle and Nerve*, vol. 34, no. 6, pp. 785–788, 2006.

[3] M. N. Ahrari, N. Zangiabadi, A. Asadi, and A. Sarafi Nejad, "Prevalence and distribution of peripheral nerve injuries in victims of Bam earthquake," *Electromyography and Clinical Neurophysiology*, vol. 46, no. 1, pp. 59–62, 2006.

[4] M. Etienne, C. Powell, and B. Faux, "Disaster relief in Haiti: a perspective from the neurologists on the USNS COMFORT," *The Lancet Neurology*, vol. 9, no. 5, pp. 461–463, 2010.

[5] S. Charuluxananan, P. Bunburaphong, L. Tuchinda, P. Vorapaluk, and O. Kyokong, "Anesthesia for Indian Ocean tsunami-affected patients at a southern Thailand provincial hospital," *Acta Anaesthesiologica Scandinavica*, vol. 50, no. 3, pp. 320–323, 2006.

[6] M. O. Hansen, D. W. Polly, K. A. McHale, and L. M. Asplund, "A prospective evaluation of orthopedic patients evacuated from Operations Desert Shield and Desert Storm: the Walter Reed experience," *Military Medicine*, vol. 159, no. 5, pp. 376–380, 1994.

[7] J. Nanobashvili, T. Kopadze, M. Tvaladze, T. Buachidze, and G. Nazvlishvili, "War injuries of major extremity arteries," *World Journal of Surgery*, vol. 27, no. 2, pp. 134–139, 2003.

[8] M. E. Kett and S. J. Mannion, "Managing the health effects of the explosive remnants of war," *Journal of The Royal Society for the Promotion of Health*, vol. 124, no. 6, pp. 262–267, 2004.

[9] H. J. Seddon, "Three types of nerve injury," *Brain*, vol. 66, no. 4, pp. 237–288, 1943.

[10] S. Sunderland, "A classification of peripheral nerve injuries producing loss of function," *Brain*, vol. 74, no. 4, pp. 491–516, 1951.

[11] S. Sunderland, "The anatomy and physiology of nerve injury," *Muscle and Nerve*, vol. 13, no. 9, pp. 771–784, 1990.

[12] S. E. Mackinnon and A. L. Dellon, "A comparison of nerve regeneration across a sural nerve graft and a vascularized pseudosheath," *Journal of Hand Surgery*, vol. 13, no. 6, pp. 935–942, 1988.

[13] B. C. Cooley, "History of vein grafting," *Microsurgery*, vol. 18, no. 4, pp. 234–236, 1998.

[14] K. L. Colen, M. Choi, and D. T. Chiu, "Nerve grafts and conduits," *Plastic and Reconstructive Surgery*, vol. 124, no. 6 supplement, pp. 386–394, 2009.

[15] N. Lago and X. Navarro, "Correlation between target reinnervation and distribution of motor axons in the injured rat sciatic nerve," *Journal of Neurotrauma*, vol. 23, no. 2, pp. 227–240, 2006.

[16] W. Z. Ray and S. E. Mackinnon, "Management of nerve gaps: autografts, allografts, nerve transfers, and end-to-side neurorrhaphy," *Experimental Neurology*, vol. 223, no. 1, pp. 77–85, 2010.

[17] S. Yoshii and M. Oka, "Collagen filaments as a scaffold for nerve regeneration," *Journal of Biomedical Materials Research*, vol. 56, no. 3, pp. 400–405, 2001.

[18] D. F. Kalbermatten, P. J. Kingham, D. Mahay et al., "Fibrin matrix for suspension of regenerative cells in an artificial nerve conduit," *Journal of Plastic, Reconstructive and Aesthetic Surgery*, vol. 61, no. 6, pp. 669–675, 2008.

[19] Y. Zhang, H. Luo, Z. Zhang et al., "A nerve graft constructed with xenogeneic acellular nerve matrix and autologous adipose-derived mesenchymal stem cells," *Biomaterials*, vol. 31, no. 20, pp. 5312–5324, 2010.

[20] L. A. Pfister, M. Papaloïzos, H. P. Merkle, and B. Gander, "Nerve conduits and growth factor delivery in peripheral nerve repair," *Journal of the Peripheral Nervous System*, vol. 12, no. 2, pp. 65–82, 2007.

[21] M. Timmer, S. Robben, and F. Muller-Ostermeyer, "Axonal regeneration across long gaps in silicone chambers filled with Schwann cells overexpressing high molecular weight FGF-2," *Cell Transplantation*, vol. 12, no. 3, pp. 265–277, 2003.

[22] B. Hood, H. B. Levene, and A. D. Levi, "Transplantation of autologous Schwann cells for the repair of segmental peripheral nerve defects," *Neurosurgical Focus*, vol. 26, no. 2, article E4, 2009.

[23] E Verdu, X Narvarro, G Gudino-Cabrera et al., "Olfactory bulb ensheathing cells enhance peripheral nerve regeneration," *Neuroreport*, vol. 10, pp. 1097–1101, 1999.

[24] S. Walsh and R. Midha, "Use of stem cells to augment nerve injury repair," *Neurosurgery*, vol. 65, no. 4, pp. A80–A86, 2009.

[25] E. Moyse, S. Segura, O. Liard, S. Mahaut, and N. Mechawar, "Microenvironmental determinants of adult neural stem cell proliferation and lineage commitment in the healthy and injured central nervous system," *Current Stem Cell Research and Therapy*, vol. 3, no. 3, pp. 163–184, 2008.

[26] P. Vodicka, K. Smetana Jr., B. Dvorankova et al., "The miniature pig as an animal model in biomedical research," *Annals of the New York Academy of Sciences*, vol. 1049, pp. 161–171, 2005.

[27] O. Liard, S. Segura, A. Pascual, P. Gaudreau, T. Fusai, and E. Moyse, "In vitro isolation of neural precursor cells from the adult pig subventricular zone," *Journal of Neuroscience Methods*, vol. 182, no. 2, pp. 172–179, 2009.

[28] P. E. Mangeot, K. Duperrier, D. Nègre et al., "High levels of transduction of human dendritic cells with optimized SIV vectors," *Molecular Therapy*, vol. 5, no. 3, pp. 283–290, 2002.

[29] D. T. W. Chiu, I. Janecka, and T. J. Krizek, "Autogenous vein graft as a conduit for nerve regeneration," *Surgery*, vol. 91, no. 2, pp. 226–233, 1982.

[30] D. T. W. Chiu and B. Strauch, "A prospective clinical evaluation of autogenous vein grafts used as a nerve conduit for distal sensory nerve defects of 3 cm or less," *Plastic and Reconstructive Surgery*, vol. 86, no. 5, pp. 928–934, 1990.

[31] G. Risitano, G. Cavallaro, T. Merrino, S. Coppolin, and F. Ruggeri, "Clinical results and thoughts on sensory nerve repair by autologous vein graft in emergency hand reconstruction," *Chirurgie de la Main*, vol. 21, no. 3, pp. 194–197, 2002.

[32] Y. Kaufman, P. Cole, and L. Hollier, "Peripheral nerve injuries of the pediatric hand: issues in diagnosis and management," *Journal of Craniofacial Surgery*, vol. 20, no. 4, pp. 1011–1015, 2009.

[33] H. I. Acar, A. Comert, H. Ozer et al., "Femoral seating position of the EndoButton in single incision anterior cruciate ligament reconstruction: an anatomical study," *Surgical and Radiologic Anatomy*, vol. 30, no. 8, pp. 639–643, 2008.

[34] B. Manasseri, S. Raimondo, S. Geuna, G. Risitano, and F. S. D'Alcontres, "Ulnar nerve repair by end-to-side neurorrhaphy on the median nerve with interposition of a vein: an experimental study," *Microsurgery*, vol. 27, no. 1, pp. 27–31, 2007.

[35] Y. H. Lee and S. J. Shieh, "Secondary nerve reconstruction using vein conduit grafts for neglected digital nerve injuries," *Microsurgery*, vol. 28, no. 6, pp. 436–440, 2008.

[36] B. A. Reynolds and S. Weiss, "Generation of neurons and astrocytes from isolated cells of the adult mammalian central nervous system," *Science*, vol. 255, no. 5052, pp. 1707–1710, 1992.

[37] S. A. Louis, R. L. Rietze, L. Deleyrolle et al., "Enumeration of neural stem and progenitor cells in the neural colony-forming cell assay," *Stem Cells*, vol. 26, no. 4, pp. 988–996, 2008.

[38] L. Bennett, M. Yang, G. Enikolopov, and L. Iacovitti, "Circumventricular organs: a novel site of neural stem cells in the adult brain," *Molecular and Cellular Neuroscience*, vol. 41, no. 3, pp. 337–347, 2009.

[39] R. Belvindrah, F. Lazarini, and P. M. Lledo, "Postnatal neurogenesis: from neuroblast migration to neuronal integration," *Reviews in the Neurosciences*, vol. 20, no. 5-6, pp. 331–346, 2009.

[40] M. Tavazoie, L. Van der Veken, V. Silva-Vargas et al., "A specialized vascular niche for adult neural stem cells," *Cell Stem Cell*, vol. 3, no. 3, pp. 279–288, 2008.

[41] J. S. Goldberg and K. K. Hirschi, "Diverse roles of the vasculature within the neural stem cell niche," *Regenerative Medicine*, vol. 4, no. 6, pp. 879–897, 2009.

[42] A. Schänzer, F. P. Wachs, D. Wilhelm et al., "Direct stimulation of adult neural stem cells in vitro and neurogenesis in vivo by vascular endothelial growth factor," *Brain Pathology*, vol. 14, no. 3, pp. 237–248, 2004.

[43] L. S. Shihabuddin, P. J. Horner, J. Ray, and F. H. Gage, "Adult spinal cord stem cells generate neurons after transplantation in the adult dentate gyrus," *Journal of Neuroscience*, vol. 20, no. 23, pp. 8727–8735, 2000.

[44] J. H. Huang, D. K. Cullen, K. D. Browne et al., "Long-term survival and integration of transplanted engineered nervous tissue constructs promotes peripheral nerve regeneration," *Tissue Engineering A*, vol. 15, no. 7, pp. 1677–1685, 2009.

[45] J. F. Bonner, T. M. Connors, W. F. Silverman, D. P. Kowalski, M. A. Lemay, and I. Fischer, "Grafted neural progenitors integrate and restore synaptic connectivity across the injured spinal cord," *The Journal of Neuroscience*, vol. 31, no. 12, pp. 4675–4686, 2011.

[46] T. Murakami, Y. Fujimoto, Y. Yasunaga et al., "Transplanted neuronal progenitor cells in a peripheral nerve gap promote nerve repair," *Brain Research*, vol. 974, no. 1-2, pp. 17–24, 2003.

[47] T. B. Seo, M. J. Oh, B. G. You et al., "ERK1/2-mediated schwann cell proliferation in the regenerating sciatic nerve by treadmill training," *Journal of Neurotrauma*, vol. 26, no. 10, pp. 1733–1744, 2009.

[48] R. Mi, Y. Luo, J. Cai, T. L. Limke, M. S. Rao, and A. Höke, "Immortalized neural stem cells differ from nonimmortalized cortical neurospheres and cerebellar granule cell progenitors," *Experimental Neurology*, vol. 194, no. 2, pp. 301–319, 2005.

[49] T. S. Johnson, A. C. O'Neill, P. M. Motarjem, J. Nazzal, M. Randolph, and J. M. Winograd, "Tumor formation following murine neural precursor cell transplantation in a rat peripheral nerve injury model," *Journal of Reconstructive Microsurgery*, vol. 24, no. 8, pp. 545–550, 2008.

[50] C. Foroni, R. Galli, B. Cipelletti et al., "Resilience to transformation and inherent genetic and functional stability of adult neural stem cells ex vivo," *Cancer Research*, vol. 67, no. 8, pp. 3725–3733, 2007.

[51] H. Zhang, Y. T. Wei, K. S. Tsang et al., "Implantation of neural stem cells embedded in hyaluronic acid and collagen composite conduit promotes regeneration in a rabbit facial nerve injury model," *Journal of Translational Medicine*, vol. 6, article no. 67, 2008.

[52] C. Y. Tseng, G. Hu, R. T. Ambron, and D. T. W. Chiu, "Histologic analysis of Schwann cell migration and peripheral nerve regeneration in the autogenous venous nerve conduit (AVNC)," *Journal of Reconstructive Microsurgery*, vol. 19, no. 5, pp. 331–339, 2003.

[53] M. Xiao, K. M. Klueber, C. Lu et al., "Human adult olfactory neural progenitors rescue axotomized rodent rubrospinal neurons and promote functional recovery," *Experimental Neurology*, vol. 194, no. 1, pp. 12–30, 2005.

[54] S. R. Chirasani, A. Sternjak, P. Wend et al., "Bone morphogenetic protein-7 release from endogenous neural precursor cells suppresses the tumourigenicity of stem-like glioblastoma cells," *Brain*, vol. 133, no. 7, pp. 1961–1972, 2010.

8

Bone-Marrow-Derived Mesenchymal Stem Cells for Organ Repair

Ming Li and Susumu Ikehara

Department of Stem Cell Disorders, Kansai Medical University, Moriguchi, Osaka 570-8506, Japan

Correspondence should be addressed to Susumu Ikehara; ikehara@takii.kmu.ac.jp

Academic Editor: Rangnath Mishra

Mesenchymal stem cells (MSCs) are prototypical adult stem cells with the capacity for self-renewal and differentiation with a broad tissue distribution. MSCs not only differentiate into types of cells of mesodermal lineage but also into endodermal and ectodermal lineages such as bone, fat, cartilage and cardiomyocytes, endothelial cells, lung epithelial cells, hepatocytes, neurons, and pancreatic islets. MSCs have been identified as an adherent, fibroblast-like population and can be isolated from different adult tissues, including bone marrow (BM), umbilical cord, skeletal muscle, and adipose tissue. MSCs secrete factors, including IL-6, M-CSF, IL-10, HGF, and PGE2, that promote tissue repair, stimulate proliferation and differentiation of endogenous tissue progenitors, and decrease inflammatory and immune reactions. In this paper, we focus on the role of BM-derived MSCs in organ repair.

1. Introduction

The shortage of donor organs and the need of lifelong immunosuppression for the thousands of patients suffering from end-stage diseases worldwide are problems that need to be resolved. The repair, replacement, and regeneration of organs can restore impaired functions and are regarded as a potential solution to allotransplantation [1]. The bone marrow (BM) is an invaluable source of adult pluripotent stem cells, including hematopoietic stem cells (HSCs), endothelial progenitor cells (EPCs), and mesenchymal stem cells (MSCs). MSCs are prototypical adult stem cells with the capacity for self-renewal and differentiation with a broad tissue distribution. MSCs have been identified as an adherent, fibroblast-like population, originally isolated from BM [2]. These multipotent cells can be differentiated *in vitro* and *in vivo* into various cell types of mesenchymal origin, such as osteoblasts, adipocytes, and chondrocytes [3, 4]. Recently, more reports have demonstrated that MSCs secrete a variety of factors that promote tissue repair, stimulate proliferation and differentiation of endogenous tissue progenitors, and decrease inflammatory and immune reactions [5–7]. Because MSCs do not evoke an immune response, they are useful for allogenic organ and tissue repair.

2. Source, Multilineage Potential and Definition of MSCs

MSCs were first isolated from BM and have since been isolated from different adult tissues, including skeletal muscle [8], adipose tissue [9], umbilical cord [10], synovium [11], the circulatory system [12], dental pulp [13], amniotic fluid [14], fetal blood [15], lung [16], liver, and BM [17]. Friedenstein and coworkers first reported the existence of adherent, fibroblast-like cells isolated from BM [2], and that these cells could differentiate into mesodermal lineage such as osteoblasts, adipocytes, and chondrocytes *in vitro* [18] and cardiomyocytes [19]. Also, MSCs have been reported to differentiate into types of cells of endodermal and ectodermal lineages, including lung [20], retinal pigment [21], skin [22], sebaceous duct cells [23], renal tubular cells [24], and neural cells [25, 26], hepatocytes [27], and pancreatic islets [28]. There has hitherto been no specific surface marker for the identification of MSCs. For the isolation of human MSCs, the International Society for Cell Therapy proposed criteria [18] that comprise (1) adherence to plastic in standard culture conditions; (2) expression of the surface molecules CD73, CD90, and CD105 in the absence of CD34, CD45, HLA-DR, CD14 or CD11b, CD79a, or CD19 surface molecules as assessed by fluorescence-activated cell sorter analysis; (3) a capacity for differentiation to osteoblasts, adipocytes, and chondroblasts *in vitro*. Similarly, murine MSCs have been shown to differ from human MSCs in terms of marker expression and behavior and have been identified as an adherent, fibroblast-like population, negative for CD45, CD11b, and CD 31, and positive for Scal1 and CD106 [29].

3. MSCs and the Immune System

MSCs have the ability to modify and influence almost all the cells of the innate and adaptive immune systems, to interfere with and affect cellular proliferation, differentiation, maturation, and function to induce an anti-inflammatory phenotype, and to modulate the immune response mediated by MSC soluble factors, including IL-6, M-CSF, IL-10, TGFβ, HGF, and PGE2 [7, 30, 31]. The innate immune cells include neutrophils, dendritic cells (DCs), natural killer (NK) cells, eosinophils, mast cells, and macrophages. MSCs modulate DC function, indirectly regulate T and B cell activities, delay and prevent the development of acute graft versus host disease (GVHD) [32], and suppress DC function during allogeneic islet transplantation [33]. MSCs have been shown to suppress these inflammatory cells [34] and to alter NK cell phenotype and suppress proliferation, cytokine secretion, and cytotoxicity against HLA class I expressing targets [35]. MSCs mediated NK cell suppression via soluble factors such as indoleamine 2,3-dioxygenase, PGE2, and TGFβ [36]. The adaptive immune system, which is composed of T and B lymphocytes generates specific immune responses to pathogens with the production of memory cells. It has been reported that MSCs upregulate anti-inflammatory Th2 cytokines, including IL-3, -5, -10, and -13, and downregulate proinflammatory Th1 cytokines, including IL-1α and β, IFNγ, and TNFα [37]. MSCs induced an alteration of DC cytokine secretion, inducing a decreased secretion of pro-inflammatory cytokines such as TNFα, IFNγ, and IL-12, and increased IL-10, which is a suppressive cytokine and inducer of reg T cells [38]. MSCs exert an inhibitory effect on B cells, but MSCs have stimulatory effect in low doses [39]. Concerning the immunomodulatory properties of MSCs in a mouse model, one report [40] has suggested that allogeneic MSCs are not intrinsically immunoprivileged, and under appropriate conditions, allogeneic MSCs induce a memory T-cell response resulting in rejection of an allogeneic stem cell graft. Another report [41] has suggested that MSCs could potentially improve experimental autoimmune encephalomyelitis in mice.

4. Homing of MSCs

Intravenously injected MSCs can migrate to the BM [42, 43] in the steady state and home to the inflammation site by migrating across the endothelium and then entering the injured organ [20, 44–47]. The fact that MSCs confer protection cannot be entirely attributed to their ability to home and engraft to the site of damage, suggesting that they are also capable of mediating protection in an endocrine manner [1]. MSCs have many chemokine receptors that assist in their migration to inflammatory sites via the SDF1/CXCR4 pathway [48]. Moreover, studies have demonstrated that platelet-derived growth factor-AB, IGF-1, and CD44 are the most potent chemoattractants for MSCs [44, 49].

5. BM-Derived MSCs (BMMSCs) and Organ Repair

Many reports have indicated that MSCs have the capacity to differentiate into endodermal, mesodermal, and ectodermal lineage cells. Recently, a report has indicated that the ability of MSCs to alter the tissue microenvironment via the secretion of soluble factors may contribute more significantly than their capacity for differentiation in tissue repair [50]. Adipose tissue and BM are the most readily available sources of MSCs because they are easy to harvest, and because of their relative abundance of progenitors and the lack of ethical concerns. Although adipose tissue-derived MSCs and BMMSCs show the same immunoregulatory and supporting hematopoiesis [51], BMMSCs have a higher degree of commitment to differentiate into chondrogenic and osteogenic lineages than adipose tissue-derived MSCs [52]. BMMSCs have been shown to ameliorate tissue damage and to improve function after lung injury [53–55], kidney disease [56, 57], diabetes [58, 59], myocardial infarction [60, 61], liver injury [62, 63], and neurological disorders [64].

5.1. BMMSCs and Lung. The lung is an organ that is highly susceptible to edema and endothelial permeability after traumatic injury. BMMSCs inhibit endothelial cell barrier permeability and preserve pulmonary endothelial cell integrity by preserving adherent junctions, tight junctions and decreasing inflammation. BMMSCs address both components of endothelial permeability and inflammation induced by hemorrhagic shock [54]. Interstitial lung diseases are characterized by epithelial injury, fibroblast proliferation, expansion of the lung matrix, and dyspnea. Of these diseases, idiopathic pulmonary fibrosis (IPF) is the most frequent and lethal. Proinflammatory cytokines IL-1 and TNF-α induce endothelial cells to express adhesion molecules and chemokines that attract other white cells from the blood to the site of injury [65]. IL-1 and TNF-α also stimulate proliferation of endothelial cells and fibroblasts that increase the blood supply at the site of injury and repair damage by the formation of scar tissue [66]. BMMSCs protect lung tissue from bleomycin-induced injury by blocking TNF-α and IL-1, two fundamental proinflammatory cytokines in the lung [53]. BMMSCs enhance the restoration of systemic oxygenation and lung compliance and decrease lung inflammation and histological lung injury. They also secrete cytokines, enhance lung repair, and attenuate the inflammatory response following ventilator-induced lung injury [55].

5.2. BMMSCs and Kidney. Acute and chronic kidney injuries after transplantation have a complex pathophysiology involving ischemic, inflammatory, and immunologic mechanisms, and adult stem cells have been used in the treatment of these kidney diseases. Adult BM stem cells and the kidney precursors have been demonstrated to have an ability to differentiate into the kidney's specialized structures [67]. Nephrons are of mesenchymal origin, and stromal cells are of crucial importance for signaling, leading to the differentiation of both nephrons and collecting ducts [67]. Ischemic acute renal failure (ARF), characterized by a sharp decline in the glomerular filtration rate, is a very common complication in hospitalized patients and particularly in patients with multiorgan failure. When BMMSCs are injected after ARF, they can histologically become located in the kidney and significantly enhance the recovery of renal function by transdifferentiation into renal tubular or vascular endothelial cells [24, 68]. A single intrarenal administration of BMMSCs 7 days after ischemia-reperfusion significantly improved renal function and modified renal remodeling. The improvement of renal function was associated with a reduction in extracellular matrix accumulation. In addition, MSC administration also reduced tubular dilation, which is a classical feature of progressive renal failure in a renal ischemia rat model [57].

5.3. BMMSCs and Pancreas.
Diabetes is caused by absolute insulin deficiency due to autoimmune destruction of insulin-secreting pancreatic β-cells (type 1 diabetes) or by relative insulin deficiency due to decreased insulin sensitivity, usually observed in overweight individuals (type 2 diabetes). In both types of the disease, an inadequate mass of functional β-cells is the major determinant for the onset of hyperglycemia and the development of overt disease. BM and BMMSCs induce the regeneration of recipient-derived pancreatic insulin-secreting cells, and MSCs inhibit T-cell-mediated immune responses against newly formed β-cells, which are able to survive in this altered immunological milieu [69].

Acute pancreatitis (AP) is characterized by a rapid onset and disease progression, with high fatality. Pancreatic acinar cells are the functional unit for the external secretion of the pancreas, which accounts for 80% of pancreatic tissue. During the process of severe AP, inflammatory mediators, metabolic products of arachidonic acid, and oxygen-derived free radicals enhance vascular permeability and cause tissue thrombosis and hemorrhage, thereby inducing necrosis of the pancreas [70]. BMMSCs can effectively relieve injury to pancreatic acinar cells and small intestinal epithelium, promote the proliferation of enteric epithelium and repair of the mucosa, and attenuate systemic inflammation in rats with severe acute peritonitis [71].

Human BM stem cells are able to differentiate into insulin-expressing cells *in vitro* by a mechanism involving several transcription factors of the β-cell developmental pathway when cultured in an appropriate microenvironment [72]. Human BMMSCs can be induced to express insulin in sufficient quantities to to reduce blood glucose in a diabetic mouse model [73] and to protect human islets from proinflammatory cytokines [74]. The use of human BMMSCs could be developed as a cell therapy for pancreatitis because of the ability, as shown in a rat model of acute pancreatitis, to reduce inflammation and damage to pancreatic tissue by reducing

levels of cytokines and inducing Foxp3(+) regulatory T cells [75].

5.4. BMMSCs and Heart.
Cardiovascular diseases are the first cause of death worldwide, and myocardial infarction (MI) is responsible for 12.8% of all deaths [76]. BMMSCs have been shown to differentiate into myogenic phenotype [77] and show a potent antifibrotic action, as their conditioned medium decreases cardiac fibroblast proliferation and the expression of collagen types I and III [78, 79] and increases the secretion of antifibrotic molecules such as matrix metalloproteinases 2, 9, and 14 [80]. BMMSCs exhibit the ability to differentiate into cardiomyocytes, smooth muscle cells, and endothelium in a swine model of chronic ischemic cardiomyopathy [81]. They have been shown to prolong survival compared with controls when hearts of Wistar rats were transplanted to Fisher 344 rats with intravenous MSC infusion [82]. Intravenous fusion of MSCs is the easiest and most practical method for delivery, though the MSCs must travel through the pulmonary circulation, where entrapment of cells is a concern [83]. Intracoronary infusion of stem cells is delivered with a standard over-the-wire balloon angioplasty catheter placed into the target coronary artery [84]. Injected BMMSCs improve cardiac function and reduce scar size in acute MI [85, 86]. Early-phase clinical trial data demonstrate that MSC therapy for post-MI is safe and has favorable effects on cardiac structure and function [87, 88].

5.5. BMMSCs and Liver.
FGF-4 is one of the most important members of the fibroblast growth factor family; it can initiate the proliferation of mesodermal and endodermal cells and improve the development of fetal liver [89]. HGF is essential for the development of several epithelial organs and has been one of the most well-characterized cytokines for the stimulation of DNA synthesis in primary hepatocyte cultures and for liver development [90]. Oncostatin M is a member of the interleukin-6 family produced by hematopoietic cells and induces the differentiation of fetal hepatic cells, conferring various metabolic activities of adult liver [91]. These three factors participate in different developmental stages of the liver. FGF4, HGF, and oncostatin M have been shown to be key cytokines for hepatic differentiation from mouse BMMSCs [92]. Transplantation of BMMSCs alleviates GalN-induced acute liver injury in rats and stimulates the recovery systems, as evidenced by an earlier surge of cellular proliferation and differentiation into functional hepatocytes. IL-6 exerts hepatoprotective and mitogenic effects by stimulating the induction of acute-phase proteins as well as by suppressing apoptosis. Transplantation of BMMSCs could ameliorate acute liver injury. It promotes cell proliferation and organ repair, and the activation of the IL-6/gp130-mediated STAT3 signaling pathway via soluble IL-6 receptor is crucial in hepatic differentiation of BMMSCs [93].

Liver fibrosis is the excessive accumulation of extracellular matrix proteins, including collagen, that occurs in most types of chronic liver disease. Advanced liver fibrosis results in cirrhosis, liver failure, and portal hypertension, and often requires liver transplantation [94]. Although liver

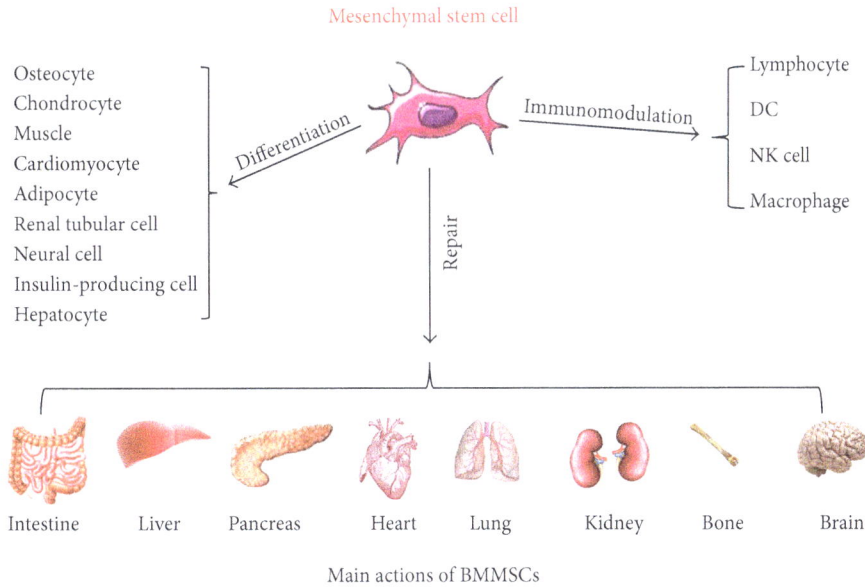

FIGURE 1: Main actions of BMMSCs.

transplantation is by far the most effective treatment for liver cirrhosis, extensive clinical application of the technique is limited by the lack of donor organ availability [95]. Cell-based hepatocyte transplantation, a potential interventional procedure, provides an effective strategy and holds great promise for the treatment of impaired livers. BMMSCs can protect against experimental liver fibrosis through promotion of IL-10 expression in CCl4- or dimethylnitrosamine-induced rats [63, 96].

5.6. BMMSCs and Brain. The development of effective treatments for human brain and spinal cord injury remains a serious challenge. In this regard, the transplantation of stem cells may help repair injured nerve tissue through the replacement of damaged cells, neuroprotection, or the creation of an environment conductive to regeneration by endogenous cells [97]. BMMSCs have been shown to promote cell proliferation and neurotrophic function of Schwann cells *in vitro* and *in vivo* [98]. Transplantation of BMMSCs can significantly reduce the behavioral abnormalities of these animals during the six weeks after engraftment [64]. Intravenously transplanted MSCs are capable of improving functional recovery and restoring neurological deficits in experimental intracerebral hemorrhage. The mechanisms are associated with enhanced survival and differentiation of neural cells and increased expression of antiapoptotic proteins and atrophic factors [99]. Human BMMSCs can improve neurological functional recovery in mice with experimental autoimmune encephalitis, possibly via a reduction of inflammatory infiltrates and areas of demyelination, stimulation of oligodendrogenesis, and by elevating brain-derived neurotrophic factor (BDNF) expression [41, 100]. Human BMMSCs transfected with the BDNF gene also showed improved functional recovery and reduced infarct size through a reduction in apoptosis [101]. Patients with Parkinson's disease transplanted with BMMSCs in

the early stages of the disease (less than 5 years) showed greater improvement than in the later stages (11–15 years) [102].

5.7. BMMSCs and Intestine. Inflammatory bowel disease comprises a spectrum of chronic and relapsing diseases, including Crohn's disease (CD) and ulcerative colitis [103]. CD is characterized by a background of mucosal T-cell dysfunction, inflammatory cell infiltration, and abnormal cytokine production leading to uncontrolled and persistent intestinal transmural inflammation. Intraperitoneally injected cryopreserved BMMSCs home to and engraft into the inflamed colon and ameliorate trinitrobenzene sulfonic acid-induced colitis in rats [104]. Similarly, the injection of adipose-derived MSCs facilitated colonic mucosal repair and reduced the infiltration of inflammatory cells in the experimental colitis model [105].

Small intestinal permeability and villi injuries were significantly reduced in an MSC-administered group compared with the control group. MSC administration accelerated the recovery of the intestinal barrier dysfunction in a rat model of ischemia/reperfusion injury [106].

5.8. BMMSCs and Bone. Bone is regarded as an organ, and small bone damage can repair spontaneously without intervention. However, bone transplantation and surgery are required when there is extensive bone damage. As adult stem cells, BMMSCs possess a number of characteristics that make them appropriate for use in promoting bone regeneration [107]. BMMSCs may differentiate into tissue cells in order to restore lost morphology as well as function and to secrete a wide spectrum of bioactive factors that help to create a repair environment through their antiapoptotic effects, immunoregulatory function, and the stimulation of endothelial progenitor cell proliferation [108]. One report shows that

BMMSCs stimulate growth with osteogenesis imperfecta when children received allogeneic BMMSCs [109].

6. Conclusion

Figure 1 summarizes the main actions of BMMSCs. The original use of BMMSCs was to accelerate hematopoiesis, since they have the potential to differentiate into various cells, and to secrete cytokines and growth factors. BMMSCs have immunomodulatory properties through paracrine and endocrine mechanisms to repair damaged tissue. Homing and immunomodulation are important aspects of MSC functioning and their clinical effects. It has been proposed that the anti-inflammatory and antiapoptotic effects of MSCs may promote tissue regeneration. The use of allogenic nonimmunogenic BMMSCs would be a more acceptable strategy clinically. The potential role of BMMSCs to promote engraftment of organs and prevent rejection may be multifactorial and might be dependent on secretion of soluble growth factors, increasing angiogenesis, suppressing alloreactive T cells, and interacting with several arms of the immune system. However, the long-term safety of transplanted BMMSCs for organ repair needs to be proven prior to their clinical application.

Conflict of Interests

None of the authors has conflict of interests to declare.

Acknowledgments

The authors would like to thank Mr. Hilary Eastwick-Field and Ms. Keiko Ando for their help in the preparation of the paper.

References

[1] B. Bi, R. Schmitt, M. Israilova, H. Nishio, and L. G. Cantley, "Stromal cells protect against acute tubular injury via an endocrine effect," *Journal of the American Society of Nephrology*, vol. 18, no. 9, pp. 2486–2496, 2007.

[2] A. J. Friedenstein, R. K. Chailakhjan, and K. S. Lalykina, "The development of fibroblast colonies in monolayer cultures of guinea-pig bone marrow and spleen cells," *Cell and Tissue Kinetics*, vol. 3, no. 4, pp. 393–403, 1970.

[3] A. J. Friedenstein, R. K. Chailakhyan, and N. V. Latsinik, "Stromal cells responsible for transferring the microenvironment of the hemopoietic tissues. Cloning in vitro and retransplantation in vivo," *Transplantation*, vol. 17, no. 4, pp. 331–340, 1974.

[4] A. I. Caplan, "Mesenchymal stem cells," *Journal of Orthopaedic Research*, vol. 9, no. 5, pp. 641–650, 1991.

[5] M. D. Nicola, C. Carlo-Stella, M. Magni et al., "Human bone marrow stromal cells suppress T-lymphocyte proliferation induced by cellular or nonspecific mitogenic stimuli," *Blood*, vol. 99, no. 10, pp. 3838–3843, 2002.

[6] L. Raffaghello, G. Bianchi, M. Bertolotto et al., "Human mesenchymal stem cells inhibit neutrophil apoptosis: a model for neutrophil preservation in the bone marrow niche," *Stem Cells*, vol. 26, no. 1, pp. 151–162, 2008.

[7] S. Aggarwal and M. F. Pittenger, "Human mesenchymal stem cells modulate allogeneic immune cell responses," *Blood*, vol. 105, no. 4, pp. 1815–1822, 2005.

[8] J. T. Williams, S. S. Southerland, J. Souza, A. F. Calcutt, and R. G. Cartledge, "Cells isolated from adult human skeletal muscle capable of differentiating into multiple mesodermal phenotypes," *American Surgeon*, vol. 65, no. 1, pp. 22–26, 1999.

[9] P. A. Zuk, M. Zhu, H. Mizuno et al., "Multilineage cells from human adipose tissue: implications for cell-based therapies," *Tissue Engineering*, vol. 7, no. 2, pp. 211–228, 2001.

[10] A. Erices, P. Conget, and J. J. Minguell, "Mesenchymal progenitor cells in human umbilical cord blood," *British Journal of Haematology*, vol. 109, no. 1, pp. 235–242, 2000.

[11] C. De Bari, F. Dell'Accio, P. Tylzanowski, and F. P. Luyten, "Multipotent mesenchymal stem cells from adult human synovial membrane," *Arthritis & Rheumatism*, vol. 44, no. 8, pp. 1928–1942, 2001.

[12] S. A. Kuznetsov, M. H. Mankani, S. Gronthos, K. Satomura, P. Bianco, and P. G. Robey, "Circulating skeletal stem cells," *Journal of Cell Biology*, vol. 153, no. 5, pp. 1133–1139, 2001.

[13] S. Gronthos, M. Mankani, J. Brahim, P. G. Robey, and S. Shi, "Postnatal human dental pulp stem cells (DPSCs) in vitro and in vivo," *Proceedings of the National Academy of Sciences of the United States of America*, vol. 97, no. 25, pp. 13625–13630, 2000.

[14] P. S. In 't Anker, S. A. Scherjon, C. Kleijburg-van der Keur et al., "Amniotic fluid as a novel source of mesenchymal stem cells for therapeutic transplantation," *Blood*, vol. 102, no. 4, pp. 1548–1549, 2003.

[15] W. A. Noort, A. B. Kruisselbrink, P. S. In't Anker et al., "Mesenchymal stem cells promote engraftment of human umbilical cord blood-derived CD_{34}^+ cells in NOD/SCID mice," *Experimental Hematology*, vol. 30, no. 8, pp. 870–878, 2002.

[16] C. G. Fan, F. W. Tang, Q. J. Zhang et al., "Characterization and neural differentiation of fetal lung mesenchymal stem cells," *Cell Transplantation*, vol. 14, no. 5, pp. 311–321, 2005.

[17] C. Campagnoli, I. A. G. Roberts, S. Kumar, P. R. Bennett, I. Bellantuono, and N. M. Fisk, "Identification of mesenchymal stem/progenitor cells in human first-trimester fetal blood, liver, and bone marrow," *Blood*, vol. 98, no. 8, pp. 2396–2402, 2001.

[18] M. Dominici, K. Le Blanc, I. Mueller et al., "Minimal criteria for defining multipotent mesenchymal stromal cells. The International Society for Cellular Therapy position statement," *Cytotherapy*, vol. 8, no. 4, pp. 315–317, 2006.

[19] S. Makino, K. Fukuda, S. Miyoshi et al., "Cardiomyocytes can be generated from marrow stromal cells in vitro," *Journal of Clinical Investigation*, vol. 103, no. 5, pp. 697–705, 1999.

[20] L. A. Ortiz, F. Gambelli, C. McBride et al., "Mesenchymal stem cell engraftment in lung is enhanced in response to bleomycin exposure and ameliorates its fibrotic effects," *Proceedings of the National Academy of Sciences of the United States of America*, vol. 100, no. 14, pp. 8407–8411, 2003.

[21] S. Arnhold, Y. Absenger, H. Klein, K. Addicks, and U. Schraermeyer, "Transplantation of bone marrow-derived mesenchymal stem cells rescue photoreceptor cells in the dystrophic retina of the rhodopsin knockout mouse," *Graefe's Archive for Clinical and Experimental Ophthalmology*, vol. 245, no. 3, pp. 414–422, 2007.

[22] H. Nakagawa, S. Akita, M. Fukui, T. Fujii, and K. Akino, "Human mesenchymal stem cells successfully improve skin-substitute wound healing," *British Journal of Dermatology*, vol. 153, no. 1, pp. 29–36, 2005.

[23] X. Fu, L. Fang, X. Li, B. Cheng, and Z. Sheng, "Enhanced wound-healing quality with bone marrow mesenchymal stem cells autografting after skin injury," *Wound Repair and Regeneration*, vol. 14, no. 3, pp. 325–335, 2006.

[24] M. Morigi, B. Imberti, C. Zoja et al., "Mesenchymal stem cells are renotropic, helping to repair the kidney and improve function in acute renal failure," *Journal of the American Society of Nephrology*, vol. 15, no. 7, pp. 1794–1804, 2004.

[25] G. C. Kopen, D. J. Prockop, and D. G. Phinney, "Marrow stromal cells migrate throughout forebrain and cerebellum, and they differentiate into astrocytes after injection into neonatal mouse brains," *Proceedings of the National Academy of Sciences of the United States of America*, vol. 96, no. 19, pp. 10711–10716, 1999.

[26] G. Muñoz-Elias, A. J. Marcus, T. M. Coyne, D. Woodbury, and I. B. Black, "Adult bone marrow stromal cells in the embryonic brain: engraftment, migration, differentiation, and long-term survival," *Journal of Neuroscience*, vol. 24, no. 19, pp. 4585–4595, 2004.

[27] R. E. Schwartz, M. Reyes, L. Koodie et al., "Multipotent adult progenitor cells from bone marrow differentiate into functional hepatocyte-like cells," *Journal of Clinical Investigation*, vol. 109, no. 10, pp. 1291–1302, 2002.

[28] D. Q. Tang, L. Z. Cao, B. R. Burkhardt et al., "In vivo and in vitro characterization of insulin-producing cells obtained from murine bone marrow," *Diabetes*, vol. 53, no. 7, pp. 1721–1732, 2004.

[29] A. Peister, J. A. Mellad, B. L. Larson, B. M. Hall, L. F. Gibson, and D. J. Prockop, "Adult stem cells from bone marrow (MSCs) isolated from different strains of inbred mice vary in surface epitopes, rates of proliferation, and differentiation potential," *Blood*, vol. 103, no. 5, pp. 1662–1668, 2004.

[30] S. Beyth, Z. Borovsky, D. Mevorach et al., "Human mesenchymal stem cells alter antigen-presenting cell maturation and induce T-cell unresponsiveness," *Blood*, vol. 105, no. 5, pp. 2214–2219, 2005.

[31] R. Ramasamy, H. Fazekasova, E. W. F. Lam, I. Soeiro, G. Lombardi, and F. Dazzi, "Mesenchymal stem cells inhibit dendritic cell differentiation and function by preventing entry into the cell cycle," *Transplantation*, vol. 83, no. 1, pp. 71–76, 2007.

[32] B. Zhang, R. Liu, D. Shi et al., "Mesenchymal stem cells induce mature dendritic cells into a novel Jagged-2 dependent regulatory dendritic cell population," *Blood*, vol. 113, no. 1, pp. 46–57, 2009.

[33] A. Aldinucci, L. Rizzetto, L. Pieri et al., "Inhibition of immune synapse by altered dendritic cell actin distribution: a new pathway of mesenchymal stem cell immune regulation," *Journal of Immunology*, vol. 185, no. 9, pp. 5102–5110, 2010.

[34] A. Uccelli, L. Moretta, and V. Pistoia, "Mesenchymal stem cells in health and disease," *Nature Reviews Immunology*, vol. 8, no. 9, pp. 726–736, 2008.

[35] P. A. Sotiropoulou, S. A. Perez, A. D. Gritzapis, C. N. Baxevanis, and M. Papamichail, "Interactions between human mesenchymal stem cells and natural killer cells," *Stem Cells*, vol. 24, no. 1, pp. 74–85, 2006.

[36] G. M. Spaggiari, A. Capobianco, H. Abdelrazik, F. Becchetti, M. C. Mingari, and L. Moretta, "Mesenchymal stem cells inhibit natural killer-cell proliferation, cytotoxicity, and cytokine production: role of indoleamine 2,3-dioxygenase and prostaglandin E2," *Blood*, vol. 111, no. 3, pp. 1327–1333, 2008.

[37] J. A. Potian, H. Aviv, N. M. Ponzio, J. S. Harrison, and P. Rameshwar, "Veto-like activity of mesenchymal stem cells: functional discrimination between cellular responses to alloantigens and recall antigens," *Journal of Immunology*, vol. 171, no. 7, pp. 3426–3434, 2003.

[38] W. Zhang, W. Ge, C. Li et al., "Effects of mesenchymal stem cells on differentiation, maturation, and function of human monocyte-derived dendritic cells," *Stem Cells and Development*, vol. 13, no. 3, pp. 263–271, 2004.

[39] A. Corcione, F. Benvenuto, E. Ferretti et al., "Human mesenchymal stem cells modulate B-cell functions," *Blood*, vol. 107, no. 1, pp. 367–372, 2006.

[40] A. J. Nauta, G. Westerhuis, A. B. Kruisselbrink, E. G. A. Lurvink, R. Willemze, and W. E. Fibbe, "Donor-derived mesenchymal stem cells are immunogenic in an allogeneic host and stimulate donor graft rejection in a nonmyeloablative setting," *Blood*, vol. 108, no. 6, pp. 2114–2120, 2006.

[41] J. Zhang, Y. Li, J. Chen et al., "Human bone marrow stromal cell treatment improves neurological functional recovery in EAE mice," *Experimental Neurology*, vol. 195, no. 1, pp. 16–26, 2005.

[42] S. M. Devine, A. M. Bartholomew, N. Mahmud et al., "Mesenchymal stem cells are capable of homing to the bone marrow of non-human primates following systemic infusion," *Experimental Hematology*, vol. 29, no. 2, pp. 244–255, 2001.

[43] R. F. Wynn, C. A. Hart, C. Corradi-Perini et al., "A small proportion of mesenchymal stem cells strongly expresses functionally active CXCR4 receptor capable of promoting migration to bone marrow," *Blood*, vol. 104, no. 9, pp. 2643–2645, 2004.

[44] M. B. Herrera, B. Bussolati, S. Bruno et al., "Exogenous mesenchymal stem cells localize to the kidney by means of CD44 following acute tubular injury," *Kidney International*, vol. 72, no. 4, pp. 430–441, 2007.

[45] A. Chapel, J. M. Bertho, M. Bensidhoum et al., "Mesenchymal stem cells home to injured tissues when co-infused with hematopoietic cells to treat a radiation-induced multi-organ failure syndrome," *Journal of Gene Medicine*, vol. 5, no. 12, pp. 1028–1038, 2003.

[46] A. Mahmood, D. Lu, M. Lu et al., "Treatment of traumatic brain injury in adult rats with intravenous administration of human bone marrow stromal cells," *Neurosurgery*, vol. 53, no. 3, pp. 697–703, 2003.

[47] D. Orlic, J. Kajstura, S. Chimenti et al., "Mobilized bone marrow cells repair the infarcted heart, improving function and survival," *Proceedings of the National Academy of Sciences of the United States of America*, vol. 98, no. 18, pp. 10344–10349, 2001.

[48] J. M. Fox, G. Chamberlain, B. A. Ashton, and J. Middleton, "Recent advances into the understanding of mesenchymal stem cell trafficking," *British Journal of Haematology*, vol. 137, no. 6, pp. 491–502, 2007.

[49] A. L. Ponte, E. Marais, N. Gallay et al., "The in vitro migration capacity of human bone marrow mesenchymal stem cells: comparison of chemokine and growth factor chemotactic activities," *Stem Cells*, vol. 25, no. 7, pp. 1737–1745, 2007.

[50] D. G. Phinney and D. J. Prockop, "Concise review: mesenchymal stem/multipotent stromal cells: the state of transdifferentiation and modes of tissue repair—current views," *Stem Cells*, vol. 25, no. 11, pp. 2896–2902, 2007.

[51] A. Poloni, G. Maurizi, P. Leoni et al., "Human dedifferentiated adipocytes show similar properties to bone marrow-derived mesenchymal stem cells," *Stem Cells*, vol. 30, no. 5, pp. 965–974, 2012.

[52] J. M. Gimble, A. J. Katz, and B. A. Bunnell, "Adipose-derived stem cells for regenerative medicine," *Circulation Research*, vol. 100, no. 9, pp. 1249–1260, 2007.

[53] L. A. Ortiz, M. DuTreil, C. Fattman et al., "Interleukin 1 receptor antagonist mediates the antiinflammatory and antifibrotic effect of mesenchymal stem cells during lung injury," *Proceedings of the National Academy of Sciences of the United States of America*, vol. 104, no. 26, pp. 11002–11007, 2007.

[54] S. Pati, M. H. Gerber, T. D. Menge et al., "Bone marrow derived mesenchymal stem cells inhibit inflammation and preserve vascular endothelial integrity in the lungs after hemorrhagic shock," *PLoS One*, vol. 6, no. 9, Article ID e25171, 2011.

[55] G. F. Curley, M. Hayes, B. Ansari et al., "Mesenchymal stem cells enhance recovery and repair following ventilator-induced lung injury in the rat," *Thorax*, vol. 67, no. 6, pp. 496–501, 2012.

[56] U. Kunter, S. Rong, Z. Djuric et al., "Transplanted mesenchymal stem cells accelerate glomerular healing in experimental glomerulonephritis," *Journal of the American Society of Nephrology*, vol. 17, no. 8, pp. 2202–2212, 2006.

[57] C. Alfarano, C. Roubeix, R. Chaaya et al., "Intraparenchymal injection of bone marrow mesenchymal stem cells reduces kidney fibrosis after ischemia-reperfusion in cyclosporine-immunosuppressed rats," *Cell Transplant*, vol. 21, no. 9, pp. 2009–2019, 2012.

[58] R. H. Lee, M. J. Seo, R. L. Reger et al., "Multipotent stromal cells from human marrow home to and promote repair of pancreatic islets and renal glomeruli in diabetic NOD/scid mice," *Proceedings of the National Academy of Sciences of the United States of America*, vol. 103, no. 46, pp. 17438–17443, 2006.

[59] Y. Si, Y. Zhao, H. Hao et al., "Infusion of mesenchymal stem cells ameliorates hyperglycemia in type 2 diabetic rats: identification of a novel role in improving insulin sensitivity," *Diabetes*, vol. 61, no. 6, pp. 1616–1625, 2012.

[60] Y. Iso, J. L. Spees, C. Serrano et al., "Multipotent human stromal cells improve cardiac function after myocardial infarction in mice without long-term engraftment," *Biochemical and Biophysical Research Communications*, vol. 354, no. 3, pp. 700–706, 2007.

[61] J. Cho, P. Zhai, Y. Maejima, and J. Sadoshima, "Myocardial injection with GSK-3β-overexpressing bone marrow-derived mesenchymal stem cells attenuates cardiac dysfunction after myocardial infarction," *Circulation Research*, vol. 108, no. 4, pp. 478–489, 2011.

[62] H. Kanazawa, Y. Fujimoto, T. Teratani et al., "Bone marrow-derived mesenchymal stem cells ameliorate hepatic ischemia reperfusion injury in a rat model," *PLoS ONE*, vol. 6, no. 4, Article ID e19195, 2011.

[63] W. Zhao, J. J. Li, D. Y. Cao et al., "Intravenous injection of mesenchymal stem cells is effective in treating liver fibrosis," *World Journal of Gastroenterology*, vol. 18, no. 10, pp. 1048–1058, 2012.

[64] M. A. Edalatmanesh, A. R. Bahrami, E. Hosseini, M. Hosseini, and S. Khatamsaz, "Bone marrow derived mesenchymal stem cell transplantation in cerebellar degeneration: a behavioral study," *Behavioural Brain Research*, vol. 225, no. 1, pp. 63–70, 2011.

[65] N. C. Kaneider, A. J. Leger, and A. Kuliopulos, "Therapeutic targeting of molecules involved in leukocyte-endothelial cell interactions," *FEBS Journal*, vol. 273, no. 19, pp. 4416–4424, 2006.

[66] M. Kolb, P. J. Margetts, D. C. Anthony, F. Pitossi, and J. Gauldie, "Transient expression of IL-1β induces acute lung injury and chronic repair leading to pulmonary fibrosis," *Journal of Clinical Investigation*, vol. 107, no. 12, pp. 1529–1536, 2001.

[67] F. Anglani, M. Forino, D. Del Prete, E. Tosetto, R. Torregrossa, and A. D'Angelo, "In search of adult renal stem cells," *Journal of Cellular and Molecular Medicine*, vol. 8, no. 4, pp. 474–487, 2004.

[68] C. Lange, F. Tögel, H. Ittrich et al., "Administered mesenchymal stem cells enhance recovery from ischemia/reperfusion-induced acute renal failure in rats," *Kidney International*, vol. 68, no. 4, pp. 1613–1617, 2005.

[69] V. S. Urbán, J. Kiss, J. Kovács et al., "Mesenchymal stem cells cooperate with bone marrow cells in therapy of diabetes," *Stem Cells*, vol. 26, no. 1, pp. 244–253, 2008.

[70] Z. H. Liu, J. S. Peng, C. J. Li et al., "A simple taurocholate-induced model of severe acute pancreatitis in rats," *World Journal of Gastroenterology*, vol. 15, no. 45, pp. 5732–5739, 2009.

[71] X. H. Tu, J. X. Song, X. J. Xue et al., "Role of bone marrow-derived mesenchymal stem cells in a rat model of severe acute pancreatitis," *World Journal of Gastroenterology*, vol. 18, no. 18, pp. 2270–2279, 2012.

[72] C. Moriscot, F. De Fraipont, M. J. Richard et al., "Human bone marrow mesenchymal stem cells can express insulin and key transcription factors of the endocrine pancreas developmental pathway upon genetic and/or microenvironmental manipulation in vitro," *Stem Cells*, vol. 23, no. 4, pp. 594–603, 2005.

[73] M. Zhao, S. A. Amiel, S. Ajami et al., "Amelioration of streptozotocin-induced diabetes in mice with cells derived from human marrow stromal cells," *PLoS ONE*, vol. 3, no. 7, Article ID e2666, 2008.

[74] T. Y. Yeung, K. L. Seeberger, T. Kin et al., "Human mesenchymal stem cells protect human islets from pro-inflammatory cytokines," *PLoS One*, vol. 7, no. 5, Article ID e38189, 2012.

[75] K. H. Jung, S. U. Song, T. Yi et al., "Human bone marrow-derived clonal mesenchymal stem cells inhibit inflammation and reduce acute pancreatitis in rats," *Gastroenterology*, vol. 140, no. 3, pp. 998–1008, 2011.

[76] M. Mazo, B. Pelacho, and F. Prósper, "Stem cell therapy for chronic myocardial infarction," *Journal of Cardiovascular Translational Research*, vol. 3, no. 2, pp. 79–88, 2010.

[77] S. Wakitani, T. Saito, and A. I. Caplan, "Myogenic cells derived from rat bone marrow mesenchymal stem cells exposed to 5-azacytidine," *Muscle and Nerve*, vol. 18, no. 12, pp. 1417–1426, 1995.

[78] L. Li, S. Zhang, Y. Zhang, B. Yu, Y. Xu, and Z. Guan, "Paracrine action mediate the antifibrotic effect of transplanted mesenchymal stem cells in a rat model of global heart failure," *Molecular Biology Reports*, vol. 36, no. 4, pp. 725–731, 2009.

[79] S. Ohnishi, H. Sumiyoshi, S. Kitamura, and N. Nagaya, "Mesenchymal stem cells attenuate cardiac fibroblast proliferation and collagen synthesis through paracrine actions," *FEBS Letters*, vol. 581, no. 21, pp. 3961–3966, 2007.

[80] C. Mias, O. Lairez, E. Trouche et al., "Mesenchymal stem cells promote matrix metalloproteinase secretion by cardiac fibroblasts and reduce cardiac ventricular fibrosis after myocardial infarction," *Stem Cells*, vol. 27, no. 11, pp. 2734–2743, 2009.

[81] H. C. Quevedo, K. E. Hatzistergos, B. N. Oskouei et al., "Allogeneic mesenchymal stem cells restore cardiac function in chronic ischemic cardiomyopathy via trilineage differentiating capacity," *Proceedings of the National Academy of Sciences of the United States of America*, vol. 106, no. 33, pp. 14022–14027, 2009.

[82] H. P. Zhou, D. H. Yi, S. Q. Yu et al., "Administration of donor-derived mesenchymal stem cells can prolong the survival of rat cardiac allograft," *Transplantation Proceedings*, vol. 38, no. 9, pp. 3046–3051, 2006.

[83] I. M. Barbash, P. Chouraqui, J. Baron et al., "Systemic delivery of bone marrow-derived mesenchymal stem cells to the infarcted myocardium: feasibility, cell migration, and body distribution," *Circulation*, vol. 108, no. 7, pp. 863–868, 2003.

[84] W. Sherman, T. P. Martens, J. F. Viles-Gonzalez, and T. Siminiak, "Catheter-based delivery of cells to the heart," *Nature Clinical Practice Cardiovascular Medicine*, vol. 3, supplement 1, pp. S57–S64, 2006.

[85] L. C. Amado, A. P. Saliaris, K. H. Schuleri et al., "Cardiac repair with intramyocardial injection of allogeneic mesenchymal stem cells after myocardial infarction," *Proceedings of the National Academy of Sciences of the United States of America*, vol. 102, no. 32, pp. 11474–11479, 2005.

[86] K. H. Schuleri, L. C. Amado, A. J. Boyle et al., "Early improvement in cardiac tissue perfusion due to mesenchymal stem cells," *American Journal of Physiology*, vol. 294, no. 5, pp. H2002–H2011, 2008.

[87] S. L. Chen, W. W. Fang, F. Ye et al., "Effect on left ventricular function of intracoronary transplantation of autologous bone marrow mesenchymal stem cell in patients with acute myocardial infarction," *American Journal of Cardiology*, vol. 94, no. 1, pp. 92–95, 2004.

[88] A. R. Williams, B. Trachtenberg, D. L. Velazquez et al., "Intramyocardial stem cell injection in patients with ischemic cardiomyopathy: functional recovery and reverse remodeling," *Circulation Research*, vol. 108, no. 7, pp. 792–796, 2011.

[89] D. A. Rappolee, C. Basilico, Y. Patel, and Z. Werb, "Expression and function of FGF-4 in peri-implantation development in mouse embryos," *Development*, vol. 120, no. 8, pp. 2259–2269, 1994.

[90] C. Schmidt, F. Bladt, S. Goedecke et al., "Scatter factor/hepatocyte growth factor is essential for liver development," *Nature*, vol. 373, no. 6516, pp. 699–702, 1995.

[91] A. Miyajima, T. Kinoshita, M. Tanaka, A. Kamiya, Y. Mukouyama, and T. Hara, "Role of oncostatin M in hematopoiesis and liver development," *Cytokine and Growth Factor Reviews*, vol. 11, no. 3, pp. 177 183, 2000.

[92] X. J. Dong, H. Zhang, R. L. Pan, L. X. Xiang, and J. Z. Shao, "Identification of cytokines involved in hepatic differentiation of mBM-MSCs under liver-injury conditions," *World Journal of Gastroenterology*, vol. 16, no. 26, pp. 3267–3278, 2010.

[93] S. P. Lam, J. M. Luk, K. Man et al., "Activation of interleukin-6-induced glycoprotein 130/signal transducer and activator of transcription 3 pathway in mesenchymal stem cells enhances hepatic differentiation, proliferation, and liver regeneration," *Liver Transplantation*, vol. 16, no. 10, pp. 1195–1206, 2010.

[94] R. Bataller and D. A. Brenner, "Liver fibrosis," *Journal of Clinical Investigation*, vol. 115, no. 2, pp. 209–218, 2005.

[95] D. S. Lee, W. H. Gil, H. H. Lee et al., "Factors affecting graft survival after living donor liver transplantation," *Transplantation Proceedings*, vol. 36, no. 8, pp. 2255–2256, 2004.

[96] D. C. Zhao, J. X. Lei, R. Chen et al., "Bone marrow-derived mesenchymal stem cells protect against experimental liver fibrosis in rats," *World Journal of Gastroenterology*, vol. 11, no. 22, pp. 3431–3440, 2005.

[97] A. M. Parr, C. H. Tator, and A. Keating, "Bone marrow-derived mesenchymal stromal cells for the repair of central nervous system injury," *Bone Marrow Transplantation*, vol. 40, no. 7, pp. 609–619, 2007.

[98] J. Wang, F. Ding, Y. Gu, J. Liu, and X. Gu, "Bone marrow mesenchymal stem cells promote cell proliferation and neurotrophic function of Schwann cells in vitro and in vivo," *Brain Research*, vol. 1262, pp. 7–15, 2009.

[99] S. P. Wang, Z. H. Wang, D. Y. Peng, S. M. Li, H. Wang, and X. H. Wang, "Therapeutic effect of mesenchymal stem cells in rats with intracerebral hemorrhage: reduced apoptosis and enhanced neuroprotection," *Molecular Medicine Reports*, vol. 6, no. 4, pp. 848–854, 2012.

[100] A. Uccelli, E. Zappia, F. Benvenuto, F. Frassoni, and G. Mancardi, "Stem cells in inflammatory demyelinating disorders: a dual role for immunosuppression and neuroprotection," *Expert Opinion on Biological Therapy*, vol. 6, no. 1, pp. 17–22, 2006.

[101] K. Kurozumi, K. Nakamura, T. Tamiya et al., "BDNF gene-modified mesenchymal stem cells promote functional recovery and reduce infarct size in the rat middle cerebral artery occlusion model," *Molecular Therapy*, vol. 9, no. 2, pp. 189–197, 2004.

[102] N. K. Venkataramana, R. Pal, S. A. Rao et al., "Bilateral transplantation of allogenic adult human bone marrow-derived mesenchymal stem cells into the subventricular zone of Parkinson's disease: a pilot clinical study," *Stem Cells International*, vol. 2012, Article ID 931902, 12 pages, 2012.

[103] D. K. Podolsky, "Inflammatory bowel disease," *The New England Journal of Medicine*, vol. 347, no. 6, pp. 417–429, 2002.

[104] M. T. Castelo-Branco, I. D. Soares, D. V. Lopes et al., "Intraperitoneal but not intravenous cryopreserved mesenchymal stromal cells home to the inflamed colon and ameliorate experimental colitis," *PLoS One*, vol. 7, no. 3, Article ID e33360, 2012.

[105] Y. Ando, M. Inaba, Y. Sakaguchi et al., "Subcutaneous adipose tissue-derived stem cells facilitate colonic mucosal recovery from 2,4,6-trinitrobenzene sulfonic acid (TNBS)-induced colitis in rats," *Inflammatory Bowel Diseases*, vol. 14, no. 6, pp. 826–838, 2008.

[106] H. Jiang, L. Qu, Y. Li et al., "Bone marrow mesenchymal stem cells reduce intestinal ischemia/reperfusion injuries in rats," *Journal of Surgical Research*, vol. 168, no. 1, pp. 127–134, 2011.

[107] E. Zomorodian and M. B. Eslaminejad, "Mesenchymal stem cells as a potent cell source for bone regeneration," *Stem Cells International*, vol. 2012, Article ID 980353, 9 pages, 2012.

[108] F. Granero-Moltó, J. A. Weis, M. I. Miga et al., "Regenerative effects of transplanted mesenchymal stem cells in fracture healing," *Stem Cells*, vol. 27, no. 8, pp. 1887–1898, 2009.

[109] E. M. Horwitz, P. L. Gordon, W. K. K. Koo et al., "Isolated allogeneic bone marrow-derived mesenchymal cells engraft and stimulate growth in children with osteogenesis imperfecta: implications for cell therapy of bone," *Proceedings of the National Academy of Sciences of the United States of America*, vol. 99, no. 13, pp. 8932–8937, 2002.

9

Effects of Intravenous Administration of Human Umbilical Cord Blood Stem Cells in 3-Acetylpyridine-Lesioned Rats

Lucía Calatrava-Ferreras,[1] **Rafael Gonzalo-Gobernado,**[1]
Antonio S. Herranz,[1] **Diana Reimers,**[1] **Teresa Montero Vega,**[2] **Adriano Jiménez-Escrig,**[3]
Luis Alberto Richart López,[4] **and Eulalia Bazán**[1, 5]

[1] *Servicio de Neurobiología, Instituto Ramón y Cajal de Investigación Sanitaria (IRYCIS), 28034 Madrid, Spain*
[2] *Servicio de Bioquímica, Instituto Ramón y Cajal de Investigación Sanitaria (IRYCIS), 28034 Madrid, Spain*
[3] *Servicio de Neurología, Hospital Universitario Ramón y Cajal, 28034 Madrid, Spain*
[4] *Centro de Transfusiones de la Comunidad de Madrid, Valdebernardo, 28030 Madrid, Spain*
[5] *Servicio de Neurobiología-Investigación, Hospital Ramón y Cajal, Carretera de Colmenar Km. 9, 1, 28034 Madrid, Spain*

Correspondence should be addressed to Eulalia Bazán, eulalia.bazan@hrc.es

Academic Editor: Oscar Gonzalez-Perez

Cerebellar ataxias include a heterogeneous group of infrequent diseases characterized by lack of motor coordination caused by disturbances in the cerebellum and its associated circuits. Current therapies are based on the use of drugs that correct some of the molecular processes involved in their pathogenesis. Although these treatments yielded promising results, there is not yet an effective therapy for these diseases. Cell replacement strategies using human umbilical cord blood mononuclear cells (HuUCBMCs) have emerged as a promising approach for restoration of function in neurodegenerative diseases. The aim of this work was to investigate the potential therapeutic activity of HuUCBMCs in the 3-acetylpyridine (3-AP) rat model of cerebellar ataxia. Intravenous administered HuUCBMCs reached the cerebellum and brain stem of 3-AP ataxic rats. Grafted cells reduced 3-AP-induced neuronal loss promoted the activation of microglia in the brain stem, and prevented the overexpression of GFAP elicited by 3-AP in the cerebellum. In addition, HuUCBMCs upregulated the expression of proteins that are critical for cell survival, such as phospho-Akt and Bcl-2, in the cerebellum and brain stem of 3-AP ataxic rats. As all these effects were accompanied by a temporal but significant improvement in motor coordination, HuUCBMCs grafts can be considered as an effective cell replacement therapy for cerebellar disorders.

1. Introduction

Cerebellar ataxias (CAs) include a heterogeneous group of infrequent diseases characterized by lack of motor coordination [1]. According to their etiology, they can be divided into sporadic forms and hereditary diseases. All of them have in common cerebellum and associated neuronal circuits dysfunction, in particular spinocerebellar afferents [2–5]. Current therapeutic approaches are based on the use of drugs that correct some of the molecular processes involved in the pathogenesis of this group of diseases [1, 6–8]. Furthermore, other studies have assayed the potential therapeutic activity of intracerebroventricular, peripheral, or intranasal administration of neurotrophic factors such as insulin-like growth factor (IGF-I), or glial-derived growth factor (GDNF), in different experimental models of cerebellar ataxia in rodents [9–13]. Although the above-mentioned treatments (drugs and trophic factors) yielded promising results, there is not yet an effective therapy for these types of diseases to date [1].

Cell replacement strategies using stem cells (SCs) as donor tissue have emerged as a promising approach for restoration of function in neurodegenerative diseases [14–19]. Hematopoietic stem cells from human umbilical cord blood (HuUCBs) have been proposed as an excellent source of embryonic SCs in regenerative therapies for the Central Nervous System [20–23]. HuUCBCs are easily accessible they retain certain properties of embryonic SCs such as the expression of transcription factors specific to embryonic antigens [24] and are well tolerated by the host due to their low immunogenicity [25]. Additionally, in vitro manipulation of HuUCBCs has shown their plasticity. Thus, after exposure to different agents, these cells are able to express antigens of diverse cellular lineages, including the neural type [26–31].

HuUCBCs were used successfully for the first time in 1989, as a bone marrow transplant in a patient with Fanconi's anemia [32]. Other studies have shown that systemic administration of HuUCBCs to different experimental models of neurodegenerative diseases improved their neurological symptoms and life expectancy [22, 23]. The beneficial effects of HuUCBCs seemed to be due to their ability to synthesize and release trophic factors involved in cell survival, rather than having a role in neuronal replacement [23, 33–36].

Stem cell-reparative approaches have been proposed for cerebellum-related disorders [37–40]. However, the type of stem cells most appropriate for future human cell therapy is not clearly defined at present [37]. Considering the possibility that HuUCBCs could be used as a therapeutic agent in CA, we analyze their potential neuroregenerative and/or neuroprotective activity in the 3-acetylpyridine (3-AP) experimental model of CA in rats. The rationale for using this CA model was because the neurotoxin 3-AP selectively lesions calbindin expressing neurons in the inferior olive [9], and this nucleus plays a key role in the control of the cerebellar function by sending glutamatergic excitatory signals to Purkinje cells [41, 42].

Here, we report that intravenous administration of HuUCB mononuclear cells (HuUCBMCs) reaches the cerebellum and brain stem of 3-AP-lesioned rats. Grafted cells reduce neuronal loss in the brain stem, prevent glial reactivity in the cerebellum, and improve motor coordination in ataxic rats. In this study, we also show that HuUCBMCs upregulate the expression of proteins that are critical for cell survival, such as phospho-Akt and Bcl-2, in the cerebellum and brain stem of 3-AP-lesioned rats. The role of activated microglia in HuUCBMCs-mediated neuronal protection in the brain stem is also discussed.

2. Materials and Methods

2.1. Experimental Model of Cerebellar Ataxia in Rats. A total of 40 female Sprague Dawley rats weighing 220–250 g were used in accordance with the European Union Council Directive (86/609/EEC). Rats received an intraperitoneal (i.p.) injection of the neurotoxine 3-AP (40 mg/kg) that selectively lesioned calbindin expressing neurons in the inferior olive [9]. This nucleus plays a key role in the control of the cerebellar function by sending glutamatergic excitatory signals to Purkinje cells (PCs) [41, 42]. From a histological point of view, PC and granule neurons of the cerebellar cortex are the most commonly affected population of neurons in CA [3].

2.2. Behavioral Testing. Motor performance was analyzed using the rotarod test. Before 3-AP lesions were produced, rats received 9 independent training sessions in the rotarod (PanLab S.L., Mod. LE 8500, Cornellá, Spain), with 4 1-minute evaluations at 40 rpm (fixed speed), and 4 1-minute evaluations at 4 to 40 rpm (accelerating rod). Those animals that withstood more than 1 minute at 40 rpm and at 4 to 40 rpm were selected for 3-AP lesions. Motor coordination was evaluated at 72 hours after lesion. Those animals resulting in mean latencies to fall on the accelerating rod of approximately 19 ± 3 s ($n = 16$) were selected for HuUCBMCs or vehicle administration. Starting 10 days after 3-AP lesion procedure, animals were monitored once a week until the end of the study period.

2.3. HuUCBMCs Isolation of Blood Cell Concentrate. Assessment, processing, and cryopreservation of HuUCBCs were carried out by the Centro de Transfusiones de la Comunidad de Madrid (Valdebernardo) in accordance with the Spanish Directive for Donors' Selection (Edition 4/May 2009/PO.CO.01). The donated units met the criteria for minimal cellularity and volume showing the following parameters: mononuclear cells (MCs): $337.8 \times 10^6 \pm 32.56$, total nucleated cells (TNCs): $910.8 \times 10^6 \pm 86.77$, and cells positives for CD34: $0.7620 \times 10^6 \pm 0.09140$.

For isolation of HuUCBMCs we followed a methodology previously described [43]. Briefly, HuUCBCs were drawn from the bag and divided into 2 Falcon tubes with half volume of Lymphoprep and centrifuged at 800 g and 20°C for 40 min to create a Ficoll gradient. The band of mononuclear cells located at the interface (2 to 7 mL) was taken and washed 3 times with PBS. An aliquot of 40 μL was used to determine the number of living cells by Trypan Blue using a Neubahuer chamber.

2.4. Cell Transplantation. At 3 days after 3-AP lesion, rats were anesthetized by inhalatory administration of Isoflurane (2%). One group of animals ($n = 14$) received a single injection of 4.5×10^6 HuUCBMNCs in 250 μL of sterile PBS into the lateral vein of the tail (3-AP + cells). Another group of 3-AP-lesioned rats ($n = 10$) received the same volume of sterile PBS (3-AP + vehicle). As controls we used a group of naïve rats that did not receive HuUCBMNCs grafts ($n = 6$). All experimental groups received cyclosporine (5 mg/kg i.p.) once a day to avoid rejection of human cells 24 hours before cell transplantation, and until the end of the study. Animals were sacrificed at 1, 7, 21 and 44 days after transplantation (4, 10, 24, and 48 days after lesion, resp.).

2.5. Tissue Processing. At 4, 10, and 21 days after lesion the animals were perfused intracardially under deep anesthesia with 50 mL of isotonic saline, followed by 250 mL of 4% paraformaldehyde. Brains were postfixed in the same solution for 24 hr at 4°C, cryoprotected and frozen, before sectioning on a cryostat. For the inferior olive 20 μm thick coronal sections were performed at three levels separated by a distance of approximately 400 μm. These levels correspond to the following coordinates of the stereotaxic atlas of Paxinos and Watson [44]: −13.30 mm from Bregma (Zone 1), −12.80 mm (zone 2) and −11.96 mm (zone 3).

For immunohistochemical analysis of the cerebellum, 20 μm thick coronal sections were obtained in the cryostat, and mounted on positively charged slides (Dako REAL Capillary Gap microscope slides).

2.6. Antibodies and Immunochemicals. The primary antibodies used in this study were rabbit antiproliferating cell nuclear antigen (PCNA, 1:75; Santa Cruz Biotechnology Inc., Santa Cruz, CA, USA), rabbit antiglial fibrillary acidic protein (GFAP, 1:200; DakoCytomation), mouse antineuronal nuclei (NeuN, 1:1000; Chemicon International Inc.), mouse anti-OX6 (1:250; AbD Serotec, Oxford, UK), rabbit antilaminin (1:25; Sigma Chemical Co., St. Louis, MO, USA), mouse anti-Bcl-2 (1:25; Santa Cruz Biotech), rabbit anticalbindin (1:500; Millipore, Temecula, CA, USA), mouse anti-human leucocyte antigen ABC (HLA-ABC 1:500; AbD Serotec, Oxford, UK), mouse anti-human nuclei protein (HuNu, 1:25; Millipore, Temecula, CA, USA), and rabbit anti-Bax (1:250; Santa Cruz Biotech). The secondary antibodies and other immunochemicals used were peroxidase-labeled isolectin B4 (IB4, 1:20; Sigma Chemical Co, St. Louis, MO, USA), biotinylated goat anti-mouse IgG (Zymed Laboratories; South San Francisco, CA, USA), streptavidin-biotin-peroxidase complex (DakoCytomation), diaminobenzidine (DAB) + substrate-chromogen system (both from DakoCytomation), Alexa Fluor-568 goat anti-mouse IgG, and Alexa Fluor-488 goat anti-rabbit IgG (1:400; all from Molecular Probes; Eugene, OR, USA), fluorescein-conjugated goat anti-mouse IgG (1:25; Jackson ImmunoResearch Laboratories Inc., West Grove, PA, USA), Cy3-conjugated donkey anti-guinea pig IgG (1:500; Jackson ImmunoResearch Laboratories Inc.), and rhodamine-conjugated goat anti-rabbit IgG (1:100, Chemicon International Inc.).

2.7. Immunohistochemistry and Morphometric Analysis. Tissue sections were treated with sodium acetate 10 mM, pH 6.0, at 95°C for 4 min, and preincubated with 5% normal goat serum (NGS) in Tris-buffered saline (TBS: 0.15 M NaCl and 0.1 M Tris HCl, pH 7.4)/0.1% Triton X-100 for 30 min. Primary antibodies were applied for 24 hr at 4°C, and most of them were visualized using immunofluorescence procedures. The slides were coverslipped in a medium containing p-phenylenediamine and bisbenzimide (Hoechst 33342; Sigma) for the detection of nuclei. Some series of sections were preincubated with 5% NGS in TBS and then processed for the histochemical detection of IB4, a marker of microglia and macrophages, by incubating for 2 hr with IB4 conjugated to peroxidase. Finally, the reaction product was detected with DAB chromogen.

For quantitative estimation of calbindin immunostaining in the inferior olive, measurements were performed in several coronal sections of the brainstem, at the three levels indicated previously (see tissue processing). The area of the olive was demarcated and measured in each zone, and the number of cells with caldindin staining was assessed using the 20X objective. Immunohistochemical results were expressed as the number of positive cells/section with the aid of the Computer-Assisted Stereology Toolbox (CAST) grid system (Olympus, Ballerup, Denmark). Fluorescence images were acquired and analyzed by confocal microscopy (Nikon C1 plus ECLIPSE Ti-e microscope).

2.8. Western Blotting Protein Analysis. After 44 days of cells transplantation, the brain stem and cerebellum of 3-AP-lesioned rats that received vehicle ($n = 8$) or cells ($n = 9$) were removed and dissected following a previously described methodology [45]. Tissue was homogenized (1:8, w/v) with homogenization buffer (20 mM Tris-HCl, pH 7.5: 140 mM potassium chloride; 5 mM magnesium acetate; 1 mM dithiothreitol, 2 mM benzamidine, 1 mM EDTA, 2 mM EGTA, 0.5% Triton X-100, 10 μg/mL pepstatin A, 10 μg/mL leupeptin, and 10 μg/mL antipain; 20 mM sodium β-glycerophosphate; 20 mM sodium molybdate; 200 mM sodium orthovanadate). Homogenates were centrifuged at 11,000 g for 20 min, and proteins were processed for Western blot analysis to determine the relative levels of several proteins. The procedures were performed at 4°C, and samples were kept at −80°C until use. Aliquots of 30 μg of protein were separated by electrophoresis on 10–15% SDS-polyacrylamide minigels and transferred to nitrocellulose filters. Membranes were soaked in blocking solution (0.1 M PBS and 5% dry skimmed milk, pH 7.4) and incubated with the following primary antibodies diluted in 0.1 M PBS and 1% dry skimmed milk, pH 7.4: mouse anti-Bcl-2 (1:400; Santa Cruz Biotechnology Inc., Burlingame, CA, USA), rabbit anti-Bax (1:300; Santa Cruz Biotechnology, Santa Cruz, CA, USA), rabbit antiproliferating cell nuclear antigen (PCNA, 1:1000; Santa Cruz Biotechnology, Santa Cruz, CA, USA), rabbit antiglial fibrillary acidic protein (GFAP, 1:5000; DakoCytomation, Denmark), rabbit anti-Glut5 (1:500; Abcam), mouse anti-OX6 (1:1000, AbD Serotec, Oxford, UK), rabbit anti-HuNu protein (1:200, Millipore, Temecula, CA, USA), rabbit anticalbindin (1:5000; Millipore, Temecula, CA, USA), rabbit anti-Akt (Ser473P) (1:2000; Cell Signaling Technology, Beverly, MA, USA), rabbit anti-Akt (1:2000; Cell Signaling Technology). After extensive washing in 0.05% PBS-Tween, membranes were incubated with the peroxidase-conjugated or alkaline-phosphatase-conjugated secondary antibodies diluted 1:2000 in blocking solution. The membranes were developed with enhanced chemiluminescence Western blotting, following the manufacturer's instructions (Amersham, Buckinghamshire, England), and were exposed to hyperfilm. Membranes were also immunolabeled for loading control using mouse anti-β actin (1:5000; Sigma Aldrich) and anti-mouse IgG alkaline phosphatase-conjugated (1:3000, Sigma Aldrich) and were developed with alkaline phosphatase reagent. The density of stained bands was scanned and quantified with the Image QuantTL software package, and the data were normalized in relation to β actin levels.

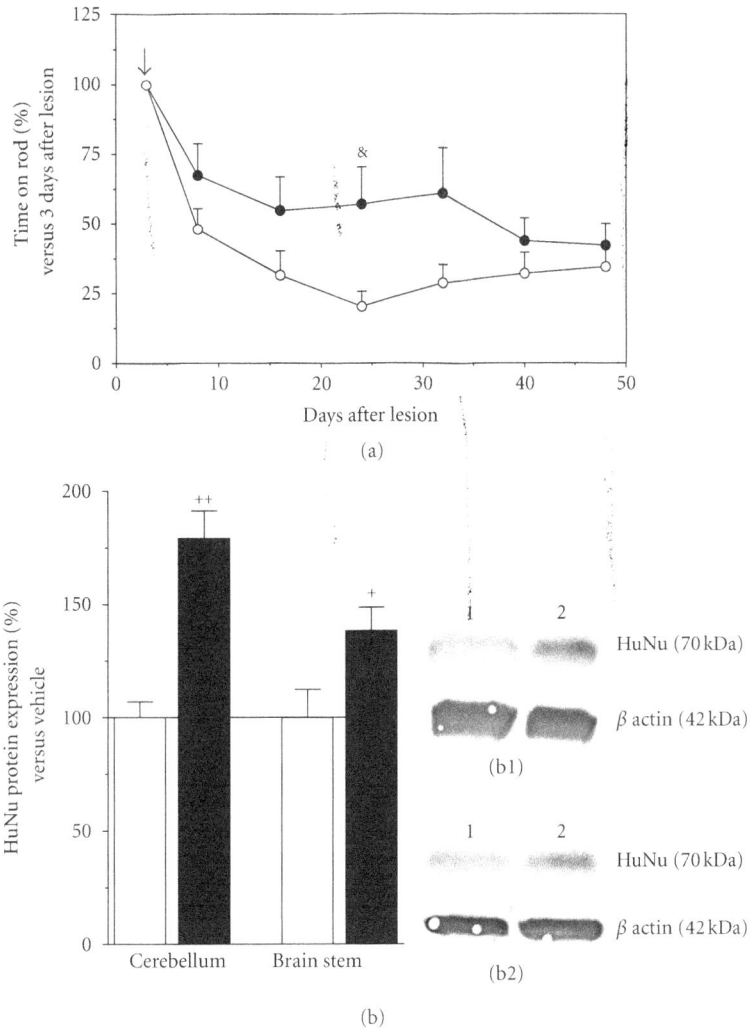

FIGURE 1: HuUCBMCs grafts improve motor coordination and reach the cerebellum and brain stem of 3-AP ataxic rats. Motor performance, as assessed by the rotarod test, shows a progressive impairment in 3-AP-lesioned rats receiving vehicle ((a) white circles) that reaches a plateau between 15 and 24 days after lesion. Motor coordination in 3-AP-lesioned rats that received HuUCBMCs grafts ((a) black circles) is significantly improved at 24 days after lesion. Time of implantation of HuUCBMCs (↓). (b) shows the detection by western blot of HuNu protein in the cerebellum and brain stem of 3-AP-lesioned rats treated with vehicle (white bars), or with HuUCBMCs (black bars). (b1) and (b2) show representative blots for HuNu protein in the cerebellum (b1) and brain stem (b2). Lane 1: 3-AP-lesioned rats treated with vehicle (3-AP + vehicle); lane 2: 3-AP-lesioned rats treated with HuUCBMCs grafts (3-AP + cells). Results represent the mean ± SEM of 4 (b) to 10 (a) individual animals. $^{\&}P \leq 0.05$ versus 3-AP + vehicle rats at 24 days after lesion, $^{+}P \leq 0.05$, $^{++}P \leq 0.01$ versus 3-AP + vehicle rats at 48 days after lesion.

2.9. Data Analysis. Results are expressed as mean ± SEM of (n) independent animals. Statistical analyses for immunohistochemical and biochemical studies were performed using one-way ANOVA followed by the Newman-Keuls multiple comparison test. For behavioral studies, a two-way ANOVA followed by Student's t-test was used. Differences were considered significant when $P \leq 0.05$.

3. Results

3.1. HuUCBMCs Grafts Ameliorate Motor Coordination in 3-AP-Lesioned Rats. To determine whether HuUCBMCs transplantation was functional in vivo, we have analyzed motor coordination using the rotarod test. Motor performance of naïve rats was relatively stable over repeated tests, resulting in mean latencies to fall on the accelerating rod of approximately 52.31 ± 2.7 s ($n = 16$). At 3 days after 3-AP lesion, the latency to fall from rotarod was reduced to 19 ± 3 sec ($n = 16$). As shown in Figure 1(a), 3-AP-lesioned rats showed a progressive impairment that reached a plateau between 15 and 24 days after lesion. By contrast, in the 3-AP + cells group of animals, motor performance was stable between 8 and 32 weeks after lesion (Figure 1(a)). Moreover, 21 days after HuUCBMCs transplantation (24 days after lesion), their motor coordination was significantly

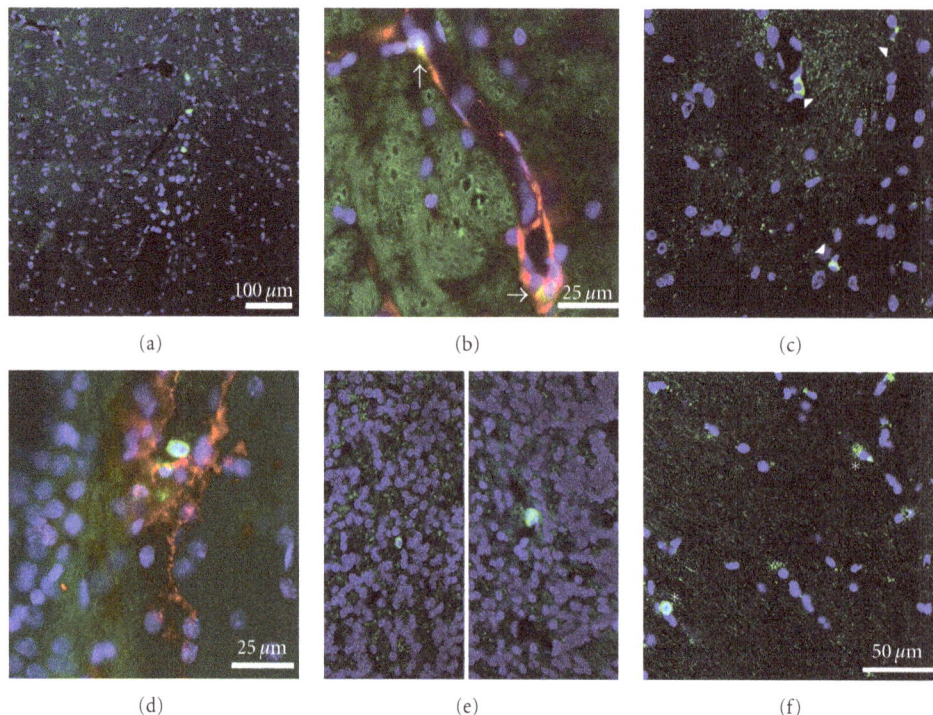

FIGURE 2: Immunodetection of human leucocyte antigen-ABC in the brain stem and cerebellum of 3-AP ataxic rats. (a) and (c) show HLA-ABC immunostaining (green) in the ventral (a) and dorsal (c) brain stem of 3-AP-lesioned rats receiving HuUCBMCs grafts. (b) Shows HLA-ABC (b, green) and laminin (b, red) immunoreactivity in the ventral brain stem. Note how HLA-ABC-positive cells are associated to laminin-positive blood vessels (b, yellow, white arrows) or integrated in the parenchyma (c, white arrowheads). In the cerebellum HLA-ABC-positive cells (d–f, green) are located near to the vermis in laminin-positive blood vessels (d, red), and in the parenchyma of the granular (e, green) and molecular layers (f, green, white stars) of the cerebellar cortex. Nuclei were counterstained with Hoechst 33342 (blue). Scale bar: 25 μm (b and d), 50 μm (c, e, and f), and 100 μm (a).

improved, to compared with 3-AP-lesioned rats receiving vehicle (Figure 1(a)).

3.2. Detection of HuUCBMCs in Brain Stem and Cerebellum of 3-AP-Lesioned Rats. Immunohistochemical analysis for the human endogenous marker HLA-ABC was performed to determine if intravenous transplanted HuUCBMCs were able to reach the brain stem and cerebellum of 3-AP-lesioned rats. Seven days after HuUCBMCs transplantation, 3-AP-lesioned rats showed HLA-ABC-positive cells in ventral (Figure 2(a)) and dorsal (Figure 2(c)) zones of the brain stem. These cells were associated to laminin-positive blood vessels (Figure 2(b)), or integrated in the parenchyma (Figure 2(c)). Similarly, the cerebellum of 3-AP + cells treated rats showed HLA-ABC immunoreactivity (Figures 2(d)–2(f)). Thus, HLA-ABC-positive cells were observed in the vermis associated to blood vessels (Figure 2(d)), and in the parenchyma of the granular (Figure 2(e)) and molecular (Figure 2(f)) layers of the cerebellar cortex. Under our experimental conditions, HLA-ABC immunoreactivity was not observed at longer periods after transplantation (i.e. 21 days). However, by western blot analysis we found that 45 days after HuUCBMCs grafts were performed (48 days after lesion), the cerebellum and brain stem of 3-AP-lesioned rats showed significant levels of the nuclear antigen expressed by

human cells HuNu, compared to 3-AP + vehicle-treated rats, where HuNu protein expression was very low in both structures (Figure 1(b)). We were unable to confirm these results by immunohistochemistry because the antibody used for HuNu detection gave a high background in rat brain slices.

3.3. HuUCBMCs Grafts Partially Prevent Neurotoxin-Induced Neuronal Loss in the Brain Stem. A single injection of 40 mg/kg 3-AP significantly ($P \leq 0.001$, $n = 6$) reduced the number of calbindin-positive neurons in zone 3 (Z3) of the inferior olive from 616 ± 22 to 220 ± 51 calbindin-positive cells/section in naïve and 3-AP-lesioned rats, respectively. A similar effect was observed in zone 1 (Z1) where calbindin-positive cells were reduced by 1.7-fold in 3-AP-lesioned rats ($P \leq 0.01$, $n = 4$). As shown in Figure 3, after 48 days after lesion calbindin immunoreactivity was slightly higher in both zones of the inferior olive of 3-AP-lesioned rats that received HuUCBMCs (Figures 3(b) and 3(d)), compared to 3-AP + vehicle-treated rats (Figures 3(a) and 3(c)). We also analyzed the expression of calbindin and NeuN, a nuclear antigen expressed by neurons, by western blot. In the brain stem of 3-AP + vehicle-treated rats calbindin (Figure 4(a)) and NeuN (Figure 4(b)) protein levels were significantly lower than those found in naïve and 3-AP + cells treated rats. The neurotoxin 3-AP also reduced calbindin and

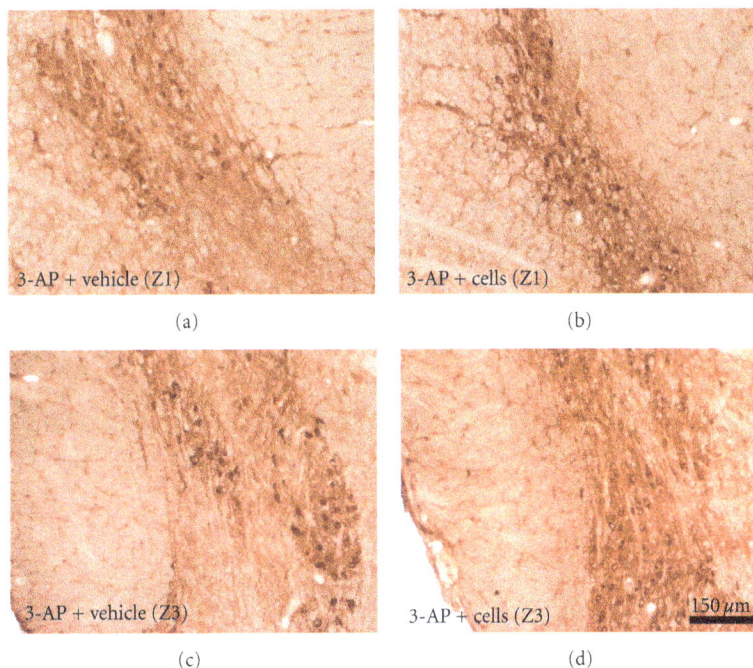

FIGURE 3: Immunodetection of calbindin in the inferior olive of 3-AP ataxic rats. (a) and (c) show calbindin immunostaining in two different levels of the inferior olive of 3-AP-lesioned rats separated by a distance of approximately 800 μm. Note how HuUCBMCs grafts increase calbindin-positive cells in both zones of the structure (b, c). Scale bar: 150 μm.

NeuN protein expression in the cerebellum, but HuUCBMCs transplantation was unable to recover the levels of both proteins in this structure (Figures 4(a) and 4(b)).

3.4. HuUCBMCs Grafts Modulate Glial Reactivity in 3-AP-Lesioned Rats.
Previously, we observed that 3-AP induced a time-dependent invasion of cells expressing the vital marker of microglia IB4 in the inferior olive, that was maintained up to 24 days after lesion [46]. In agreement with those studies, the inferior olive of 3-AP + vehicle-treated rats showed a higher number of IB4-positive cells at 10 days after lesion than 48 hours after 3-AP was injected (Figures 5(a) and 5(b)). Moreover, IB4 labeling was increased in the inferior olive of 3-AP + vehicle-treated rats, as compared with 3-AP lesioned rats that received HuUCBMCs (Figures 5(b) and 5(c)). At 48 days after lesion, western blot analysis for the glucose transporter expressed by microglia GLUT5 gave similar results. Thus, GLUT5 protein expression was significantly raised in the brain stem of 3-AP + vehicle group of animals, compared to naïve and 3-AP + cells-treated rats (Figure 6(a)).

The anti-OX6 antibody recognizes a histocompatiblility Class II antigen expressed by activated microglia. As shown in Figure 6(b), OX6 protein levels were raised by 1.76-fold in the brain stem of 3-AP + cell-treated rats. Similarly, OX6 immunoreactivity was increased in the inferior olive of 3-AP + cells rats (Figure 5(f)), compared to naïve (Figure 5(d)), and 3-AP + vehicle-treated animals (Figure 5(e)). Proliferation is another feature of microglial activation. HuUCBMCs transplantation upregulated PCNA protein expression by 1.6-fold in brain stem (**$P \leq 0.01$ and +$P \leq 0.05$ versus

naïve and 3-AP + vehicle rats, resp.). In addition, some of the OX6-positive cells were PCNA positive in the inferior olive of 3-AP + cell-treated rats (Figure 5(g)).

In the cerebellum, neither GLUT5 (Figure 6(a)), or OX6 (Figure 6(b)), nor PCNA protein levels were affected by HuUCBMCs transplantation, compared to naïve and 3-AP + vehicle-treated rats. However, the intravenous injection of HuUCBMCs prevented the increase in GFAP protein expression induced by 3-AP (Figure 6(c)). Besides, the cerebellum of 3-AP + cell-treated rats showed lower GFAP immunoreactivity than the cerebellum of 3-AP + vehicle rats (Figures 5(h)–5(j)).

3.5. HuUCBMCs Grafts Stimulate Bcl-2 Protein Expression and Phosphorylation of Akt.
Several studies have proposed a neuroprotective role for HuUCBMCs [23]. Using western blot analysis, we studied the effects of HuUCBMCs grafts in the expression of proteins involved in cell survival. The Bcl-2 family comprise proteins that have either antiapoptotic (such as Bcl-2), or proapoptotic (such as Bax) effects [47–49]. In the cerebellum of 3-AP + cell-treated rats, the ratio Bcl-2/Bax was significantly raised compared to naïve rats and 3-AP + vehicle-treated animals (Figure 7(a)). This effect was due to the increase by 1.6-fold observed in Bcl-2 protein levels (*$P \leq 0.05$ and +$P \leq 0.05$ versus naïve and 3-AP + vehicle rats, resp.), while Bax levels remained unchanged in all experimental conditions studied (Figure 7(a1)). Neither 3-AP + vehicle rats, nor 3-AP + cell-treated animals showed significant changes in Bcl-2 and Bax protein expression in the brain stem (Figure 7(a)).

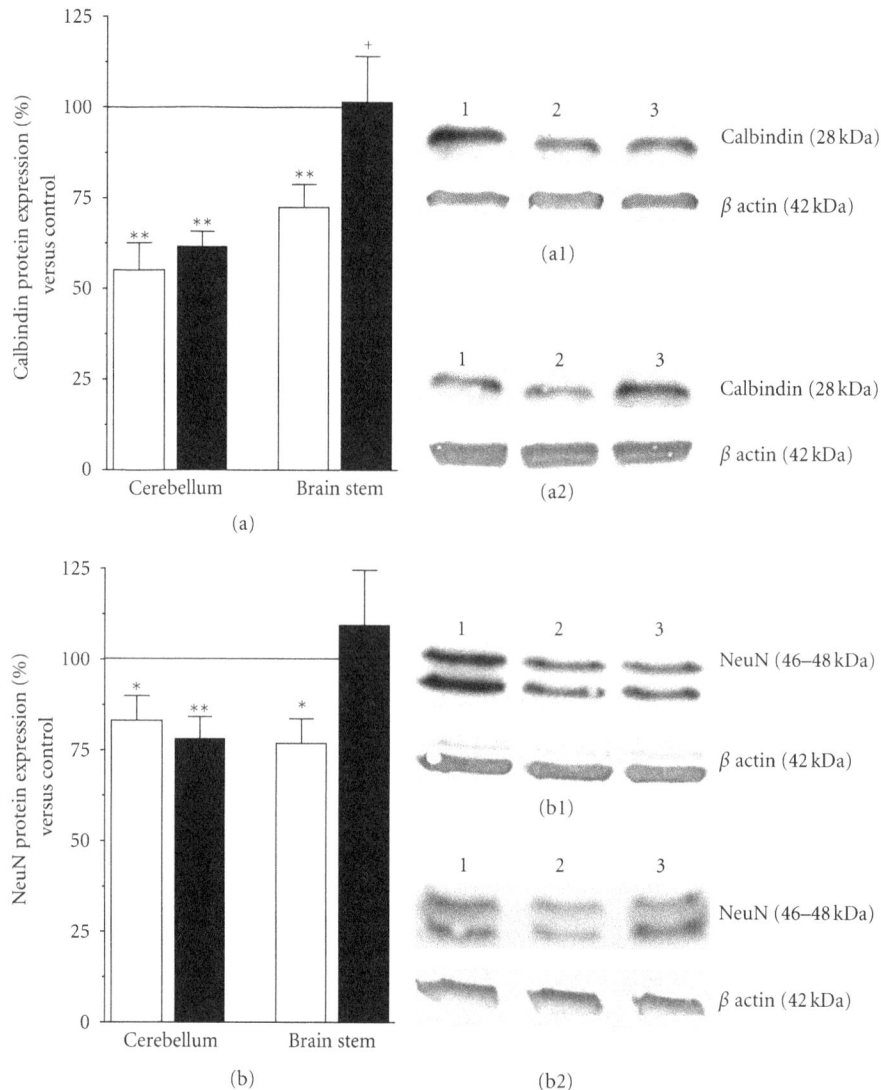

FIGURE 4: HuUCBMCs grafts partially prevent 3-AP-induced neuronal loss in the brain stem. (a) and (b) show the detection by western blot of calbindin (a) and neuronal nuclei (b, NeuN) in the cerebellum and brain stem of 3-AP-lesioned rats receiving vehicle (3-AP + vehicle rats, white bars) or HuUCBMCs grafts (3-AP + cells rats, black bars). (a1) and (a2) Show representative blots for calbindin, and (b1) and (b2) for NeuN in the cerebellum (a1, b1) and brain stem (a2, b2). Lane 1: naïve rats (control); lane 2: 3-AP + vehicle; lane 3: 3-AP + cells. Results represent the mean ± SEM of 6 to 9 individual animals. $*P \leq 0.05$, $**P \leq 0.01$ versus naïve rats, $+P \leq 0.05$ versus 3-AP + vehicle rats.

The protein Akt is a key downstream effector of the PI3K/Akt-signaling pathway which phosphorylation plays a critical role in the regulation of neuronal survival [24, 50–54]. As shown in Figure 7(b), the ratio phospho-Akt/Akt was significantly increased in the cerebellum and brain stem of 3-AP + cells rats. HuUCBMCs grafts did not modify total Akt protein expression in both structures, but upregulated phospho-Akt levels in the cerebellum and brain stem of 3-AP-lesioned rats by 2- and 1.4-fold, respectively ($*P < 0.05$ versus naïve cerebellum and $+P < 0.05$ versus 3-AP + vehicle brain stem).

4. Discussion

In the present study we show that intravenous administered HuUCBMCs were able to reach the cerebellum and brain stem of 3-AP-lesioned rats. Implanted cells partially blocked the loss of neurons induced by the neurotoxin in the brain stem, prevented the overexpression of GFAP in cerebellum, and stimulated the expression of proteins involved in cell survival in both structures. All these effects were accompanied by a temporal but significant improvement in motor coordination, suggesting the potentiality of HuUCBMCs grafts as a cell replacement therapy for cerebellar disorders.

HuUCBMCs are considered an excellent source of stem cells that can be used for cell replacement therapies in neurodegeneration [20, 22, 23]. However, to our knowledge there are only two studies using HuUCBCs for the treatment of CA [39, 40]. By using an anti-HLA-ABC antibody, we found that intravenous administered HuUCBMCs reached the cerebellum and brain stem of 3-AP-lesioned rats. Under our experimental conditions, HLA-ABC immunostaining

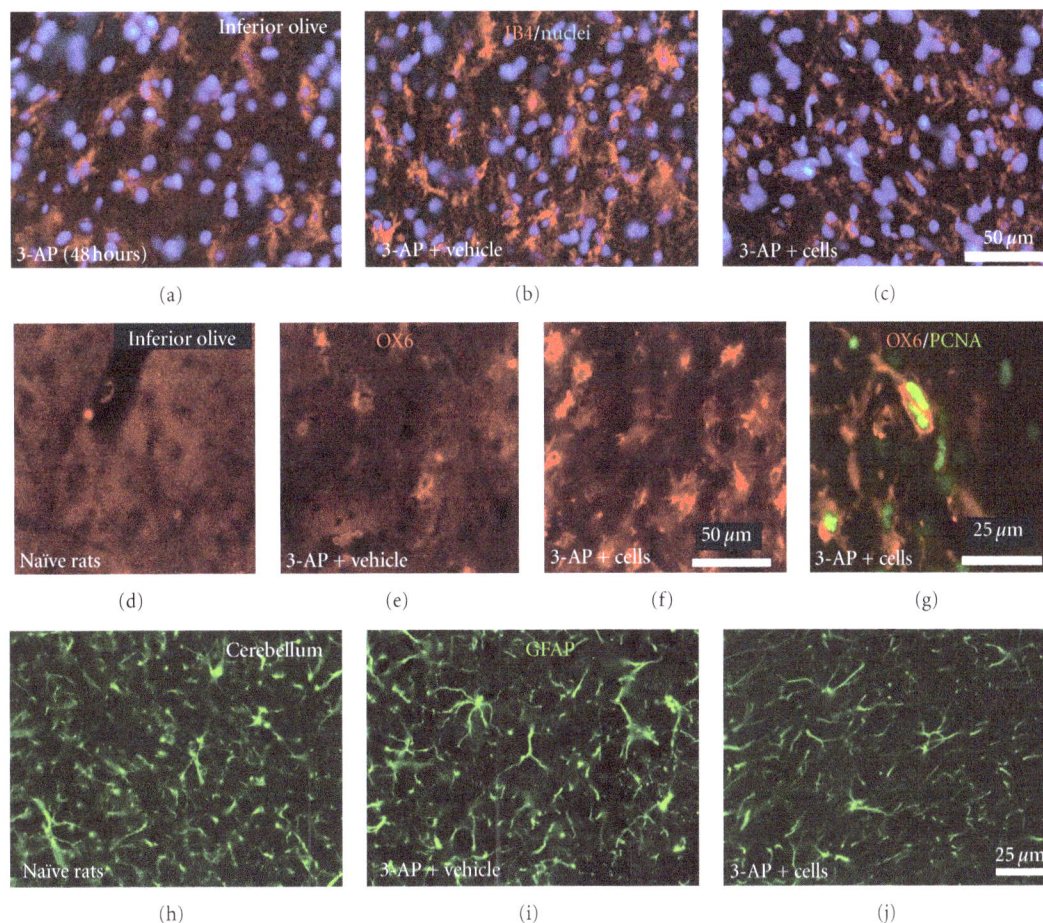

FIGURE 5: Immunodetection of glial cells in the inferior olive and cerebellum of 3-AP ataxic rats. (a) and (b) show the histochemical detection of isolectin B4 (IB4, red) in the inferior olive of 3-AP-lesioned rats 48 hours (a) and 10 days (b, c) after lesion. Note how 3-AP lesioned rats that received HuUCBMCs grafts (c, red) show lower IB4 staining at 10 days after lesion than ataxic rats treated with vehicle (b, red). (d) to (g) show OX6 immunostaining in the inferior olive of naïve rats (d, red) and 3-AP-lesioned rats treated with vehicle (e, red) or HuUCBMCs (f, red). Cell transplantation increases OX6 immunoreactivity (f, red). (g) shows double immunolabeling for OX6 (red) and PCNA (green) in the inferior olive of 3-AP + cells-treated rats. (h) to (j) show GFAP immunoreactivity in the cerebellum. Note how HuUCBMCs grafts reduce GFAP immunolabeling in this structure (j, green). Nuclei were counterstained with Hoechst 33342 (blue). Scale bar: 25 μm (g, h, I, and j), 50 μm (a, b, c, d, e, and f).

was only observed during the first three weeks of transplantation. However, western blot analysis showed HuNu protein expression in the cerebellum and brain stem of 3-AP + cell-treated rats two months after the administration of HuUCBMCs. These apparently contradictory results could be explained by a potential reduction in the expression of HLA-ABC at two months of transplantation.

In vitro and in vivo studies have demonstrated that HuUCBMCs are able to differentiate into neurons [31, 34, 43, 55, 56]. In ataxic rats HuUCBMCs implantation slightly recovered calbindin-positive neurons from 3-AP neurotoxicity in the inferior olive and restored calbindin and NeuN levels in brain stem. Although we found HLA-ABC-positive cells in the brain stem of 3-AP + cells-treated rats, none of these cells were located in the inferior olive. For this reason, we may infer that HuUCBMCs did not differentiate in calbindin-positive neurons in this structure. However, from our studies we cannot exclude the possibility

that HuUCBMCs are able to differentiate in neurons in the brain stem as we were unable to detect HLA-ABC-positive cells after one month of transplantation.

Increasing evidence strengthens the hypothesis that the beneficial role of transplanted HuUCBMCs is associated with the production of neuroprotective factors [14, 33, 36, 40, 57]. We did not analyze the expression of neurotrophins or cytokines and chemokines with anti-inflammatory properties, but we found that HuUCBMCs grafts potentiated the activation of microglia in the inferior olive and the brain stem of 3-AP-lesioned rats, as analyzed by OX6 and PCNA immunohistochemistry and immunoblot. Although activated microglia have been associated with the pathogenesis of several neurodegenerative diseases [58, 59], these cells could play a key role in neuroprotection through the production and release of neurotrophic factors [60, 61]. A recent study associated the therapeutic benefits of HuUCBMCs transplantation in a rat model of neonatal

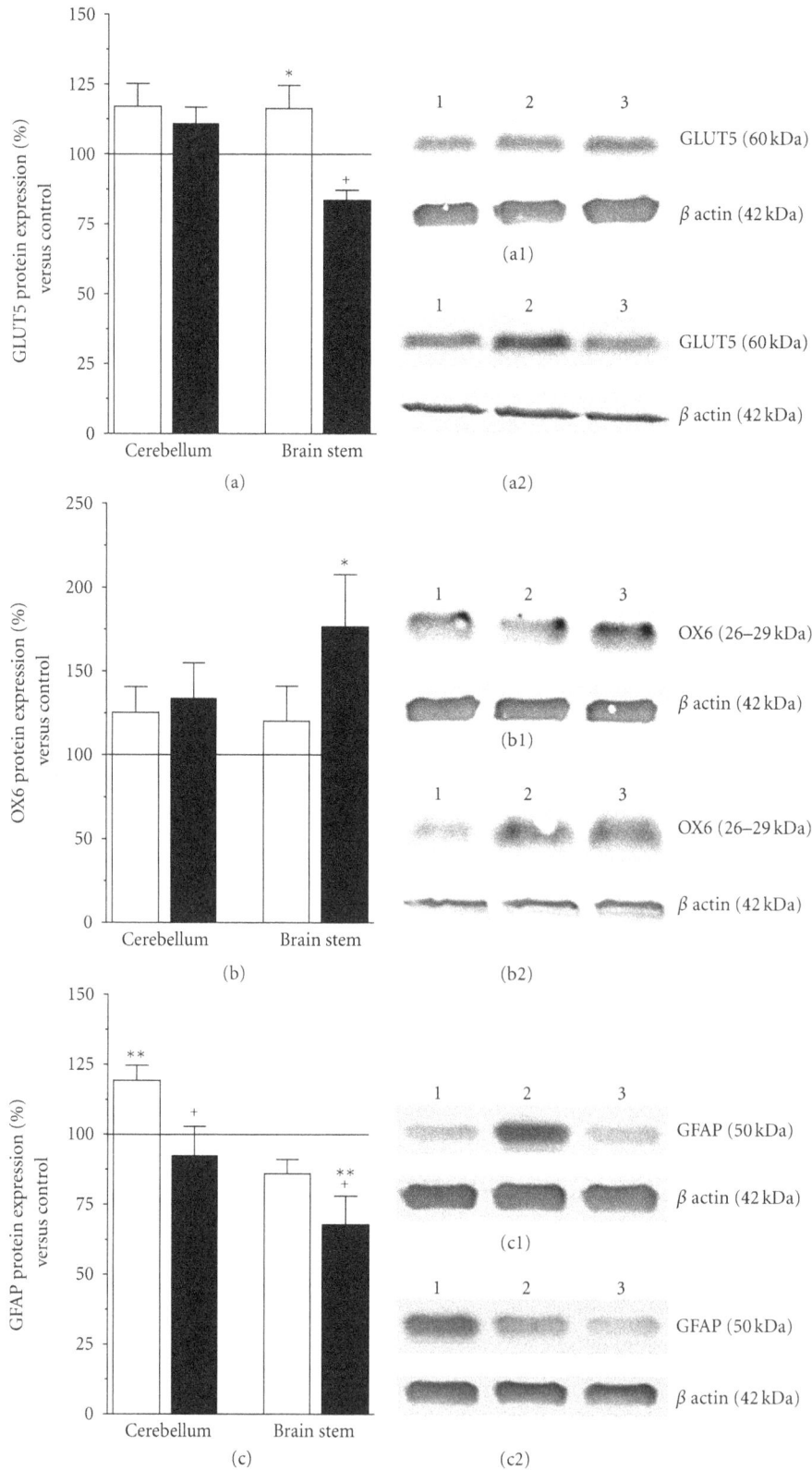

FIGURE 6: HuUCBMCs grafts modulate glial reactivity in 3-AP ataxic rats. (a), (b), and (c) show GLUT5 (a), OX6 (b), and GFAP (c) protein levels in the cerebellum and brain stem of 3-AP-lesioned rats receiving vehicle (3-AP + vehicle rats, white bars) or HuUCBMCs grafts (3-AP + cells rats, black bars). Note how HuUCBMCs transplantation upregulates OX6 protein expression in the brain stem and reduces GFAP protein levels in the cerebellum of 3-AP-lesioned rats. (a1) and (a2) show representative blots for GLUT5, (b1) and (b2) for OX6, and (c1) and (c2) for GFAP in the cerebellum (a1, b1, and c1) and brain stem (a2, b2, and c2). Lane 1: naïve rats (control); lane 2: 3-AP + vehicle; lane 3: 3-AP + cells. Results represent the mean ± SEM of 9 to 15 individual animals. $^{*}P \leq 0.05$, $^{**}P \leq 0.01$ versus naïve rats, $^{+}P \leq 0.05$ versus 3-AP + vehicle rats.

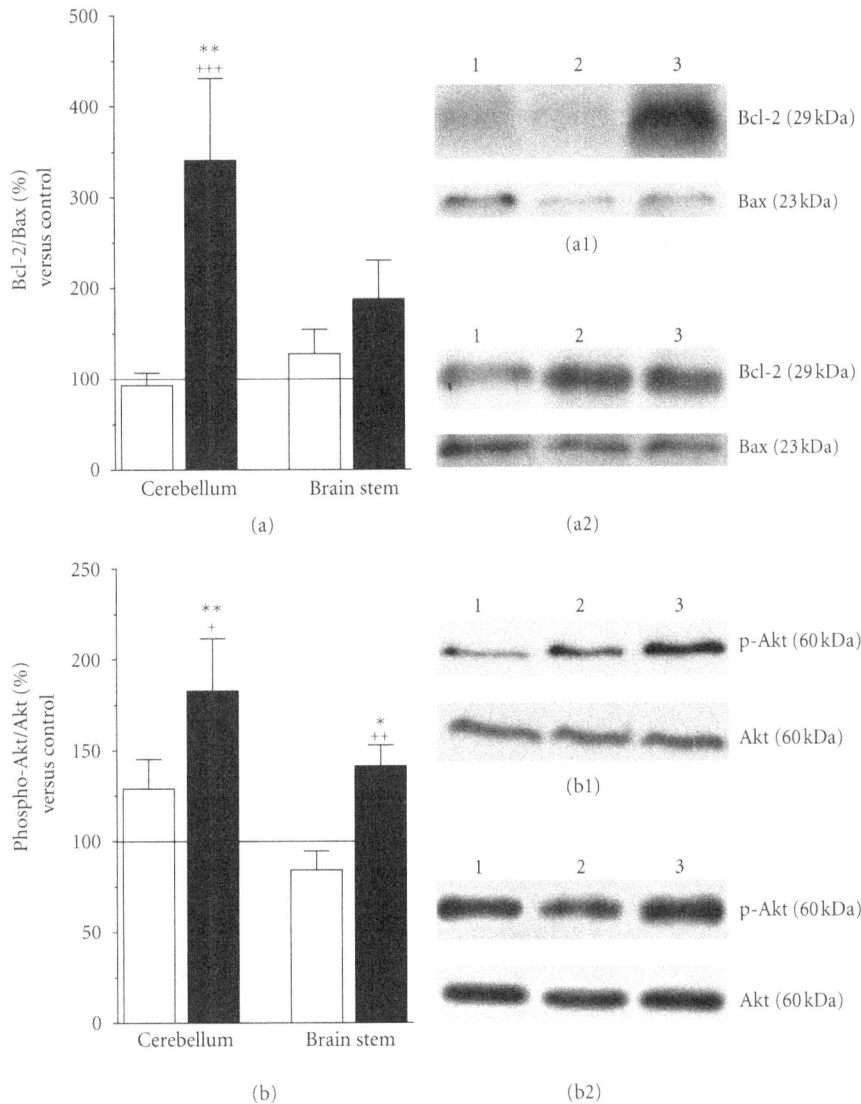

FIGURE 7: HuUCBMCs grafts upregulate Bcl-2 and phospho-Akt protein levels in the cerebellum and brain stem of 3-AP ataxic rats. HuUCBMCs transplantation raises the ratio Bcl2/Bax in the cerebellum of 3-AP-lesioned rats (a, black bars). Note how this effect is due to an increase in the expression of the antiapoptotic protein Bcl-2 (a1). HuUCBMCs also upregulate the ratio phospho-Akt/Akt in the cerebellum and brain stem of 3-AP ataxic rats (b, black bars). In both structures cell transplantation significantly enhances phospho-Akt levels (b1, b2), which is a protein involved in neuronal survival. (a1) and (a2) show representative blots for Bcl-2 and Bax, and (b1) and (b2) for phospho-Akt and Akt in the cerebellum (a1, b1) and brain stem (a2, b2). Lane 1: naïve rats (control); lane 2: 3-AP-lesioned rats treated with vehicle (3-AP + vehicle); lane 3: 3-AP-lesioned rats treated with HuUCBMCs grafts (3-AP + cells). Results represent the mean ± SEM of 9 to 15 individual animals. $*P \leq 0.05$, $**P \leq 0.01$ versus naïve rats, $^{+}P \leq 0.05$, $^{++}P \leq 0.01$, $^{+++}P \leq 0.001$ versus 3-AP + vehicle rats.

hypoxia with a transient up-regulation of microglial activity [62]. By contrast, the blockage of microglia activation enhanced neuroprotection and functional recovery induced by HuUCBMCs grafts in cortical ischemia [63]. Whether HuUCBMCs-driven activated microglia mediates the up-regulation of neuronal markers in the brain stem of 3-AP-lesioned rats or not, will be analyzed in the near future by blocking microglia activation with agents such as minocycline.

Up-regulation of GFAP is a feature of reactive astrocytes that was reported in the cerebellum of ataxic rats [64, 65], and patients suffering from progressive ataxia [66]. In

agreement with those studies, we found increased GFAP protein levels in the cerebellum of 3-AP ataxic rats. This overexpression of GFAP could be the consequence of glial activation induced by a loss of neurons, as has been reported in several diseases and neuropathologies [67–69]. Although we did not analyze the number of neurons in the cerebellum, we found that 3-AP significantly decreased the expression of the neuronal markers calbindin and NeuN.

Rat umbilical cord stem cells grafts prevented reactive astrogliosis and rendered neuronal protection in the hippocampus of ischemic rats [70]. In our study, HuUCBMCs transplantation reduced GFAP protein levels and immunoreactivity, but was unable to prevent the fall in calbindin and NeuN levels due to 3-AP neurotoxicity in the cerebellum. These results suggest that grafted cells could be involved in the modulation of astrogliosis, but they are not enough efficient to prevent neuronal damage in the cerebellum of 3-AP-ataxic rats.

An interesting finding was that HuUCBMCs transplantation modulated the expression of proteins involved in cell survival. As shown here, intravenous administration of HuUCBMCs significantly raised the phospho-Akt/Akt ratio in the cerebellum and brain stem of 3-AP + cell-treated rats. This effect was due to an increase in phospho-Akt levels, while total Akt remained unchanged in both structures. As other studies have shown that phospho-Akt plays a critical role in the regulation of neuronal survival induced by HuUCBMCs [71, 72], we may consider that this protein could mediate the neuroprotective activity of HuUCBMCs grafts observed in the brain stem. Phospho-Akt also contributes to glial cells survival [72–74]. However, there are no reports showing its possible role in preventing astrogliosis to our knowledge. The PI3K/Akt-signaling pathway regulates the expression of the antiapoptotic factor Bcl-2 [69, 75–77]. Here we found that HuUCBMCs grafts upregulated Bcl-2 protein expression in the cerebellum of 3-AP-lesioned rats. Bcl-2 overexpression enhanced the survival of different types of neurons [69, 77, 78], including those of the granular layer of the cerebellum [79]. Additionally, Bcl-2 may contribute to the maintenance of grafted cells in the cerebellum of 3-AP ataxic rats. In fact, Bcl-2 overexpression mediated the survival of human hematopoietic precursors during fetal life [80] and prolonged the survival of myoblasts transplantation in acute myocardial infarction [81] and chronic heart failure [82].

Finally, our results show that HuUCBMCs implantation ameliorates motor coordination in 3-AP-lesioned rat. This beneficial effect was probably due to neuronal protection elicited by the graft in the brain stem. In addition, HuUCBMCs could modulate neuronal activity in ataxic rats. In this respect, our preliminary studies have detected increased levels of glutamate and GABA in the brain stem of 3-AP-lesioned rats that were significantly reduced to basal levels in those animals receiving HuUCBMCs grafts (our unpublished observations). Under our experimental conditions, functional improvement was not maintained up to one month after transplantation. Recent studies have reported that repeated injections of HuUCBCs improved motor skills in ataxic mice and functional symptoms in patients with hereditary ataxia for longer periods of time [39, 40]. We administered a single intravenous injection of 4.5×10^6 cells/rat, so further experiments are needed to determine the effectiveness of the repeated application of HuUCBMCs in the 3-AP-experimental model of cerebellar ataxia.

5. Conclusions

In summary, our results show that intravenous administered HuUCBMCs reach the cerebellum and brain stem of 3-AP-lesioned rats. Implanted cells stimulate the expression of proteins involved in cell survival in both structures. These proteins could mediate the survival of grafted cells, and the neuroprotective effect observed in the brain stem of ataxic rats. As HuUCBMCs grafts also ameliorate motor coordination in 3-AP-lesioned rats, they can be considered as a potential source of cells useful for cerebellar disorders treatment.

Author Contributions

L. Calatrava-Ferreras, R. Gonzalo-Gobernado, A. S. Herranz, and D. Reimers made the experimental design. L. Calatrava-Ferreras, R. Gonzalo-Gobernado, A. S. Herranz, D. Reimers, T. Montero Vega, L. A. R. López, and E. Bazán contributed in experimental realization. L. Calatrava-Ferreras, R. Gonzalo-Gobernado, A. S. Herranz, D. Reimers, and E. Bazán carried out data analysis. L. Calatrava-Ferreras, R. Gonzalo-Gobernado, A. S. Herranz, D. Reimers, A. Jiménez-Escrig, and E. Bazán wrote the paper.

Acknowledgments

This work was funded by Agencia Pedro Laín Entralgo (NDG7/09) and Fundación Ataxias en Movimiento. L. Calatrava-Ferreras and R. Gonzalo-Gobernado were the recipients of Agencia Pedro Laín Entralgo fellowship and Contrato de Personal de Apoyo a la Investigación (Fondo de Investigaciones Sanitarias), respectively. We are grateful to Maria José Asensio and Judit Muñoz for technical help and Kerry Davis for her paper.

References

[1] D. Marmolino and M. Manto, "Past, present and future therapeutics for cerebellar ataxias," *Current Neuropharmacology*, vol. 8, no. 1, pp. 41–61, 2010.

[2] A. M. Fernandez, E. M. Carro, C. Lopez-Lopez, and I. Torres-Aleman, "Insulin-like growth factor I treatment for cerebellar ataxia: addressing a common pathway in the pathological cascade?" *Brain Research Reviews*, vol. 50, no. 1, pp. 134–141, 2005.

[3] T. Klockgether, "Ataxias," *Parkinsonism & Related Disorders*, vol. 13, supplement 3, pp. S391–S394, 2007.

[4] T. Klockgether, "Update on degenerative ataxias," *Current Opinion in Neurology*, vol. 24, no. 4, pp. 339–345, 2011.

[5] M. Manto and D. Marmolino, "Cerebellar ataxias," *Current Opinion in Neurology*, vol. 22, no. 4, pp. 419–429, 2009.

[6] F. Lim, G. M. Palomo, C. Mauritz et al., "Functional recovery in a Friedreich's ataxia mouse model by frataxin gene transfer using an HSV-1 amplicon vector," *Molecular Therapy*, vol. 15, no. 6, pp. 1072–1078, 2007.

[7] M. Pandolfo, "Drug Insight: antioxidant therapy in inherited ataxias," *Nature Clinical Practice Neurology*, vol. 4, no. 2, pp. 86–96, 2008.

[8] M. Voncken, P. Ioannou, and M. B. Delatycki, "Friedreich ataxia—update on pathogenesis and possible therapies," *Neurogenetics*, vol. 5, no. 1, pp. 1–8, 2004.

[9] A. M. Fernandez, A. G. de la Vega, and I. Torres-Aleman, "Insulin-like growth factor I restores motor coordination in a rat model of cerebellar ataxia," *Proceedings of the National*

Academy of Sciences of the United States of America, vol. 95, no. 3, pp. 1253–1258, 1998.

[10] D. L. Tolbert and B. R. Clark, "GDNF and IGF-I trophic factors delay hereditary Purkinje cell degeneration and the progression of gait ataxia," *Experimental Neurology*, vol. 183, no. 1, pp. 205–219, 2003.

[11] P. J. Vig, S. H. Subramony, D. R. D'Souza, J. Wei, and M. E. Lopez, "Intranasal administration of IGF-I improves behavior and Purkinje cell pathology in SCA1 mice," *Brain Research Bulletin*, vol. 69, no. 5, pp. 573–579, 2006.

[12] A. M. Fernandez, A. G. de la Vega, B. Planas, and I. Torres-Aleman, "Neuroprotective actions of peripherally administered insulin-like growth factor I in the injured olivo-cerebellar pathway," *European Journal of Neuroscience*, vol. 11, no. 6, pp. 2019–2030, 1999.

[13] J. Zhong, J. Deng, J. Phan et al., "Insulin-like growth factor-I protects granule neurons from apoptosis and improves ataxia in weaver mice," *Journal of Neuroscience Research*, vol. 80, no. 4, pp. 481–490, 2005.

[14] P. Bigini, P. Veglianese, G. Andriolo et al., "Intracerebroventricular administration of human umbilical cord blood cells delays disease progression in two murine models of motor neuron degeneration," *Rejuvenation Research*, vol. 14, no. 6, pp. 623–639, 2011.

[15] S. Erceg, M. Ronaghi, I. Zipancic et al., "Efficient differentiation of human embryonic stem cells into functional cerebellar-like cells," *Stem Cells and Development*, vol. 19, no. 11, pp. 1745–1756, 2010.

[16] D. H. Park, D. J. Eve, Y. G. Chung, and P. R. Sanberg, "Regenerative medicine for neurological disorders," *The Scientific World Journal*, vol. 10, pp. 470–489, 2010.

[17] S. Pluchino, L. Zanotti, M. Deleidi, and G. Martino, "Neural stem cells and their use as therapeutic tool in neurological disorders," *Brain Research Reviews*, vol. 48, no. 2, pp. 211–219, 2005.

[18] D. Reimers, C. Osuna, R. Gonzalo-Gobernado et al., "Liver growth factor promotes the survival of grafted neural stem cells in a rat model of Parkinson's disease," *Current Stem Cell Research & Therapy*, vol. 7, no. 1, pp. 15–25, 2012.

[19] J. Sharp and H. S. Keirstead, "Stem cell-based cell replacement strategies for the central nervous system," *Neuroscience Letters*, vol. 456, no. 3, pp. 107–111, 2009.

[20] J. Dalous, J. Larghero, and O. Baud, "Transplantation of umbilical cord-derived mesenchymal stem cells as a novel strategy to protect the central nervous system: technical aspects, preclinical studies, and clinical perspectives," *Pediatric Research*, vol. 71, no. 4, part 2, pp. 482–490, 2012.

[21] D. T. Harris, "Cord blood stem cells: a review of potential neurological applications," *Stem Cell Reviews*, vol. 4, no. 4, pp. 269–274, 2008.

[22] A. S. Herranz, R. Gonzalo-Gobernado, D. Reimers, M. J. Asensio, M. Rodríguez-Serrano, and E. Bazán, "Applications of human umbilical cord blood cells in central nervous system regeneration," *Current Stem Cell Research & Therapy*, vol. 5, no. 1, pp. 17–22, 2010.

[23] P. R. Sanberg, D. J. Eve, A. E. Willing et al., "The treatment of neurodegenerative disorders using umbilical cord blood and menstrual blood-derived stem cells," *Cell Transplantation*, vol. 20, no. 1, pp. 85–94, 2011.

[24] Y. Zhao, H. Wang, and T. Mazzone, "Identification of stem cells from human umbilical cord blood with embryonic and hematopoietic characteristics," *Experimental Cell Research*, vol. 312, no. 13, pp. 2454–2464, 2006.

[25] P. Rubinstein, C. Carrier, A. Scaradavou et al., "Outcomes among 562 recipients of placental-blood transplants from unrelated donors," *The New England Journal of Medicine*, vol. 339, no. 22, pp. 1565–1577, 1998.

[26] A. R. Bicknese, H. S. Goodwin, C. O. Quinn, V. C. D. Henderson, S. N. Chien, and D. A. Wall, "Human umbilical cord blood cells can be induced to express markers for neurons and glia," *Cell Transplantation*, vol. 11, no. 3, pp. 261–264, 2002.

[27] L. Buzańska, E. K. Machaj, B. Zabłocka, Z. Pojda, and K. Domańskka-Janik, "Human cord blood-derived cells attain neuronal and glial features *in vitro*," *Journal of Cell Science*, vol. 115, part 10, pp. 2131–2138, 2002.

[28] N. Chen, J. E. Hudson, P. Walczak et al., "Human umbilical cord blood progenitors: the potential of these hematopoietic cells to become neural," *Stem Cells*, vol. 23, no. 10, pp. 1560–1570, 2005.

[29] A. Habich, M. Jurga, I. Markiewicz, B. Lukomska, U. Bany-Laszewicz, and K. Domanska-Janik, "Early appearance of stem/progenitor cells with neural-like characteristics in human cord blood mononuclear fraction cultured *in vitro*," *Experimental Hematology*, vol. 34, no. 7, pp. 914–925, 2006.

[30] J. R. Sanchez-Ramos, S. Song, S. G. Kamath et al., "Expression of neural markers in human umbilical cord blood," *Experimental Neurology*, vol. 171, no. 1, pp. 109–115, 2001.

[31] T. Zigova, S. Song, A. E. Willing et al., "Human umbilical cord blood cells express neural antigens after transplantation into the developing rat brain," *Cell Transplantation*, vol. 11, no. 3, pp. 265–274, 2002.

[32] E. Gluckman, H. E. Broxmeyer, A. D. Auerbach et al., "Hematopoietic reconstitution in a patient with Fanconi's anemia by means of umbilical-cord blood from an HLA-identical sibling," *The New England Journal of Medicine*, vol. 321, no. 17, pp. 1174–1178, 1989.

[33] H. Arien-Zakay, S. Lecht, M. M. Bercu et al., "Neuroprotection by cord blood neural progenitors involves antioxidants, neurotrophic and angiogenic factors," *Experimental Neurology*, vol. 216, no. 1, pp. 83–94, 2009.

[34] N. Chen, S. Kamath, J. Newcomb et al., "Trophic factor induction of human umbilical cord blood cells *in vitro* and *in vivo*," *Journal of Neural Engineering*, vol. 4, no. 2, pp. 130–145, 2007.

[35] W. V. Nikolic, H. Hou, T. Town et al., "Peripherally administered human umbilical cord blood cells reduce parenchymal and vascular β-amyloid deposits in Alzheimer mice," *Stem Cells and Development*, vol. 17, no. 3, pp. 423–439, 2008.

[36] I. Zwart, A. J. Hill, F. Al-Allaf et al., "Umbilical cord blood mesenchymal stromal cells are neuroprotective and promote regeneration in a rat optic tract model," *Experimental Neurology*, vol. 216, no. 2, pp. 439–448, 2009.

[37] S. Erceg, V. Moreno-Manzano, M. Garita-Hernandez, M. Stojkovic, and S. S. Bhattacharya, "Concise review: stem cells for the treatment of cerebellar-related disorders," *Stem Cells*, vol. 29, no. 4, pp. 564–569, 2011.

[38] K. Kemp, E. Mallam, K. Hares, J. Witherick, N. Scolding, and A. Wilkins, "Mesenchymal stem cells restore frataxin expression and increase hydrogen peroxide scavenging enzymes in Friedreich ataxia fibroblasts," *PLoS ONE*, vol. 6, no. 10, Article ID e26098, 2011.

[39] W. Z. Yang, Y. Zhang, F. Wu et al., "Human umbilical cord blood-derived mononuclear cell transplantation: case series of 30 subjects with hereditary ataxia," *Journal of Translational Medicine*, vol. 9, article 65, 2011.

[40] M. J. Zhang, J. J. Sun, L. Qian et al., "Human umbilical mesenchymal stem cells enhance the expression of neurotrophic factors and protect ataxic mice," *Brain Research*, vol. 1402, pp. 122–131, 2011.

[41] H. Aoki and I. Sugihara, "Morphology of single olivocerebellar axons in the denervation-reinnervation model produced by subtotal lesion of the rat inferior olive," *Brain Research*, vol. 1449, pp. 24–37, 2012.

[42] S. Ausim Azizi, "And the olive said to the cerebellum: organization and functional significance of the olivo-cerebellar system," *The Neuroscientist*, vol. 13, no. 6, pp. 616–625, 2007.

[43] S. Garbuzova-Davis, A. E. Willing, T. Zigova et al., "Intravenous administration of human umbilical cord blood cells in a mouse model of amyotrophic lateral sclerosis: distribution, migration, and differentiation," *Journal of Hematotherapy and Stem Cell Research*, vol. 12, no. 3, pp. 255–270, 2003.

[44] G. Paxinos and C. Watson, *The Rat Brain in Stereotaxic Coordinates*, 1997.

[45] A. Carlsson and M. Lindqvist, "Effect of ethanol on the hydroxylation of tyrosine and tryptophan in rat brain *in vivo*," *Journal of Pharmacy and Pharmacology*, vol. 25, no. 6, pp. 437–440, 1973.

[46] L. Calatrava, R. Gonzalo-Gobernado, D. Reimers et al., "Acción Neuroprotectora del Factor de Crecimiento del Higado (LGF) en un modelo experimental de ataxia cerebelosa," in *Proceedings of the XIV Congreso Nacional de la Sociedad Española de Neurociencia*, Salamanca, Spain, September 2011.

[47] K. Frebel and S. Wiese, "Signalling molecules essential for neuronal survival and differentiation," *Biochemical Society Transactions*, vol. 34, part 6, pp. 1287–1290, 2006.

[48] A. Gross, J. M. McDonnell, and S. J. Korsmeyer, "BCL-2 family members and the mitochondria in apoptosis," *Genes and Development*, vol. 13, no. 15, pp. 1899–1911, 1999.

[49] S. I. Lee, B. G. Kim, D. H. Hwang, H. M. Kim, and S. U. Kim, "Overexpression of Bcl-XL in human neural stem cells promotes graft survival and functional recovery following transplantation in spinal cord injury," *Journal of Neuroscience Research*, vol. 87, no. 14, pp. 3186–3197, 2009.

[50] N. Noshita, A. Lewén, T. Sugawara, and P. H. Chan, "Evidence of phosphorylation of Akt and neuronal survival after transient focal cerebral ischemia in mice," *Journal of Cerebral Blood Flow and Metabolism*, vol. 21, no. 12, pp. 1442–1450, 2001.

[51] K. Chakrabarty, T. Serchov, S. A. Mann, I. D. Dietzel, and R. Heumann, "Enhancement of dopaminergic properties and protection mediated by neuronal activation of Ras in mouse ventral mesencephalic neurones," *European Journal of Neuroscience*, vol. 25, no. 7, pp. 1971–1981, 2007.

[52] E. J. Sanders, E. Parker, and S. Harvey, "Growth hormone-mediated survival of embryonic retinal ganglion cells: signaling mechanisms," *General and Comparative Endocrinology*, vol. 156, no. 3, pp. 613–621, 2008.

[53] P. Shah, B. B. Nankova, S. Parab, and E. F. La Gamma, "Short chain fatty acids induce TH gene expression via ERK-dependent phosphorylation of CREB protein," *Brain Research*, vol. 1107, no. 1, pp. 13–23, 2006.

[54] W. H. Zheng and R. Quirion, "Insulin-like growth factor-1 (IGF-1) induces the activation/phosphorylation of Akt kinase and cAMP response element-binding protein (CREB) by activating different signaling pathways in PC12 cells," *BMC Neuroscience*, vol. 7, article 51, 2006.

[55] J. Y. Lim, S. I. Park, J. H. Oh et al., "Brain-derived neurotrophic factor stimulates the neural differentiation of human umbilical cord blood-derived mesenchymal stem cells and survival of differentiated cells through MAPK/ERK and PI3K/Akt-dependent signaling pathways," *Journal of Neuroscience Research*, vol. 86, no. 10, pp. 2168–2178, 2008.

[56] C. B. Low, Y. C. Liou, and B. L. Tang, "Neural differentiation and potential use of stem cells from the human umbilical cord for central nervous system transplantation therapy," *Journal of Neuroscience Research*, vol. 86, no. 8, pp. 1670–1679, 2008.

[57] C. V. Borlongan, M. Hadman, C. D. Sanberg, and P. R. Sanberg, "Central nervous system entry of peripherally injected umbilical cord blood cells is not required for neuroprotection in stroke," *Stroke*, vol. 35, no. 10, pp. 2385–2389, 2004.

[58] M. Czeh, P. Gressens, and A. M. Kaindl, "The yin and yang of microglia," *Developmental Neuroscience*, vol. 33, no. 3-4, pp. 199–209, 2011.

[59] E. Polazzi and A. Contestabile, "Reciprocal interactions between microglia and neurons: from survival to neuropathology," *Reviews in the Neurosciences*, vol. 13, no. 3, pp. 221–242, 2002.

[60] S. Rivest, "The promise of anti-inflammatory therapies for CNS injuries and diseases," *Expert Review of Neurotherapeutics*, vol. 11, no. 6, pp. 783–786, 2011.

[61] W. J. Streit, "Microglia as neuroprotective, immunocompetent cells of the CNS," *GLIA*, vol. 40, no. 2, pp. 133–139, 2002.

[62] S. H. Bae, T. H. Kong, H. S. Lee et al., "Long-lasting paracrine effects of human cord blood cells (hUCBCs) on damaged neocortex in an animal model of cerebral palsy," *Cell Transplantation*. In press.

[63] E. C. Franco, M. M. Cardoso, A. Gouveia, A. Pereira, and W. Gomes-Leal, "Modulation of microglial activation enhances neuroprotection and functional recovery derived from bone marrow mononuclear cell transplantation after cortical ischemia," *Neuroscience Research*, vol. 73, no. 2, pp. 122–132, 2012.

[64] A. M. Fernandez, J. Garcia-Estrada, L. M. Garcia-Segura, and I. Torres-Aleman, "Insulin-like growth factor I modulates c-Fos induction and astrocytosis in response to neurotoxic insult," *Neuroscience*, vol. 76, no. 1, pp. 117–122, 1996.

[65] J. Shi, Y. Ma, M. Zheng et al., "Effect of sub-acute exposure to acrylamide on GABAergic neurons and astrocytes in weaning rat cerebellum," *Toxicology and Industrial Health*, vol. 28, no. 1, pp. 10–20, 2012.

[66] M. Mittelbronn, J. Schittenhelm, G. Bakos et al., "CD8+/perforin+/granzyme B+ effector cells infiltrating cerebellum and inferior olives in gluten ataxia," *Neuropathology*, vol. 30, no. 1, pp. 92–96, 2010.

[67] A. Buffo, C. Rolando, and S. Ceruti, "Astrocytes in the damaged brain: molecular and cellular insights into their reactive response and healing potential," *Biochemical Pharmacology*, vol. 79, no. 2, pp. 77–89, 2010.

[68] A. Chvatal, M. Anderova, H. Neprasova et al., "Pathological potential of astroglia," *Physiological Research*, vol. 57, supplement 3, pp. S101–S110, 2008.

[69] D. Zhang, X. Hu, L. Qian, J. P. O'Callaghan, and J. S. Hong, "Astrogliosis in CNS pathologies: is there a role for microglia?" *Molecular Neurobiology*, vol. 41, no. 2-3, pp. 232–241, 2010.

[70] A. C. Hirko, R. Dallasen, S. Jomura, and Y. Xu, "Modulation of inflammatory responses after global ischemia by transplanted umbilical cord matrix stem cells," *Stem Cells*, vol. 26, no. 11, pp. 2893–2901, 2008.

[71] V. R. Dasari, D. G. Spomar, L. Li, M. Gujrati, J. S. Rao, and D. H. Dinh, "Umbilical cord blood stem cell mediated downregulation of fas improves functional recovery of rats

after spinal cord injury," *Neurochemical Research*, vol. 33, no. 1, pp. 134–149, 2008.

[72] V. R. Dasari, K. K. Veeravalli, K. L. Saving et al., "Neuroprotection by cord blood stem cells against glutamate-induced apoptosis is mediated by Akt pathway," *Neurobiology of Disease*, vol. 32, no. 3, pp. 486–498, 2008.

[73] B. Gabryel, A. Pudelko, and A. Malecki, "Erk1/2 and Akt kinases are involved in the protective effect of aniracetam in astrocytes subjected to simulated ischemia *in vitro*," *European Journal of Pharmacology*, vol. 494, no. 2-3, pp. 111–120, 2004.

[74] D. D. Rowe, C. C. Leonardo, J. A. Recio, L. A. Collier, A. E. Willing, and K. R. Pennypacker, "Human umbilical cord blood cells protect oligodendrocytes from brain ischemia through Akt signal transduction," *The Journal of Biological Chemistry*, vol. 287, no. 6, pp. 4177–4187, 2012.

[75] T. K. Creson, P. Yuan, H. K. Manji, and G. Chen, "Evidence for involvement of ERK, PI3K, and RSK in induction of Bcl-2 by valproate," *Journal of Molecular Neuroscience*, vol. 37, no. 2, pp. 123–134, 2009.

[76] M. Tamatani, Y. H. Che, H. Matsuzaki et al., "Tumor necrosis factor induces Bcl-2 and Bcl-x expression through NFκB activation in primary hippocampal neurons," *The Journal of Biological Chemistry*, vol. 274, no. 13, pp. 8531–8538, 1999.

[77] H. Matsuzaki, M. Tamatani, N. Mitsuda et al., "Activation of Akt kinase inhibits apoptosis and changes in Bcl-2 and Bax expression induced by nitric oxide in primary hippocampal neurons," *Journal of Neurochemistry*, vol. 73, no. 5, pp. 2037–2046, 1999.

[78] T. Sasaki, K. Kitagawa, Y. Yagita et al., "Bcl2 enhances survival of newborn neurons in the normal and ischemic hippocampus," *Journal of Neuroscience Research*, vol. 84, no. 6, pp. 1187–1196, 2006.

[79] L. Lossi, G. Gambino, F. Ferrini, S. Alasia, and A. Merighi, "Posttranslational regulation of BCL2 levels in cerebellar granule cells: a mechanism of neuronal survival," *Developmental Neurobiology*, vol. 69, no. 13, pp. 855–870, 2009.

[80] A. Bonati, R. Albertini, D. Garau et al., "BCL2 oncogene protein expression in human hematopoietic precursors during fetal life," *Experimental Hematology*, vol. 24, no. 3, pp. 459–465, 1996.

[81] K. Kitabayashi, A. Siltanen, T. Pätilä et al., "Bcl-2 expression enhances myoblast sheet transplantation therapy for acute myocardial infarction," *Cell Transplantation*, vol. 19, no. 5, pp. 573–588, 2010.

[82] A. Siltanen, K. Kitabayashi, T. Pätilä et al., "Bcl-2 improves myoblast sheet therapy in rat chronic heart failure," *Tissue Engineering A*, vol. 17, no. 1-2, pp. 115–125, 2011.

10

Gas7 Is Required for Mesenchymal Stem Cell-Derived Bone Development

Chuck C.-K. Chao, Feng-Chun Hung, and Jack J. Chao

Department of Biochemistry and Molecular Biology and Institute of Biomedical Sciences, College of Medicine, Chang Gung University, Taoyuan 333, Taiwan

Correspondence should be addressed to Chuck C.-K. Chao; cckchao@mail.cgu.edu.tw

Academic Editor: Gaël Y. Rochefort

Mesenchymal stem cells (MSCs) can differentiate into osteoblasts and lead to bone formation in the body. Osteoblast differentiation and bone development are regulated by a network of molecular signals and transcription factors induced by several proteins, including BMP2, osterix, and Runx2. We recently observed that the growth-arrest-specific 7 gene (Gas7) is upregulated during differentiation of human MSCs into osteoblasts. Downregulation of Gas7 using short-hairpin RNA decreased the expression of Runx2, a master regulator of osteogenesis, and its target genes (alkaline phosphatase, type I collagen, osteocalcin, and osteopontin). In addition, knockdown of Gas7 decreased the mineralization of dexamethasone-treated MSCs in culture. Conversely, ectopic expression of Gas7 induced Runx2-dependent transcriptional activity and gene expression leading to osteoblast differentiation and matrix mineralization. Genetic mutations of the Gas7 gene increased body fat levels and decreased bone density in mice. These results showed that Gas7 plays a role in regulating the pathways which are essential for osteoblast differentiation and bone development. In this review, we summarize the involvement of Gas7 in MSC-based osteogenesis and osteoporosis and describe the possible mechanisms responsible for the maintenance of cellular homeostasis in MSCs and osteoblasts.

1. Gas7: A *Pombe* Cdc15 Homology Protein

The Gas7 protein is part of the Pombe Cdc 15 homology (PCH) family which belongs to the proline, serine, threonine-rich phosphatase interacting protein (PSTPIP) subfamily [1, 2]. Gas7 was initially identified as an upregulated gene in NIH3T3 cells cultured without serum, and the structure of the encoded protein showed homology to Oct2 and synapsins, proteins involved, respectively, in neuron development, and neurotransmitter release [3, 4]. Gas7 is selectively expressed in mature cerebellar neurons, cerebral cortical neurons, and hippocampal neurons [4, 5]. The human Gas7 gene is located on chromosome 17p12 (based on information provided by Ensembl and UDB/GeneLoc). Open reading frame analysis of the 412 amino acid-coding Gas7 gene predicted the production of a 47,266-Da protein. Gas7a and Gas7b protein isoforms, which are obtained by alternative splicing, have also been described [6].

Several studies have been performed to examine the physiological functions of Gas7 in humans and rodents [3, 7].

These studies have shown that Gas7 is mainly expressed in the brain and is involved in morphological differentiation and neuritogenesis [3, 5–7]. These observations are consistent with the observed Gas7 expression pattern in normal human tissues based on the quantification of expressed sequence tags (ESTs) from various tissues in Unigene clusters. Gas7 isoforms also appear to be differentially expressed and regulated in the brain of rats after hippocampal neuron injury [5]. Recently, the neurite outgrowth of hippocampal neurons was shown to require the binding of Gas7 to N-WASP [8]. This binding required WW-Pro domains—unique to the PCH protein family—and was largely of the SH3-Pro type. These observations indicate that the binding between Gas7 and N-WASP may lead to formation of membrane protrusions, possibly via recruitment of the Arp2/3 complex and independently of Cdc42 [8]. Controlled expression of Gas7 also appears to be critical for tissue development since MLL-GAS7 translocations were detected in individuals suffering of treatment-related acute myeloid leukemia [9]. Other authors showed that Gas7b binds to the WW domain of Tau and that

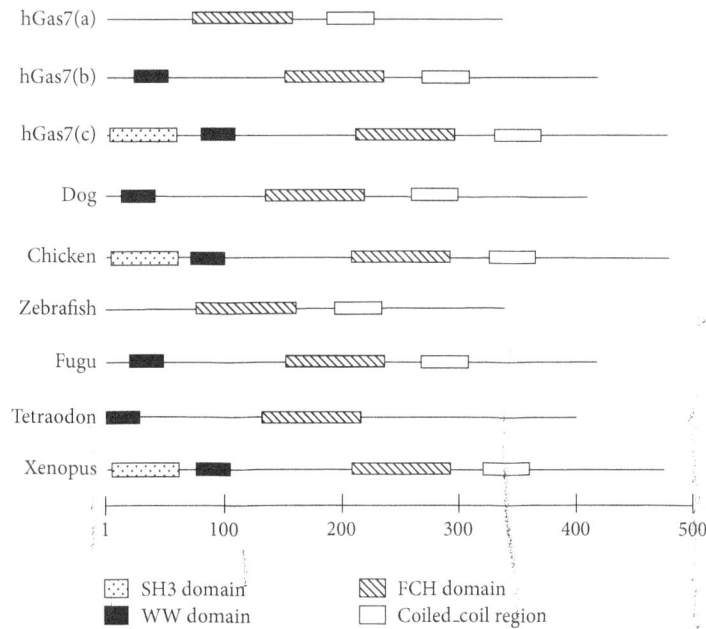

FIGURE 1: Domain structure of Gas7 protein isoforms. The Gas7 isoform b found in mammals possesses WW, Fes/CIP4 homology (FCH), and coiled-coil domains the Gas7 isoform c possesses an additional SH3 domain at the N-terminus. The number of amino acids for the proteins is indicated.

the Gas7b/Tau complex binds to microtubules in Neuro2A cells, a process which promotes tubulin polymerization [10]. Gas7b downregulation was shown to protect neuroblast cells against apoptosis in vitro [11]. Similar Gas7 genes have been identified in other organisms. Comparison of the predicted Gas7 proteins in these various organisms confirmed the conservation of unique protein domains (Figure 1).

These results illustrate that Gas7 is implicated in several cellular processes that are evolutionarily conserved in various species. Earlier, we also found a functional link between the expression of Gas7 and the processes of chondrogenesis and osteogenesis in human bone marrow-derived human MSCs [12, 13].

2. Mesenchymal Stem Cells

MSCs represent nonhematopoietic stem cells with the capacity to differentiate into various lineages, including osteoblastic, chondrogenic, and adipogenic lineages. Recent studies have shown that MSCs may also differentiate into other lineages, including neuronal and cardiomyogenic ones. Extracellular stimuli enable efficient initiation of mechanotransductive signaling which regulate stem cell fate. Examples include the effects of stereotopography and matrix stiffness on the fate of MSCs [14, 15]. Following their initial detection and isolation from bone marrow, MSCs have been harvested from many other tissues, including adipose tissue, muscles, tendons, placenta, liver, cartilage, spleen, and thymus. Our group has previously demonstrated that density gradient media is an efficient method to isolate marrow-derived human MSCs with osteogenic potential [16]. Their easy isolation and ex vivo expansion along with their immune-privileged nature make MSCs popular candidates for stem

cell-based regenerative therapies [17]. MSCs can alter disease pathophysiology in various ways, including by differentiating into various lineages, by leading to cytokine secretion and immune modulation, and by interacting with damaged and diseased tissues. The main characteristics of MSC biology, such as culture, differentiation capabilities, and homing mechanisms, have been extensively reviewed [18]. MSCs found in bone marrow and adipose tissue represent the common precursor which can differentiate into osteoblasts and adipocytes. Several transcription factors and extracellular and intracellular signals regulating adipogenesis and osteoblastogenesis have been identified. For instance, the Wnt/β-catenin pathway was shown to induce osteoblastogenesis and to inhibit adipogenesis, whereas the peroxisome proliferator activated receptor-γ (PPAR-γ) is a potent inducer of adipogenesis and inhibitor of osteoblastogenesis [19].

3. Gas7 in MSC-Based Osteogenesis

Over the last two decades, many factors have been identified that regulate cell differentiation. Runx2/Cbfa1 [20, 21], osterix [22], Msh homeobox 2 [23], BMP2 [24], Wnt, and Hedgehog [25] have all been shown to play a role in osteoblastogenesis [26, 27]. Similarly, PPAR-γ, CCAAT/enhancer binding protein (C/EBP) α and β, glucocorticoid receptor (GR), insulin, and Kruppel-like factor 5 (KLF5) have been identified as critical regulators of adipogenesis [28]. Notably, the primary inducer of adipogenesis, PPAR-γ, may inhibit osteoblastogenesis [29]. Functional crosstalk between Wnt and PPAR-γ signaling pathways regulating MSC differentiation have been discussed in detail [19]. Bone is a special tissue where calcium, osteocalcin, and amino acids represent extracellular signals regulating mineralization. Runx2, for example, represents an

(a)

(b)

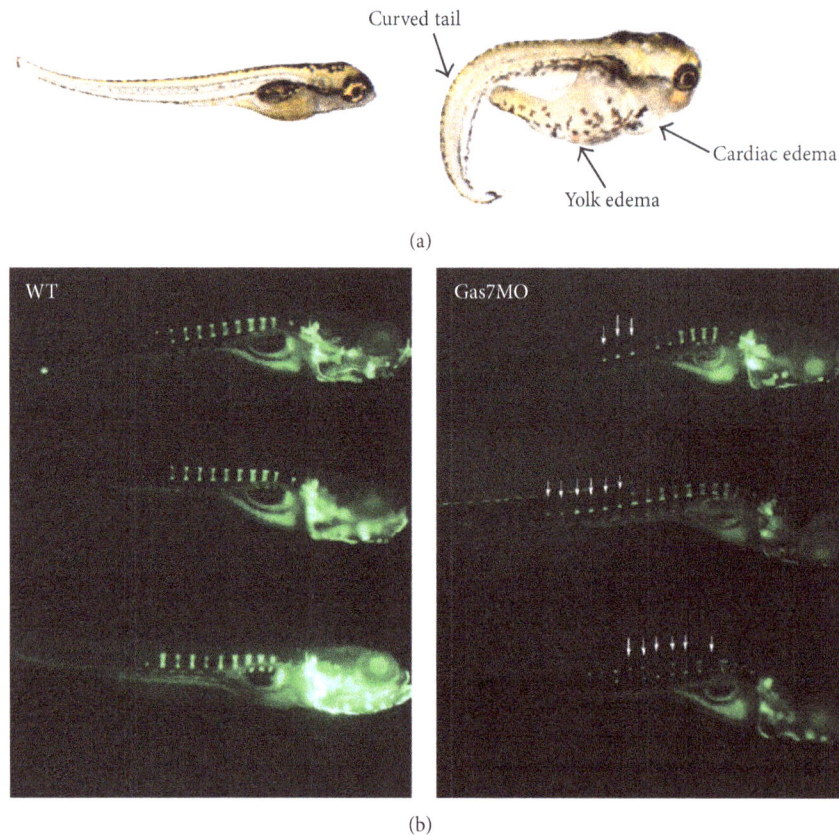

FIGURE 2: Abnormal bone structure and phenotypes in zebrafish embryos following Gas7 knockdown (Gas7MO). (a) Representative embryos with Gas7MO or control treatment (WT). (b) Abnormal bone structure in embryos with Gas7MO as revealed by fluorescence-labeled bone component.

essential transcription factor controlling osteoblast differentiation as seen from the observation that Runx2-deficient mice do not form bones due to the lack of osteoblasts [21, 30]. Consistent with these results, Runx2 mutations have been found in patients with cleidocranial dysplasia, a disease characterized by deformities in the collarbone and skull [31]. Following the commitment to osteogenesis mediated by Runx2, development of the bone cell phenotype is reinforced by osterix; accordingly, osterix-deficient preosteoblasts only express chondrocyte gene markers [22]. In addition, Runx2-overepressing mice produce abnormal osteoblasts showing impaired matrix production and mineralization [32, 33]. Therefore, Runx2 plays a critical role in controlling the commitment of multipotent mesenchymal cells to the osteoblastic lineage during bone formation. Several in vitro studies have shown that Runx2 can upregulate bone matrix gene expression, including bone sialoprotein, fibronectin, osteocalcin, osteopontin, and type I collagen [20, 27]. The role of Runx2-dependent transcriptional activation has been demonstrated through analysis of osteocalcin and type I collagen gene promoters [34, 35].

Recently, we observed that Gas7 represents a novel regulator of MSC-based osteogenesis [13]. Gas7 controls the differentiation of human MSCs into functional osteoblasts by enhancing Runx2-dependent gene expression. We observed that Gas7, specifically the b isoform (Gas7b), was upregulated during dexamethasone-induced differentiation of MSCs into osteoblasts. Downregulation of Gas7 using shRNA reduced the expression of Runx2 and its target genes alkaline phosphatase, osteocalcin, osteopontin, and type I collagen. In addition, knockdown of Gas7 reduced matrix mineralization of dexamethasone-treated MSCs in vitro. In contrast, overexpression of Gas7 induced gene expression associated with osteoblast differentiation and matrix mineralization, and also induced the mineralization of MSCs in vitro. Moreover, by using a gene reporter assay to monitor osteocalcin expression in human MSCs, we showed that Runx2-dependent transcriptional activity was enhanced by ectopic expression of Gas7. These observations demonstrated that Gas7 enhances Runx2-dependent gene expression and represents an endogenous regulator of osteogenic differentiation in human MSCs. The importance of Gas7 in early development was also observed in zebrafish [36]. Gas7 knockdown with Morpholino (MO) antisense oligonucleotides reduced bone density, shortened the vertebral column, and produced a curved body shape in laboratory animals (Figure 2). Gas7 knockdown caused defects that could be rescued by overexpression of Gas7 of either zebrafish or human origin. Further studies are under way to determine whether the regulatory effects of Gas7 require other protein partners.

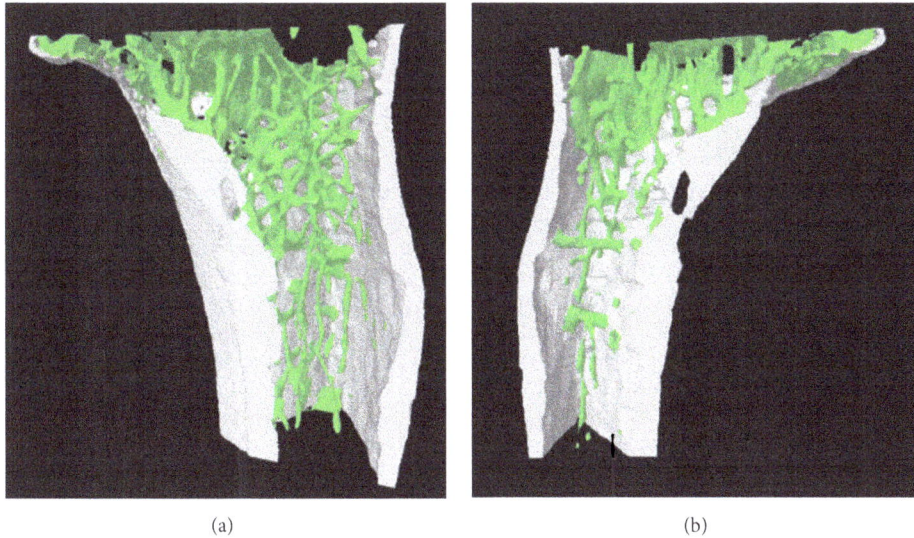

(a)   (b)

FIGURE 3: Reduced tibia bone density in gas7-knockout mouse. Volumetric images of trabecular and cortical bone were reconstructed using a commercial surface rendering program from series of micro-CT images. The images support the mass reduction in trabecular bone in gas7-knockout mice (b) compared to the wild-type group (a).

4. Gas7 in Osteoporosis

In a recent study, we provided a detailed account of the creation and characterization of Gas7-deficient mice that express a labile Gas7 mutant protein with the same properties of wild-type Gas7 [37]. Our data showed that Gas7 is involved in motor neuron function associated with muscle strength maintenance. Gas7 protein expression was not detected in bone-marrow MSCs prepared from Gas7 mutant mice. Notably, these mutant MSCs showed impaired osteogenesis (unpublished observations). Bone density in wild-type and Gas7 mutant mice was determined (Figure 3). Volumetric images of trabecular and cortical bone for each group were reconstructed using a commercial surface rendering program from series of micro-X-ray computed topography (CT) images. Other calculations of trabecular bone mass and fractal dimension in tibia bones also supported the observations of mass reduction in trabecular bones in male Gas7 mutant mice compared to the wild-type group. Consistent with our findings, other authors have reported that perturbation of Gas7, Me1, or Gpx3 leads to significant changes in mouse obesity-related traits [38]. Among the newly validated genes, Gas7 is thought to be involved in fat metabolism and other pathways, such as the insulin signaling pathway. Given that PPAR-γ, C/EBP α and β, GR, insulin, and KLF5 have been identified as essential regulators of adipogenesis [28], whether and how Gas7 functionally interacts with these transcription factors or their downstream gene products will be an interesting topic in future studies.

5. Concluding Remarks

Two signaling pathways that determine the differentiation of MSCs into adipocytes or osteoblasts by suppressing the transactivation function of PPAR-γ have been described. These signaling cascades promote osteoblastic differentiation from MSCs via two distinct modes of PPAR-γ transrepression. Recent studies indicate that certain differentiation factors may affect the biological activity of other regulators. For instance, differentiation factors regulating osteoblastogenesis inhibit adipogenesis and vice versa. Runx2-dependent gene expression and the differentiation of MSCs into osteoblasts enhance bone formation. Gas7 also plays a role in regulating the pathways, which are essential for osteoblast differentiation and bone development, probably through the induction of undetermined factors that interact with Runx2. The role of Gas7 in regulating these pathways is under intense investigation and may lead to novel therapies. Current therapies for osteoporosis are mainly based on the prevention of bone resorption by treatment with bisphosphonates and selective estrogen receptor modulators [39]. However, serious side effects have been reported for these drugs, particularly an increased incidence of breast and ovarian cancers [40]. Induction of osteoblastogenesis may prove to be beneficial for the treatment of osteoporosis. We expect that shifting the focus from inhibition of bone resorption to stimulation of bone formation may lead to the development of better strategies to prevent and treat osteoporosis.

Acknowledgments

The authors would like to thank the members of their research group for helpful discussions and Dr. S. J. Tu for help with micro-CT imaging analysis. This review is based on studies supported in part by the National Science Council (Taiwan), Chang Gung University and Chang Gung Memorial Hospital (Linkou, Taiwan), and the Foundation for the Advancement of Outstanding Scholarship.

References

[1] V. Chitu and E. R. Stanley, "Pombe Cdc15 homology (PCH) proteins: coordinators of membrane-cytoskeletal interactions," *Trends in Cell Biology*, vol. 17, no. 3, pp. 145–156, 2007.

[2] K. Tsujita, S. Suetsugu, N. Sasaki, M. Furutani, T. Oikawa, and T. Takenawa, "Coordination between the actin cytoskeleton and membrane deformation by a novel membrane tubulation domain of PCH proteins is involved in endocytosis," *The Journal of Cell Biology*, vol. 172, no. 2, pp. 269–279, 2006.

[3] Y.-T. Ju, A. C. Y. Chang, B.-R. She et al., "gas7: a gene expressed preferentially in growth-arrested fibroblasts and terminally differentiated Purkinje neurons affects neurite formation," *Proceedings of the National Academy of Sciences of the United States of America*, vol. 95, no. 19, pp. 11423–11428, 1998.

[4] P. P. Moorthy, A. A. Kumar, and H. Devaraj, "Expression of the gas7 gene and Oct4 in embryonic stem cells of mice," *Stem Cells and Development*, vol. 14, no. 6, pp. 664–670, 2005.

[5] P.-Y. Chang, J.-T. Kuo, S. Lin-Chao, and C. C.-K. Chao, "Identification of rat Gas7 isoforms differentially expressed in brain and regulated following kainate-induced neuronal injury," *Journal of Neuroscience Research*, vol. 79, no. 6, pp. 788–797, 2005.

[6] C. C.-K. Chao, P.-Y. Chang, and H. H.-P. Lu, "Human Gas7 isoforms homologous to mouse transcripts differentially induce neurite outgrowth," *Journal of Neuroscience Research*, vol. 81, no. 2, pp. 153–162, 2005.

[7] C. C.-K. Chao, L.-J. Su, N.-K. Sun, Y.-T. Ju, J. C.-J. Lih, and S. Lin-Chao, "Involvement of gas7 in nerve growth factor-independent and dependent cell processes in PC12 cells," *Journal of Neuroscience Research*, vol. 74, no. 2, pp. 248–254, 2003.

[8] J.-J. You and S. Lin-Chao, "Gas7 functions with N-WASP to regulate the neurite outgrowth of hippocampal neurons," *The Journal of Biological Chemistry*, vol. 285, no. 15, pp. 11652–11666, 2010.

[9] M. D. Megonigal, N.-K. V. Cheung, E. F. Rappaport et al., "Detection of leukemia-associated MLL-GAS7 translocation early during chemotherapy with DNA topoisomerase II inhibitors," *Proceedings of the National Academy of Sciences of the United States of America*, vol. 97, no. 6, pp. 2814–2819, 2000.

[10] H. Akiyama, A. Gotoh, R.-W. Shin et al., "A novel role for hGas7b in microtubular maintenance: possible implication in Tau-associated pathology in Alzheimer disease," *The Journal of Biological Chemistry*, vol. 284, no. 47, pp. 32695–32699, 2009.

[11] F.-C. Hung and C. C.-K. Chao, "Knockdown of growth-arrest-specific gene 7b (gas7b) using short-hairpin RNA desensitizes neuroblastoma cells to cisplatin: Implications for preventing apoptosis of neurons," *Journal of Neuroscience Research*, vol. 88, no. 16, pp. 3578–3587, 2010.

[12] Y. Chang, S. W. N. Ueng, S. Lin-Chao, and C. C.-K. Chao, "Involvement of Gas7 along the ERK1/2 MAP kinase and SOX9 pathway in chondrogenesis of human marrow-derived mesenchymal stem cells," *Osteoarthritis and Cartilage*, vol. 16, no. 11, pp. 1403–1412, 2008.

[13] F.-C. Hung, Y. Chang, S. Lin-Chao, and C. C.-K. Chao, "Gas7 mediates the differentiation of human bone marrow-derived mesenchymal stem cells into functional osteoblasts by enhancing Runx2-dependent gene expression," *Journal of Orthopaedic Research*, vol. 29, no. 10, pp. 1528–1535, 2011.

[14] S.-W. Kuo, H.-I. Lin, J. Hui-Chun Ho et al., "Regulation of the fate of human mesenchymal stem cells by mechanical and stereo-topographical cues provided by silicon nanowires," *Biomaterials*, vol. 33, no. 20, pp. 5013–5022, 2012.

[15] Y.-R. V. Shih, K.-F. Tseng, H.-Y. Lai, C.-H. Lin, and O. K. Lee, "Matrix stiffness regulation of integrin-mediated mechanotransduction during osteogenic differentiation of human mesenchymal stem cells," *Journal of Bone and Mineral Research*, vol. 26, no. 4, pp. 730–738, 2011.

[16] Y. Chang, P.-H. Hsieh, and C. C.-K. Chao, "The efficiency of using density gradient media in isolation of marrow-derived human mesenchymal stem cells with osteogenic potential," *Chang Gung Medical Journal*, vol. 32, no. 3, pp. 264–275, 2009.

[17] A. Arthur, A. Zannettino, and S. Gronthos, "The therapeutic applications of multipotential mesenchymal/stromal stem cells in skeletal tissue repair," *Journal of Cellular Physiology*, vol. 218, no. 2, pp. 237–245, 2009.

[18] F. Rastegar, D. Shenaq, J. Huang et al., "Mesenchymal stem cells: molecular characteristics and clinical applications," *World Journal of Stem Cells*, vol. 2, pp. 67–80, 2010.

[19] I. Takada, A. P. Kouzmenko, and S. Kato, "Molecular switching of osteoblastogenesis versus adipogenesis: implications for targeted therapies," *Expert Opinion on Therapeutic Targets*, vol. 13, no. 5, pp. 593–603, 2009.

[20] P. Ducy, R. Zhang, V. Geoffroy, A. L. Ridall, and G. Karsenty, "Osf2/Cbfa1: a transcriptional activator of osteoblast differentiation," *Cell*, vol. 89, no. 5, pp. 747–754, 1997.

[21] T. Komori, H. Yagi, S. Nomura et al., "Targeted disruption of Cbfa1 results in a complete lack of bone formation owing to maturational arrest of osteoblasts," *Cell*, vol. 89, no. 5, pp. 755–764, 1997.

[22] K. Nakashima, X. Zhou, G. Kunkel et al., "The novel zinc finger-containing transcription factor Osterix is required for osteoblast differentiation and bone formation," *Cell*, vol. 108, no. 1, pp. 17–29, 2002.

[23] D. A. Towler, S. J. Rutledge, and G. A. Rodan, "Msx-2/Hox 8.1: a transcriptional regulator of the rat osteocalcin promoter," *Molecular Endocrinology*, vol. 8, no. 11, pp. 1484–1493, 1994.

[24] T. Katagiri, A. Yamaguchi, T. Ikeda et al., "The non-osteogenic mouse pluripotent cell line, C3H10T1/2, is induced to differentiate into osteoblastic cells by recombinant human bone morphogenetic protein-2," *Biochemical and Biophysical Research Communications*, vol. 172, no. 1, pp. 295–299, 1990.

[25] B. Lanske, A. C. Karaplis, K. Lee et al., "PTH/PTHrP receptor in early development and Indian hedgehog-regulated bone growth," *Science*, vol. 273, no. 5275, pp. 663–666, 1996.

[26] T. Komori, "Regulation of bone development and maintenance by Runx2," *Frontiers in Bioscience*, vol. 13, no. 3, pp. 898–903, 2008.

[27] H. Harada, S. Tagashira, M. Fujiwara et al., "Cbfa1 isoforms exert functional differences in osteoblast differentiation," *The Journal of Biological Chemistry*, vol. 274, no. 11, pp. 6972–6978, 1999.

[28] S. Gesta, Y.-H. Tseng, and C. R. Kahn, "Developmental origin of fat: tracking obesity to Its source," *Cell*, vol. 131, no. 2, pp. 242–256, 2007.

[29] T. Akune, S. Ohba, S. Kamekura et al., "PPARγ insufficiency enhances osteogenesis through osteoblast formation from bone marrow progenitors," *The Journal of Clinical Investigation*, vol. 113, no. 6, pp. 846–855, 2004.

[30] F. Otto, A. P. Thornell, T. Crompton et al., "Cbfa1, a candidate gene for cleidocranial dysplasia syndrome, is essential for osteoblast differentiation and bone development," *Cell*, vol. 89, no. 5, pp. 765–771, 1997.

[31] S. Mundlos, F. Otto, C. Mundlos et al., "Mutations involving the transcription factor CBFA1 cause cleidocranial dysplasia," *Cell*, vol. 89, no. 5, pp. 773–779, 1997.

[32] V. Geoffroy, M. Kneissel, B. Fournier, A. Boyde, and P. Matthias, "High bone resorption in adult aging transgenic mice over-expressing Cbfa1/Runx2 in cells of the osteoblastic lineage," *Molecular and Cellular Biology*, vol. 22, no. 17, pp. 6222–6233, 2002.

[33] W. Liu, S. Toyosawa, T. Furuichi et al., "Overexpression of Cbfa1 in osteoblasts inhibits osteoblast maturation and causes osteopenia with multiple fractures," *The Journal of Cell Biology*, vol. 155, no. 1, pp. 157–166, 2001.

[34] M. H. Lee, A. Javed, H. J. Kim et al., "Transient upregulation of CBFA1 in response to bone morphogenetic protein-2 and transforming growth factor beta1 in C2C12 myogenic cells coincides with suppression of the myogenic phenotype but is not sufficient for osteoblast differentiation," *Journal of Cellular Biochemistry*, vol. 73, pp. 114–125, 1999.

[35] B. Kern, J. Shen, M. Starbuck, and G. Karsenty, "Cbfa1 contributes to the osteoblast-specific expression of type I collagen genes," *The Journal of Biological Chemistry*, vol. 276, no. 10, pp. 7101–7107, 2001.

[36] F. C. Hung, Y. C. Cheng, N. K. Sun, and C. C. Chao, "Identification and characterization of zebrafish gas7 gene in early development," *Journal of Neuroscience Research*, vol. 91, pp. 51–61, 2013.

[37] B. T. Huang, P. Y. Chang, C. H. Su, C. C. Chao, and S. Lin-Chao, "Gas7-deficient mouse reveals roles in motor function and muscle fiber composition during aging," *PLoS ONE*, vol. 7, no. 5, Article ID e37702, 2012.

[38] X. Yang, J. L. Deignan, H. Qi et al., "Validation of candidate causal genes for obesity that affect shared metabolic pathways and networks," *Nature Genetics*, vol. 41, no. 4, pp. 415–423, 2009.

[39] T. V. Nguyen, J. R. Center, and J. A. Eisman, "Pharmacogenetics of osteoporosis and the prospect of individualized prognosis and individualized therapy," *Current Opinion in Endocrinology, Diabetes and Obesity*, vol. 15, no. 6, pp. 481–488, 2008.

[40] K. Dahlman-Wright, V. Cavailles, and S. A. Fuqua, "International union of pharmacology. LXIV. Estrogen receptors," *Pharmacological Reviews*, vol. 58, no. 4, pp. 773–781, 2006.

11

Small Molecules Greatly Improve Conversion of Human-Induced Pluripotent Stem Cells to the Neuronal Lineage

Sally K. Mak, Y. Anne Huang, Shifteh Iranmanesh, Malini Vangipuram,
Ramya Sundararajan, Loan Nguyen, J. William Langston, and Birgitt Schüle

Basic Research Department, The Parkinson's Institute, 675 Almanor Ave, Sunnyvale, CA 94085, USA

Correspondence should be addressed to Birgitt Schüle, bschuele@thepi.org

Academic Editor: Mahendra Rao

Efficient *in vitro* differentiation into specific cell types is more important than ever after the breakthrough in nuclear reprogramming of somatic cells and its potential for disease modeling and drug screening. Key success factors for neuronal differentiation are the yield of desired neuronal marker expression, reproducibility, length, and cost. Three main neuronal differentiation approaches are stromal-induced neuronal differentiation, embryoid body (EB) differentiation, and direct neuronal differentiation. Here, we describe our neurodifferentiation protocol using small molecules that very efficiently promote neural induction in a 5-stage EB protocol from six induced pluripotent stem cells (iPSC) lines from patients with Parkinson's disease and controls. This protocol generates neural precursors using Dorsomorphin and SB431542 and further maturation into dopaminergic neurons by replacing sonic hedgehog with purmorphamine or smoothened agonist. The advantage of this approach is that all patient-specific iPSC lines tested in this study were successfully and consistently coaxed into the neural lineage.

1. Introduction

The advent of nuclear reprogramming of somatic cells into induced pluripotent stem cells (iPSCs) for *in vitro* disease modeling also accelerated the field of differentiation into specialized cell types. Differentiation into specific lineages had its primary place to provide a resource for cell replacement therapies [1]. These specialized differentiated cells were in general derived from a small number of "approved" human embryonic stem cell lines [2, 3].

Patient-specific iPSC-derived differentiated cells have now become an attractive tool to study disease mechanisms on a human background and are a vanguard into a new era of science and potentially personalized medicine. In particular for monogenic forms of disease, patient-derived iPSCs have already been shown to recapitulate known disease mechanisms, as shown in spinal muscular atrophy [4], fragile X syndrome [5], progeria syndrome [6], and several genetic forms of Parkinson disease (PD) like LRRK2 [7], PINK1 [8], SNCA [9], and GBA [10]. This novel approach of disease modeling becomes very attractive for drug screening and discovery [11, 12].

One of the challenges is to differentiate these patient-derived iPSCs into the desired specialized cell type of interest. For neuronal differentiation, there were three main approaches developed in the last decade to derive dopaminergic neurons [13–15]. The first method is stromal-induced neuronal differentiation, termed stromal cell-derived inducing activity (SDIA) [16, 17]. The concept is that mouse stromal cells such as PA6 or MS5 or midbrain astrocytes were used to coax the regionalization of stem cells. The disadvantage of this method is the variability of stromal cells and unknown factors; furthermore, this protocol is overall lengthy and takes about 40–60 days *in vitro*. The second main approach is embryoid body (EB)/neurosphere-mediated differentiation [18, 19], caveats are clonal expansion of subgroup of cells and potential forebrain specification. However, the usefulness of neuronal precursors (NPCs) is that they can be expanded, cryopreserved, and be a starting pool for final maturation. NPCs are also important for scientific questions of developmental phenotypes related to disease. The third approach of direct neuronal differentiation utilizes high-density monolayer ESC/iPSC cultures via floor-plate formation which gives the promise of shortening the time for neuronal development while reaching high differentiation efficiency of midbrain dopaminergic neurons [15] and show excellent survival and functional benefit which gives hope for regenerative therapies in Parkinson's disease [20].

Here, we describe a 5-stage EB differentiation approach using small molecules to enhance neural induction consistently in patient and control iPSC lines. In addition, we substituted sonic hedgehog (Shh) with purmorphamine (Pur) and/or smoothened agonist (SAG) to reduce cost for the final maturation and have shown comparable results between Shh and these small molecules. We have made considerable progress in consistency and reproducibility of this process; however, there is still a challenge of improving the overall yield of region-specific dopaminergic neurons.

2. Materials and Methods

2.1. Skin Biopsies of Patient and Control Subjects. Skin punch biopsies (4-mm circular) were taken from all individuals employing a standard punch biopsy [21]. All biopsies were taken from the upper inner arm, an area that is mostly unexposed to direct sunlight. We used a standard skin explant culture technique by cutting the biopsy tissue into 12–15 pieces and placed 2-3 pieces into one well of a gelatinized 6-well plate in 1 mL of high-glucose DMEM, 20% fetal bovine serum, 1x nonessential aminoacids (NEAA), 1x penicillin streptomycin (P/S), 1x L-glutamine (Glu) (all were purchased from Invitrogen, Carlsbad, CA). Outgrowth of keratinocytes was first noted 2–5 days after plating. Cells were expanded using standard tissue culture techniques, cells were passaged upon confluency using trypsin/EDTA (Invitrogen) and 15–20 million cells. Miocells were cryopreserved for banking. This study and protocol had Institutional Review Board approval and all subjects gave written informed consent for this study. Clinical information on the patients is provided in Supplementary Table 1 (see supplementary materials available at doi:10.1155/2012/140427).

2.2. Generation of iPSC. All iPSCs were derived using a retroviral system to deliver four genes encoding OCT4, KLF4, SOX2 and cMYC (from Addgene plasmids 17217, 17218, 17219, 17220, http://www.addgene.org/) using published protocols [22, 23]. All lines have been characterized for pluripotency, differentiation potential into three germ layers, are karyotypically normal and genotype-match the parental fibroblasts, (see Supplementary Table 2). IPSC line 1761 was previously described and characterized in Nguyen et al. 2011 [7].

2.3. iPSC Maintenance and Propagation. iPSCs were cultured and maintained on mitomycin C inactivated mouse embryonic fibroblasts (iMEF) (EMD Millipore Cat. No. PMEF-CF) in hESC media containing DMEM/F12, 20% knockout serum replacement (Invitrogen, Cat. No. 10828028), 1x NEAA, 1x P/S, 0.1% β-Mercaptoethanol (Invitrogen, Cat. No. 21985023), 0.5x L-Glu and 6 ng/mL of basic fibroblast growth factor (FGF2) (Cat. No. 233-FB, R&D Systems,

Minneapolis, MN). Cells were split every week manually without enzymatic treatment.

2.4. Generation and Maintenance of Neural Progenitor Cells (NPCs). To derive NPCs, iPSC colonies were harvested using 1 mg/mL of collagenase IV (Invitrogen, Cat. No. 174104019). After about 1 hr, when all colonies lifted up completely from culture dish, colonies were transferred to 10 cm bacterial petri dishes (BD Bioscience, Bedford, MA). Forming embryoid bodies (EB) was cultured in suspension with agitation on rocker (Rocker II Model 260350, Boekel Scientific, Feasterville, PA) for 4 days in EB media, which consisted of hESC media minus FGF2 with or without 5 μM dorsomorphin (Dor) (Sigma, St Louis, MO, Cat. No. P5499) and 10 μM SB431542 (SB) (Tocris Bioscience, Ellisville, MO, Cat. No. 1614).

Next, EBs were cultured for additional 2-3 days with agitation in neural induction media (NIM) consisting of DMEM/F12 (Invitrogen, Cat. No. 12500, powder form), 1x NEAA, 0.5x L-Glu, and freshly made and sterile filtered N2, which contained 1.55 g/L glucose (Sigma, Cat. No. G7021), 2 g/L sodium bicarbonate (Sigma, Cat. No. S5761), 100 μM putrescine (Sigma, Cat. No. P5780), 30 nM sodium selenite (Sigma, Cat. No. S9133), 20 nM progesterone (Sigma, Cat. No. P8783), 0.1 mg/mL transferrin (Sigma, Cat. No. T0665), 0.025 mg/mL insulin (Sigma, Cat. No. I6634) and FGF2 (20 ng/mL). Cell culture plates were coated with Geltrex (Invitrogen, Cat. No. 12760021), media changed every day. Neural rosettes were formed in 2–5 days in adherent culture.

To obtain a pure population of NPCs, rosettes were manually isolated using No. 15 scalpel cutting in squares with distance to edges of colonies (Figure 3(F)). Dissected pieces of rosettes were lifted using a pipette, replated onto Geltrex-coated culture dishes and maintained in neural progenitor cell media (NPC media) containing neurobasal media (Invitrogen, Cat. No. 21103049), 1x NEAA, 1x L-Glu, 1x P/S, 1x B27 supplement (Invitrogen, Cat. No. 17504044), and FGF2 (20 ng/mL). Manual isolation of rosettes as described above was repeated once to obtain more pure population of NPCs. Approximately 5–10 pieces of rosettes were dissociated into single cells using Accutase (MP Biomedicals, Solon, OH, Cat. No. 0910004). Cells were treated with Accutase for 2–5 minutes until cells became round in shape, then the cells were collected, centrifuged, resuspended in NPC media, and plated onto one 96-well coated with Geltrex and cultured at 37°C and 5% CO_2. When confluent, NPCs were split at a ratio of 1 : 2 in single wells with larger surface area such as 48-well, 24-well, 12-well, and so forth in NPC media.

2.5. NPC Enrichment Using Anti PSA-NCAM Microbeads. For magnetic bead sorting, NPCs were treated with Accutase, collected, and passed through 30 μm nylon mesh (pre-separation filters, 30 μm, Miltenyi Biotec Auburn, CA, Cat. No. 130-041-407). The total cell number was approximately 10^7. Cell suspension was centrifuged at 300 $\times$g for 10 minutes. Supernatant was aspirated completely and cell pellet was resuspended in 60 μL of buffer (1x PBS, 2 mM EDTA (Ambion Inc, Austin, TX, Cat. No. AM9260G) and

	Stage I	Stage II	Stage III	Stage IV	Stage V	
	Expansion of iPSCs $\longrightarrow$	Embryoid body formation $\longrightarrow$	Neural rosette formation $\longrightarrow$	Expansion of neural progenitor cells $\longrightarrow$	Dopaminergic maturation	
Media name		EB	NIM	NPC	DA1	DA2
Basal media		DMEM/F12	DMEM/F12	Neurobasal medium	Neurobasal medium	
Media supplements		β-mercaptoethanol	Putrescine sodium selenite progesterone transferrin insulin FGF2	B27 FGF2	B27 FGF8	B27 BDNF GDNF
Test components		Dorsomor phine SB431524			Purmorphamine SAG Sonic hedgehog	
Dish coating			Geltrex™	Geltrex™	Geltrex™ or polyornithine/ laminin	

(a)

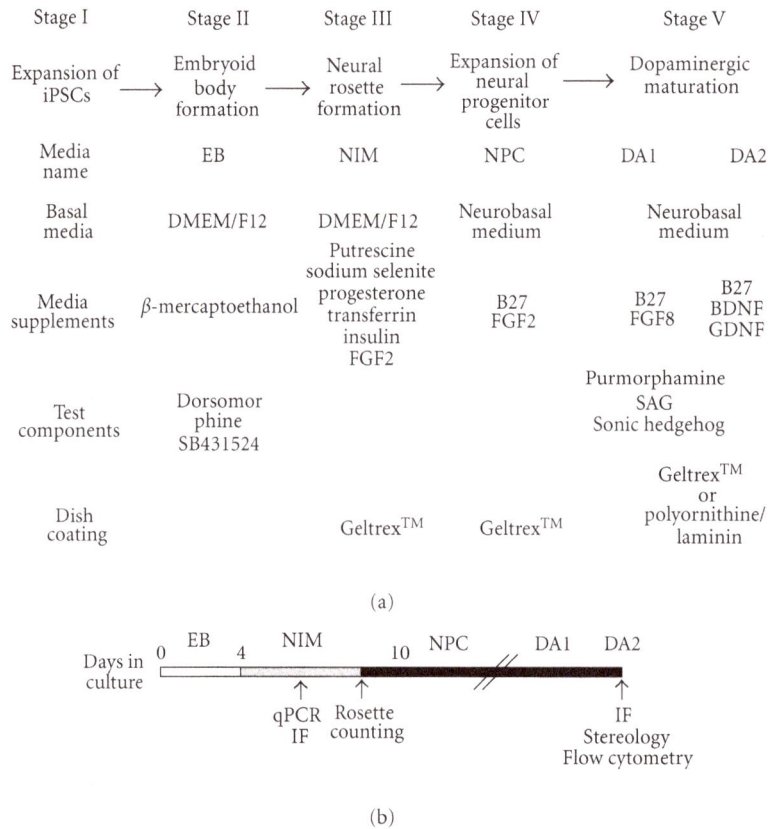

(b)

FIGURE 1: Schematic summary of the differentiation conditions used in the generation of dopaminergic neurons (a) Schematic diagram illustrating the different stages of NPC generation and dopaminergic neuronal differentiation. The abbreviations are. Dor/SB: Dorsomorphin and SB431542, EB: EB media, NIM: neural induction media, NPC: neural progenitor cell media, and DA1/DA2: medium for dopaminergic differentiation. (b) Timeline shows the medium used at different stages of NPCs and dopaminergic maturation and displays the sampling dates for performing gene expression studies, such as qPCR, marker characterization (immunofluorescence: IF), to analyze efficiency of rosette formation and for quantitative studies of TUJ1 and TH immunoreactivity using stereology and flow cytometry.

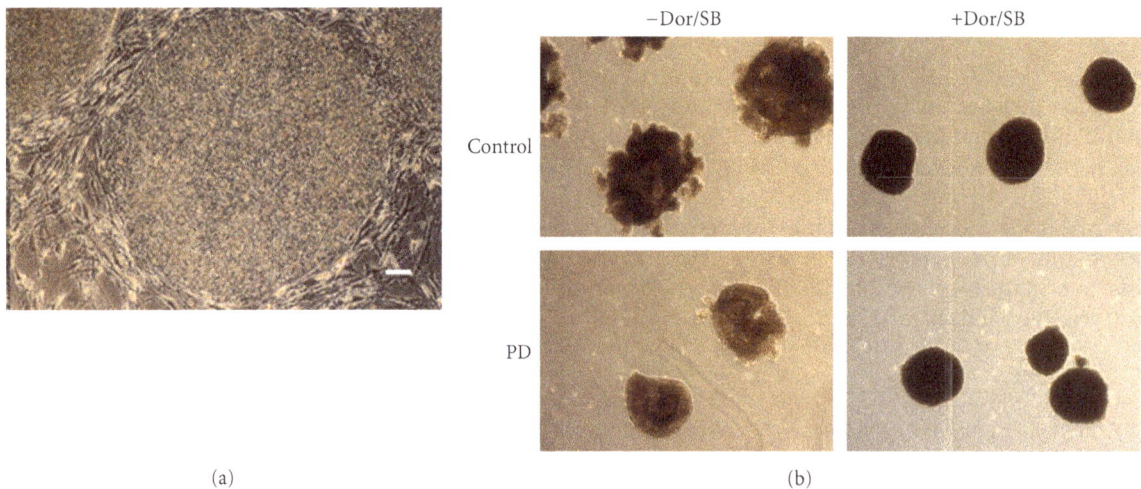

(a)   (b)

FIGURE 2: (a) Representative image of the quality of iPSC colonies used to produce EBs: distinct border with little to no differentiation. The recommended size for EB formation should be double the size as the depicted colony, approximately 2 mm in diameter. Scale bar 100 μm (b) In-control and PD-specific cell lines (Control and PD), EBs were lacking that compact structure and round borders when cultured without Dor/SB; EBs were found to be round, uniform in the presence of Dor/SB.

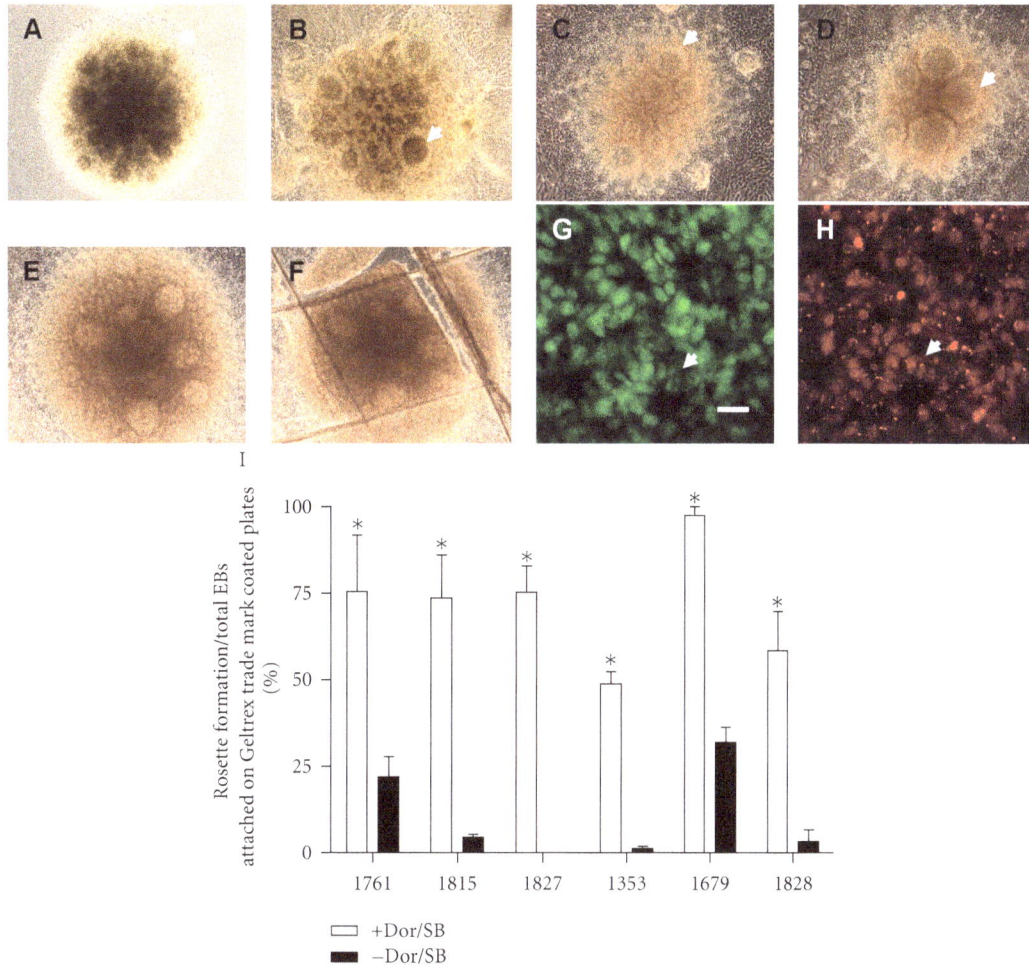

FIGURE 3: Representative images of neural rosettes at different stages (A–D). Neural rosettes after Dor/SB treatment at days 7–12, stage III of the differentiation protocol (5x magnification). Arrows indicate boundary lines in the early and late stages of rosettes. (E) and (F) Manual dissection of rosettes using scalpel are illustrated before (E) and after (F) cutting. (G and H) Arrows indicate the positions of neural rosettes that were immunoreactive with Pax6 (green) (E) and Sox1 (red) (F). Scale bar represents 20 μm. (i) There is a significant difference in neural rosette formation in all control and PD-specific EBs treated with Dor/SM compared to those with no Dor/SB treatment during stage II (*P < 0.01). Data are presented as mean + standard error of the mean (SEM) compared to the controls (n = 3, except 1679, n = 2). P value of each study was assessed by one-way ANOVA along with Newman-Keuls post-*hoc* analysis.

0.5% albumin from bovine serum (BSA) (Sigma, Cat. No. A3294). Cells were mixed well and incubated for 10 minutes in the refrigerator (2−8°C). Then, 20 μL of anti-PSA-NCAM microbeads (Miltenyi Biotech, Auburn, CA, Cat. No. 130-092-966) were added to the mixture, mixed well with pipetting up and down, and incubated for 15 minutes in the refrigerator (2−8°C). Cells were washed by adding 2 mL of buffer and centrifuged at 300 ×g for 10 minutes. Supernatant was aspirated completely and cell pellet was resuspended up to 10^8 cells in 500 μL of buffer. A MS column (Miltenyi Biotec, Cat. No. 130-042-201) was placed in the magnetic field of a miniMACS separator (Miltenyi Biotec, Cat. No. 130-042-102), rinsed with 500 μL of buffer three times. Cell suspension was applied onto the column. The column was washed with 500 μL of buffer three times again. New buffer was added when the column reservoir was empty. The column was removed from the separator and

placed on a 15 mL BD Falcon conical tube (BD Bioscience, 352097). One mL of buffer was added onto the column and magnetically labeled cells were flushed out by firmly pushing the plunger into the column. The eluted fraction was directly enriched over a second column and the magnetic separation procedure was repeated once by using a new MS column. One mL of NPC media was added onto the column to flush out the magnetically labeled cells. Then another 1 mL of NPC media was added and cell suspension was transferred to a 35 mm Geltrex-coated culture dish.

2.6. Dopaminergic Differentiation of NPCs. Dopaminergic differentiation was initiated by culturing NPCs on Geltrex-coated culture dishes or glass coverslips (Fisher Scientific, Pittsburg, PA, Cat. No. 12-545-80-12CIR-1) coated with poly-L-ornithine (20 μg/mL) (Sigma, Cat. No. P4957)

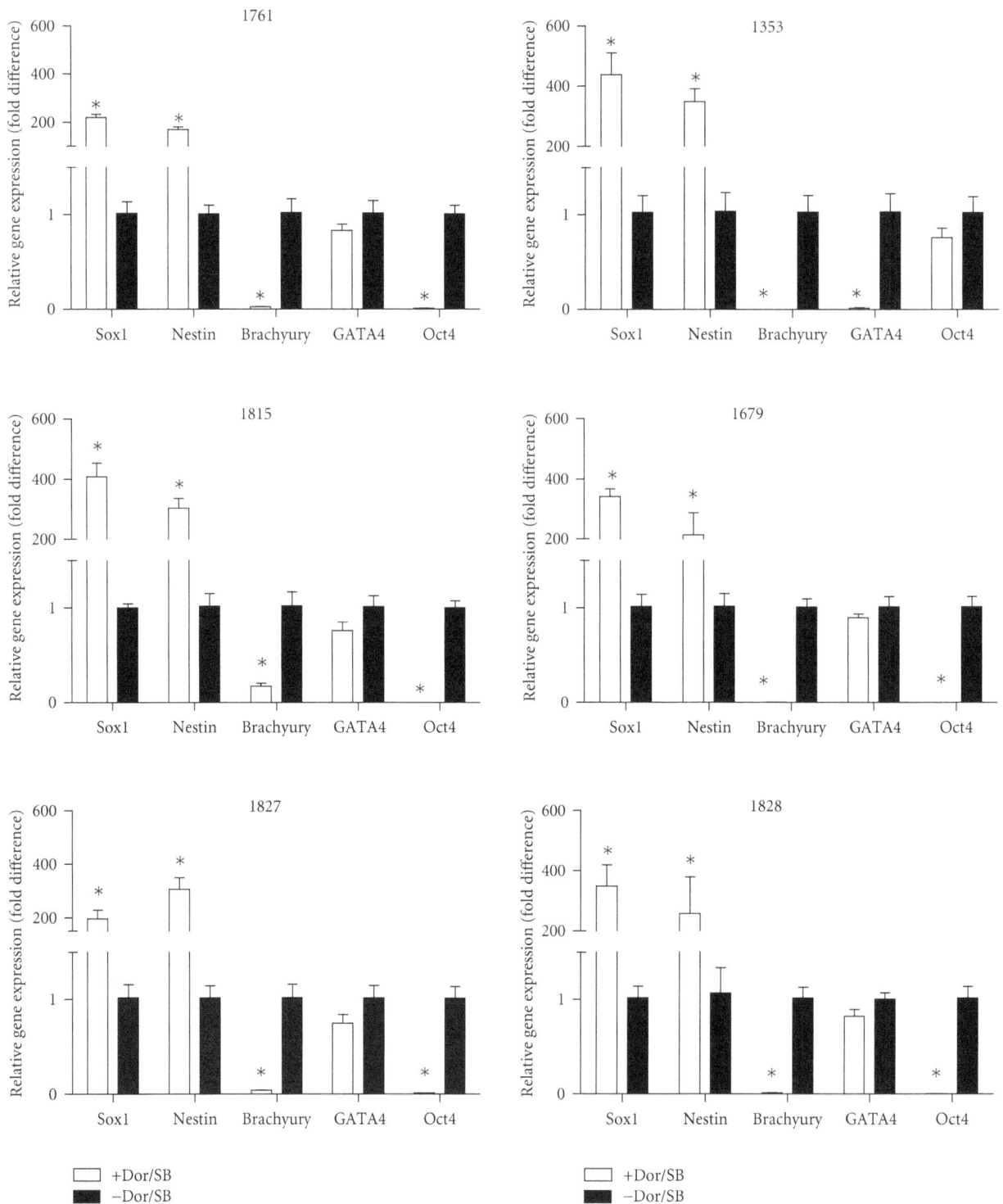

FIGURE 4: Quantitative gene expression analysis of PD and control lines with and without Dor/SB. Expression levels of neuroectoderm (Sox1 and Nestin), mesoderm (Brachyury), endoderm (GATA4), and pluripotent markers (Oct4) were assessed by quantitative PCR. The y-axis represents means + SEM of relative expression levels of each gene in the EBs with Dor/SB relative to no Dor/SB treatment ($*P < 0.01$). Left panel depicts lines from healthy donors; right panels depicts cell lines derived from patients with PD. Data are presented as mean + SEM compared to the controls ($n = 3$, except 1679, $n = 2$). P-value of each study was assessed by one-way ANOVA along with Newman-Keuls post-hoc analysis.

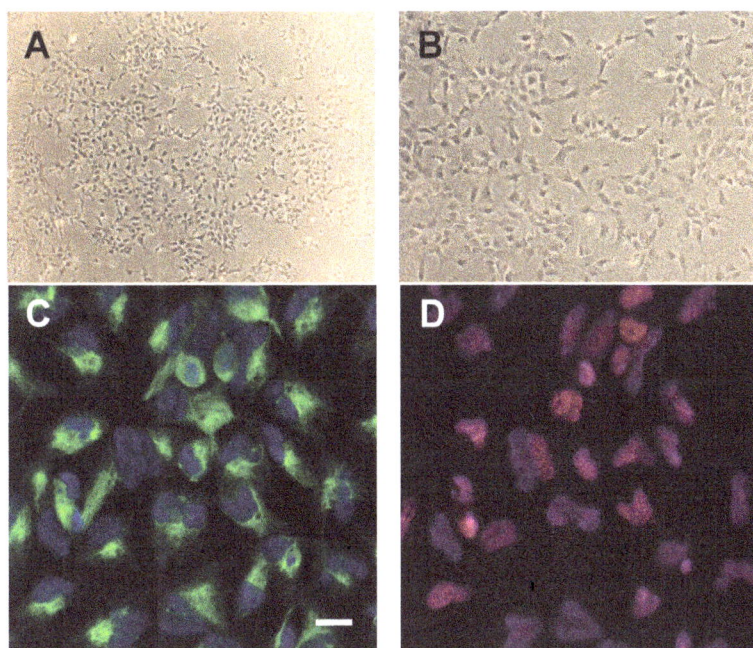

FIGURE 5: Characterization of NPCs. (A) and (B) NPC morphology was observed under phase-contrast microscopy with 5x (A and 10x (B) magnification. (C and D) NPCs expressed Nestin (green) (C) and Sox1 (red). (D) Nuclei were counterstained with DAPI (blue). Scale bar represents 20 μm.

at 37°C for 4 hrs and laminin (Sigma Cat. No. L2020) (20 μg/mL) at 4°C overnight.

Dopaminergic differentiation in defined media was initiated by culturing ∼0.5 × 10⁶ NPCs (in 35 mm culture dish) in DA1 media for 10 days in Neurobasal media supplemented with 1x NEAA, 1x L-Glu, 1x P/S, 1x B27, FGF8b (100 ng/mL) (R&D Systems, Cat. No. 423-F8) and tested with either 2 μM Purmorphamine (Pur) (EMD Chemicals, Cat. No. 540220), Gibbstown, NJ), 0.4 mM SAG (Enzo Life Sciences, Farmingdale, NY, Cat. No. ALX-270-426-M001) or 200 ng/mL Sonic Hedgehog, C24II (Shh) (R&D Systems, Cat. No. 1845-SH). During these 10 days, when cells grew confluent, they were passaged with Accutase as described above and replated onto a Geltrex-coated plates at cell density of ∼80%. Lower density led to cell death.

Final maturation into dopaminergic neurons was carried out in DA2 media containing neurobasal media supplemented with 1x NEAA, 1x L-Glutamine, 1x B27 supplement, 1x Penicillin-Streptomycin, 20 ng/mL BDNF (R&D Systems, Cat. No. 248-BD), 20 ng/mL GDNF (R&D Systems, Cat. No. 212-GD), and 1 mM dibutyryl cAMP (Sigma, Cat. No. D0627) for 20–30 days. Cells were not continued to passage in DA2 media when the processes formed. Cells were analyzed on day 30 of the maturation process.

2.7. Quantitative PCR (qPCR). EBs were collected on day 6 of EB formation before plating down for rosette formation. Total RNA was extracted using a RNeasy Micro kit (Qiagen, Valencia, CA) and 500 ng RNA was used for reverse-transcription into cDNA using the iScript cDNA Synthesis Kit (BioRad, Hercules, CA). Total reaction volume was 20 μL;

the resulting cDNA sample was diluted with 80 μL of ultra-pure water, and 5 μL of the diluted cDNA sample was used as template for qPCR amplification. qPCR was performed using ABI PRISM 7000 Sequence Detection System (Applied Biosystems, Foster City, CA). All reactions were run in 20 μL reactions volume using SYBR Green PCR Master Mix (Applied Biosystems) and 30 pmol of each primer. qPCR parameters were as follows: 2 min at 50°C; 10 min at 95°C; 40 cycles at 95°C for 15 sec, and at 60°C for 1 min. Data were collected at 60°C. All data were normalized to *β-actin* expression and plotted as fold changes over samples from EBs without Dor/SB. Primers of genes used in this study: Sox1 (5′-GAGATTCATCTCAGGATTGAGATTCTA-3′ and 5′-GGCCTACTGTAATCTTTTCTCCAC-3′); Nestin (5′-TGCGGGCTACTGAAAAGTTC-3′ and 5′-AGGCTGAGG-GACATCTTGAG-3′); Brachyury (5′-AGGTACCCAACC-CTGAGGA-3′ and 5′-GCAGGTGAGTTGTCAGAATAG-GT-3′); GATA4 (5′-GTCATCTCACTACGGGCACA-3′ and 5′-CTTCAGGGCCGAGAGGAC-3′); Oct4 (5′-TGGGCT-CGAGAAGGATGTG-3′ and 5′-GCATAGTCGCTGCTT-GATCG-3′) and *β-actin* (5′-CTGAACCCCAAGGCCAAC-3′ and 5′-TAGCACAGCCTGGATAGCAA-3′).

2.8. Immunocytochemistry. EBs and NPCs were fixed with 4% paraformaldehyde (PFA) (Electron Microscopy Sciences, Hatfield, PA) at room temperature for 10 minutes. Neurons were fixed carefully by adding equal volume of 8% PFA into wells to equal volume of medium and incubated at room temperature for 10 minutes. Fixed cells were permeabilized with 0.3% Triton X-100 (Sigma, Cat. No. X100) for 5 minutes and were blocked in blocking buffer (5% normal

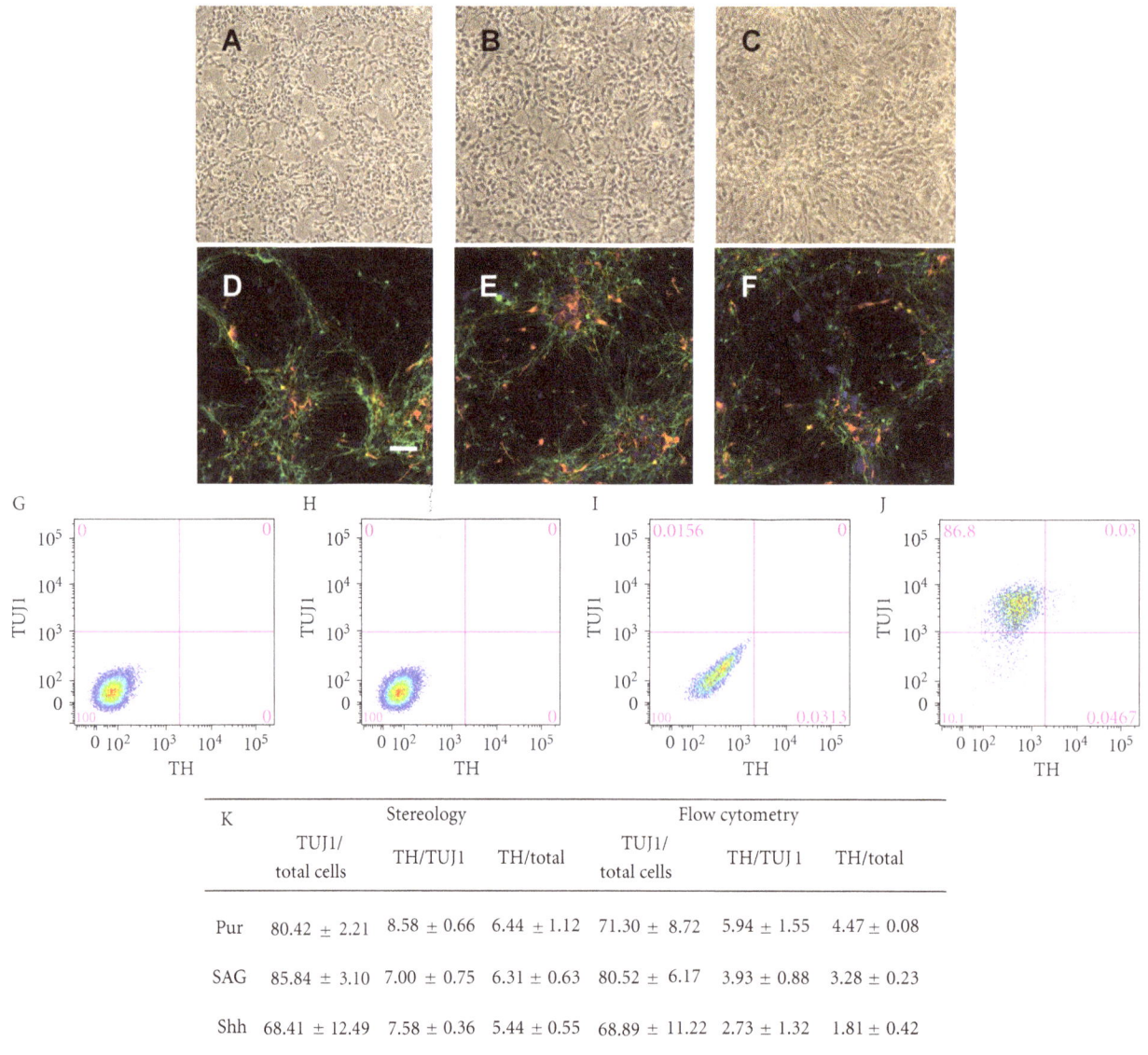

FIGURE 6: Analysis of number of TH+ and TUJ+ neurons (A)–(C). Image under phase-contrast microscopy showed plating density of NPCs at day 1 in DA1 media (5x magnification) (A), cell morphology at day 12 (arrows indicate the formation of processes) (B) 10x magnification) and neurons at day 30 during dopaminergic maturation (C) 10x magnification. (D)–(F), Neurons treated with Pur (D), SAG (E) and Shh (F) were characterized by immunostaining with TUJ1 (green) and TH (red) and counterstained with DAPI (blue). Scale bar represents 200 μm. (G)–(J) Flow cytometry: No TUJ1 and TH immunoreactive NPCs were detected (H), which is comparable to unstained NPCs (G). In contrast to the population of unstained differentiated neurons (I), differentiated cells showed positive immunoreactivity to TUJ1 and TH (j). (k) Table illustrates percentage of TUJ1 relative to total cells, TH immunoreactive neurons relative to TUJ1 immunoreactive neurons, and also relative to total cells quantified using stereology and flow cytometry in control NPCs after dopaminergic maturation.

goat serum, Vector Labs, Burlingame, CA) in 1x Phosphate buffered saline (PBS) (Sigma, Cat. No. P5493) and followed by incubation with the primary antibody at 4°C overnight in 5% normal goat serum and PBS. The following primary antibodies were used: Nestin (EMD Millipore, Billerica, MA, Cat. No. MAB5326), 1:200; Sox1 (EMD Millipore, Cat. No. AB15766), 1:100; Tyrosine Hydroxylase (TH) (PelFreez Biologicals, Rogers, AR, Cat. No. P40101-0), 1:300; Pax6 (Developmental Studies Hybridoma Bank, Iowa City, IA, Cat. No. Pax6), 1:20; neuronal class III β-Tubulin (TUJ1)

(Covance, Princeton, NJ, Cat. No. MMS-435P), 1:500, and secondary antibodies were Alexa Fluor 488 Goat Anti-Mouse, Alexa Fluor 555 Goat Anti-Mouse, Alexa Fluor 488 Goat Anti-Rabbit, Alexa Fluor 555 Goat Anti-Rabbit (Invitrogen) at 1:300. Coverslips were mounted with Vectashield Mounting Medium with DAPI (Vector Labs). Fluorescent images were captured on an Eclipse Ti inverted fluorescence microscope (Nikon Instruments Inc, Melville, NY). Phase contrast images were taken with a Zeiss Axiovert 25 Inverted Microscope (Carl Zeiss AG, Oberkochen, Germany).

2.9. Stereological Analysis. Stereological analysis was performed using an Olympus BH2 microscope (Olympus, Center Valley, PA) with a motorized X-Y stage linked to a computer-assisted stereological system (Olympus America Inc.). This comprises a color video camera (CCD-Iris, Sony), a PC with a high-resolution SVGA monitor, a microcator (VRZ 401, Heidenhain), and Stereo Investigator (MBF Bioscience, Williston, VT). Immunostained coverslips were delineated at 4x magnification. From a random start position, a counting frame was superimposed on the image, and cells were systematically sampled using a 40x objective lens (Olympus), with DAPI stained nucleus used as the sampling unit. A minimum of 200 cells was sampled according to the rules of the optical dissector [24], and the coefficient of error for each stereological estimate was between 0.07 and 0.1 [25].

2.10. Flow Cytometry. After dopaminergic differentiation, cells were dissociated with TrypLE Express (Invitrogen, Cat. No. 12605-028) at 37°C for 5 minutes, washed with PBS, centrifuged, resuspended in PBS, and strained through a 70 μm cell strainer (BD Biosciences, Cat No. 352350), centrifuged, resuspended, and fixed in 4% PFA in PBS at room temperature for 10 minutes. Then they were centrifuged, resuspended, and permeabilized with 0.3% saponin (Sigma, Cat. No. 47036), incubated with TUJ1 (Covance, 1 : 100) and TH (Pel Freez Biologicals, 1 : 100) on ice for 30 minutes and washed with washing buffer (PBS and 0.03% saponin) once. Then cells were incubated with APC-conjugated anti mouse IgG antibody (BD Biosciences, Cat. No. 550826) and PE-conjugated anti rabbit IgG antibody (BD Biosciences, Cat. No. 558416) on ice for 30 minutes, washed with washing buffer, and resuspended in PBS. All sorting procedures were carried out using BD Digital Vantage (BD Biosciences) with a 80 μm nozzle. Data were analyzed by FlowJo flow cytometry software (Version 7.6.4, Tree Star Inc, Ashland, OR). We compared cell suspension of unstained NPCs and unstained differentiated cells as negative control to determine the threshold for detection of immunofluorescence.

2.11. Statistical Analysis. Statistical analysis was performed using GraphPad Prism (Version 4, GraphPad Software, San Diego, CA). Data were analyzed by one-way analysis of variance (ANOVA). Newman-Keuls post hoc analysis was employed when differences were observed in ANOVA testing ($P < 0.05$). Data were presented as the means + standard error of the mean (SEM). All results were derived from at least three independent experiments, except results of cell line 1679 in Figure 1 and flow cytometry data in Figure 6 were derived from two independent experiments.

3. Results and Discussion

3.1. Neuronal Differentiation Using a 5-Stage Embryoid Body Approach. The majority of published neuronal differentiation methods describe selected human embryonic stem cell (hESC) lines such as H9 or I6 and these protocols were optimized around these cell lines. Despite general

reproducibility across multiple hESC lines, in patient-specific human iPSCs consistent reproducibility has not been demonstrated, posing a challenge for disease modeling and drug screening. [26–29]. One recent publication points towards specific markers such as miR-371-3 and FoxA2 that could predict a priori the differentiation potential of iPSCs or ESCs into the neuronal lineage, which can be relevant for downstream applications [30].

Our goal was to develop a reliable protocol reproducible across various patient-specific iPSC lines. We tested a 5-stage protocol for neuronal dopaminergic differentiation that was originally introduced by Lee and Studer in mouse embryonic stem cells [18] and subsequently further developed [28, 29]. This protocol involves EB formation for four days, neural rosette formation, isolation of neural rosettes, and expansion and PSA-NCAM enrichment using magnetic bead sorting of neuroprogenitors. A final maturation stage utilizes FGF8 and sonic hedgehog (Shh) for the first ten days followed by BDNF, GDNF, B27, and dcAMP in Neurobasal media for another 20–50 days (Figure 1(a)). We reason that this 5-stage protocol generating EBs has several advantages in generating neural precursors that can be easily expanded without loss of differentiation potential [31]. Thus, this protocol is suitable for studying disease-mechanisms at the neuroprogenitor stage and maintaining potential for derivation of other CNS cell types [28].

In a control iPSC line, EBs incubated for 4 days in EB media showed a similar result of neural rosette formation as described by Swistowski et al., 2009 [28] (data not shown). When we attempted to derive NPCs from additional iPSCs derived from controls and patients affected with PD we observed very little neural rosette formation. Furthermore, these rosettes were not expandable as NPCs.

Small molecules have been reported to improve directing ESC/iPSCs into neural lineage [32, 33]. We tested a combination of small molecules: Dor and SB, both of which have been described for SMAD inhibition. The synergistic mode of action of inhibitors of SMAD signaling, Noggin and SB431542, has been reported to rapidly induce neural conversion of hESCs [15, 34]. Noggin, a bone morphogenetic protein (BMP) antagonist, and the small molecule Dor have similar activities which selectively inhibit the BMP type I receptors: ALK2, ALK3, and ALK6 and block SMAD1/5/8 phosphorylation [35]. SB has been shown to be a selective inhibitor of activin receptor-like kinase receptors ALK4, ALK5, and ALK7 [36].

For successful generation of NPCs, it is crucial to start with pristine, undifferentiated iPSC cultures. IPSC colonies should be densely packed show low nucleus to cytoplasma ratios and have discrete borders and no differentiation along the peripheries and/or in the centers of the colonies. In this protocol, we found that 2 mm diameter sized colonies yield the best results for neural rosette formation (Figure 2(a)).

3.2. Combination of Dorsomorphin and SB431542 Improved Neural Induction. IPSC colonies were enzymatically treated with collagenase. After detachment, half of the colonies in a dish were exposed to 5 μM Dor/10 μM SB. The other half was left untreated. The colonies were then cultured for 4 days in EB media with or without Dor/SB. EBs cultured in EB media alone showed loose, less compact, and irregular shapes (Figure 2(b)) while the majority of EBs treated with Dor/SB demonstrated compact, solid and round shaped aggregates and had an average size of $350\,\mu m$ in diameter (Figure 2(b)). On day 4, media was changed to NIM media containing N2 media which was freshly made of different individual components. None of the commercially available N2 supplements showed consistent results (data not shown). EBs were then plated onto Geltrex-coated culture dishes on day 6. During days 6–10, neural rosettes were detected by their characteristic morphology of radially arranged cells (Figures 3(A)–3(D)). In the early stages of NIM incubation (approximately days 8–10), neural rosettes showed darker centers of "flower-shaped" structures with indiscrete boundary lines (Figures 3(A) and 3(B)). In the latter incubation with NIM, "flower-shaped" morphologies were more distinct and edges more clearly defined, shown in Figures 3(C) and 3(D). Dissected rosettes (Figures 3(E) and 3(F)) that are replated and manually isolated a second time generate NPC populations of higher purity.

We evaluated neural differentiation of EBs on day 10 (Figure 1(b)) via immunocytochemistry. Neural markers Pax6 and Sox1 were used as well as the pluripotent cell marker Oct4. Pax6 and Sox1 showed positive staining in attached EB (Figures 3(G) and 3(H)), however, Oct4 showed no immunoreactivity (data not shown). At the same time point, the percentage of neural rosettes formed with and without addition of Dor/SB was quantified by manually counting the colonies containing neural rosettes divided by total colonies attached on the culture dish (Figures 1(b) and 3(I)). Without Dor/SB, we observed low rosette formation between 0% and 31.9%, and we were not able to derive expandable NPCs. The combination of Dor/SB, on the other hand, increased the neural rosette formation substantially to 48% to 97.5% of EBs in both control and PD-specific cell lines. Overall, we did not notice a difference in the efficiency of rosette formation between PD lines and control lines.

At day 6, we performed gene expression analysis of multiple markers in attached EBs. In all six lines we studied neuroectodermal markers Sox1 and Nestin, mesodermal marker Brachyury, endodermal marker GATA4 and pluripotent marker Oct4. Surprisingly, there was a striking difference of >150-fold in the gene expressions of neuroectodermal markers Sox1 and Nestin in Dor-/SB-treated EBs compared to EBs without small molecules (Figure 4). This suggests that the two small molecules very efficiently modulate the SMAD signaling pathway leading to this enormous increase in neuroectodermal markers. This increase was consistent in all six iPSC lines tested, and differences in neuronal differentiation were not observed between patient and control lines. Endo and mesodermal markers GATA4 and Brachyury as well as pluripotency marker Oct 4 were all lower compared to the untreated, normalized NPC lines.

Neural rosettes were manually cut and replated as pieces to produce a population of NPCs of higher purity. Rosettes were manually isolated once again, collected, enzymatically

treated with Accutase, and plated and expanded in NPC media. Manual passaging and expansion of NPCs still yielded approximately 10% undifferentiated Oct4-positive cells in NPC cultures, which upon further expansion showed iPSC morphology (data not shown). Therefore, we used magnetic bead sorting with a neural cell adhesion molecule antibody against polysialic acid neural cell adhesion molecule (PSA-NCAM or CD56) (Figures 5(A) and 5(B)). We observed an approximately 20% cell loss after magnetic bead sorting. We characterized NPCs after sorting by immunocytochemistry with defined markers Nestin and Sox1. We detected >90% Nestin and Sox1 immunoreactive NPCs in all iPSC cell lines taken through this protocol (Figures 5(C) and 5(D)). NPCs were readily expandable at a passaging ratio of 1 : 2 to 1 : 3 with Accutase. Cultures grew well when media was prepared freshly every 2 to 3 days and B27 added freshly to NPC media, before media changes. We expanded NPC cultures for >15 passages after derivation and did not observe any changes in morphology or expression of Nestin and Sox1.

With this new approach for neural induction using small molecules, we have dramatically increased reproducibility and efficiency of neural rosette stage/NPC generation. This is invaluable when using patient-derived iPSCs for disease modeling, which may have an intrinsic disadvantage in culture when carrying potential disease-related deficiencies. Since NPCs can be easily expanded, this could become a suitable cell type for high throughput screening where a very large number of starting material is needed.

3.3. Substitution of Small Molecules Purmorphamine or Smoothened Agonist for Sonic Hedgehog Had Similar Effects on Neuronal Maturation. We investigated the substitution of sonic hedgehog (Shh) for small molecules purmorphamine (Pur) or smoothened agonist (SAG) during dopaminergic maturation. These chemicals that are considerably less expensive, have minimal lot-to-lot variabilities, and have longer shelf-life compared to recombinant proteins.

For final dopaminergic maturation, we used a 2-step approach. For the first ten days, we cultured NPCs in FGF8 and tested two small molecules SAG and Pur as substitutes for Shh in control and patient cell lines. At day 1 in DA1 media, the plating density of the NPCs should be approximately 60% to 70% (Figure 6(A)). During this 10-day protocol, cells were split at 100% confluency using Accutase and replated at a cell density of approximately 80%. When cells were plated at a lower cell density (<50%), we observed remarkable cell death and low rates of cell attachment. After ten days, we switched to Neurobasal media supplemented with BDNF, GDNF, dcAMP, and B27 every second day, but added B27 daily preventing cell death. Cells were split until they began growing out processes (Figure 6(B)). After day 30 of dopaminergic maturation, cells were fixed, immunostained with TUJ1 and TH, and counterstained with DAPI (Figures 6(C)–6(F)).

To measure the efficiency of the neuronal differentiation, we evaluated the percentage of TH and TUJ1 expressing neurons relative to total cells using two approaches: stereology with systematic random sampling and flow cytometry. Flow cytometry was employed to minimize bias. The challenges of accurate counting of these cultures are the dense "patches" of neurons and the majority of TH immunoreactive neurons localized in these "patches" [37].

In the scatter plots for flow cytometry, (Figures 6(G)–6(J)), undifferentiated NPCs did not show immunoreactivity for TUJ1 and TH (Figure 6(H)) and had a similar pattern in the scatter plot to unstained NPCs (Figure 6(G)). Differentiated neurons were immunoreactive for TUJ1 and TH (Figure 6(I)) and were compared to the total number of unstained differentiated neurons (Figure 6(J)).

Both approaches, stereology and flow cytometry, showed no significant differences among the three different components Shh, SAG, or Pur used in dopaminergic differentiation in terms of the ratio of TUJ1/total, TH/TuJ1, and TH/total cells (Figure 6(K)). Data from flow cytometry was slightly lower than those from the stereological approach. We suspect that we lost neurons during the handling process such as dissociation and passaging through a cell strainer to filter clumps from cell suspension before flow cytometry was performed.

Some studies have shown that with an extension of culturing time by up to 60 days, more neurons convert to TH-positive as well as become electrophysiologically mature [37, 38]. Other studies showed a higher percentage of TH-positive neurons, however, different quantification approaches may have introduced bias toward a higher percentage of neuronal yields.

4. Discussion: Small Molecules for Efficient Neuronal Differentiation

Over the last few years, there has been an enormous push to optimize differentiation protocols with different small molecules and screens to identify new factors that would modulate and improve neuronal differentiation and maturation.

Other small molecules and compounds have been identified for the enhancement of neuronal differentiation. Glycogen synthase kinase-3 (GSK-3) inhibitors such as kenpaullone or SB-216763 have been shown to positively impact the neuronal differentiation of neural progenitor cells without changing cell cycle exit or cell survival [39]. Furthermore, GSK-3 inhibitors showed protection against excitotoxicity, mediated by NMDA and non-NMDA receptor agonists, in cultured rat primary cerebellar granule neuronal cultures from the cerebellum and hippocampus [40].

(+)-Cholesten-3-one but not cholesterol has been shown to effectively promote the activity of the TH promoter. (+)-Cholesten-3-one has also been shown to induce differentiation of neuroprogenitors into dopaminergic neurons monitored by expression of TH, dopamine transporter, dopa decarboxylase, and higher levels of dopamine secretion [41].

Neurosteroids are thought to affect neuronal survival, neurite outgrowth, and neurogenesis both *in vivo* and *in vitro* [42], that is, progesterone [43] and estradiol [44]. Progesterone added at the neural proliferation stage increased the number of dopaminergic neurons, whereas progesterone added during final differentiation did not induce significant changes in the number of dopaminergic neurons generated. Interestingly, this effect was not mediated by the activation of progesterone receptors because RU 486 did not block the effects of progesterone on dopaminergic differentiation [43]. It has also been shown that estradiol can increase the generation of dopaminergic precursors expressing Lmx1a and can induce formation of a higher percentage of mature dopaminergic neurons [44].

In addition, polyunsaturated fatty acids such as arachidonic acid (ARA) and docosahexaenoic acid (DHA) have been shown to have critical roles in brain development and function and can promote neurogenesis [45]. Specifically, DHA, a ligand for the RXR/Nurr1 heterodimer, can activate the Nurr1 gene in iPSCs. It has been shown that DHA facilitates iPSC differentiation into TH-positive neurons *in vitro* as well as *in vivo* [46].

Through a peptide library screen a novel small synthetic peptide Cripto BP was discovered to block Cripto, a glycosylphosphatidylinositol-anchored coreceptor. It has been shown that this receptor binds Nodal and the ALK-4 receptors and promotes cardiac differentiation. The deletion or inhibition of Cripto leads to a promotion of neuronal and midbrain differentiation of mouse embryonic stem cells. The synthetic peptide Cripto BP can mimic this effect [47].

5. Conclusion

Small molecules can enhance various steps of neuronal differentiation into dopaminergic neurons and can replace expensive recombinant proteins that were initially used in the pioneering protocols. However, there is still a need for improvement of differentiation protocols that increase the number and region-specificity of mature region specific dopaminergic neurons, but selective inhibitors and other small molecules might change the field and reduce the cost.

Conflict of Interests

The authors declare they have no conflict of interests.

Acknowledgments

The authors are indebted to all patients, family members, spouses, and healthy volunteers participating in this study for "putting their skin in the game". This study was sponsored by the California Institute for Regenerative Medicine, Parkinson Alliance, Blume Foundation, Brin Wojcicki Foundation. The author thank Drs. Andrezj Swistowski and Xianmin Zeng for technical training and advice on their original 5-stage neuronal differentiation protocol. We were delighted to receive the HUF5/1761 iPSC line from Dr. Renee Reijo Pera's lab as a control iPSC line. The author thank Drs. Theo Palmer and Alexandre de la Cruz for thoughtful discussions about *in vitro* and *in vivo* neuronal differentiation. The author also thank Martha Isla for technical advice on stereology and all staffs in the Stanford University FACS facility for technical support on flow cytometry analysis.

References

[1] L. E. Allan, G. H. Petit, and P. Brundin, "Cell transplantation in Parkinson's disease: problems and perspectives," *Current Opinion in Neurology*, vol. 23, no. 4, pp. 426–432, 2010.

[2] R. SoRelle, "Two-thirds of Bush-approved stem-cell lines too immature for research, Thompson says; NIH access to some assured," *Circulation*, vol. 104, no. 12, pp. E9027–9028, 2001.

[3] E. A. Zerhouni and J. F. Battey, "National Institutes of Health (NIH)—progress on stem cell research," *Stem Cell Reviews*, vol. 1, no. 2, pp. 83–85, 2005.

[4] A. D. Ebert, J. Yu, F. F. Rose et al., "Induced pluripotent stem cells from a spinal muscular atrophy patient," *Nature*, vol. 457, no. 7227, pp. 277–280, 2009.

[5] A. Urbach, O. Bar-Nur, G. Q. Daley, and N. Benvenisty, "Differential modeling of fragile X syndrome by human embryonic stem cells and induced pluripotent stem cells," *Cell Stem Cell*, vol. 6, no. 5, pp. 407–411, 2010.

[6] J. Zhang, Q. Lian, G. Zhu et al., "A Human iPSC model of Hutchinson Gilford progeria reveals vascular smooth muscle and mesenchymal stem cell defects," *Cell Stem Cell*, 2010.

[7] H. N. Nguyen, B. Byers, B. Cord et al., "LRRK2 mutant iPSC-derived da neurons demonstrate increased susceptibility to oxidative stress," *Cell Stem Cell*, vol. 8, no. 3, pp. 267–280, 2011.

[8] P. Seibler, J. Graziotto, H. Jeong, F. Simunovic, C. Klein, and D. Krainc, "Mitochondrial parkin recruitment is impaired in neurons derived from mutant PINK1 induced pluripotent stem cells," *Journal of Neuroscience*, vol. 31, no. 16, pp. 5970–5976, 2011.

[9] M. J. Devine, M. Ryten, P. Vodicka et al., "Parkinson's disease induced pluripotent stem cells with triplication of the α-synuclein locus," *Nature Communications*, vol. 2, no. 1, article 440, 2011.

[10] J. R. Mazzulli, Y. -H. Xu, Y. Sun et al., "Gaucher disease gluco-cerebrosidase and α-synuclein form a bidirectional pathogenic loop in synucleinopathies," *Cell*, vol. 146, no. 1, pp. 37–52, 2011.

[11] A. D. Ebert and C. N. Svendsen, "Human stem cells and drug screening: opportunities and challenges," *Nature Reviews Drug Discovery*, vol. 9, no. 5, pp. 367–372, 2010.

[12] B. Schüle, R. A. R. Pera, and J. W. Langston, "Can cellular models revolutionize drug discovery in Parkinson's disease?" *Biochimica et Biophysica Acta*, vol. 1792, no. 11, pp. 1043–1051, 2009.

[13] A. L. Perrier and L. Studer, "Making and repairing the mammalian brain—*in vitro* production of dopaminergic neurons," *Seminars in Cell and Developmental Biology*, vol. 14, no. 3, pp. 181–189, 2003.

[14] S. Kriks and L. Studer, "Protocols for generating ES cell-derived dopamine neurons," *Advances in Experimental Medicine and Biology*, vol. 651, pp. 101–111, 2009.

[15] S. M. Chambers, C. A. Fasano, E. P. Papapetrou, M. Tomishima, M. Sadelain, and L. Studer, "Highly efficient neural conversion of human ES and iPS cells by dual inhibition of SMAD signaling," *Nature Biotechnology*, vol. 27, no. 3, pp. 275–280, 2009.

[16] H. Kawasaki, K. Mizuseki, S. Nishikawa et al., "Induction of midbrain dopaminergic neurons from ES cells by stromal cell-derived inducing activity," *Neuron*, vol. 28, no. 1, pp. 31–40, 2000.

[17] T. Vazin, J. Chen, C. T. Lee, R. Amable, and W. J. Freed, "Assessment of stromal-derived inducing activity in the generation of dopaminergic neurons from human embryonic stem cells," *Stem Cells*, vol. 26, no. 6, pp. 1517–1525, 2008.

[18] S. H. Lee, N. Lumelsky, L. Studer, J. M. Auerbach, and R. D. McKay, "Efficient generation of midbrain and hindbrain neurons from mouse embryonic stem cells," *Nature Biotechnology*, vol. 18, no. 6, pp. 675–679, 2000.

[19] S. C. Zhang, M. Wernig, I. D. Duncan, O. Brüstle, and J. A. Thomson, "In vitro differentiation of transplantable neural precursors from human embryonic stem cells," *Nature Biotechnology*, vol. 19, no. 12, pp. 1129–1133, 2001.

[20] S. Kriks, J. -W. Shim, J. Piao et al., "Dopamine neurons derived from human ES cells efficiently engraft in animal models of Parkinson's disease," *Nature*, vol. 480, no. 7378, pp. 547–551, 2011.

[21] T. J. Zuber, "Punch biopsy of the skin," *American Family Physician*, vol. 65, no. 6, pp. 1155–1167, 2002.

[22] K. Takahashi, K. Tanabe, M. Ohnuki et al., "Induction of pluripotent stem cells from adult human fibroblasts by defined factors," *Cell*, vol. 131, no. 5, pp. 861–872, 2007.

[23] I. H. Park, P. H. Lerou, R. Zhao, H. Huo, and G. Q. Daley, "Generation of human-induced pluripotent stem cells," *Nature Protocols*, vol. 3, no. 7, pp. 1180–1186, 2008.

[24] M. J. West, L. Slomianka, and H. J. Gundersen, "Unbiased stereological estimation of the total number of neurons in the subdivisions of the rat hippocampus using the optical fractionator," *The Anatomical Record*, vol. 231, pp. 482–497, 1991.

[25] H. J. Gundersen and E. B. Jensen, "The efficiency of systematic sampling in stereology and its prediction," *Journal of Microscopy*, vol. 147, pp. 229–263, 1987.

[26] X. Zeng, J. Cai, J. Chen et al., "Dopaminergic differentiation of human embryonic stem cells," *Stem Cells*, vol. 22, no. 6, pp. 925–940, 2004.

[27] A. Swistowski, J. Peng, Q. Liu et al., "Efficient generation of functional dopaminergic neurons from human induced pluripotent stem cells under defined conditions," *Stem Cells*, vol. 28, no. 10, pp. 1893–1904, 2010.

[28] A. Swistowski, J. Peng, Y. Han, A. M. Swistowska, M. S. Rao, and X. Zeng, "Xeno-free defined conditions for culture of human embryonic stem cells, neural stem cells and dopaminergic neurons derived from them," *PLoS One*, vol. 4, no. 7, Article ID e6233, 2009.

[29] S. Colleoni, C. Galli, S. G. Giannelli et al., "Long-term culture and differentiation of CNS precursors derived from anterior human neural rosettes following exposure to ventralizing factors," *Experimental Cell Research*, vol. 316, no. 7, pp. 1148–1158, 2010.

[30] H. Kim, G. Lee, Y. Ganat et al., "miR-371-3 expression predicts neural differentiation propensity in human pluripotent stem cells," *Cell Stem Cell*, vol. 8, no. 6, pp. 695–706, 2011.

[31] S. Chung, B. S. Shin, M. Hwang et al., "Neural precursors derived from embryonic stem cells, but not those from fetal ventral mesencephalon, maintain the potential to differentiate into dopaminergic neurons after expansion *in vitro*," *Stem Cells*, vol. 24, no. 6, pp. 1583–1593, 2006.

[32] D. S. Kim, J. S. Lee, J. W. Leem et al., "Robust enhancement of neural differentiation from human ES and iPS cells regardless of their innate difference in differentiation propensity," *Stem Cell Reviews and Reports*, vol. 6, no. 2, pp. 270–281, 2010.

[33] A. Morizane, D. Doi, T. Kikuchi, K. Nishimura, and J. Takahashi, "Small-molecule inhibitors of bone morphogenic protein and activin/nodal signals promote highly efficient neural induction from human pluripotent stem cells," *Journal of Neuroscience Research*, vol. 89, no. 2, pp. 117–126, 2011.

[34] S. M. Chambers, Y. Mica, L. Studer, and M. J. Tomishima, "Converting human pluripotent stem cells to neural tissue and neurons to model neurodegeneration," *Methods in Molecular Biology*, vol. 793, pp. 87–97, 2011.

[35] P. B. Yu, C. C. Hong, C. Sachidanandan et al., "Dorsomorphin inhibits BMP signals required for embryogenesis and iron metabolism," *Nature Chemical Biology*, vol. 4, no. 1, pp. 33–41, 2008.

[36] G. J. Inman, F. J. Nicolás, J. F. Callahan et al., "SB-431542 is a potent and specific inhibitor of transforming growth factor-β superfamily type I activin receptor-like kinase (ALK) receptors ALK4, ALK5, and ALK7," *Molecular Pharmacology*, vol. 62, no. 1, pp. 65–74, 2002.

[37] G. S. Belinsky, A. R. Moore, S. M. Short, M. T. Rich, and S. D. Antic, "Physiological properties of neurons derived from human embryonic stem cells using a dibutyryl cyclic AMP-based protocol," *Stem Cells and Development*, vol. 20, no. 10, pp. 1733–1746, 2011.

[38] G. Lepski, J. Maciaczyk, C. E. Jannes, D. Maciaczyk, J. Bischof-berger, and G. Nikkhah, "Delayed functional maturation of human neuronal progenitor cells in vitro," *Molecular and Cellular Neuroscience*, vol. 47, no. 1, pp. 36–44, 2011.

[39] C. Lange, E. Mix, J. Frahm et al., "Small molecule GSK-3 inhibitors increase neurogenesis of human neural progenitor cells," *Neuroscience Letters*, vol. 488, no. 1, pp. 36–40, 2011.

[40] L. Facci, D. A. Stevens, and S. D. Skaper, "Glycogen synthase kinase-3 inhibitors protect central neurons against excitotoxi-city," *NeuroReport*, vol. 14, no. 11, pp. 1467–1470, 2003.

[41] D. F. Chen, L. J. Meng, S. H. Du et al., "(+)-Cholesten-3-one induces differentiation of neural stem cells into dopaminergic neurons through BMP signaling," *Neuroscience Research*, vol. 68, no. 3, pp. 176–184, 2010.

[42] I. Charalampopoulos, E. Remboutsika, A. N. Margioris, and A. Gravanis, "Neurosteroids as modulators of neurogen-esis and neuronal survival," *Trends in Endocrinology and Metabolism*, vol. 19, no. 8, pp. 300–307, 2008.

[43] N. F. Díaz, N. E. Díaz-Martínez, I. Velasco, and I. Camacho-Arroyo, "Progesterone increases dopamine neurone number in differentiating mouse embryonic stem cells," *Journal of Neuroendocrinology*, vol. 21, no. 8, pp. 730–736, 2009.

[44] N. F. Díaz, N. E. Díaz-Martínez, I. Camacho-Arroyo, and I. Velasco, "Estradiol promotes proliferation of dopaminergic precursors resulting in a higher proportion of dopamine neu-rons derived from mouse embryonic stem cells," *International Journal of Developmental Neuroscience*, vol. 27, no. 5, pp. 493–500, 2009.

[45] N. Sakayori, M. Maekawa, K. Numayama-Tsuruta, T. Katura, T. Moriya, and N. Osumi, "Distinctive effects of arachidonic acid and docosahexaenoic acid on neural stem/progenitor cells," *Genes to Cells*, vol. 16, no. 7, pp. 778–790, 2011.

[46] Y. L. Chang et al., "Docosahexaenoic acid promotes dopamin-ergic differentiation in induced pluripotent stem cells and inhibits teratoma formation in rats with Parkinson-like Pathology," *Cell Transplantation*, vol. 21, no. 1, pp. 313–32, 2012.

[47] E. Lonardo, C. L. Parish, S. Ponticelli et al., "A small synthetic cripto blocking peptide improves neural induction, dopaminergic differentiation, and functional integration of mouse embryonic stem cells in a rat model of Parkinson's disease," *Stem Cells*, vol. 28, no. 8, pp. 1326–1337, 2010.

12

Bench to Bedside of Neural Stem Cell in Traumatic Brain Injury

Solomon O. Ugoya and Jian Tu

Australian School of Advanced Medicine, Macquarie University, 2 Technology Place, North Ryde, Sydney, NSW 2109, Australia

Correspondence should be addressed to Jian Tu, james.tu@mq.edu.au

Academic Editor: Rocio E. Gonzalez-Castaneda

Traumatic brain injury (TBI) is one of the leading causes of major disability and death worldwide. Neural stem cells (NSCs) have recently been shown to contribute to the cellular remodelling that occurs following TBI and attention has been drawn to the area of neural stem cell as possible therapy for TBI. The NSCs may play an important role in the treatment of TBI by replacing the damaged cells and eventual remyelination. This paper summarized a critical assessment of recent data and developed a view comprising of six points to possible quality translation of NSCs in TBI.

1. Introduction

Traumatic brain injury (TBI) has remained a major cause of mortality, morbidity and leading cause of large-scale disabilities worldwide. TBI results in a large number of deaths and a cause of permanent disabilities with enormous losses to individuals, families, and communities [1]. World Health Organization (WHO), in 2004, has estimated that 25% of road traffic collisions requiring admission to a hospital suffered TBI [1–3].

Moreover, WHO has introduced the new metric tool, the disability-adjusted life year (DALY), which quantifies the burden of diseases, injuries and risk factors. The worldwide leading causes of TBI include road traffic accidents that were estimated being 41.2 million DALYs in 2008, violence being responsible for 21.7 million DALYs, and self-inflicted injuries being 19.6 million DALYs, respectively. All these will leave disability associated with TBI in survivors [2, 3].

However, no effective therapy or program is available for treatment of individuals with TBI; nonetheless, researchers had tried some therapeutic agents like levodopa/carbidopa and some neurotrophic factors in brain injury with persistent vegetative state with the aim of augmenting and slowing the progression from persistent vegetative state into some degree of consciousness. This still needs experimentation to confirm if these dopamine precursors and other neurotrophic factors have any role in TBI. Several other therapeutic agents like cannabinoid dexanabinol, erythropoietin, and gamma-glutamylcysteine ethyl ester have all shown to have neuroprotective effect in human at experimental stage with remarkable improvement in post-TBI outcome [4–8].

Recently, more attention has been drawn to the area of stem cell therapy, largely due to advanced knowledge about stem cells. The stem cells may play an important role in the treatment of TBI by replacing damaged cells, and helping functional recovery. The search for stem cell therapy for TBI is progressing. Since the pathophysiology of TBI is largely unknown, it makes a search for an effective stem cell therapy difficult. This is because multiple cell types like neuronal cells, glial, and endothelial cells are usually involved in TBI. Furthermore, cerebral vasculature, especially the blood brain barrier (BBB), may be affected in TBI; this injury may be focal or diffuse axonal injury (DAI). Taming these burgeoning effects of TBI will require NSCs which can differentiate into neurons and glial cells. It has been reported that progenitor cells differentiated into neurons and glial in adult brain, and an increase in astrocytic progeny is forming reactive astrocytes to primarily limit cyst enlargement in posttraumatic syringomyelia [9–12].

This review is an optional extra to see if we can achieve the translation of basic knowledge of neural stem cells into therapeutic options in persons with TBI by enhancing and integrating these neural progenitor cells (NPCs) unto neurogenesis and directing these cells to the specified targets or through multipotency where the transplanted cells can differentiate into glial cells, neurons, and endothelial cells, as the injuries are not always selective but diffuse and we may need to induce these transplanted cells into appropriate phenotype. This is a critical review of existing current literature on neural stem cell research and proposing an approach for quality clinical translation in TBI. We will look at the pathophysiology of TBI and proposing the "six-point schematic approach" to achieve standard and quality bench to bedside in neural stem cell of TBI. We also highlighted the need for suitable clinical translation, coordination, and administration of research in the field of neural stem cell therapy of TBI.

2. Pathophysiology of TBI

Pathophysiology of TBI involves two main phases: these are primary injury following the trauma, and the secondary injury which is mediated by inflammatory response to trauma.

2.1. Primary Injury. Pathophysiology of initial injury has been postulated to include acceleration, deceleration, and rotational forces which may or may not be as a result of the trauma. This flow of events leads to initiation of inertia which is both acceleration and rotational head movements. This impact on the cortical and subcortical brain structures causes focal or diffuse axonal injury (DAI) and these inertial forces will disrupt the BBB [13]. The primary events also involve massive ionic influx referred to as traumatic depolarization. The major inflammatory neurotransmitters released are excitatory amino acids. This may explain the pathophysiology of DAI in TBI. This is followed by cerebral edema with associated increase in intracranial pressure, which usually forms the major immediate consequences of TBI. Brain edema may come from astrocyte swelling and disruption of the BBB [14, 15]. The BBB is disrupted in acute phase of severe TBI. The expression of high levels of glucose transporter 1 (GLUT 1) was observed in capillaries from acutely injured brain, which occurs in association with compromised BBB function. Vascular endothelial growth factor also plays a role in neuronal tissue disruption and increases the permeability of the BBB via the synthesis and release of nitric oxide [16]. Figure 1 depicts the pathophysiology of the primary injury.

2.2. Secondary Injury. The secondary events are a complex association of the inflammatory response initiated by the trauma leading to diffuse neuronal degeneration of neurons, glial, axonal tearing, and genetic predisposition (Figure 2). Furthermore, excitatory amino acid release, oxygen radical reactions, and nitric oxide production will lead to activation of N-Methyl-D-aspartate (NMDA), 2-amino-3-(5-methyl-3-oxo-1,2-oxazol-4-yl)propanoic acid (AMPA), alpha-7 nicotinic receptor (α7), and nicotinic acetylcholine receptor (nACR) [17–19] and subsequent calcium influx. All these cascades of events will cause mitochondrial disruption and

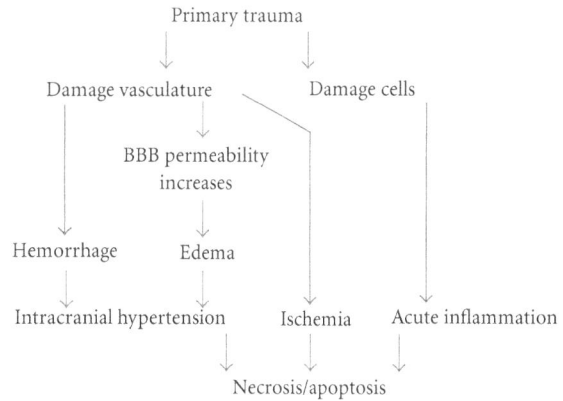

FIGURE 1: Sequential events of primary injury in TBI. Initial impact is usually by directing trauma to the head either open or closed head injury. This trauma will cause mechanical damage to neurons, axons, glia, and blood vessels by shearing, tearing, or stretching. Blood vessel ruptures cause hemorrhage. Even in unruptured blood vessels, BBB permeability increases resulting in edema. Hemorrhage and edema often lead to intracranial hypertension. Following hemorrhage, ischemia could occur in brain tissue. TBI-caused cell damage induces macrophage and lymphocytes migrant to the injury site releasing inflammatory mediators that triggers a cascade of events towards necrosis and/or apoptosis. Necrosis and/or apoptosis also can be a consequence of hemorrhage and ischemia.

free radical release with eventual tissue peroxidation. One theory is that excitatory amino acid release leads to calcium influx into neurons and other brain cells which promote oxygen-free radical reactions. High calcium and the presence of free-radical molecules create an unstable environment in the cell that may lead to increased production and release of nitric oxide and excitatory amino acids (e.g., glutamate). Nitric oxide may participate in oxygen radical reactions and lipid peroxidation in neighboring cells [20]. A summary is shown in Figure 2. The secondary injury plays a major role in the outcome of TBI. Therapeutic interventions should target this phase as it is the major determinant of morbidity and mortality in TBI [16]. Genes implicated to influence the outcome of TBI include *apoe*. *Apoe* multifactorially affects the clinicopathological consequences of TBI [21]. *Apoe* is associated with increased amyloid deposition, amyloid angiopathy, larger intracranial hematomas, and more severe contusional injury. *Comt* and *drd2* are genes which may influence dopamine-dependent cognitive processes, such as executive or frontal lobe functions. The *ace* gene may affect TBI outcome *via* alteration of cerebral blood flow and/or autoregulation and the *cacna1a* gene may exert an influence *via* the calcium channel pathways and its effect on delayed cerebral edema [22]. Increased signal transducers and activator of transcription (STAT) 3 signaling has been reported in a rat model of TBI [23]. Although several potential genes that may influence the outcomes following TBI have been identified, future investigations are needed to validate these genetic studies and identify new genes that might contribute to the outcomes following TBI.

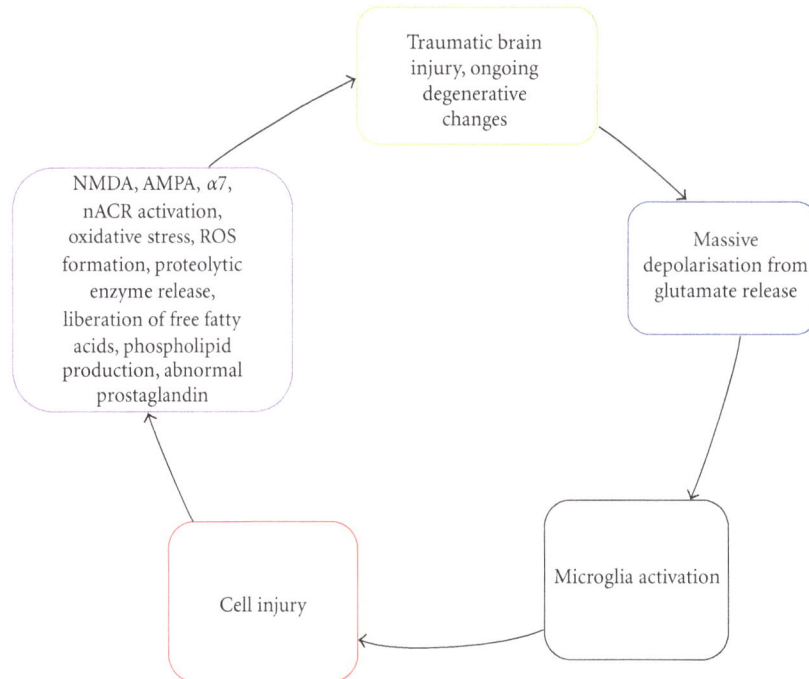

FIGURE 2: Sequential events of secondary injury in TBI. This includes variety of processes such as depolarization, disruption of ionic homeostasis and release of neurotransmitters, lipid degradation, and oxidative stress. These events are a result of interaction between the excitatory amino acid released with an influx of oxygen-free radicals that ultimately set up NMDA, AMPA, α7, and nACR to sustain the unstable environment for cell injury and degenerative changes.

3. Application of NSCs in TBI

There are at least two possible strategies involving neural stem cells (NSCs) to repair injured brain. They are transplantation of exogenous NSCs and stimulation of endogenous NSCs.

3.1. Transplantation of Exogenous NSCs. There have been attempts to transplant various types of cells, such as neurons and neural stem cells to repair damaged brain. The main objectives of these transplantation experiments are (1) growth facilitation: the transplant fills the lesion site and serves as a cellular bridge; (2) new neurons: the transplant can provide new neurons, which in turn provide new targets and sources of innervations and thus repair the damaged neural circuits; (3) factor secretion: the transplant can produce a variety of substances, such as neurotrophic factors, that may aid in the repair process [24]. Several characteristics of NSCs make them potentially suitable for repair after TBI. Firstly, they can serve as a renewable supply of transplantable cells by clonally expansion in culture. Secondly, they are of CNS origin and the cells generated from the grafts have neural characteristics. Thirdly, NSCs can be manipulated by genetic engineering methods to produce specific proteins, such as neurotrophins, neurotransmitters, and enzymes [25].

It has been reported that autologous-cultured cells harvested at time of emergency surgery from patients with TBI and subsequently engrafted into damaged part of the brain can be detected using MRI [26]. The efficacy of transplantation largely depends on a grafting method

that optimizes the survival of the transplanted cells and minimizes the graft-induced lesion. Most transplantation studies involved intraparenchymal injection into the CNS, in which cells were grafted directly into or adjacent to the lesion [27–29]. The optimal time for transplantation may not be immediately after injury. The levels of various inflammatory cytokines (TNFα, IL-1α, IL-1β, and IL-6) in the injured brain peak 6–12 hours after injury remain elevated until the 4th day. Although these inflammatory cytokines are known to have both neurotoxic and neurotrophic actions, they are believed to be neurotoxic within a week after injury, which causes the microenvironment to be unsuitable for survival of the grafted cells [30]. However, if too much time passes after the injury, glial scar forms a barrier around the lesion site and inhibits local blood circulation which is needed for graft survival. Thus, it is considered that those 7 to 14 days after injury are the optimal time for transplantation [31, 32].

3.2. Stimulation of Endogenous NPCs. Since the description of endogenous neurogenesis in adult brain by Luskin in 1997 [33] and Alvarez-Buylla and co-workers in 2000 [34], several publications have confirmed their findings. They demonstrated the presence of NSCs in adult rodent ventricular zone (VZ) that migrated to the olfactory bulb and integrated into the neuronal network called the rostral migratory stream (RMS).

However, the potential success of stimulating endogenous NPCs is hinged on delivery of various growth factors. More so, this seems to be the most common way to stimulate NPCs. The following growth factors have been reported: EGF, FGF-2 [35–37], bFGF [38], aFGF [39], BDNF [40], NGF, NT-3 [40, 41], VEGF [42], GDNF [43], IGF-1 [42], and SDF-1 alpha [44]. They were administrated by intraventricular [35], intraparenchymal [40, 42, 45] or intrathecal [36–38, 43] injection. They were reported not only to enhance the proliferation, migration, and gliogenesis of NPCs [35–37, 44] but also to protect the spinal cord from further damage [41, 42]. In addition, these growth factors facilitated the regrowth of axons and remyelination [39, 40, 46]. Functional recovery was also reported after they were delivered into injured spinal cord [35–37, 39]. However, the details of functionary recovery are still not clear.

Not only growth factors, other molecules, were shown to stimulate endogenous NPCs. Proliferation of endogenous NPCs was demonstrated when the sodium channel blocker tetrodotoxin and the glycoprotein molecule sonic hedgehog were injected into the parenchyma [47, 48]. Imitola and colleagues reported that cognate chemokine receptor type 4 (CXCR4) expressed by NSCs can regulate their proliferation and direct their migration towards the injury site [44]. In addition, antibodies blocking IL-6 receptors were reported to not only inhibit differentiation of endogenous NSCs into astroglia *in vivo* and *in vitro*, but also to promote functionary recovery [49, 50]. Okano and colleagues assumed that the functionary recovery is probably due to blocking IL-6 and consequently inhibiting the formation of glial scars and promoting axonal regeneration [49, 51]. Notably, studies of ATP-binding cassette (ABC) transporters have emerged as a new field of investigation. ABC transporters (especially ABCA2, ABCA3, ABCB1, and ABCG2) are found to play an important role in proliferation and differentiation of NSCs [45, 52–56].

In contrast to transplantation of exogenous NPCs, stimulation of endogenous NPCs to repair damaged spinal cord has three main advantages: (1) there is no ethical issue of embryonic and foetal cells, (2) it is usually less invasive, and (3) no immunogenicity; it avoids immunorejection that observed in transplantation of exogenous NPCs [57].

Like adult NPCs transplantation studies in SCI, no neurogenesis has been reported from the stimulation of endogenous NPCs. Yamamoto and colleagues reported that lack of neuronal differentiation is related to upregulation of the Notch signal pathways [58]. The increased level of various cytokines within the microenviroment surrounding the area of injury may also cause a lack of trophic support for differentiation into neuronal lineage [59–62].

Recently, more attention has been drawn to CBP/p300-phosphorylated Smad complex. It was found that CBP/p300-phosphorylated Smad complex can be bound in NSCs, which may decide the differentiation of NSCs. If the complex is bound with phosphorylated STAT 3, the NSCs differentiate into astroglia lineage cells. On the other hand, if the complex is bound with proneural-type of the basic helix-loop-helix (bHLH) factor, such as neurogenin 1 and 2, they differentiate into the neuronal lineage [51, 63, 64]. Apart from that, Peveny and Placzek reported that *SOX* gene may also play an important role in neural differentiation [65].

Once NSCs decide to differentiate into neuronal lineage, a cascade of hundreds of genes is regulated over time to lead the immature neuron into its mature phenotype. Many of these neural genes are controlled by RE1-silencing transcription factor (REST). REST acts as a repressor of neural genes in nonneural cells, while regulation of REST activates large networks of genes required for neural differentiation [66–68].

4. Bench to Bedside Translation of Stem Cell Therapy

The main purpose of scientific studies is to put our discoveries into daily clinical practice. The basic science laboratory takes its observations obtained at cellular or molecular levels in a cutting edge condition and implements this into acceptable practice clinically to the benefit of the public. However, this is always met with a lot of challenges, such as ethics, governmental regulations, funding constraints, paucity of adequate collaboration among clinical and basic science, and the challenges of conducting a clinical study.

The authors, nonetheless, propose six-point schema for improving bench to bedside translation of stem cell therapy (Figure 3(a)) involving a rigorous network of six stakeholders: basic researchers, pharmaceutical companies, patient or general public participating in clinical trials, regulatory bodies or agencies for grant approval, collaborative research between basic and clinical scientist with the plan of developing biomarkers for potential drug targets, and creating a concerted network of groups that identifies some of the medical problems relating to TBI. We are still faced with the need to formulate hypothesis both at experimental and clinical epidemiologic levels and implementing these into clinical practice while the translational researcher serves to collaborate and coordinate all these strategies.

Indeed, communication and dissemination (Figure 3(b)) which are patient centeredness will not only impact on the public, but will also help to tame the ethical problems in this field. Communication will involve both patients and other clinicians involved in conducting randomized clinical trials (RCTs). With strong feedback on outcomes, pharmacovigilance, and health promotion, education of the populace in form of scientific advocacy is so paramount as this will impact on improved scientific collaboration, quality public control, and increased transparency among researchers and may improve funding of research work [69].

Research in neural stem cell is still a grey area and much knowledge needs to be gained, to actually close the gaps. There is inadequate understanding of secondary injury process, insufficient preclinical testing in diffuse axonal injury models, species differences, and lack of understanding of the mechanism of drug-receptor interactions. Smith and colleagues had suggested the need to use gyrencephalic models for proper translation of TBI [70]. There is need for increased linkages and networking between academician, researchers, and clinicians for greater reward of what is being generated.

Methodological disparities between experimental models of TBI and clinical studies cannot be overemphasized.

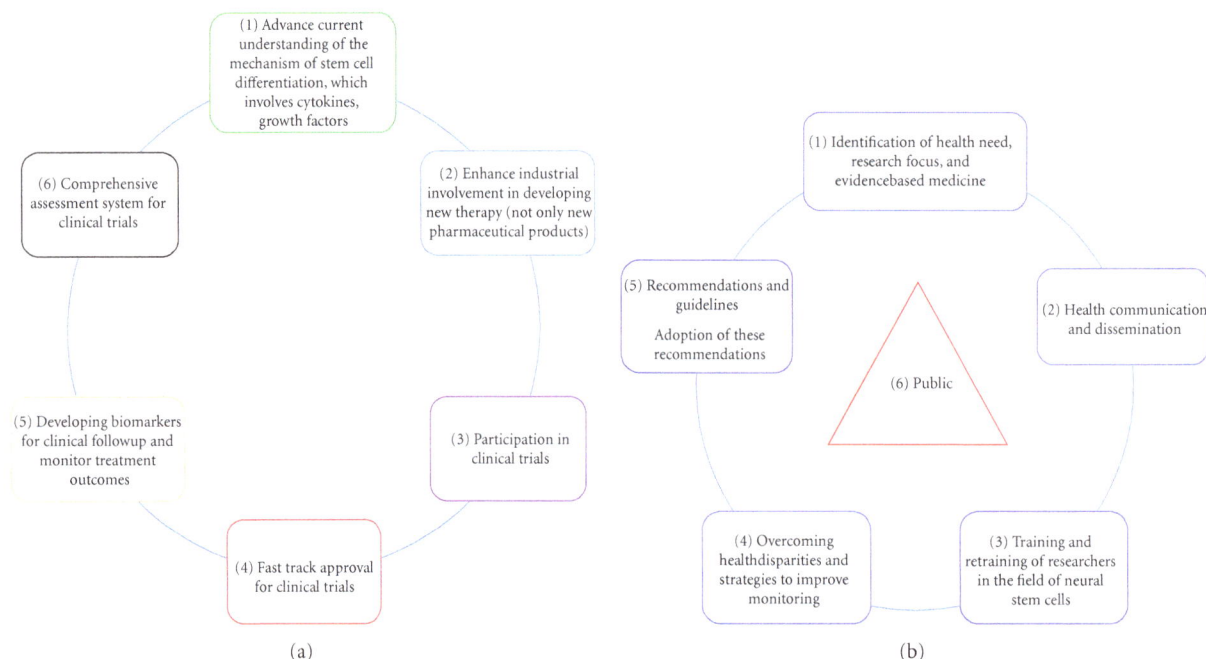

FIGURE 3: (a) Proposed schema for effective translation involving concerted effort of multilevel strategies of six main stakeholders. (b) Proposed framework for the reinforcement of the multi-level strategies effective bench to bedside translation of NSCs in TBI.

The intent to treat models, differences in statistical analysis as a result of differences in sample size, and different behaviours between human and animals. Injury severities in animals differ from humans; while they are well defined in animals, they could take any direction in human. The need to improve study quality score has recently being called for by stroke therapy academic industry roundtable (STAIR), which was recently updated and this includes the following recommendations: (1) elimination of randomizations and assessment bias, (2) use of a priori definitions of inclusion/exclusion criteria, (3) inclusion of appropriate power and sample size calculations, (4) full disclosure of potential conflict of interest, (5) evaluation of therapies in male and female animals across the spectrum of ages, and with comorbid conditions such as hypertension and/or diabetes. Furthermore, some researchers had also expanded on these proposed recommendations for improved clinical trials in brain injury with special focus on neuroprotective therapies in TBI [70, 71]. Nonadherence was the single most important determinant of trial failure in the past.

Finally, the International Mission on Prognosis and Clinical Trial Design in TBI (IMPACT) proposed ways of overcoming the above disparities and challenges. The recommendations include a robust inclusion criteria and recommendations for general research in TBI [70]. The six-point schema is an overview recommendation with the public, patient, or the society as the core and the fulcrum of all activities of research and if implemented may yield quality research outcome in neural stem cells translation in TBI.

5. Conclusions

Mortality and disability from TBI are projected to rise globally. Neural stem cell therapy is a strategy that offers

hope in the future for treatment of brain injury. In addition, we are now able to monitor autologous neural stem cells in vivo, cell migration and clearly demonstrate that neural stem cells could selectively target injured brain or spinal cord tissue and undergo neurogenesis. Finally, the proposed six-points cyclical schema should be implemented with determined effort of all stakeholders for effective bench to bedside translation of neural stem cell therapy in TBI.

Conflict of Interests

The authors declare that they have no conflict of interests.

Acknowledgments

S. O. Ugoya is a recipient of International Macquarie University Research Excellence Scholarship.

References

[1] J. D. Corrigan, A. W. Selassie, and J. A. Orman, "The epidemiologyo of traumatic brain injury," Journal of Head Trauma Rehabilitation, vol. 25, no. 2, pp. 72–80, 2010.

[2] Atlas, "country resources for neurological disorders home page," http://www.whoint/mental_health/neurology/epidemiology/en/index.html, 2012.

[3] Global burden of disease estimates, http://www.who.int/healthinfo/bodestimates/en/index.html, 2012.

[4] S. Nori, O. Tsuji, Y. Okada, Y. Toyama, H. Okano, and M. Nakamura, "Therapeutic potential of induced pluripotent stem cells for spinal cord injury," Brain Nerve, vol. 64, no. 1, pp. 17–27, 2012.

[5] S. O. Ugoya and R. O. Akinyemi, "The place of l-dopa/carbidopa in persistent vegetative state," *Clinical Neuropharmacology*, vol. 33, no. 6, pp. 279–284, 2010.

[6] A. Biegon, "Cannabinoids as neuroprotective agents in traumatic brain injury," *Current Pharmaceutical Design*, vol. 10, no. 18, pp. 2177–2183, 2004.

[7] J. Lok, W. Leung, S. Zhao et al., "Gamma-glutamylcysteine ethyl ester protects cerebral endothelial cells during injury and decreases blood-brain barrier permeability after experimental brain trauma," *Journal of Neurochemistry*, vol. 118, no. 2, pp. 248–255, 2011.

[8] A. I. R. Maas, "Neuroprotective agents in traumatic brain injury," *Expert Opinion on Investigational Drugs*, vol. 10, no. 4, pp. 753–767, 2001.

[9] A. Mammis, T. K. McIntosh, and A. H. Maniker, "Erythropoietin as a neuroprotective agent in traumatic brain injury," *Surgical Neurology*, vol. 71, no. 5, pp. 527–531, 2009.

[10] B. Stoica, K. Byrnes, and A. I. Faden, "Multifunctional drug treatment in neurotrauma," *Neurotherapeutics*, vol. 6, no. 1, pp. 14–27, 2009.

[11] J. Tu, J. Liao, M. A. Stoodley, and A. M. Cunningham, "Differentiation of endogenous progenitors in an animal model of post-traumatic Syringomyelia," *Spine*, vol. 35, no. 11, pp. 1116–1121, 2010.

[12] J. Tu, J. Liao, M. A. Stoodley, and A. M. Cunningham, "Reaction of endogenous progenitor cells in a rat model of post-traumatic syringomyelia: laboratory investigation," *Journal of Neurosurgery*, vol. 14, no. 5, pp. 573–582, 2011.

[13] C. Albert-Weissenberger, C. Varrallyay, F. Raslan, C. Kleinschnitz, and A. L. Siren, "An experimental protocol for mimicking pathomechanisms of traumatic brain injury in mice," *Experimental & Translational Stroke Medicine*, vol. 4, no. 1, 2012.

[14] J. T. Povlishock, "Traumatically induced axonal injury: pathogenesis and pathobiological implications," *Brain Pathology*, vol. 2, no. 1, pp. 1–12, 1992.

[15] M. W. Greve and B. J. Zink, "Pathophysiology of traumatic brain injury," *Mount Sinai Journal of Medicine*, vol. 76, no. 2, pp. 97–104, 2009.

[16] H. Nawashiro, K. Shima, and H. Chigasaki, "Blood-brain barrier, cerebral blood flow, and cerebral plasma volume immediately after head injury in the rat," *Acta Neurochirurgica, Supplement*, vol. 60, pp. 440–442, 1994.

[17] J. M. Hinzman, T. C. Thomas, J. E. Quintero, G. A. Gerhardt, and J. Lifshitz, "Disruptions in the regulation of extracellular glutamate by neurons and glia in the rat striatum two days after diffuse brain injury," *Journal of Neurotrauma*, vol. 29, no. 6, pp. 1197–1208, 2012.

[18] P. B. Goforth, E. F. Ellis, and L. S. Satin, "Enhancement of AMPA-mediated current after traumatic injury in cortical neurons," *Journal of Neuroscience*, vol. 19, no. 17, pp. 7367–7374, 1999.

[19] M. L. Kelso and J. H. Oestreich, "Traumatic brain injury: Central and peripheral role of $\alpha 7$ nicotinic acetylcholine receptors," *Current Drug Targets*, vol. 13, no. 5, pp. 631–636, 2012.

[20] M. Stoffel, M. Rinecker, N. Plesnila, J. Eriskat, and A. Baethmann, "Role of nitric oxide in the secondary expansion of a cortical brain lesion from cold injury," *Journal of Neurotrauma*, vol. 18, no. 4, pp. 425–434, 2001.

[21] A. A. Potapov, M. M. Iusupova, V. D. Tendieva, A. G. Nikitin, and V. V. Nosikov, "Clinical and prognostic significance of genetic markers of ApoE gene in traumatic brain injury," *Zhurnal voprosy neĭrokhirurgii imeni N N Burdenko*, no. 3, pp. 54–62, 2010.

[22] B. D. Jordan, "Genetic influences on outcome following traumatic brain injury," *Neurochemical Research*, vol. 32, no. 4-5, pp. 905–915, 2007.

[23] A. A. Oliva, Y. Kang, J. Sanchez-Molano, C. Furones, and C. M. Atkins, "STAT3 signaling after traumatic brain injury," *Journal of Neurochemistry*, vol. 120, no. 5, pp. 710–720, 2012.

[24] K. Barami and F. G. Diaz, "Cellular transplantation and spinal cord injury," *Neurosurgery*, vol. 47, no. 3, pp. 691–700, 2000.

[25] D. W. Pincus, R. R. Goodman, R. A. R. Fraser, M. Nedergaard, and S. A. Goldman, "Neural stem and progenitor cells: a strategy for gene therapy and brain repair," *Neurosurgery*, vol. 42, no. 4, pp. 858–868, 1998.

[26] M. Nakamura, R. A. Houghtling, L. MacArthur, B. M. Bayer, and B. S. Bregman, "Differences in cytokine gene expression profile between acute and secondary injury in adult rat spinal cord," *Experimental Neurology*, vol. 184, no. 1, pp. 313–325, 2003.

[27] S. Y. Chow, J. Moul, C. A. Tobias et al., "Characterization and intraspinal grafting of EGF/bFGF-dependent neurospheres derived from embryonic rat spinal cord," *Brain Research*, vol. 874, no. 2, pp. 87–106, 2000.

[28] Q. L. Cao, Y. P. Zhang, R. M. Howard, W. M. Walters, P. Tsoulfas, and S. R. Whittemore, "Pluripotent stem cells engrafted into the normal or lesioned adult rat spinal cord are restricted to a glial lineage," *Experimental Neurology*, vol. 167, no. 1, pp. 48–58, 2001.

[29] P. Jendelová, V. Herynek, L. Urdzíková et al., "Magnetic resonance tracking of transplanted bone marrow and embryonic stem cells labeled by iron oxide nanoparticles in rat brain and spinal cord," *Journal of Neuroscience Research*, vol. 76, no. 2, pp. 232–243, 2004.

[30] J. Zhu, L. Zhou, and F. XingWu, "Tracking neural stem cells in patients with brain trauma," *The New England Journal of Medicine*, vol. 355, no. 22, pp. 2376–2378, 2006.

[31] Y. Ogawa, K. Sawamoto, T. Miyata et al., "Transplantation of in vitro-expanded fetal neural progenitor cells results in neurogenesis and functional recovery after spinal cord contusion injury in adult rats," *Journal of Neuroscience Research*, vol. 69, no. 6, pp. 925–933, 2002.

[32] H. Okano, Y. Ogawa, M. Nakamura, S. Kaneko, A. Iwanami, and Y. Toyama, "Transplantation of neural stem cells into the spinal cord after injury," *Seminars in Cell and Developmental Biology*, vol. 14, no. 3, pp. 191–198, 2003.

[33] M. B. Luskin, T. Zigova, B. J. Soteres, and R. R. Stewart, "Neuronal progenitor cells derived from the anterior subventricular zone of the neonatal rat forebrain continue to proliferate in vitro and express a neuronal phenotype," *Molecular and Cellular Neurosciences*, vol. 8, no. 5, pp. 351–366, 1996.

[34] A. Alvarez-Buylla, D. G. Herrera, and H. Wichterle, "The subventricular zone: Source of neuronal precursors for brain repair," *Progress in Brain Research*, vol. 127, pp. 1–11, 2000.

[35] D. J. Martens, R. M. Seaberg, and D. Van der Kooy, "In vivo infusions of exogenous growth factors into the fourth ventricle of the adult mouse brain increase the proliferation of neural progenitors around the fourth ventricle and the central canal of the spinal cord," *European Journal of Neuroscience*, vol. 16, no. 6, pp. 1045–1057, 2002.

[36] A. Kojima and C. H. Tator, "Epidermal growth factor and fibroblast growth factor 2 cause proliferation of ependymal precursor cells in the adult rat spinal cord in vivo," *Journal of Neuropathology and Experimental Neurology*, vol. 59, no. 8, pp. 687–697, 2000.

[37] A. Kojima and C. H. Tator, "Intrathecal administration of epidermal growth factor and fibroblast growth factor 2 promotes ependymal proliferation and functional recovery after spinal cord injury in adult rats," *Journal of Neurotrauma*, vol. 19, no. 2, pp. 223–238, 2002.

[38] A. G. Rabchevsky, I. Fugaccia, A. F. Turner, D. A. Blades, M. P. Mattson, and S. W. Scheff, "Basic fibroblast growth factor (bFGF) enhances functional recovery following severe spinal cord injury to the rat," *Experimental Neurology*, vol. 164, no. 2, pp. 280–291, 2000.

[39] Y. S. Lee, C. Y. Lin, R. T. Robertson, I. Hsiao, and V. W. Lin, "Motor recovery and anatomical evidence of axonal regrowth in spinal cord-repaired adult rats," *Journal of Neuropathology and Experimental Neurology*, vol. 63, no. 3, pp. 233–245, 2004.

[40] J. Namiki, A. Kojima, and C. H. Tator, "Effect of brain-derived neurotrophic factor, nerve growth factor, and neurotrophin-3 on functional recovery and regeneration after spinal cord injury in adult rats," *Journal of Neurotrauma*, vol. 17, no. 12, pp. 1219–1231, 2000.

[41] J. Widenfalk, A. Lipson, M. Jubran et al., "Vascular endothelial growth factor improves functional outcome and decreases secondary degeneration in experimental spinal cord contusion injury," *Neuroscience*, vol. 120, no. 4, pp. 951–960, 2003.

[42] H. S. Sharma, "Neurotrophic factors attenuate microvascular permeability disturbances and axonal injury following trauma to the rat spinal cord," *Acta Neurochirurgica*, no. 86, pp. 383–388, 2003.

[43] C. Iannotti, Y. Ping Zhang, C. B. Shields, Y. Han, D. A. Burke, and X. M. Xu, "A neuroprotective role of glial cell line-derived neurotrophic factor following moderate spinal cord contusion injury," *Experimental Neurology*, vol. 189, no. 2, pp. 317–332, 2004.

[44] J. Imitola, K. Raddassi, K. I. Park et al., "Directed migration of neural stem cells to sites of CNS injury by the stromal cell-derived factor 1α/CXC chemokine receptor 4 pathway," *Proceedings of the National Academy of Sciences of the United States of America*, vol. 101, no. 52, pp. 18117–18122, 2004.

[45] G. Li, P. Shi, and Y. Wang, "Evolutionary dynamics of the ABCA chromosome 17q24 cluster genes in vertebrates," *Genomics*, vol. 89, no. 3, pp. 385–391, 2007.

[46] J. M. Gensert and J. E. Goldman, "Endogenous progenitors remyelinate demyelinated axons in the adult CNS," *Neuron*, vol. 19, no. 1, pp. 197–203, 1997.

[47] L. J. Rosenberg, L. J. Zai, and J. R. Wrathall, "Chronic alterations in the cellular composition of spinal cord white matter following contusion injury," *GLIA*, vol. 49, no. 1, pp. 107–120, 2005.

[48] N. C. Bambakidis, R. Z. Wang, L. Franic, and R. H. Miller, "Sonic hedgehog-induced neural precursor proliferation after adult rodent spinal cord injury," *Journal of Neurosurgery*, vol. 99, no. 1, pp. 70–75, 2003.

[49] S. Okada, M. Nakamura, Y. Mikami et al., "Blockade of interleukin-6 receptor suppresses reactive astrogliosis and ameliorates functional recovery in experimental spinal cord injury," *Journal of Neuroscience Research*, vol. 76, no. 2, pp. 265–276, 2004.

[50] M. Nakamura, S. Okada, Y. Toyama, and H. Okano, "Role of IL-6 in spinal cord injury in a mouse model," *Clinical Reviews in Allergy and Immunology*, vol. 28, no. 3, pp. 197–203, 2005.

[51] H. Okano, S. Okada, M. Nakamura, and Y. Toyama, "Neural stem cells and regeneration of injured spinal cord," *Kidney International*, vol. 68, no. 5, pp. 1927–1931, 2005.

[52] T. Lin, O. Islam, and K. Heese, "ABC transporters, neural stem cells and neurogenesis—a different perspective," *Cell Research*, vol. 16, no. 11, pp. 857–871, 2006.

[53] P. D. W. Eckford and F. J. Sharom, "P-glycoprotein (ABCB1) interacts directly with lipid-based anti-cancer drugs and platelet-activating factors," *Biochemistry and Cell Biology*, vol. 84, no. 6, pp. 1022–1033, 2006.

[54] D. F. P. Leite, J. Echevarria-Lima, J. B. Calixto, and V. M. Rumjanek, "Multidrug resistance related protein (ABCC1) and its role on nitrite production by the murine macrophage cell line RAW 264.7," *Biochemical Pharmacology*, vol. 73, no. 5, pp. 665–674, 2007.

[55] T. Saito, K. Yamada, Y. Wang et al., "Expression of ABCA2 protein in both non-myelin-forming and myelin-forming Schwann cells in the rodent peripheral nerve," *Neuroscience Letters*, vol. 414, no. 1, pp. 35–40, 2007.

[56] A. Tamura, K. Wakabayashi, Y. Onishi et al., "Genetic polymorphisms of human ABC transporter ABCG2: development of the standard method for functional validation of SNPs by using the Flp recombinase system," *Journal of Experimental Therapeutics and Oncology*, vol. 6, no. 1, pp. 1–11, 2006.

[57] P. Mohapel and P. Brundin, "Harnessing endogenous stem cells to treat neurodegenerative disorders of the basal ganglia," *Parkinsonism and Related Disorders*, vol. 10, no. 5, pp. 259–264, 2004.

[58] S. I. Yamamoto, M. Nagao, M. Sugimori et al., "Transcription factor expression and notch-dependent regulation of neural progenitors in the adult rat spinal cord," *Journal of Neuroscience*, vol. 21, no. 24, pp. 9814–9823, 2001.

[59] J. Frisén, C. B. Johansson, C. Török, M. Risling, and U. Lendahl, "Rapid, widespread, and longlasting induction of nestin contributes to the generation of glial scar tissue after CNS injury," *Journal of Cell Biology*, vol. 131, no. 2, pp. 453–464, 1995.

[60] C. B. Johansson, S. Momma, D. L. Clarke, M. Risling, U. Lendahl, and J. Frisén, "Identification of a neural stem cell in the adult mammalian central nervous system," *Cell*, vol. 96, no. 1, pp. 25–34, 1999.

[61] H. Okano, Y. Ogawa, M. Nakamura, S. Kaneko, A. Iwanami, and Y. Toyama, "Transplantation of neural stem cells into the spinal cord after injury," *Seminars in Cell and Developmental Biology*, vol. 14, no. 3, pp. 191–198, 2003.

[62] J. Widenfalk, K. Lundströmer, M. Jubran, S. Brené, and L. Olson, "Neurotrophic factors and receptors in the immature and adult spinal cord after mechanical injury or kainic acid," *Journal of Neuroscience*, vol. 21, no. 10, pp. 3457–3475, 2001.

[63] Y. Sun, M. Nadal-Vicens, S. Misono et al., "Neurogenin promotes neurogenesis and inhibits glial differentiation by independent mechanisms," *Cell*, vol. 104, no. 3, pp. 365–376, 2001.

[64] K. Nakashima, M. Yanagisawa, H. Arakawa et al., "Synergistic signaling in fetal brain by STAT3-Smad1 complex bridged by p300," *Science*, vol. 284, no. 5413, pp. 479–482, 1999.

[65] L. Pevny and M. Placzek, "SOX genes and neural progenitor identity," *Current Opinion in Neurobiology*, vol. 15, no. 1, pp. 7–13, 2005.

[66] F. H. Gage and A. K. M, "Neuronal and glial cell biology," *Current Opinion in Neurobiology*, vol. 15, no. 5, pp. 497–499, 2005.

[67] N. Ballas, C. Grunseich, D. D. Lu, J. C. Speh, and G. Mandel, "REST and its corepressors mediate plasticity of neuronal gene chromatin throughout neurogenesis," *Cell*, vol. 121, no. 4, pp. 645–657, 2005.

[68] N. Ballas and G. Mandel, "The many faces of REST oversee epigenetic programming of neuronal genes," *Current Opinion in Neurobiology*, vol. 15, no. 5, pp. 500–506, 2005.

[69] N. C. Keramaris, N. K. Kanakaris, C. Tzioupis, G. Kontakis, and P. V. Giannoudis, "Translational research: from benchside to bedside," *Injury*, vol. 39, no. 6, pp. 643–650, 2008.

[70] D. J. Loane and A. I. Faden, "Neuroprotection for traumatic brain injury: translational challenges and emerging therapeutic strategies," *Trends in Pharmacological Sciences*, vol. 31, no. 12, pp. 596–604, 2010.

[71] M. Fisher, G. Feuerstein, D. W. Howells et al., "Update of the stroke therapy academic industry roundtable preclinical recommendations," *Stroke*, vol. 40, no. 6, pp. 2244–2250, 2009.

13

The Flatworm *Macrostomum lignano* Is a Powerful Model Organism for Ion Channel and Stem Cell Research

Daniil Simanov,[1] **Imre Mellaart-Straver,**[1] **Irina Sormacheva,**[2] **and Eugene Berezikov**[1,3]

[1] *Hubrecht Institute, KNAW, University Medical Center Utrecht, 3584 CT Utrecht, The Netherlands*
[2] *Institute of Cytology and Genetics SB RAS, 630090 Novosibirsk, Russia*
[3] *European Research Institute for the Biology of Ageing and University Medical Center Groningen, University of Groningen, 9713 AV Groningen, The Netherlands*

Correspondence should be addressed to Eugene Berezikov, e.berezikov@umcg.nl

Academic Editor: Michael Levin

Bioelectrical signals generated by ion channels play crucial roles in many cellular processes in both excitable and nonexcitable cells. Some ion channels are directly implemented in chemical signaling pathways, the others are involved in regulation of cytoplasmic or vesicular ion concentrations, pH, cell volume, and membrane potentials. Together with ion transporters and gap junction complexes, ion channels form steady-state voltage gradients across the cell membranes in nonexcitable cells. These membrane potentials are involved in regulation of such processes as migration guidance, cell proliferation, and body axis patterning during development and regeneration. While the importance of membrane potential in stem cell maintenance, proliferation, and differentiation is evident, the mechanisms of this bioelectric control of stem cell activity are still not well understood, and the role of specific ion channels in these processes remains unclear. Here we introduce the flatworm *Macrostomum lignano* as a versatile model organism for addressing these topics. We discuss biological and experimental properties of *M. lignano*, provide an overview of the recently developed experimental tools for this animal model, and demonstrate how manipulation of membrane potential influences regeneration in *M. lignano*.

1. Introduction

Ion channels represent a diverse family of pore-forming proteins. They are crucial for establishing voltage gradients across plasma membranes by allowing the flow of inorganic ions (such as Na^+, K^+, Ca^{2+}, or Cl^-) down their electrochemical gradients. Ionic flux through the channels provides the foundation for membrane excitability, which is essential for the proper functioning of neurons, cardiac, and muscle cells [1]. At the same time, ion channels serve many functions apart from electrical signal transduction. For example, Ca^{2+} is an important messenger, and changes in its intracellular concentrations influence numerous cellular processes in virtually all types of nonexcitable cells [2–4], including stem cells [5–7]. Besides, a number of ion channels are known

to be directly involved in chemical signaling pathways in different cell types [8, 9]. As a result, mutations in genes encoding ion channel proteins have been associated with many disorders (so-called "channelopathies"), caused by dysfunction of both excitable (epilepsy, hypertension, cardiac arrhythmia) and nonexcitable (diabetes, osteopetrosis, and cystic fibrosis) cells [10]. Here we briefly describe the crucial role ion channels play in maintenance, proliferation, and differentiation of stem cells on the level of single cell and the whole organism. We discuss the importance of animal model systems, such as flatworms, for studying bioelectric signaling in complex morphogenesis during development and regeneration. Finally, we introduce the new flatworm model, *Macrostomum lignano*, and discuss its experimental potential for dissecting the roles of ion channels in stem cell regulation.

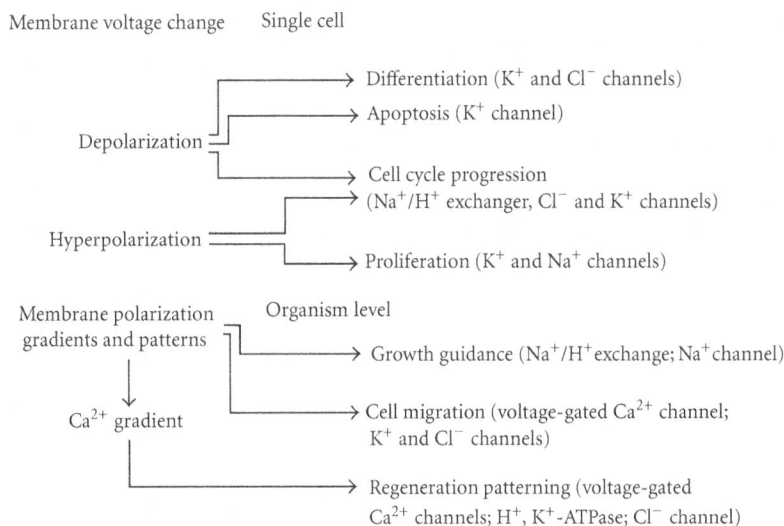

FIGURE 1: Ion channels and membrane voltage during regeneration. Changes of membrane potentials can directly affect different aspects of cell behavior and large-scale morphogenetic processes during regeneration. Ion channels and transporters implicated in these processes are mentioned in brackets.

2. Ion Channels and Membrane Potential in Stem Cells

Numerous ion channels and pumps together with gap junction complexes form transmembrane voltage gradients. While quick changes of these membrane potentials (V_{mem}) are best described in neurons, muscle, and cardiac cells, long-term steady-state V_{mem} levels are present in all other cells [11, 12]. Membrane potentials strongly correlate with the mitotic ability of different cell types, with the high resting potential associated with differentiated nondividing cells [13]. V_{mem} fluctuations during progression through the cell cycle have been reported in a number of cell types, and changes of membrane potential appear to be required for both G1/S and G2/S phase transitions [14–16]. Modulation of V_{mem} through applied electric fields or by inhibition of ion channels leads to cell cycle arrest in dividing cells [17–20], and artificial membrane hyperpolarization induces differentiation of mesenchymal stem cells [21]. On the other hand, electroporation (supposedly followed by membrane depolarization) activates cell hyperproliferation and de-differentiation [22].

On the level of multicellular organism, progression through the cell cycle should be strictly regulated and synchronized during such processes as development and regeneration in order to achieve a proper body patterning. Accordingly, stable and reproducible membrane polarization patterns have been recently described in various model organisms. Artificial modulation of these patterns during development or regeneration has a large impact on left-right asymmetry and anterior-posterior identity [23–27]. The role of bioelectric signaling in regeneration is comprehensively reviewed in [28] and schematically shown in Figure 1. Finally, modulations of membrane voltage have

been observed in a large number of oncological disorders, and ion channels were proposed as cancer treatment targets [29, 30].

Thus, bioelectric signaling is an important mechanism of cell regulation, including stem cell maintenance, proliferation and differentiation. Recent findings suggest this control system to be well conserved in a wide range of animal phyla. However, the mechanisms linking membrane potential to the cell cycle, proliferation and differentiation, and the role of specific ion channels in this process remain largely unclear. The picture becomes even more complicated on the level of multicellular organism. Our understanding of the ways cells produce and receive bioelectric signals and translate them into positional information during development and regeneration is still fairly poor. While considerable knowledge about the role of membrane potential in stem cells was gathered recently from different species, the number of models used in this field is still limited. Expanding the range of model organisms used for functional studies of bioelectric signaling is crucial for better understanding of this control system and its role in complex morphogenesis.

3. Planarian Models in Ion Channel Research

Planarian flatworms are long-established models for stem cell and regeneration research. The adult stem cell system and regeneration capacity of the species *Planaria maculata* and *Planaria lugubris* were described by Morgan as early as in the end of 19th century [31, 32]. In our days the favorite planarian species for research in the regeneration field are *Schmidtea mediterranea* and *Dugesia japonica* [33, 34]. Planaria were also one of the first species in which stable membrane potential patterns were described, and their role in regeneration postulated. In 1940s and 1950s Marsh and Beams were able to specifically control establishing of anterior-posterior axis by providing bioelectrical signals to regenerating planaria fragments [35–37].

In the last 5 years considerable work was done in planaria on understanding the molecular and genetic mechanisms that allow cells to establish and maintain long-term membrane potential patterns and transduce bioelectric signals into proliferation and differentiation decisions. The importance of gap junction signaling in establishing anterior-posterior polarity during regeneration was shown [38], and the specific innexin gene, *Smedinx-11*, responsible for blastema (regenerating tissue) formation and stem cell maintenance identified [39].

The role of ion channels and pumps in the establishment of anterior-posterior axis during regeneration of planaria *D. japonica* was recently highlighted by groups of Michael Levin and Jonathan Marchant. *D. japonica*, which can regenerate an entire animal from a small part of a cut worm, has highly depolarized cell membranes in the head region, and highly polarized in the posterior part. In the cut worm this pattern is reestablished rapidly, regardless of the cutting plane [26]. After the wound is closed, blastema at all anterior-facing wounds gives origin to heads, while tails are regenerated from the posterior-facing wounds. The polarization pattern is altered by highly specific drugs against different ion channels and transporters, such as SCH-28080 (inhibitor of H^+, K^+-ATPase), ivermectin (IVM, activator of the invertebrate GluCl channels), or praziquantel (PZQ, activator of voltage-operated Ca^{2+}-channels). Remarkably, induced depolarization itself is sufficient to drive ectopic anterior (head) regeneration even in posterior-facing blastemas, whereas membrane polarization of anterior-facing wounds blocks the head regeneration [25, 26]. The role of specific voltage-operated Ca^{2+} channels in regenerative patterning was addressed in the followup experiments [27].

Thus, planarian flatworms can be successfully used for ion channel and stem cell studies. Fascinating regeneration capacity of these animals, together with a wide range of research techniques established and optimized over the last 100 years, make planaria a very attractive model for studying bioelectric signaling during regenerative morphogenesis. However, due to inefficient sexual reproduction under laboratory conditions, classical genetic methods are not available in planarians, and reverse genetics methods are limited to RNA interference. Since genetic manipulation of these animals is difficult, no reproducible transgenesis methods are available for planaria [40].

4. Experimental Properties of the Flatworm *Macrostomum lignano*

During the last decade another flatworm, *Macrostomum lignano*, has emerged as a complementary model organism for regeneration research [41–44]. This marine free-living basal flatworm is about 1.5 mm long and consists of roughly 25000 cells. *M. lignano* is easy to culture in laboratory conditions, and populations of this animal are continuously maintained in the number of laboratories for over a

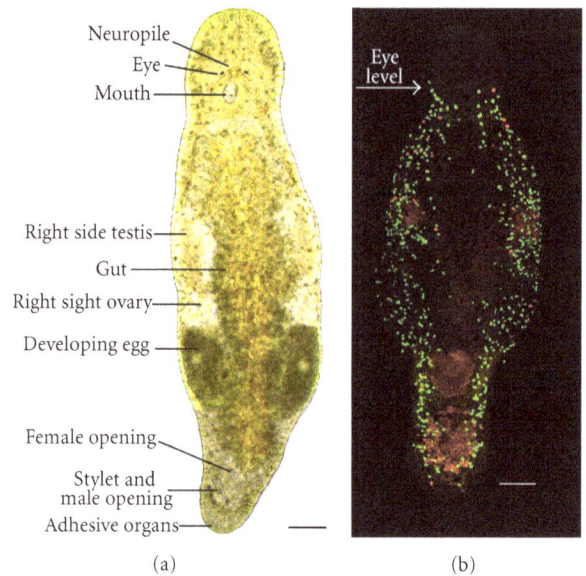

FIGURE 2: *Macrostomum lignano* as a model organism. (a) Bright field image of a living specimen. (b) Confocal projection of BrdU and phospho-histone H3 immunostaining after 30 minutes BrdU pulse in an adult worm (green: S-phase cells, red: mitotic cells). Scalebar 100 μm.

decade. The generation time of the flatworm is short, with about two weeks of postembryonic development to sexually mature adult. Both juvenile and adult worms have clear morphology and are highly transparent (Figure 2(a)), greatly facilitating phenotyping and both fluorescent and nonfluorescent staining. The regeneration capacity of *M. lignano* is provided by roughly 1600 neoblasts (adult stem cells) located mesodermally. Proliferation activity of these cells can be easily studied using BrdU labeling, performed by simple soaking [43, 45] (Figure 2(b)). Importantly, *M. lignano* is nonself fertilizing hermaphrodite and has exclusively sexual reproduction. Well-fed adult animals generate a lot of embryos all year through (one animal lies on average one egg a day), making it accessible for genetic manipulation. *In situ* hybridization [43] and RNA interference (by soaking) [45] protocols are established and optimized for *M. lignano*, and a number of tissue-specific monoclonal antibodies are available [41]. Basic culturing and experimental properties of *M. lignano* are summarized in Table 1.

Considerable progress has been made in the past three years towards establishing *M. lignano* as versatile stem cell research model for the genomics era. The work on *M. lignano* genome assembly and annotation is in progress (Berezikov and colleagues), and draft genome and transcriptome assemblies are publicly available at http://www.macgenome.org/. Comparing transcriptome data obtained from irradiated (neoblast-depleted) and control worms provided the insight into the role of a number of genes in regeneration, while stage-specific transcriptome data showed the temporal expression of *Macrostomum* genes through development

TABLE 1: Biological and experimental properties of *M. lignano*.

Size	1 mm
Total cell number	±25.000
Neoblasts	±1600
Transparency	Highly transparent
Culturing media	f/2 (sea water based)
Feeding	Diatom algae (*Nitzschia curvilineata*)
Embryogenesis	5 days
Generation time	18 days
Nervous, muscle system, and gonads	Simple
Stem cell system	Pluripotent
BrdU/H3 staining	Yes (easy by soaking)
RNA interference	Yes (easy by soaking)
Accessibility to eggs	Single eggs (one egg/day per animal)
Transgenics	Possible, by injection into eggs

(Simanov et al., in preparation). Most importantly, proof-of-principle for transgenesis in *M. lignano* has been demonstrated and first stable transgenic GFP-expressing lines of *M. lignano* have been established (Demircan, De Mulder, Berezikov et al., in preparation). Thus, biological and experimental properties of *M. lignano*, combined with its rapidly expanding experimental toolbox, make this animal an attractive and powerful model organism for stem cell and regeneration research. Its astonishing ability to resist γ-irradiation and recover after being exposed to it makes the neoblast system of this animal exceptional even for flatworms [46]. Moreover, fascinating but yet poorly understood link between regeneration and rejuvenation provides an exciting opportunity of using *M. lignano* as a model for ageing research [47].

5. Ion Channels and Regeneration in *M. lignano*

Unlike planarian flatworm species, *M. lignano* is unable to regenerate the head under normal circumstances. Posterior-facing blastemas give origin to fully functioning tails with all its organs and structures, whereas anterior-facing wounds develop blastema layer but the actual regeneration can only happen if the worm was amputated in front of the brain (at the very tip of the head). Thus, anterior fragments of the worm, having a functional head, can regenerate the whole body in 2-3 weeks, while posterior fragments normally die 5–10 days after losing the head [42]. These differences in the head regeneration capacity between *M. lignano* and planarians, and the ability to induce ectopic head regeneration in *D. japonica* by the manipulation of membrane voltage gradients, prompted us to investigate how these findings in planarians translate into *M. lignano*.

DiBAC$_4$(3) voltage-reporting dye stainings (as described in [48]) showed that membrane voltage pattern in *M. lignano* is similar to the one observed in *D. japonica* [26]—the anterior part is highly depolarized, while the tail is relatively polarized. In the cut worms this pattern is quickly reestablished in the anterior head-containing fragments, while the posterior headless fragments do not show any

clear anterior-posterior polarization gradient and do not regenerate (Figure 3(a)). Just like in planarians, membrane polarization patterns in *M. lignano* can be altered using drugs against ion channels. IVM induces depolarization of the membranes of intact and cut worms, both in anterior and posterior regions (Figure 3(b)). Posterior-facing blastemas still regenerate the tails after treatment, though the full regeneration takes longer than normally. Anterior-facing wounds treated with IVM develop blastema, and some tissue growth is often observed within a week after wound closure. IVM-treated headless fragments always move more actively and survive longer comparing to control fragments. Strikingly, 1.5% of posterior fragments after IVM treatment are able to regenerate head-specific structures and, in a few cases, a fully functional head (Figures 3(c) and 3(c′)). PZQ causes the same depolarization effect but does not have any effect on regeneration patterning at tested concentrations (data not shown). Intact animals exposed to high doses of IVM or PZQ display phenotypes that in planarian flatworms are stereotypically associated with stem cell loss or disorder [49–52]. *M. lignano* animals treated with 2 μM IVM gradually lose anterior identity, with no head-specific structures left 7–9 days after treatment (Figure 3(d)). After exposure to higher doses of IVM (3-4 μM), worms develop characteristic square head due to partial tissue loss in the most anterior part of the body, get paralyzed and die 3-4 days after treatment (Figure 3(d′)). High concentration of PZQ in culturing media causes formation of bulges, mainly in the posterior part of the body (Figure 3(d″)). This phenotype is completely different from the one observed after IVM treatment, suggesting specific action of the drugs.

These pilot experimental results show that *M. lignano* can be successfully used as a model for ion channel and stem cell studies. The complete transcriptome and established *in situ* hybridization and RNA interference methods, in combination with chemical treatment make it possible to address the function of specific ion channels in development, tissue turnover, and regeneration. For example, comparison of transcriptome data from irradiated (stem cell-deficient) and nonirradiated animals (Simanov et al., in preparation)

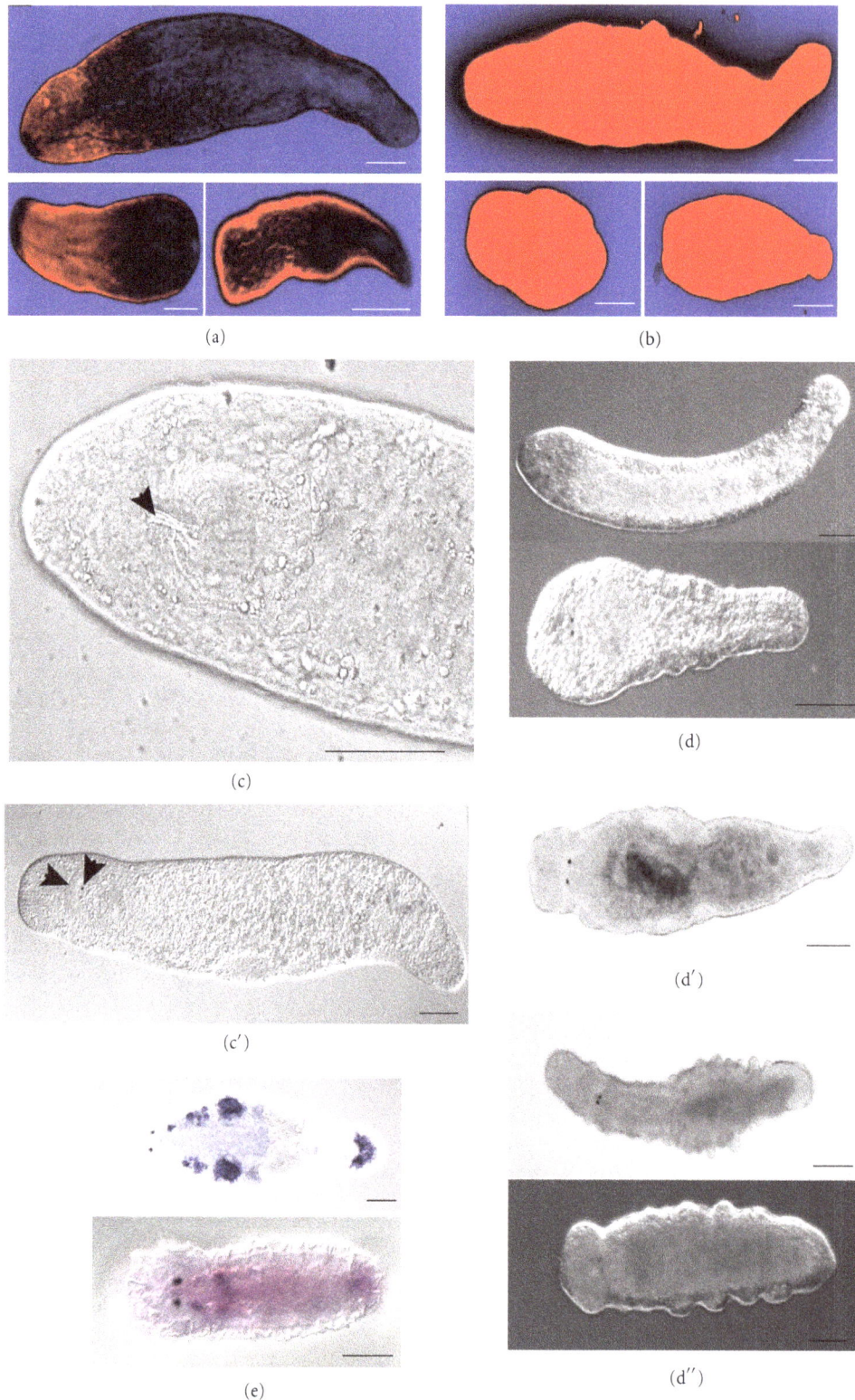

FIGURE 3: Bioelectric signaling and stem cells in *M. lignano*. (a-b) DiBAC$_4$(3) staining of intact worm (top), anterior (left bottom) and posterior (right bottom) fragments. (a) control worm, (b) worm treated with 1 μM IVM. Blue is more polarized than black, black is more polarized than red. (c-c′) Regeneration of head-specific structures after 1 μM IVM treatment. Arrowheads in (c) indicate regenerated pharynx, in (c′) regenerated eye and half of the brain. (d-d″) intact worms exposed to high doses of IVM (2 μM in d and 4 μM in d′) and PZQ (150 μM in d″). (d) head regression; (d′) square head; (d″) bulges and outgrowth. (e) *In situ* hybridization results in adult (top) and juvenile (bottom) animals with the probe against RNA815_5834 transcript from ML110815 transcriptome assembly (voltage-gated sodium channel). In juvenile worm this gene is expressed almost ubiquitously, and in adults expression is only detected in gonads and (likely) in somatic stem cells. Strong signal in the adhesive glands in the tail is likely a common artifact.

TABLE 2: Major categories of ion channel genes conserved between *H. sapiens* and *M. lignano*.

GO term	Description	*H*	*M*	Human genes
GO:0004889	Acetylcholine-activated cation-selective channel activity	13	132	CHRNA4, CHRNE, CHRNA10, CHRNB1, CHRNB3, CHRNA6, CHRNA3, CHRND, CHRNB2, CHRNB4, CHRNA9, CHRNA2, CHRNA7
GO:0004931	Extracellular ATP-gated cation channel activity	5	15	P2RX6, P2RX7, P2RX5, P2RX4, P2RX2
GO:0004970	Ionotropic glutamate receptor activity	12	67	GRIN1, GRIA4, GRIN2A, GRIK2, GRIK1, GRIA1, GRIK4, GRIA2, GRIK3, GRID1, GRIN3A, GRIK5
GO:0005216	Ion channel activity	6	23	PKD1L2, MCOLN3, MCOLN2, PKD2L2, PKD2L1, PKDREJ
GO:0005221	Intracellular cyclic nucleotide activated cation channel activity	2	5	KCNA10, CNGA3
GO:0005222	Intracellular cAMP activated cation channel activity	1	2	HCN4
GO:0005223	Intracellular cGMP activated cation channel activity	1	1	CNGB3
GO:0005229	Intracellular calcium activated chloride channel activity	2	3	ANO1, ANO2
GO:0005232	Serotonin-activated cation-selective channel activity	2	3	HTR3B, HTR3A
GO:0005237	Inhibitory extracellular ligand-gated ion channel activity	2	3	GABRA6, GABRB2
GO:0005242	Inward rectifier potassium channel activity	6	26	KCNH6, KCNJ12, KCNK6, KCNJ8, KCNQ5, KCNH7
GO:0005245	Voltage-gated calcium channel activity	8	27	CACNA1C, CATSPER1, CACNG7, CACNG5, CACNB1, CACNA1B, CACNB2, CACNA1E
GO:0005247	Voltage-gated chloride channel activity	6	14	CLCN7, CLCN4, CLIC1, CLIC4, CLIC6, CLCN3
GO:0005248	Voltage-gated sodium channel activity	8	19	SCN3A, SCN2A, SCN4A, PKD2, SCN8A, SCN5A, SCN9A, SCN11A
GO:0005249	Voltage-gated potassium channel activity	23	75	KCTD12, KCTD21, KCNH3, KCTD10, KCTD3, KCTD6, KCNAB3, KCTD2, KCTD15, KCTD7, KCNH4, KCNB1, KCTD9, KCNH8, KCNC3, KCNC2, KCTD16, KCND1, KCNC1, KCNV2, KCNH5, KCTD1, KCTD20
GO:0005250	A-type (transient outward) potassium channel activity	3	11	KCNIP2, KCND3, KCND2
GO:0005251	Delayed rectifier potassium channel activity	8	26	KCNA3, KCNB2, KCNH2, KCNA1, KCNA5, KCNQ1, KCNA2, KCNH1
GO:0005254	Chloride channel activity	17	55	CLCA1, ANO3, GABRB3, GABRA2, GABRB1, ANO7, ANO9, ANO4, GABRG2, CLCA4, CLCC1, ANO6, GABRQ, GABRG1, ANO10, GABRA4, GABRG3
GO:0005261	Cation channel activity	7	33	TRPM3, TRPV4, TRPM6, TRPC7, TMEM38A, TRPV1, HCN2
GO:0005262	Calcium channel activity	7	51	TRPM1, TRPM7, TRPM8, TRPV5, TRPM5, TRPM4, TRPV6

TABLE 2: Continued.

GO term	Description	H	M	Human genes
GO:0005267	Potassium channel activity	13	27	KCNC4, KCNK16, KCNK10, KCNG1, KCNK2, KCNK5, KCNK3, KCNK12, KCNQ4, KCNK17, KCNIP1, KCNIP4, KCNK9
GO:0005272	Sodium channel activity	4	40	HCN1, NALCN, ACCN4, TRPM2
GO:0008308	Voltage-gated anion channel activity	2	3	VDAC1, VDAC2
GO:0008331	High voltage-gated calcium channel activity	7	38	CACNA1A, CACNA2D4, CACNA1D, CACNA2D1, CACNA1S, CACNA2D3, CACNA2D2
GO:0008332	Low voltage-gated calcium channel activity	3	18	CACNA1H, CACNA1I, CACNA1G
GO:0015269	Calcium-activated potassium channel activity	9	49	KCNMA1, KCNN1, KCNT2, KCNN2, KCNT1, KCNU1, KCNMB2, KCNK18, KCNN3
GO:0015276	Ligand-gated ion channel activity	2	4	CLCA2, CNGB1
GO:0015279	Store-operated calcium channel activity	5	40	TRPC4, TRPC6, ORAI1, TRPA1, TRPC3
GO:0015280	Ligand-gated sodium channel activity	8	97	SCNN1B, SCNN1G, ACCN1, ACCN3, SCNN1A, ACCN5, ACCN2, SCNN1D
GO:0022824	Transmitter-gated ion channel activity	4	34	GLRA2, GLRA4, GLRA1, GLRA3
GO:0030171	Voltage-gated proton channel activity	1	3	HVCN1
GO:0072345	NAADP-sensitive calcium-release channel activity	2	3	TPCN1, TPCN2
	Total	199	947	
	Total number of genes in these GO categories	390		

H: number of different ion channel genes in human with homologs in *M. lignano*. M: number of transcripts in *M. lignano de novo* transcriptome assembly ML110815 with homology to ion channel genes in human. Note that alternatively spliced transcripts are counted separately in the *M. lignano* transcriptome assembly, hence the total reported number of transcripts is higher than the number of corresponding human genes. For this classification, genes were assigned to the least frequent available GO term within predefined list of ion channel-related GO terms (molecular function domain).

highlights a number of ion channel genes expressed specifically in dividing cells (Figure 3(e)), and future elaborated studies of such genes may provide novel insights into the role of bioelectric signaling in stem cell maintenance and differentiation. Importantly, a significant number of ion channels are well-conserved between *M. lignano* and human (Table 2), increasing the relevance of findings in flatworms to understanding ion channels and stem cells in human situation.

6. Future Directions

We advocate that *Macrostomum lignano* has great potential as a model for ion channel and stem cell research. The genetic toolbox available for this organism is already useful enough to address a wide range of scientific problems, and more methods and approaches will be optimized and used in this flatworm in the near future. *M. lignano* is a small animal and it is cultured in water, which makes it easy to apply different chemicals to the worms. Another major advantage of the animal is its high transparency. Phenotypic changes,

fluorescent signals or certain transgene expression can be observed in any part of the body, as well is on the whole organism scale. For example, various fluorescent reporter dyes can be just added to culturing media in order to enable real-time *in vivo* monitoring of membrane potentials, pH, and ion flows [53]. Short generation time and efficient reproduction of *M. lignano* make logistics of large-scale experiments, such as drug screens, feasible in this animal.

As a model, *M. lignano* offers an exciting opportunity to bridge the gap between bioelectric signaling and genetic pathways involved in stem cell functions. The expression pattern and function of any gene can be determined by *in situ* hybridization and RNAi protocols, but it is transgenics that can bring such studies to the whole new level. Transgenic reporter lines expressing pH-sensitive or Ca^{2+}-sensitive fluorescent proteins [54, 55] would make a perfect tool to visualize bioelectric phenotypes during drug- or RNAi-screens. Overexpression of ion channels or even certain subunits would help to better understand their functions and interactions. Targeted genome editing by Zinc Finger Nucleases have not been tested yet in this animal but should

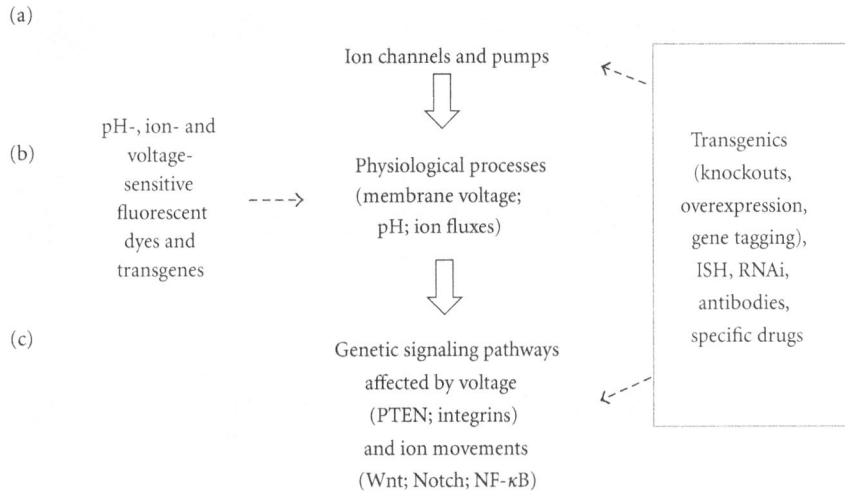

FIGURE 4: Approaches to study the roles of ion channels in regulation of stem cells in *M. lignano*. (a) Expression, localization, and function of ion channels and pumps that give rise to bioelectric signals can be addressed in *M. lignano* by established methods such as RNAi or *in situ* hybridization (ISH) in combination with specific drugs, antibodies, and transgenics. (b) Changes in ion flows, pH and membrane voltage caused by these channels and pumps can be detected with sensitive fluorescent dyes or followed *in vivo* in mutants expressing pH- or ion-sensitive forms of fluorescent proteins. (c) These processes affect known (and possibly unknown) genetic signaling pathways via different mechanisms including changes of Ca^{2+} concentrations, voltage-sensing domains of proteins, and voltage-gated transport of signaling molecules. These pathways and functional links between genetic and epigenetic mechanisms of stem cell function regulation can be studied in transgenic mutant lines with the help of RNAi and ISH techniques.

be also feasible and potentially can be used to generate ion channel knockout and knock-in lines [56, 57]. The same method allows fluorescent tagging of genes of interest and analysis of their expression, localization, and functions at the endogenous level [58]. Sexual reproduction and lack of self-fertilization make possible crossing different lines of *M. lignano* and hence to use the power of classical genetics approaches in this animal. Taken all together, we are convinced that *M. lignano* is poised to become a productive model to study relations between ion channels and stem cell regulation (Figure 4).

Acknowledgments

The authors thank S. Mouton and T. Demircan for critical comments on the paper, and S. Mouton for providing the image of the BrdU-labeled *M. lignano* animal.

References

[1] B. Hille, *Ion Channels of Excitable Membranes*, Sinauer, Sunderland, Mass, USA, 2001.

[2] C. Fewtrell, "Ca^{2+} oscillations in non-excitable cells," *Annual Review of Physiology*, vol. 55, pp. 427–454, 1993.

[3] A. P. Thomas, G. S. T. J. Bird, G. Hajnóczky, L. D. Robb-Gaspers, and J. W. Putney, "Spatial and temporal aspects of cellular calcium signaling," *The FASEB Journal*, vol. 10, no. 13, pp. 1505–1517, 1996.

[4] S. Schuster, M. Marhl, and T. Höfer, "Modelling of simple and complex calcium oscillations from single-cell responses to intercellular signalling," *European Journal of Biochemistry*, vol. 269, no. 5, pp. 1333–1355, 2002.

[5] F. M. Tonelli, A. K. Santos, D. A. Gomes et al., "Stem cells and calcium signaling," *Advances in Experimental Medicine and Biology*, vol. 740, pp. 891–916, 2012.

[6] A. Apáti, K. Pászty, Z. Erdei, K. Szebényi, L. Homolya, and B. Sarkadi, "Calcium signaling in pluripotent stem cells," *Molecular and Cellular Endocrinology*, vol. 353, pp. 57–67, 2012.

[7] E. J. Paredes-Gamero, C. M. Barbosa, and A. T. Ferreira, "Calcium signaling as a regulator of hematopoiesis," *Frontiers in Bioscience*, vol. 4, pp. 1375–1384, 2012.

[8] M. Sheng and D. T. S. Pak, "Ligand-gated ion channel interactions with cytoskeletal and signaling proteins," *Annual Review of Physiology*, vol. 62, pp. 755–778, 2000.

[9] A. Arcangeli and A. Becchetti, "Complex functional interaction between integrin receptors and ion channels," *Trends in Cell Biology*, vol. 16, no. 12, pp. 631–639, 2006.

[10] C. A. Hübner and T. J. Jentsch, "Ion channel diseases," *Human Molecular Genetics*, vol. 11, no. 20, pp. 2435–2445, 2002.

[11] A. Pandiella, M. Magni, D. Lovisolo, and J. Meldolesi, "The effects of epidermal growth factor on membrane potential. Rapid hyperpolarization followed by persistent fluctuations," *Journal of Biological Chemistry*, vol. 264, no. 22, pp. 12914–12921, 1989.

[12] F. Lang, F. Friedrich, E. Kahn et al., "Bradykinin-induced oscillations of cell membrane potential in cells expressing the Ha-ras oncogene," *Journal of Biological Chemistry*, vol. 266, no. 8, pp. 4938–4942, 1991.

[13] R. Binggeli and R. C. Weinstein, "Membrane potentials and sodium channels: hypotheses for growth regulation and

cancer formation based on changes in sodium channels and gap junctions," *Journal of Theoretical Biology*, vol. 123, no. 4, pp. 377–401, 1986.

[14] C. D. Cone, "Electroosmotic interactions accompanying mitosis initation in sarcoma cells in vitro," *Transactions of the New York Academy of Sciences*, vol. 31, no. 4, pp. 404–427, 1969.

[15] B. D. Freedman, M. A. Price, and C. J. Deutsch, "Evidence for voltage modulation of IL-2 production in mitogen-stimulated human peripheral blood lymphocytes," *Journal of Immunology*, vol. 149, no. 12, pp. 3784–3794, 1992.

[16] D. J. Blackiston, K. A. McLaughlin, and M. Levin, "Bioelectric controls of cell proliferation: ion channels, membrane voltage and the cell cycle," *Cell Cycle*, vol. 8, no. 21, pp. 3519–3528, 2009.

[17] T. E. DeCoursey, K. G. Chandy, S. Gupta, and M. D. Cahalan, "Voltage-gated K^+ channels in human T lymphocytes: a role in mitogenesis?" *Nature*, vol. 307, no. 5950, pp. 465–468, 1984.

[18] S. Y. Chiu and G. F. Wilson, "The role of potassium channels in Schwann cell proliferation in Wallerian degeneration of explant rabbit sciatic nerves," *Journal of Physiology*, vol. 408, pp. 199–222, 1989.

[19] S. Amigorena, D. Choquet, J. L. Teillaud, H. Korn, and W. H. Fridman, "Ion channel blockers inhibit B cell activation at a precise stage of the G1 phase of the cell cycle. Possible involvement of K^+ channels," *Journal of Immunology*, vol. 144, no. 6, pp. 2038–2045, 1990.

[20] E. Wang, Y. Yin, M. Zhao, J. V. Forrester, and C. D. McCaig, "Physiological electric fields control the G1/S phase cell cycle checkpoint to inhibit endothelial cell proliferation," *The FASEB Journal*, vol. 17, no. 3, pp. 458–460, 2003.

[21] S. Sundelacruz, M. Levin, and D. L. Kaplan, "Membrane potential controls adipogenic and osteogenic differentiation of mesenchymal stem cells," *PLoS ONE*, vol. 3, no. 11, Article ID e3737, 2008.

[22] D. L. Atkinson, T. J. Stevenson, E. J. Park, M. D. Riedy, B. Milash, and S. J. Odelberg, "Cellular electroporation induces dedifferentiation in intact newt limbs," *Developmental Biology*, vol. 299, no. 1, pp. 257–271, 2006.

[23] D. S. Adams, K. R. Robinson, T. Fukumoto et al., "Early, H^+-V-ATPase-dependent proton flux is necessary for consistent left-right patterning of non-mammalian vertebrates," *Development*, vol. 133, no. 9, pp. 1657–1671, 2006.

[24] D. S. Adams, A. Masi, and M. Levin, "H^+ pump-dependent changes in membrane voltage are an early mechanism necessary and sufficient to induce *Xenopus* tail regeneration," *Development*, vol. 134, no. 7, pp. 1323–1335, 2007.

[25] T. Nogi, D. Zhang, J. D. Chan, and J. S. Marchant, "A novel biological activity of praziquantel requiring voltage-operated Ca^{2+} channel β subunits: subversion of flatworm regenerative polarity," *PLoS Neglected Tropical Diseases*, vol. 3, no. 6, article e464, 2009.

[26] W. S. Beane, J. Morokuma, D. S. Adams, and M. Levin, "A chemical genetics approach reveals H,K-ATPase-mediated membrane voltage is required for planarian head regeneration," *Chemistry and Biology*, vol. 18, no. 1, pp. 77–89, 2011.

[27] D. Zhang, J. D. Chan, T. Nogi, and J. S. Marchant, "Opposing roles of voltage-gated Ca^{2+} channels in neuronal control of regenerative patterning," *The Journal of Neuroscience*, vol. 31, pp. 15983–15995, 2011.

[28] M. Levin, "Bioelectric mechanisms in regeneration: unique aspects and future perspectives," *Seminars in Cell and Developmental Biology*, vol. 20, no. 5, pp. 543–556, 2009.

[29] K. Kunzelmann, "Ion channels and cancer," *Journal of Membrane Biology*, vol. 205, no. 3, pp. 159–173, 2005.

[30] A. Arcangeli, O. Crociani, E. Lastraioli, A. Masi, S. Pillozzi, and A. Becchetti, "Targeting ion channels in cancer: a novel frontier in antineoplastic therapy," *Current Medicinal Chemistry*, vol. 16, no. 1, pp. 66–93, 2009.

[31] T. H. Morgan, "Experimental studies of the regeneration of *Planaria maculata*," *Archiv für Entwickelungsmechanik der Organismen*, vol. 7, no. 2-3, pp. 364–397, 1898.

[32] T. H. Morgan, "Growth and regeneration in *Planaria lugubris*," *Archiv Für Entwicklungsmechanik der Organismen*, vol. 13, pp. 1179–2212, 1901.

[33] A. Sánchez Alvarado, "Regeneration and the need for simpler model organisms," *Philosophical Transactions of the Royal Society B*, vol. 359, no. 1445, pp. 759–763, 2004.

[34] K. Agata, E. Nakajima, N. Funayama, N. Shibata, Y. Saito, and Y. Umesono, "Two different evolutionary origins of stem cell systems and their molecular basis," *Seminars in Cell and Developmental Biology*, vol. 17, no. 4, pp. 503–509, 2006.

[35] G. Marsh and H. W. Beams, "Electrical control of growth polarity in regenerating *Dugesia tigrina*," *Federation Proceedings*, vol. 6, article 163, 1947.

[36] G. Marsh and H. W. Beams, "Electrical control of morphogenesis in regenerating *Dugesia tigrina*. I. Relation of axial polarity to field strength," *Journal of Cellular Physiology*, vol. 39, pp. 191–213, 1952.

[37] J. Dimmitt and G. Marsh, "Electrical control of morphogenesis in regenerating *Dugesia tigrina*. II. Potential gradient vs. current density as control factors," *Journal of Cellular Physiology*, vol. 40, no. 1, pp. 11–23, 1952.

[38] T. Nogi and M. Levin, "Characterization of innexin gene expression and functional roles of gap-junctional communication in planarian regeneration," *Developmental Biology*, vol. 287, no. 2, pp. 314–335, 2005.

[39] N. J. Oviedo and M. Levin, "Smedinx-11 is a planarian stem cell gap junction gene required for regeneration and homeostasis," *Development*, vol. 134, no. 17, pp. 3121–3131, 2007.

[40] K. D. Poss, "Advances in understanding tissue regenerative capacity and mechanisms in animals," *Nature Reviews Genetics*, vol. 11, no. 10, pp. 710–722, 2010.

[41] P. Ladurner, D. Pfister, C. Seifarth et al., "Production and characterisation of cell- and tissue-specific monoclonal antibodies for the flatworm *Macrostomum* sp.," *Histochemistry and Cell Biology*, vol. 123, no. 1, pp. 89–104, 2005.

[42] B. Egger, P. Ladurner, K. Nimeth, R. Gschwentner, and R. Rieger, "The regeneration capacity of the flatworm *Macrostomum lignano*—on repeated regeneration, rejuvenation, and the minimal size needed for regeneration," *Development Genes and Evolution*, vol. 216, no. 10, pp. 565–577, 2006.

[43] D. Pfister, K. De Mulder, I. Philipp et al., "The exceptional stem cell system of *Macrostomum lignano*: screening for gene expression and studying cell proliferation by hydroxyurea treatment and irradiation," *Frontiers in Zoology*, vol. 4, article 9, 2007.

[44] K. De Mulder, D. Pfister, G. Kuales et al., "Stem cells are differentially regulated during development, regeneration and homeostasis in flatworms," *Developmental Biology*, vol. 334, no. 1, pp. 198–212, 2009.

[45] D. Pfister, K. De Mulder, V. Hartenstein et al., "Flatworm stem cells and the germ line: developmental and evolutionary implications of macvasa expression in *Macrostomum lignano*," *Developmental Biology*, vol. 319, no. 1, pp. 146–159, 2008.

[46] K. De Mulder, G. Kuales, D. Pfister et al., "Potential of *Macrostomum lignano* to recover from γ-ray irradiation," *Cell and Tissue Research*, vol. 339, no. 3, pp. 527–542, 2010.

[47] S. Mouton, M. Willems, B. P. Braeckman et al., "The free-living flatworm *Macrostomum lignano*: a new model organism for ageing research," *Experimental Gerontology*, vol. 44, no. 4, pp. 243–249, 2009.

[48] N. J. Oviedo, C. L. Nicolas, D. S. Adams, and M. Levin, "Live imaging of planarian membrane potential using $DiBAC_4(3)$," *Cold Spring Harbor Protocols*, vol. 2008, Article ID pdb.prot5055, 2008.

[49] P. W. Reddien, N. J. Oviedo, J. R. Jennings, J. C. Jenkin, and A. Sánchez Alvarado, "Developmental biology: SMEDWI-2 is a PIWI-like protein that regulates planarian stem cells," *Science*, vol. 310, no. 5752, pp. 1327–1330, 2005.

[50] T. Guo, A. H. F. M. Peters, and P. A. Newmark, "A bruno-like gene is required for stem cell maintenance in planarians," *Developmental Cell*, vol. 11, no. 2, pp. 159–169, 2006.

[51] B. J. Pearson and A. S. Alvarado, "A planarian p53 homolog regulates proliferation and self-renewal in adult stem cell lineages," *Development*, vol. 137, no. 2, pp. 213–221, 2010.

[52] M. W. Cowles, A. Hubert, and R. M. Zayas, "A Lissencephaly-1 homologue is essential for mitotic progression in the planarian *Schmidtea mediterranea*," *Developmental Dynamics*, vol. 241, pp. 901–910, 2012.

[53] C. Wolff, B. Fuks, and P. Chatelain, "Comparative study of membrane potential-sensitive fluorescent probes and their use in ion channel screening assays," *Journal of Biomolecular Screening*, vol. 8, no. 5, pp. 533–543, 2003.

[54] M. J. Mahon, "pHluorin2: an enhanced, ratiometric, pH-sensitive green florescent protein," *Advances in Bioscience and Biotechnology*, vol. 2, pp. 132–137, 2011.

[55] Y. Zhao, S. Araki, J. Wu et al., "An expanded palette of genetically encoded Ca^{2+} indicators," *Science*, vol. 333, pp. 1888–1891, 2011.

[56] P. Q. Liu, E. M. Chan, G. J. Cost et al., "Generation of a triple-gene knockout mammalian cell line using engineered zinc-finger nucleases," *Biotechnology and Bioengineering*, vol. 106, no. 1, pp. 97–105, 2010.

[57] J. Wang, G. Friedman, Y. Doyon et al., "Targeted gene addition to a predetermined site in the human genome using a ZFN-based nicking enzyme," *Genome Research*, vol. 22, no. 7, pp. 1316–1326, 2012.

[58] J. B. Doyon, B. Zeitler, J. Cheng et al., "Rapid and efficient clathrin-mediated endocytosis revealed in genome-edited mammalian cells," *Nature Cell Biology*, vol. 13, no. 3, pp. 331–337, 2011.

14

Stem Cells and Gene Therapy for Cartilage Repair

Umile Giuseppe Longo,[1,2] **Stefano Petrillo,**[1,2] **Edoardo Franceschetti,**[1,2]
Alessandra Berton,[1,2] **Nicola Maffulli,**[3] **and Vincenzo Denaro**[1,2]

[1] Department of Orthopaedic and Trauma Surgery, Campus Bio-Medico University, Via Alvaro del Portillo 200, Trigoria,
    00128 Rome, Italy
[2] Centro Integrato di Ricerca (CIR), Università Campus Bio-Medico, Via Alvaro del Portillo, 21, 00128, Rome, Italy
[3] Centre for Sports and Exercise Medicine, Barts and The London School of Medicine and Dentistry, Mile End Hospital,
    275 Bancroft Road, London E1 4DG, UK

Correspondence should be addressed to Umile Giuseppe Longo, g.longo@unicampus.it

Academic Editor: Wasim S. Khan

Cartilage defects represent a common problem in orthopaedic practice. Predisposing factors include traumas, inflammatory conditions, and biomechanics alterations. Conservative management of cartilage defects often fails, and patients with this lesions may need surgical intervention. Several treatment strategies have been proposed, although only surgery has been proved to be predictably effective. Usually, in focal cartilage defects without a stable fibrocartilaginous repair tissue formed, surgeons try to promote a natural fibrocartilaginous response by using marrow stimulating techniques, such as microfracture, abrasion arthroplasty, and Pridie drilling, with the aim of reducing swelling and pain and improving joint function of the patients. These procedures have demonstrated to be clinically useful and are usually considered as first-line treatment for focal cartilage defects. However, fibrocartilage presents inferior mechanical and biochemical properties compared to normal hyaline articular cartilage, characterized by poor organization, significant amounts of collagen type I, and an increased susceptibility to injury, which ultimately leads to premature osteoarthritis (OA). Therefore, the aim of future therapeutic strategies for articular cartilage regeneration is to obtain a hyaline-like cartilage repair tissue by transplantation of tissues or cells. Further studies are required to clarify the role of gene therapy and mesenchimal stem cells for management of cartilage lesions.

1. Introduction

Hyaline articular cartilage is a highly specialized tissue. The function of cartilage is to protect the bones of diarthrodial joints from friction, forces associated with load bearing and impact [1, 2]. The peculiar problem of this tissue is its durability. Once articular cartilage is injured or degenerated, it has very limited capacities for self-repair and regeneration. In partial thickness lesions, in whom the defect is completely contained within the articular cartilage, there is no involvement of the vasculature. Consequently, chondroprogenitor cells from marrow or blood cannot reach the damaged region to repair the lesion or contribute to the healing of the tissue. The most considerable consequence of cartilage avascularity is that articular chondrocytes are not able to migrate towards the lesion and to produce reparative matrix to fill the defect.

As such, the defect is not repaired and remains permanently [1, 2].

Full thickness cartilage lesions result in the damage of the chondral layer and subchondral bone plate. The rupture of blood vessels promotes the formation of the hematoma at the injury site. In this condition, the repair response is promoted and the defect is filled with fibrocartilaginous tissue within weeks [1, 2].

Usually, in focal cartilage defects without a stable fibrocartilaginous repair tissue formed, surgeons try to promote a natural fibrocartilaginous response by using marrow stimulating techniques, such as microfracture, abrasion arthroplasty, and Pridie drilling with the aim of reducing swelling and pain and improving joint function of the patients. These procedures have demonstrated to be clinically useful and are usually considered as first-line treatment for focal cartilage defects [3–5].

However, fibrocartilage presents inferior mechanical and biochemical properties compared to normal hyaline articular cartilage, characterized by poor organization, significant amounts of collagen type I, and an increased susceptibility to injury, which ultimately leads to premature osteoarthritis (OA).

Therefore, as outlined in the modern literature on the subject, the aim of future therapeutic strategies for articular cartilage regeneration is to obtain a hyaline-like cartilage repair tissue by transplantation of tissues or cells [2, 3, 6–8].

Tissue transplantation procedures such as periosteum, perichondrium, or osteochondral grafts have shown positive results for a limited number of patients, especially in the short term, but long-term clinical results are uncertain, with tissue availability for transplant that seems to be the major limitation, especially in large cartilage defects [2, 3, 6–8]. The autologous chondrocyte transplantation (ACT) procedure has been performed since 1987 in combination with a periosteal cover to treat chondral or osteochondral lesions of the knee, reporting good clinical results [9–11].

Recently, several authors improved this procedure embedding chondrocytes in a three-dimensional matrix before transplantation into cartilage defects [4, 12, 13].

Good results have also been obtained especially regarding clinical symptoms, such as pain relief and joint motion, but none of the current treatment options has proved the capacity to reproduce the biochemical properties of articular hyaline cartilage [3, 10, 14].

Moreover, in the last years, tissue engineering approaches have been investigated with the aim to produce cartilage grafts *in vitro* to facilitate regeneration of articular cartilage *in vivo*. While promising *in vitro* data have been obtained compared to current cartilage repair options, various problems remain unresolved for a successful repair associated with the formation of hyaline cartilage *in vivo* [2, 7, 15, 16].

2. Gene Therapy

The gene transfer to articular tissues was firstly described and performed by Evans et al., as a method to treat patient with rheumatoid arthritis [17, 18]. Initial successful experiments in several animal models using retroviral-mediated gene delivery promoted subsequent clinical trials to evaluate the safety and feasibility of using gene therapy for rheumatoid arthritis [17, 18]. The study was performed on 9 patients without any complications; all the nine participants tolerated the treatment and, in addition, in all the treated joints, intra-articular gene transfer and expression was observed [17, 18]. The relative success of these studies suggests that this new treatment option can be used in major articular disorders for which only unsatisfactory treatment options are currently available.

Nowadays research and recent results indicate that the design of a successful genetic treatment for cartilage repair and restoration includes a refined strategy of gene delivery that takes into account the complexities of treating this particular tissue.

For the purpose of cartilage repair, potentially useful complementary DNAs (cDNAs) include members of the transforming growth factor- (TGF-) β superfamily, including TGF-βs 1, 2, and 3, a number of bone morphogenetic proteins (BMPs), insulin-like growth factor- (IGF-) 1, fibroblast growth factors (FGFs), and epidermal growth factor (EGF).

Alternatively, to support production and maintenance of the proper hyaline cartilage matrix, delivery, and expression of cDNAs encoding specific extracellular matrix (ECM) components such as collagen type II, tenascin, or cartilage oligomeric matrix protein (COMP) may also be used [19].

Another class of biologics that may be useful in cartilage repair is represented by transcription factors that promote chondrogenesis or the maintenance of the chondrocyte phenotype. SOX9 and related transcription factors (i.e., LSOX5) and SOX6 have been identified as essential for chondrocyte differentiation and cartilage formation [20].

Signal transduction molecules, such as SMADs, are also known to be important regulators of chondrogenesis [21]. However, since these molecules function completely in the intracellular environment, gene transfer may represent the only way to harness these factors for repair, as they cannot be delivered in soluble form.

Other secreted proteins, such as indian hedgehog (IHH) or sonic hedgehog (SHH), play key roles in regulating chondrocyte hypertrophy [22] and could be beneficial for modulating the chondrocytic phenotype of grafted cells.

Prevention or treatment of cartilage loss may also require the inhibition of the activity of certain proinflammatory cytokines, such as interleukin- (IL-) 1 and tumor necrosis factor- (TNF-) α, as these are important mediators of cartilage matrix degradation and apoptosis after trauma and disease. Therefore, anti-inflammatory or immunmodulatory mediators, such as interleukin-1 receptor antagonist (IL-1Ra), soluble receptors for TNF (sTNFR) or IL-1 (sIL-1R), IL-4 or IL-10, inhibitors of matrix metalloproteinases, and others, may be administered to effectively reduce loss of repair cells and matrix [23].

Inhibitors of apoptosis or senescence, such as Bcl-2, Bcl-XL, hTERT, i(NOS) and others, may also be beneficially employed to maintain cell populations which are capable of favourable repair responses at the injury site [24, 25]. Different candidate cDNAs may also be administered in combination, especially when favouring complementary therapeutic responses. For example, the combined administration of an anabolic growth factor (e.g., IGF-1) together with an inhibitor of the catabolic action of inflammatory cytokines (i.e., IL-1Ra) has the potential both to control the matrix degradation and to allow partial restoration of the damaged cartilage matrix [26, 27].

There are two general modes of intra-articular gene delivery, a direct *in vivo* and an indirect *ex vivo* approach. The direct *in vivo* approach involves the application of the vector directly into the joint space, whereas the *ex vivo* approach involves the genetic modification of cells outside the body, followed by retransplantation of the modified cells into the body.

The choice of which gene transfer method as to be used depends on several considerations, including the gene to be delivered, and the vector used. In general, *in vivo* and *ex vivo* delivery can be performed using adenovirus, herpes simplex virus, adenoassociated virus vectors, lentivirus, and nonviral vectors. Due to their inability to infect nondividing cells, retroviral vectors are more appropriate for *ex vivo* use. While *ex vivo* transfer methods are generally more invasive, expensive, and technically wearisome, they finally allow control of the transduced cells and safety testing prior to transplantation. *In vivo* approaches are simpler, cheaper, and less invasive, but these methods require the introduction of viruses directly into the body, which limits safety testing [28].

Towards the treatment of damaged articular cartilage, the three primary candidate cell types to target genetic modification are synovial lining cells, chondrocytes, and mesenchymal stem cells.

Direct intra-articular injection of a recombinant vector [29–31] represents the most straightforward strategy for gene delivery to diseased joints. Cartilage and synovium are the two primary tissues to be considered for this application.

Within articular cartilage, chondrocytes are present at a low density and are located at varying depths within the dense matrix. Due to this situation, it has not been possible to achieve an efficient genetic modification of chondrocytes *in situ* [32–35]. Conversely, gene delivery within the synovium tissue has resulted much more feasible since it is usually characterized by a thin lining of cells that covers all internal surfaces of the joint except that of cartilage. Also, because of its relatively large surface area, the synovium represents the predominant site of vector interaction. Both the implant of modified cells and direct intra-articular injection of vector promote the synthesis and release of therapeutic proteins into the joint space, which then bathe all available tissues, including cartilage.

Substantial progress has been made in defining the parameters that are critical for effective gene transfer to synovium and prolonged intra-articular expression by using different types of vectors in *ex vivo* and *in vivo* approaches. Through research conducted in the field of rheumatoid arthritis, the effectiveness of synovial gene transfer of various transgenes has been well documented [23]. *Ex vivo* gene delivery to joints has been taken into phase I clinical trial and shown to be feasible and safe in humans with rheumatoid arthritis [17, 36]. Data relevant to direct intra-articular gene delivery are beginning to emerge, although to date most of the work in this field has been focused towards the study and treatment of rheumatoid arthritis, mainly because of the potential of this approach in treating OA [37], and also to expand repair methods of focal cartilage defects [28, 38–40].

For example, encouraging results have been reported for adenovirally delivered IGF-1 or IL-1Ra using animal models for OA and localized cartilage injury [32, 41].

Through both direct and *ex vivo* gene transfer to synovium, it is possible to obtain biologically considerable levels of transgene expression while for delivery of certain growth factors, this approach is not compatible. In fact, it was observed that adenoviral mediated delivery of TGF-β1 or BMP-2 to the synovial lining determined osteophytes, cartilage degeneration, joint fibrosis, and significant swelling

[42–45]. In the perspective of cartilage repair, these results suggest that synovial gene transfer may be more appropriate for the delivery of chondroprotective agents rather than strong anabolic transgenes with pleiotropic effects of their products. It has been shown that this property is common to many anti-inflammatory cytokines.

For the gene-based delivery of certain intracellular proteins or growth factors, it appears that a strategy based on increased localization of the transgenes with the gene products contained in the lesion of the cartilage may be more practical. To achieve this goal, the most direct approach may be represented by implantation into a defect of a three-dimensional matrix preloaded with a gene delivery vehicle, allowing infiltrating cells to acquire the vector and secrete the stimulating transgene products locally [37, 46].

In order to increase the healing of ligaments and bones, cartilage implants, activated genetically, have been designed [47–52]. For example, it has been seen that hydrated collagen-glycosaminoglycan matrices containing adenoviral vectors stimulate localized reporter gene expression *in vivo* for at least 21 days, after implantation into osteochondral defects localized in rabbit knees [50].

However, it is not known yet if this type of approach can promote an adequate biological response for repair due to the limited cell supply commonly present at the site of the cartilage lesion. To increase the graft cellularity, while preserving the feasibility of the procedure within one operative setting, autologous cells which are intraoperatively readily available, such as cells from bone marrow aspirates, could be mixed together with the genetically activated matrix. This genetically enhanced approach for tissue engineering would allow both the reduction of costs and execution time, while avoiding a significant effort for the *ex vivo* culture of cells [49, 50]. Nevertheless, the lack of control over gene transfer following implantation represents a limitation for their use.

Through the use of genetically modified chondrocytes, attempts have been made to further improve the quality of repaired tissue. Although chondrocytes have shown a certain resistance to transfection with plasmid DNA, it has been observed that some lipid-based formulations increase the efficiency of DNA uptake [53]. However, viral-based vectors are capable of producing far higher levels of transgene expression with enhanced persistence. It was found that transfection of monolayer-expanded chondrocytes with viral vectors such as Moloney Murine Leukemia Virus (MLV), lentivirus, adenovirus, and AAV occurs promptly. It has also been shown that adenoviral-mediated delivery of various transgenes, such as TGF-β1, BMP-2, IGF-1, or BMP-7, stimulates the production of a cartilage-specific matrix rich in proteoglycans and collagen type II and reduces tendency towards dedifferentiation [54–58].

It has been seen that following transfer of cDNA encoding matrix molecules, such as the collagen type II minigene, an increased extracellular matrix production occurs in human fetal chondrocytes [37].

Collagen type II expression of chondrocytes in three-dimensional culture *in vitro* has shown to be increased following transduction with the transcription factor SOX-9 [59, 60], whereas overexpression of the transcription factor Runx-2 (Cbfa-1) promotes chondrocyte maturation and determines a hypertrophic phenotype, expressing high levels of collagen types II and X, alkaline phosphatase, and osteogenic marker genes [61, 62].

Since it has been found that chondrocyte biology can be positively influenced by genetic modification, attention of research has focused on their efficient delivery to cartilage defects. The delivery of genetically modified chondrocytes in suspension has represented the first approach. Several studies demonstrated that after engraftment onto cartilage explants *in vitro,* genetically modified chondrocytes have the ability of expressing transgene products at functional levels [63].

Compared to transplanted control cells, in these systems, genetic modification with IGF-1 [64], FGF-2 [65], or SOX9 [66] resulted in a considerable resurfacing and thicker tissue containing increased levels of proteoglycans and collagen type II [53]. Moreover, adenoviral-mediated IL-1Ra gene transfer to chondrocytes led to resistance to IL-1-induced proteoglycan degradation after engraftment [67].

Genetically modified chondrocytes have also been used as an alternative to delivery in suspension with the aim of enhancing tissue engineering procedures. This approach requires the transduction/transfection in monolayer cells subsequently seeded into a matrix for further transplantation into chondral or osteochondral lesions. Several transgenes including TGF β1, BMP-2, -4, -7, IGF-1, SOX9, among others have shown promising results in these three-dimensional culture systems due to their ability to maintain and stimulate the chondrogenic phenotype *in vitro* [16, 28, 40].

Initial studies highlighted that following genetic modifications with adenoviral, AAV, retroviral, or plasmid vectors, chondrocytes had the ability to efficiently express reporter genes in chondral and osteochondral lesions, and that when the genetically modified chondrocytes were seeded in three-dimensional matrices, transgene expression was extended over several weeks [68–71].

The results of efficacy studies demonstrating the effects of genetically modified chondrocytes in cartilage defects *in vivo* have just started to be reported.

In an *ex vivo* approach, adenovirally transduced chondrocytes expressing BMP-7 [54], integrated in a matrix of autogenous fibrin, were implanted into full thickness articular cartilage lesions in horses [54]. An enhanced tissue volume with increased production of a proteoglycan and collagen type II rich matrix was detected 4 weeks after surgery in the BMP-7-treated lesions, compared to control lesions treated with unrelated marker genes.

After 8 months, the mechanical features of the treated lesions as well as the levels of collagen type II and proteoglycan were however similar compared to the controls. This finding was attributed to some extent to the reduction of the number of allografted chondrocytes that persisted after 8 months in the lesions [54]. Nevertheless, these findings remain encouraging since they suggest that genetically modified chondrocytes can be used to increase a cartilage repair process in a large animal model.

3. Mesenchymal Stem Cells

Until recently, scientists have mainly focused on research involving two types of stem cells from humans and animals: nonembryonic "somatic" or "adult" stem cells and embryonic stem cells.

Embryonic stem cells are present in the blastocyst while adult stem cells are found in adult tissues. The normal turnover of organs that have a high intrinsic regenerative ability which include blood, skin, and intestinal epithelium is maintained by adult stem cells. Adult stem cells are generally unipotent or multipotent and they can be found in adults as well as adolescents and children.

Adult pluripotent stem cells are normally found in small numbers since they are very rare. However, they are present in several tissues including umbilical cord blood. The adult stem cells studied most extensively to date are the multipotent stem cells which are commonly referred to by their tissue origin (i.e., hematopoietic stem cells that differentiate into platelets erythrocytes, white blood cells, etc.) and the bone marrow stromal cells (also known as MSCs) [72, 73], which have the capacity to differentiate into connective tissue cells.

MSCs have the potential to differentiate into cells of connective tissue lineages [74] including bone [75–77], cartilage [77–79], ligament [80–82], muscle [78], fat [78, 83], and IVD [81, 82, 84]. It has been detected that these cells are also capable of differentiation along myogenic and neurogenic lineages, although these are not the common pathways used to prove multipotentiality of isolated MSCs.

Originally, adult MSCs were isolated from bone marrow by Pittenger et al. in 1999 [74], who demonstrated the potential for multilineage differentiation of these cells. Subsequently, a number of studies allowed to demonstrate the presence of stem cells in various adult tissues, including synovial fluid, articular cartilage, synovial membrane, periosteum, dermis, muscle, and adipose tissue.

To date, research has allowed for MSC-like progenitor cells isolation from trabecular bone, periosteum, synovium, skeletal muscle, adipose tissue, deciduous teeth [78, 80], and bone marrow [85].

Since no definitive markers of MSCs are available, a range of cell surface markers are normally used. These include immunopositivity for STRO-1, CD73, CD105, CD106, CD145, and CD166, associated with negative immunoreactivity for CD11b, CD31, CD34, CD45, and CD117.

Compared to the previous methods based on either density-gradient centrifugation or even simple plastic adherence, these markers allow to identify a more homogeneous population of cells.

Due to general heterogeneity of bone marrow cell populations, variable results can be obtained; however, MSCs have commonly shown the ability to differentiate along the adipogenic, chondrogenic, and osteogenic pathways. Research conducted by several authors suggests that MSCs are capable of differentiation to chondrocytes, osteoblasts, and nucleus pulposus (NP) cells of the IVD [84, 86–88]. However, since no definitive markers of NP cells are available, a number of chondrocyte markers, with which they share a large phenotypic similarity, are typically used.

After Pittenger et al. [74] demonstrated the chondrogenic potential of MSCs, a number of approaches promoting MSC chondrogenesis [60] such as agarose [89] and alginate [90] gels have been described and more recently a range of tissue engineering biomaterials which allow or promote chondrogenesis have also been reported.

One of the most commonly used growth factors is TGF-b [74, 91], which has shown to promote chondrogenesis in addition to inhibiting adipogenic and osteogenic differentiation [92, 93].

Growth factors of the BMP family, principally BMP-7, and IGF-1 have also demonstrated the ability to promote chondrogenesis of MSCs and it has also been suggested that expansion of monolayer MSCs in medium containing FGF-2 induces chondrogenesis following transfer to a 3D culture environment [94–97].

However, with the *in vitro* differentiation approaches, the complexity of the signaling pathways involved in chondrogenesis represents one of the major problems, compared to the simplicity of culture systems.

Several studies have demonstrated the importance of cell-cell contact for MSC differentiation to either NP cells or chondrocytes [73] and pellet cultures mimic the mesenchymal compression that occurs during embryogenesis.

Similarly it is known that differentiation and matrix formation are induced by anabolic growth factors that exert their activity through a number of pathways, primarily the Smad and MAPKinase pathways [92, 96, 98].

The routine assessment of successful chondrogenesis is performed by the induction of SOX-9, which subsequently promotes the production of type II collagen as well as the enhanced expression of the PG aggrecan [99, 100]. Based on the similarities in the phenotype of NP cells of the IVD and articular chondrocytes [101], these markers are also used routinely to identify NP-like cells since no validated and highly specific NP marker genes are available. However, in standard *in vitro* culture systems MSC differentiation has shown to be unstable and it commonly leads to the expression of hypertrophic markers such as alkaline phosphatase and type X collagen [91, 102].

In terms of clinical application, the likelihood that chondrogenic differentiation may cause hypertrophy represents a problem since healthy surface and mid zone chondrocytes and NP cells do not express alkaline phosphatase nor type X collagen [103, 104].

This was demonstrated by Pelttari et al. [105] in pellet cultures comparing MSCs and chondrocytes, who reported that following implantation into SCID mice, the MSCs showed high levels of alkaline phosphatase and type X collagen expression which induced vascular invasion and calcification, while chondrocytes produced a cartilaginous matrix.

Improved differentiation or terminal differentiation inhibition may be induced with a number of growth factors. For example, it has been observed that the addition of PTHrP to TGF-b3-stimulated MSCs in poly-glycolic acid scaffolds also inhibits the expression of type X collagen of these cells

and suppresses their terminal differentiation [106]. Also, the combination of TGF-b3 with BMP-2 has shown improved chondrogenic differentiation of MSCs compared to either growth factor alone or the combination of TGF-b3 with either BMP-4 or BMP-6 [107].

4. Conclusions

Hyaline articular cartilage is a highly specialized tissue. The peculiar problem of this tissue is that once articular cartilage is injured or degenerated, it has very limited capacities for self-repair and regeneration.

Usually, in focal cartilage defects without a stable fibrocartilaginous repair tissue formed, surgeons try to promote a natural fibrocartilaginous response by using marrow stimulating techniques, such as microfracture, abrasion arthroplasty, and Pridie drilling [108–111].

However, fibrocartilage presents inferior mechanical and biochemical properties compared to normal hyaline articular cartilage, characterized by poor organization, significant amounts of collagen type I, and an increased susceptibility to injury, which ultimately leads to premature OA [112–114].

The implementation of gene transfer techniques may allow to overcome the limitations of the current treatments for articular cartilage lesions. It has been shown that various approaches could be appropriate for an efficient transfer of exogenous cDNAs to cartilage lesions *in vivo* and for achieving sustained expression of the related gene products.

Initial efficacy studies have proven that gene-transfer techniques represent potent tools able to promote a significant biological response *in vivo*. However, the safety of gene transfer approaches for cartilage repair is also of particular importance because cartilage injuries are not life-threatening. Therefore the application of this technology for clinical use is strongly dependent on the use of safe and efficient delivery systems vectors and transgenes.

Although a number of animal models for OA and other types of arthritis are available, none of them allow to predict the equivalent disease in humans and most them are linked with problems. Further studies are required to establish the role of stem cells and gene therapy for cartilage repair.

References

[1] J. A. Buckwalter and H. J. Mankin, "Articular cartilage: tissue design and chondrocyte-matrix interactions," *Instructional course lectures*, vol. 47, pp. 477–486, 1998.

[2] E. B. Hunziker, "Articular cartilage repair: basic science and clinical progress. A review of the current status and prospects," *Osteoarthritis and Cartilage*, vol. 10, no. 6, pp. 432–463, 2002.

[3] J. A. Buckwalter and H. J. Mankin, "Articular cartilage repair and transplantation," *Arthritis and Rheumatism*, vol. 41, no. 8, pp. 1331–1342, 1998.

[4] T. Minas, "The role of cartilage repair techniques, including chondrocyte transplantation, in focal chondral knee damage," *Instructional course lectures*, vol. 48, pp. 629–643, 1999.

[5] J. R. Steadman, W. G. Rodkey, and K. K. Briggs, "Microfracture to treat full-thickness chondral defects: surgical

technique, rehabilitation, and outcomes," *The journal of knee surgery*, vol. 15, no. 3, pp. 170–176, 2002.

[6] S. J. M. Bouwmeester, J. M. H. Beckers, R. Kuijer, A. J. Van Der Linden, and S. K. Bulstra, "Long-term results of rib perichondrial grafts for repair of cartilage defects in the human knee," *International Orthopaedics*, vol. 21, no. 5, pp. 313–317, 1997.

[7] A. I. Caplan, M. Elyaderani, Y. Mochizuki, S. Wakitani, and V. M. Goldberg, "Principles of cartilage repair and regeneration," *Clinical Orthopaedics and Related Research*, no. 342, pp. 254–269, 1997.

[8] L. Hangody and P. Füles, "Autologous osteochondral mosaic-plasty for the treatment of full-thickness defects of weight-bearing joints: ten years of experimental and clinical experience," *Journal of Bone and Joint Surgery A*, vol. 85, no. 1, pp. 25–32, 2003.

[9] M. Brittberg, A. Lindahl, A. Nilsson, C. Ohlsson, O. Isaksson, and L. Peterson, "Treatment of deep cartilage defects in the knee with autologous chondrocyte transplantation," *New England Journal of Medicine*, vol. 331, no. 14, pp. 889–895, 1994.

[10] T. Minas and S. Nehrer, "Current concepts in the treatment of articular cartilage defects," *Orthopedics*, vol. 20, no. 6, pp. 525–538, 1997.

[11] L. Peterson, T. Minas, M. Brittberg, and A. Lindahl, "Treatment of osteochondritis dissecans of the knee with autologous chondrocyte transplantation: results at two to ten years," *Journal of Bone and Joint Surgery A*, vol. 85, no. 1, pp. 17–24, 2003.

[12] P. Behrens, U. Bosch, J. Bruns et al., "Recommendations for indication and application of ACT of the joined advisory board of the German Societies for Traumatology (DGU) and Orthopaedic Surgery (DGOOC)," *Zeitschrift fur Orthopadie und Ihre Grenzgebiete*, vol. 142, no. 5, pp. 529–539, 2004.

[13] S. Marlovits, P. Zeller, P. Singer, C. Resinger, and V. Vécsei, "Cartilage repair: generations of autologous chondrocyte transplantation," *European Journal of Radiology*, vol. 57, no. 1, pp. 24–31, 2006.

[14] L. Peterson, M. Brittberg, I. Kiviranta, E. L. Åkerlund, and A. Lindahl, "Autologous chondrocyte transplantation: biomechanics and long-term durability," *American Journal of Sports Medicine*, vol. 30, no. 1, pp. 2–12, 2002.

[15] C. K. Kuo, W. J. Li, R. L. Mauck, and R. S. Tuan, "Cartilage tissue engineering: its potential and uses," *Current Opinion in Rheumatology*, vol. 18, no. 1, pp. 64–73, 2006.

[16] R. Tuli, W. J. Li, and R. S. Tuan, "Current state of cartilage tissue engineering," *Arthritis Research and Therapy*, vol. 5, no. 5, pp. 235–238, 2003.

[17] C. H. Evans, H. J. Mankin, A. B. Ferguson et al., "Clinical trial to assess the safety, feasibility, and efficacy of transferring a potentially anti-arthritic cytokine gene to human joints with rheumatoid arthritis," *Human Gene Therapy*, vol. 7, no. 10, pp. 1261–1280, 1996.

[18] C. H. Evans, P. D. Robbins, S. C. Ghivizzani et al., "Gene transfer to human joints: progress toward a gene therapy of arthritis," *Proceedings of the National Academy of Sciences of the United States of America*, vol. 102, no. 24, pp. 8698–8703, 2005.

[19] R. M. Dharmavaram, G. Liu, R. S. Tuan, D. G. Stokes, and S. A. Jiménez, "Stable transfection of human fetal chondrocytes with a type II procollagen minigene: expression of the mutant protein and alterations in the structure of the extracellular matrix in vitro," *Arthritis and Rheumatism*, vol. 42, no. 7, pp. 1433–1442, 1999.

[20] V. Lefebvre, R. R. Behringer, and B. De Crombrugghe, "L-Sox5, Sox6 and SOx9 control essential steps of the chondrocyte differentiation pathway," *Osteoarthritis and Cartilage*, vol. 9, pp. S69–S75, 2001.

[21] A. Hoffmann and G. Gross, "BMP signaling pathways in cartilage and bone formation," *Critical Reviews in Eukaryotic Gene Expression*, vol. 11, no. 1–3, pp. 23–45, 2001.

[22] A. Vortkamp, "Interaction of growth factors regulating chondrocyte differentiation in the developing embryo," *Osteoarthritis and Cartilage*, vol. 9, pp. S109–S117, 2001.

[23] P. D. Robbins, C. H. Evans, and Y. Chernajovsky, "Gene therapy for arthritis," *Gene Therapy*, vol. 10, no. 10, pp. 902–911, 2003.

[24] D. D. D'Lima, S. Hashimoto, P. C. Chen, C. W. Colwell Jr., and M. K. Lotz, "Impact of mechanical trauma on matrix and cells," *Clinical Orthopaedics and Related Research*, no. 391, pp. S90–S99, 2001.

[25] D. D. D'Lima, S. Hashimoto, P. C. Chen, M. K. Lotz, and C. W. Colwell Jr., "Cartilage injury induces chondrocyte apoptosis," *Journal of Bone and Joint Surgery A*, vol. 83, no. 2, pp. 19–21, 2001.

[26] J. L. Haupt, D. D. Frisbie, C. W. McIlwraith et al., "Dual transduction of insulin-like growth factor-I and interleukin-1 receptor antagonist protein controls cartilage degradation in an osteoarthritic culture model," *Journal of Orthopaedic Research*, vol. 23, no. 1, pp. 118–126, 2005.

[27] A. J. Nixon, J. L. Haupt, D. D. Frisbie et al., "Gene-mediated restoration of cartilage matrix by combination insulin-like growth factor-I/interleukin-1 receptor antagonist therapy," *Gene Therapy*, vol. 12, no. 2, pp. 177–186, 2005.

[28] A. F. Steinert, U. Nöth, and R. S. Tuan, "Concepts in gene therapy for cartilage repair," *Injury*, vol. 39, no. 1, pp. 97–113, 2008.

[29] S. C. Ghivizzani, E. R. Lechman, R. Kang et al., "Direct adenovirus-mediated gene transfer of interleukin 1 and tumor necrosis factor α soluble receptors to rabbit knees with experimental arthritis has local and distal anti-arthritic effects," *Proceedings of the National Academy of Sciences of the United States of America*, vol. 95, no. 8, pp. 4613–4618, 1998.

[30] S. C. Ghivizzani, E. R. Lechman, C. Tio et al., "Direct retrovirus-mediated gene transfer to the synovium of the rabbit knee: implications for arthritis gene therapy," *Gene Therapy*, vol. 4, no. 9, pp. 977–982, 1997.

[31] S. C. Ghivizzani, T. J. Oligino, J. C. Glorioso, P. D. Robbins, and C. H. Evans, "Direct gene delivery strategies for the treatment of rheumatoid arthritis," *Drug Discovery Today*, vol. 6, no. 5, pp. 259–267, 2001.

[32] M. Cucchiarini, H. Madry, C. Ma et al., "Improved tissue repair in articular cartilage defects in vivo by rAAV-mediated overexpression of human fibroblast growth factor 2," *Molecular Therapy*, vol. 12, no. 2, pp. 229–238, 2005.

[33] E. Gouze, R. Pawliuk, C. Pilapil et al., "In vivo gene delivery to synovium by lentiviral vectors," *Molecular Therapy*, vol. 5, no. 4, pp. 397–404, 2002.

[34] T. Tomita, H. Hashimoto, N. Tomita et al., "In vivo direct gene transfer into articular cartilage by intraarticular injection mediated by HVJ (Sendai virus) and liposomes," *Arthritis and Rheumatism*, vol. 40, no. 5, pp. 901–906, 1997.

[35] Q. Yao, J. C. Glorioso, C. H. Evans et al., "Adenoviral mediated delivery of FAS ligand to arthritic joints causes extensive apoptosis in the synovial lining," *Journal of Gene Medicine*, vol. 2, no. 3, pp. 210–219, 2000.

[36] C. H. Evans, E. Gouze, J. N. Gouze, P. D. Robbins, and S. C. Ghivizzani, "Gene therapeutic approaches-transfer in vivo,"

Advanced Drug Delivery Reviews, vol. 58, no. 2, pp. 243–258, 2006.

[37] C. H. Evans, J. N. Gouze, E. Gouze, P. D. Robbins, and S. C. Ghivizzani, "Osteoarthritis gene therapy," *Gene Therapy*, vol. 11, no. 4, pp. 379–389, 2004.

[38] M. Cucchiarini and H. Madry, "Gene therapy for cartilage defects," *Journal of Gene Medicine*, vol. 7, no. 12, pp. 1495–1509, 2005.

[39] K. Gelse and H. Schneider, "Ex vivo gene therapy approaches to cartilage repair," *Advanced Drug Delivery Reviews*, vol. 58, no. 2, pp. 259–284, 2006.

[40] S. B. Trippel, S. C. Ghivizzani, and A. J. Nixon, "Gene-based approaches for the repair of articular cartilage," *Gene Therapy*, vol. 11, no. 4, pp. 351–359, 2004.

[41] D. D. Frisbie, S. C. Ghivizzani, P. D. Robbins, C. H. Evans, and C. W. McIlwraith, "Treatment of experimental equine osteoarthritis by in vivo delivery of the equine interleukin-1 receptor antagonist gene," *Gene Therapy*, vol. 9, no. 1, pp. 12–20, 2002.

[42] A. C. Bakker, L. A. B. Joosten, O. J. Arntz et al., "Prevention of murine collagen-induced arthritis in the knee and ipsilateral paw by local expression of human interleukin-1 receptor antagonist protein in the knee," *Arthritis and Rheumatism*, vol. 40, no. 5, pp. 893–900, 1997.

[43] K. Gelse, Q. J. Jiang, T. Aigner et al., "Fibroblast-mediated delivery of growth factor complementary DNA into mouse joints induces chondrogenesis but avoids the disadvantages of direct viral gene transfer," *Arthritis and Rheumatism*, vol. 44, no. 8, pp. 1943–1953, 2001.

[44] K. Gelse, K. Von der Mark, T. Aigner, J. Park, and H. Schneider, "Articular cartilage repair by gene therapy using growth factor-producing mesenchymal cells," *Arthritis and Rheumatism*, vol. 48, no. 2, pp. 430–441, 2003.

[45] Z. Mi, S. C. Ghivizzani, E. Lechman, J. C. Glorioso, C. H. Evans, and P. D. Robbins, "Adverse effects of adenovirus-mediated gene transfer of human transforming growth factor beta 1 into rabbit knees," *Arthritis Res Ther*, vol. 5, no. 3, pp. R132–R139, 2003.

[46] J. Bonadio, "Tissue engineering via local gene delivery: update and future prospects for enhancing the technology," *Advanced Drug Delivery Reviews*, vol. 44, no. 2-3, pp. 185–194, 2000.

[47] J. Bonadio, E. Smiley, P. Patil, and S. Goldstein, "Localized, direct plasmid gene delivery in vivo: prolonged therapy results in reproducible tissue regeneration," *Nature Medicine*, vol. 5, no. 7, pp. 753–759, 1999.

[48] Q. Dai, L. Manfield, Y. Wang, and G. A. C. Murrell, "Adenovirus-mediated gene transfer to healing tendon—enhanced efficiency using a gelatin sponge," *Journal of Orthopaedic Research*, vol. 21, no. 4, pp. 604–609, 2003.

[49] C. H. Evans, "Gene therapies for osteoarthritis," *Current rheumatology reports*, vol. 6, no. 1, pp. 31–40, 2004.

[50] A. Pascher, G. D. Palmer, A. Steinert et al., "Gene delivery to cartilage defects using coagulated bone marrow aspirate," *Gene Therapy*, vol. 11, no. 2, pp. 133–141, 2004.

[51] A. Pascher, A. F. Steinert, G. D. Palmer et al., "Enhanced repair of the anterior cruciate ligament by in situ gene transfer: evaluation in an in vitro model," *Molecular Therapy*, vol. 10, no. 2, pp. 327–336, 2004.

[52] R. E. Samuel, C. R. Lee, S. C. Ghivizzani et al., "Delivery of plasmid DNA to articular chondrocytes via novel collagen-glycosaminoglycan matrices," *Human Gene Therapy*, vol. 13, no. 7, pp. 791–802, 2002.

[53] H. Madry and S. B. Trippel, "Efficient lipid-mediated gene transfer to articular chondrocytes," *Gene Therapy*, vol. 7, no. 4, pp. 286–291, 2000.

[54] C. Hidaka, L. R. Goodrich, C. T. Chen, R. F. Warren, R. G. Crystal, and A. J. Nixon, "Acceleration of cartilage repair by genetically modified chondrocytes over expressing bone morphogenetic protein-7," *Journal of Orthopaedic Research*, vol. 21, no. 4, pp. 573–583, 2003.

[55] A. J. Nixon, L. A. Fortier, J. Williams, and H. Mohammed, "Enhanced repair of extensive articular defects by insulin-like growth factor-I-laden fibrin composites," *Journal of Orthopaedic Research*, vol. 17, no. 4, pp. 475–487, 1999.

[56] A. J. Nixon, R. A. Saxer, and B. D. Brower-Toland, "Exogenous insulin-like growth factor-I stimulates an autoinductive IGF-I autocrine/paracrine response in chondrocytes," *Journal of Orthopaedic Research*, vol. 19, no. 1, pp. 26–32, 2001.

[57] F. D. Shuler, H. I. Georgescu, C. Niyibizi et al., "Increased matrix synthesis following adenoviral transfer of a transforming growth factor $\beta 1$ gene into articular chondrocytes," *Journal of Orthopaedic Research*, vol. 18, no. 4, pp. 585–592, 2000.

[58] P. Smith, F. D. Shuler, H. I. Georgescu et al., "Genetic enhancement of matrix synthesis by articular chondrocytes: comparison of different growth factor genes in the presence and absence of interleukin-1," *Arthritis and Rheumatism*, vol. 43, no. 5, pp. 1156–1164, 2000.

[59] L. Ying, S. R. Tew, A. M. Russell, K. R. Gonzalez, T. E. Hardingham, and R. E. Hawkins, "Transduction of passaged human articular chondrocytes with adenoviral, retroviral, and lentiviral vectors and the effects of enhanced expression of SOX9," *Tissue Engineering*, vol. 10, no. 3-4, pp. 575–584, 2004.

[60] S. R. Tew, Y. Li, P. Pothancharoen, L. M. Tweats, R. E. Hawkins, and T. E. Hardingham, "Retroviral transduction with SOX9 enhances re-expression of the chondrocyte phenotype in passaged osteoarthritic human articular chondrocytes," *Osteoarthritis and Cartilage*, vol. 13, no. 1, pp. 80–89, 2005.

[61] H. Enomoto, M. Enomoto-Iwamoto, M. Iwamoto et al., "Cbfa1 is a positive regulatory factor in chondrocyte maturation," *Journal of Biological Chemistry*, vol. 275, no. 12, pp. 8695–8702, 2000.

[62] M. Iwamoto, J. Kitagaki, Y. Tamamura et al., "Runx2 expression and action in chondrocytes are regulated by retinoid signaling and parathyroid hormone-related peptide (PTHrP)," *Osteoarthritis and Cartilage*, vol. 11, no. 1, pp. 6–15, 2003.

[63] P. J. Doherty, H. Zhang, L. Tremblay, V. Manolopoulos, and K. W. Marshall, "Resurfacing of articular cartilage explants with genetically-modified human chondrocytes in vitro," *Osteoarthritis and Cartilage*, vol. 6, no. 3, pp. 153–160, 1998.

[64] H. Madry, D. Zurakowski, and S. B. Trippel, "Overexpression of human insulin-like growth factor-I promotes new tissue formation in an ex vivo model of articular chondrocyte transplantation," *Gene Therapy*, vol. 8, no. 19, pp. 1443–1449, 2001.

[65] H. Madry, G. Emkey, D. Zurakowski, and S. B. Trippel, "Overexpression of human fibroblast growth factor 2 stimulates cell proliferation in an ex vivo model of articular chondrocyte transplantation," *Journal of Gene Medicine*, vol. 6, no. 2, pp. 238–245, 2004.

[66] M. Cucchiarini, T. Thurn, A. Weimer, D. Kohn, E. F. Terwilliger, and H. Madry, "Restoration of the extracellular matrix in human osteoarthritic articular cartilage by overexpression

of the transcription factor SOX9," *Arthritis and Rheumatism*, vol. 56, no. 1, pp. 158–167, 2007.

[67] V. M. Baragi, R. R. Renkiewicz, H. Jordan, J. Bonadio, J. W. Hartman, and B. J. Roessler, "Transplantation of transduced chondrocytes protects articular cartilage from interleukin 1-induced extracellular matrix degradation," *Journal of Clinical Investigation*, vol. 96, no. 5, pp. 2454–2460, 1995.

[68] V. M. Baragi, R. R. Renkiewicz, L. Qiu et al., "Transplantation of adenovirally transduced allogeneic chondrocytes into articular cartilage defects in vivo," *Osteoarthritis and Cartilage*, vol. 5, no. 4, pp. 275–282, 1997.

[69] T. Ikeda, T. Kubo, Y. Arai et al., "Adenovirus mediated gene delivery to the joints of guinea pigs," *Journal of Rheumatology*, vol. 25, no. 9, pp. 1666–1673, 1998.

[70] R. Kang, T. Marui, S. C. Ghivizzani et al., "Ex vivo gene transfer to chondrocytes in full-thickness articular cartilage defects: a feasibility study," *Osteoarthritis and Cartilage*, vol. 5, no. 2, pp. 139–143, 1997.

[71] H. Madry, M. Cucchiarini, U. Stein et al., "Sustained transgene expression in cartilage defects in vivo after transplantation of articular chondrocytes modified by lipid-mediated gene transfer in a gel suspension delivery system," *Journal of Gene Medicine*, vol. 5, no. 6, pp. 502–509, 2003.

[72] S. M. Richardson, J. M. Curran, R. Chen et al., "The differentiation of bone marrow mesenchymal stem cells into chondrocyte-like cells on poly-l-lactic acid (PLLA) scaffolds," *Biomaterials*, vol. 27, no. 22, pp. 4069–4078, 2006.

[73] S. M. Richardson, R. V. Walker, S. Parker et al., "Intervertebral disc cell-mediated mesenchymal stem cell differentiation," *Stem Cells*, vol. 24, no. 3, pp. 707–716, 2006.

[74] M. F. Pittenger, A. M. Mackay, S. C. Beck et al., "Multilineage potential of adult human mesenchymal stem cells," *Science*, vol. 284, no. 5411, pp. 143–147, 1999.

[75] T. L. Arinzeh, "Mesenchymal stem cells for bone repair: preclinical studies and potential orthopedic applications," *Foot and Ankle Clinics*, vol. 10, no. 4, pp. 651–665, 2005.

[76] L. Hong, A. Colpan, and I. A. Peptan, "Modulations of 17-β estradiol on osteogenic and adipogenic differentiations of human mesenchymal stem cells," *Tissue Engineering*, vol. 12, no. 10, pp. 2747–2753, 2006.

[77] D. Noël, F. Djouad, and C. Jorgensen, "Regenerative medicine through mesenchymal stem cells for bone and cartilage repair," *Current Opinion in Investigational Drugs*, vol. 3, no. 7, pp. 1000–1004, 2002.

[78] F. P. Barry and J. M. Murphy, "Mesenchymal stem cells: clinical applications and biological characterization," *International Journal of Biochemistry and Cell Biology*, vol. 36, no. 4, pp. 568–584, 2004.

[79] A. I. Caplan, "Adult mesenchymal stem cells for tissue engineering versus regenerative medicine," *Journal of Cellular Physiology*, vol. 213, no. 2, pp. 341–347, 2007.

[80] W. Sonoyama, Y. Liu, D. Fang et al., "Mesenchymal stem cell-mediated functional tooth regeneration in Swine," *PLoS One*, vol. 1, no. 1, article no. e79, 2006.

[81] O. Trubiani, R. Di Primio, T. Traini et al., "Morphological and cytofluorimetric analysis of adult mesenchymal stem cells expanded ex vivo from periodontal ligament," *International Journal of Immunopathology and Pharmacology*, vol. 18, no. 2, pp. 213–221, 2005.

[82] O. Trubiani, G. Orsini, S. Caputi, and A. Piattelli, "Adult mesenchymal stem cells in dental research: a new approach for tissue engineering," *International Journal of Immunopathology and Pharmacology*, vol. 19, no. 3, pp. 451–460, 2006.

[83] M. N. Helder, M. Knippenberg, J. Klein-Nulend, and P. I. J. M. Wuisman, "Stem cells from adipose tissue allow challenging new concepts for regenerative medicine," *Tissue Engineering*, vol. 13, no. 8, pp. 1799–1808, 2007.

[84] S. M. Richardson, A. Mobasheri, A. J. Freemont, and J. A. Hoyland, "Intervertebral disc biology, degeneration and novel tissue engineering and regenerative medicine therapies," *Histology and histopathology*, vol. 22, no. 9, pp. 1033–1041, 2007.

[85] A. E. Grigoriadis, J. N. M. Heersche, and J. E. Aubin, "Differentiation of muscle, fat, cartilage, and bone from progenitor cells present in a bone-derived clonal cell population: effect of dexamethasone," *Journal of Cell Biology*, vol. 106, no. 6, pp. 2139–2151, 1988.

[86] C. Csaki, N. Keshishzadeh, K. Fischer, and M. Shakibaei, "Regulation of inflammation signalling by resveratrol in human chondrocytes in vitro," *Biochemical Pharmacology*, vol. 75, no. 3, pp. 677–687, 2008.

[87] C. Csaki, U. Matis, A. Mobasheri, and M. Shakibaei, "Co-culture of canine mesenchymal stem cells with primary bone-derived osteoblasts promotes osteogenic differentiation," *Histochemistry and Cell Biology*, vol. 131, no. 2, pp. 251–266, 2009.

[88] A. Mobasheri, C. Csaki, A. L. Clutterbuck, M. Rahmanzadeh, and M. Shakibaei, "Mesenchymal stem cells in connective tissue engineering and regenerative medicine: applications in cartilage repair and osteoarthritis therapy," *Histology and Histopathology*, vol. 24, no. 3, pp. 347–366, 2009.

[89] T. Fukumoto, J. W. Sperling, A. Sanyal et al., "Combined effects of insulin-like growth factor-1 and transforming growth factor-β1 on periosteal mesenchymal cells during chondrogenesis in vitro," *Osteoarthritis and Cartilage*, vol. 11, no. 1, pp. 55–64, 2003.

[90] H.-L. Ma, S.-C. Hung, S.-Y. Lin, Y.-L. Chen, and W.-H. Lo, "Chondrogenesis of human mesenchymal stem cells encapsulated in alginate beads," *Journal of Biomedical Materials Research A*, vol. 64, no. 2, pp. 273–281, 2003.

[91] B. Johnstone, T. M. Hering, A. I. Caplan, V. M. Goldberg, and J. U. Yoo, "In vitro chondrogenesis of bone marrow-derived mesenchymal progenitor cells," *Experimental Cell Research*, vol. 238, no. 1, pp. 265–272, 1998.

[92] H. Jian, X. Shen, I. Liu, M. Semenov, X. He, and X. F. Wang, "Smad3-dependent nuclear translocation of β-catenin is required for TGF-β1- induced proliferation of bone marrow-derived adult human mesenchymal stem cells," *Genes and Development*, vol. 20, no. 6, pp. 666–674, 2006.

[93] S. Zhou, K. Eid, and J. Glowacki, "Cooperation between TGF-β and Wnt pathways during chondrocyte and adipocyte differentiation of human marrow stromal cells," *Journal of Bone and Mineral Research*, vol. 19, no. 3, pp. 463–470, 2004.

[94] M. Chiou, Y. Xu, and M. T. Longaker, "Mitogenic and chondrogenic effects of fibroblast growth factor-2 in adipose-derived mesenchymal cells," *Biochemical and Biophysical Research Communications*, vol. 343, no. 2, pp. 644–652, 2006.

[95] M. Knippenberg, M. N. Helder, B. Zandieh Doulabi, P. I. J. M. Wuisman, and J. Klein-Nulend, "Osteogenesis versus chondrogenesis by BMP-2 and BMP-7 in adipose stem cells," *Biochemical and Biophysical Research Communications*, vol. 342, no. 3, pp. 902–908, 2006.

[96] L. Longobardi, L. O'Rear, S. Aakula et al., "Effect of IGF-I in the chondrogenesis of bone marrow mesenchymal stem cells in the presence or absence of TGF-β signaling," *Journal of Bone and Mineral Research*, vol. 21, no. 4, pp. 626–636, 2006.

[97] L. A. Solchaga, K. Penick, J. D. Porter, V. M. Goldberg, A. I. Caplan, and J. F. Welter, "FGF-2 enhances the mitotic and chondrogenic potentials of human adult bone marrow-derived mesenchymal stem cells," *Journal of Cellular Physiology*, vol. 203, no. 2, pp. 398–409, 2005.

[98] S. Murakami, M. Kan, W. L. McKeehan, and B. De Crombrugghe, "Up-regulation of the chondrogenic Sox9 gene by fibroblast growth factors is mediated by the mitogen-activated protein kinase pathway," *Proceedings of the National Academy of Sciences of the United States of America*, vol. 97, no. 3, pp. 1113–1118, 2000.

[99] S. R. Tew, P. Pothacharoen, T. Katopodi, and T. E. Hardingham, "SOX9 transduction increases chondroitin sulfate synthesis in cultured human articular chondrocytes without altering glycosyltransferase and sulfotransferase transcription," *Biochemical Journal*, vol. 414, no. 2, pp. 231–236, 2008.

[100] H. Tsuchiya, H. Kitoh, F. Sugiura, and N. Ishiguro, "Chondrogenesis enhanced by overexpression of sox9 gene in mouse bone marrow-derived mesenchymal stem cells," *Biochemical and Biophysical Research Communications*, vol. 301, no. 2, pp. 338–343, 2003.

[101] J. I. Sive, P. Baird, M. Jeziorsk, A. Watkins, J. A. Hoyland, and A. J. Freemont, "Expression of chondrocyte markers by cells of normal and degenerate intervertebral discs," *Molecular Pathology*, vol. 55, no. 2, pp. 91–97, 2002.

[102] J. U. Yoo, T. S. Barthel, K. Nishimura et al., "The chondrogenic potential of human bone-marrow-derived mesenchymal progenitor cells," *Journal of Bone and Joint Surgery A*, vol. 80, no. 12, pp. 1745–1757, 1998.

[103] N. Boos, A. G. Nerlich, I. Wiest, K. Von Der Mark, and M. Aebi, "Immunolocalization of type X collagen in human lumbar intervertebral discs during ageing and degeneration," *Histochemistry and Cell Biology*, vol. 108, no. 6, pp. 471–480, 1997.

[104] J. C. Gan, P. Ducheyne, E. J. Vresilovic, W. Swaim, and I. M. Shapiro, "Intervertebral disc tissue engineering I: characterization of the nucleus pulposus," *Clinical Orthopaedics and Related Research*, no. 411, pp. 305–314, 2003.

[105] K. Pelttari, A. Winter, E. Steck et al., "Premature induction of hypertrophy during in vitro chondrogenesis of human mesenchymal stem cells correlates with calcification and vascular invasion after ectopic transplantation in SCID mice," *Arthritis and Rheumatism*, vol. 54, no. 10, pp. 3254–3266, 2006.

[106] Y.-J. Kim, H.-J. Kim, and G.-I. Im, "PTHrP promotes chondrogenesis and suppresses hypertrophy from both bone marrow-derived and adipose tissue-derived MSCs," *Biochemical and Biophysical Research Communications*, vol. 373, no. 1, pp. 104–108, 2008.

[107] I. Sekiya, B. L. Larson, J. T. Vuoristo, R. L. Reger, and D. J. Prockop, "Comparison of effect of BMP-2, -4, and -6 on in vitro cartilage formation of human adult stem cells from bone marrow stroma," *Cell and Tissue Research*, vol. 320, no. 2, pp. 269–276, 2005.

[108] F. Franceschi, U. G. Longo, L. Ruzzini, A. Marinozzi, N. Maffulli, and V. Denaro, "Simultaneous arthroscopic implantation of autologous chondrocytes and high tibial osteotomy for tibial chondral defects in the varus knee," *Knee*, vol. 15, no. 4, pp. 309–313, 2008.

[109] W. S. Khan and U. G. Longo, "ACI and MACI procedures for cartilage repair utilise mesenchymal stem cells rather than chondrocytes," *Medical Hypotheses*, vol. 77, no. 2, p. 309, 2011.

[110] U. G. Longo, F. Forriol, N. Maffulli, and V. Denaro, "Evaluation of histological scoring systems for tissue-engineered, repaired and osteoarthritic cartilage," *Osteoarthritis and Cartilage*, vol. 18, no. 7, p. 1001, 2010.

[111] U. G. Longo, A. Berton, S. Alexander, N. Maffulli, A. L. Wallace, and V. Denaro, "Biological resurfacing for early osteoarthritis of the shoulder," *Sports Medicine and Arthroscopy Review*, vol. 19, no. 4, pp. 380–394, 2011.

[112] C. Becher, A. Driessen, T. Hess, U. G. Longo, N. Maffulli, and H. Thermann, "Microfracture for chondral defects of the talus: maintenance of early results at midterm follow-up," *Knee Surgery, Sports Traumatology, Arthroscopy*, vol. 18, no. 5, pp. 656–663, 2010.

[113] F. Forriol, U. G. Longo, E. Alvarez et al., "Scanty integration of osteochondral allografts cryopreserved at low temperatures with dimethyl sulfoxide," *Knee Surgery, Sports Traumatology, Arthroscopy*, vol. 19, no. 7, pp. 1184–1191, 2011.

[114] U. G. Longo, F. Franceschi, L. Ruzzini, C. Rabitti, M. Nicola, and V. Denaro, "Foreign-body giant-cell reaction at the donor site after autologous osteochondral transplant for cartilaginous lesion. A case report," *Journal of Bone and Joint Surgery A*, vol. 91, no. 4, pp. 945–949, 2009.

15

Long-Term Cultured Human Term Placenta-Derived Mesenchymal Stem Cells of Maternal Origin Displays Plasticity

Vikram Sabapathy,[1] Saranya Ravi,[1] Vivi Srivastava,[2] Alok Srivastava,[1,3] and Sanjay Kumar[1]

[1] Center for Stem Cell Research, Christian Medical College, Bagayam, Vellore 632002, India
[2] Department of Cytogenetics, Christian Medical College, Bagayam, Vellore 632002, India
[3] Department of Hematology, Christian Medical College, Bagayam, Vellore 632002, India

Correspondence should be addressed to Sanjay Kumar, skumar@cmcvellore.ac.in

Academic Editor: Rajarshi Pal

Mesenchymal stem cells (MSCs) are an alluring therapeutic resource because of their plasticity, immunoregulatory capacity and ease of availability. Human BM-derived MSCs have limited proliferative capability, consequently, it is challenging to use in tissue engineering and regenerative medicine applications. Hence, placental MSCs of maternal origin, which is one of richest sources of MSCs were chosen to establish long-term culture from the cotyledons of full-term human placenta. Flow analysis established bonafied MSCs phenotypic characteristics, staining positively for CD29, CD73, CD90, CD105 and negatively for CD14, CD34, CD45 markers. Pluripotency of the cultured MSCs was assessed by in vitro differentiation towards not only intralineage cells like adipocytes, osteocytes, chondrocytes, and myotubules cells but also translineage differentiated towards pancreatic progenitor cells, neural cells, and retinal cells displaying plasticity. These cells did not significantly alter cell cycle or apoptosis pattern while maintaining the normal karyotype; they also have limited expression of MHC-II antigens and are Naive for stimulatory factors CD80 and CD 86. Further soft agar assays revealed that placental MSCs do not have the ability to form invasive colonies. Taking together all these characteristics into consideration, it indicates that placental MSCs could serve as good candidates for development and progress of stem-cell based therapeutics.

1. Introduction

The term Mesenchymal stem cells (MSCs) was coined by Caplan in 1991 [1]. MSCs are defined as the class of stem cells that has the potential to self-renew and differentiate into multiple cell lineages [2, 3]. The presence of mesenchymal stem cells in the bone marrow was hypothesized by Cohnheim in 1860s [4]. In 1920s, Maximow postulated the importance of the marrow stromal tissue in supporting the development and maintenance of blood and hematopoietic organs [5]. In 1960s, Friedenstein was the first to demonstrate stromal cells could be isolated from whole bone marrow aspirate based on differentiation adhesion to tissue culture plastic dishes [6]. In addition, MSCs secrete proangiogenic [7] and antiapoptotic cytokines and possess immunosuppressive properties [8]. Bone marrow MSCs are most commonly used and primary source of MSCs [9]. However, due to invasive nature of bone marrow aspiration and limited proliferative capacity, efforts are underway to identify abundant and reliable sources of MSCs for clinical applications [9]. Mesenchymal stem cells can be broadly grouped into two different subgroups adult MSCs and fetal MSCs. Adult MSCs are isolated from bone marrow, peripheral blood. Fetal MSCs are isolated from Placenta, amniotic fluid, umbilical cord and umbilical cord blood [10]. Placenta provides one of the most reliable and abundant source of MSCs [11]. Term placental tissues are discarded after birth, hence these tissues can be effectively utilized for research as well as clinical application without much ethical concern. In this paper, we systematically characterize the term placental MSCs isolated from cotyledons and validated that the isolated MSCs fulfill the genotypic and functional criteria laid out for a proper MSC [11, 12]. We have demonstrated that these MSCs have the ability to rapidly expand up to even 25–30 passages without compromising the chromosomal number, cell cycle or apoptosis pattern, phenotypic characteristics, pluripotency-associated endogenous gene expression profile, and differentiation capacity. Placental MSCs were able to transdifferentiate into other cell lineages thus exhibiting their inherent plasticity.

2. Materials and Methods

2.1. Collection of the Human Placenta Samples. The ethical committee of Christian Medical College (CMC), Vellore, approved the study. Following the written consent term placental samples were collected from donors after elective caesarean.

2.2. Cell Isolation. Term human placental MSCs were isolated from cotyledons present towards the maternal side of the placenta. The placental membrane from the maternal side of the placenta was cut open and about 80 g of cotyledons was exercised. The cotyledons was thoroughly washed with PBS and cut into small pieces. The blood clots present in the cotyledons were mechanically removed. The minced placental was once again washed with physiological saline and subjected to sequential digestion with trypsin and collagenase I. The tissues were incubated with 0.25% trypsin for 1 hour at 37°C. After trypsin digestion, the sample was filtered through 250 μm metal sieve. The retentate was collected and subjected to second digestion with12.5 U/mL collagenase I for 1 hour at 37°C. Collagenase I digested tissue sample was passed first through 250 μm metal sieve and filtrate collected was passed through 100 μm cell strainer. The filtrate containing cell suspension after dual filtration stages were subjected to centrifugation at 300 g for 10 minutes. The cell pellet was resuspended in RBC lysis buffer and centrifuged at 300 g for 10 minutes. Finally, the cell pellet was resuspended in Mesenchymal expansion medium (αMEM + 10% FBS + 50 u/mL penicillin + 50 μg/mL streptomycin + 1 mM L-glutamine) and plated into two 75 cm² flasks.

2.3. Antibodies. Information on primary and secondary antibodies used for flow-cytometry and immunostaining experiments is provided in Supplementary Table 1 is available online at doi: 10.1155/2012/174328.

2.4. Flow Cytometry. Cells after trypsinization was equally aliquoted (1×10^5 cells per reaction) into FACS tubes and stained on live cells with respective antibody. Unstained antibody and cells stained with isotype antibody acted as controls. Antibodies were added to the cells in dark to avoid bleaching. After addition of the antibody, the sample was incubated at room temperature in dark for 20 minutes. Cells were washed with 1 mL of DPBS without calcium and magnesium and centrifuged at 300 g for 5 min. The pelleted cells were resuspended in 300 μL DPBS w/o calcium

and magnesium and analyzed with a flow cytometer (FACS Calibur; Becton Dickinson). A minimum of 10^4 gated events was acquired from each sample for analysis using cell quest.

2.5. Cytogenetic Analysis. Karyotyping of human placental MSCs was carried at Passages 5 and 25 to verify the chromosomal integrity. Metaphase chromosomal preparations were performed according to standard procedures at a 400–550 GTG band level. Zeiss axioplan microscope was used to identify and analyse the chromosomes. Images were analyzed with a photometrics charged coupled device camera and controlled with smart capture imaging software.

2.6. Immunostaining. The cells cultured in 6-well plates were blocked with PBS (without Ca^{2+} and Mg^{2+}) containing 0.1% BSA, fixed with 4% paraformaldehyde and permeabilized using 0.2% Triton X-100. If using unconjugated antibody, samples were first incubated with primary antibody, blocked with PBS containing 0.1% BSA and subsequently incubated with fluorescent dye conjugated secondary antibody. All cell samples were additionally counterstained with Hoechst 33342. Images were taken using leica DMI6000B (Leica) equipped with DFC360FX digital camera and analyzed with Lecia AF imaging software (Leica).

2.7. Total RNA Isolation and Reverse Transcription Polymerase Chain Reaction (RT-PCR). Total RNA isolation was carried out using Trizol (Invitrogen). cDNA was prepared with superscript III reverse transcriptase enzyme. The primer sequences and their respective annealing temperature are presented in supplementary entary Table 2. PCR conditions were initial denaturation at 94°C for 2 min, followed by denaturation at 94°C for 1 min, annealing for 1 min, extension at 72°C for 2 min for 35 cycles, and final extension was carried out at 72°C for 5 min. Glyceraldehyde 3 phosphate dehydrogenase (GAPDH) RNA was used as a control for normalization of RNAs. PCR products were analyzed using ethidium bromide stained 2% agarose gels. Analysis of the gel images was carried out (Supplementary Table 2).

2.8. QPCR. Total RNA was extracted with Trizol (Invitrogen) according to the manufacturer's protocol. cDNA synthesis was carried out using Superscript III First-Strand synthesis system (Invitrogen). qRT-PCRs were carried out with SYBR Green master mix and AB real-time thermocycler (AB 7500). Primer sequences for the analysis of endogenous pluripotency gene expression are mentioned in the table below. The expression levels of individual genes were normalized against β-Actin (Supplementary Table 2).

2.9. Cell Cycle Analysis. For cell cycle analysis [13], cells were fixed with cold methanol, treated with RNase A 10 μg/mL, stained with Propidium Iodide 50 μg/mL, and analyzed by flowcytometer.

2.10. Apoptosis Analysis. Apoptosis analysis was carried by following the manufacturer's instructions (BD Pharmingen Annexin V). The cells were subjected to live staining with Annexin V and 7-AAD and analyzed the cells through flowcytometer.

2.11. Oligo-Lineage Differentiation Analysis. Placental MSCs at various passages were subjected intra- and translineage differentiation protocol to analyze the plasticity of the cells. After differentiation, cells were stained with appropriate stains and examined microscopically under Leica microscope.

2.12. Adipogenic Differentiation. Placental MSCs at 5×10^4 cells were seeded onto 24-well plate (corning) containing adipogenic differentiation medium (Invitrogen) for 30 days, fresh medium added every 48 hours. Oil red O staining was carried out to visualize the presence of fat droplets. Cells were fixed with 4% paraformaldehyde, washed with sterile water, and incubated with 60% isopropanol at room temperature. Fixed cells were stained with 0.5% oil red O in isopropanol for 20 minutes at room temperature. After staining, cells were first washed with 60% isopropanol later rinsed with sterile water before observing under the microscope for imaging.

2.13. Chondrogenic Differentiation. Chondrogenic differentiation was carried out using falcon25 static cell culture system (specially fabricated in our lab for chondrocyte differentiation). Cells were subjected to micromass cell culture conditions to induce the chondrocyte differentiation under chondrocyte differentiation medium (Invitrogen) for 30 days. One million MSCs were pelleted at 300 g and chondrocyte differentiation medium was added without disturbing the pellet. Media was changed every 48 hrs. After differentiation, cells were fixed with 10% formalin, stained with merchrome, and embedded in paraffin. Staining on deparaffinized 5 μm sections staining for proteoglycans was carried out using saffranin O and 3% alcian blue. After staining, sections were rinsed with distilled water, air dried at room temperature, immersed in xylene, and mounted using DPX before observing under microscopy.

2.14. Osteogenic Differentiation. For osteogenic differentiation, 5×10^4 cells were seeded per well in 24-well plate containing osteogenic induction medium (Invitrogen) for 30 days, with media change every 48 hrs. After differentiation, presence of extracellular calcium was confirmed by VonKossa staining. For vonkossa staining, the cells were fixed in precooled methanol. After fixing, the cells were washed with DPBS (W/O Ca^{2+} and Mg^{2+}), treated with 5% silver nitrate solution in water, and exposed to UV light for 1 hour under the laminar hood. Stained cells were washed with water and incubated with 5% sodium thiosulphate in water for 2 min at room temperature. Finally, sample was rinsed with sterile water and observed under the microscope for imaging.

2.15. Myotubule Differentiation. For myotubule differentiation [14], 5×10^4 placental MSCs were seeded in 25 cm² flask

containing mesenchymal expansion medium with 3 μM 5-azacytidine. The cells were cultured for 21 days with media changes every 7 days. The cells were stained with Hoechst 33342 (5 μg/mL), incubated at 37°C for 30 minutes before observing under the microscope for imaging.

2.16. Tubular Assay. Matrigel (BD) was thawed at 4°C for overnight. 50 μL of matrigel was aliquoted per well of 96 well plate using precooled tips. The plate was centrifuged at 300 g for 5 min, 4°C. Allowed to polymerize at 37°C for 30 min. MSCs at 1×10^5 cells/well were seeded in mesenchymal expansion medium. Cells were incubated at 37°C under hypoxic condition for 6 hours before observing under the microscope for imaging [15].

2.17. Neural Differentiation. To induced neuronal differentiation [16], 5×10^5 placental MSCs were seeded onto serum-free α-MEM containing 5 mM β-mercaptoethanol and cultured for 6–9 hrs. The cells after induction were fixed for immunostaining analysis.

2.18. Retinal Cell Differentiation. For Retinal differentiation [17], 1×10^5 cells were seeded into media containing Mesenchymal expansion medium supplemented with 50 μM Taurine with 1 mM Beta-mercaptoethanol. The cells, were cultured for 4 days with media changes every 4 days. After retinal induction cells were collected in trizol for RT-PCR analysis or fixed for immunostaining.

2.19. Pancreatic Progenitor Cell Differentiation. For pancreatic differentiation [12, 18, 19], 25 cm² flasks were treated with gelatin and 5×10^5 cells were seeded onto gelatinized dish containing mesenchymal expansion medium with 10 mM nicotinamide and 1 mM β-Mercaptoethanol for 24 hrs. Following preinduction, cells were treated with Mesenchymal expansion medium without FBS but containing 10 mM nicotinamide and 1 mM β-Mercaptoethanol for 6 hours, and for following 18 hrs cells were treated with induction media containing FBS. After differentiation, cells were collected in trizol and subjected to RT-PCR analysis or fixed for immunostaining.

2.20. Soft Agar Assay. For Soft agar assay [20], 0.6% agar containing MEM was layered on the surface of 35 mm dish (corning) and incubated in laminar hood for 30 min. Later, 2 $\times 10^4$ MSCs were mixed with 0.3% agar containing MEM and overlayed on the top of 0.6% agar layer. Plate was incubated in hood for 20 minutes. Following incubation, 500 μL of Mesenchymal expansion medium was added and incubated for 21 days. To the dish, 500 μL of fresh media was added every 7 days once. HeLa cells were used as a positive control.

2.21. Dithizone Staining. For Dithizone (STZ) Staining, the cells were incubated with DTZ solution 100 μg/mL in α-MEM media for 20 minutes at 37°C. After staining, the cells were rinsed with twice with PBS and examined under microscope [21].

2.22. Cell Population Doubling Time (Gt). Population doubling time indicates the growth rate of the placental MSCs [22], population doubling (PD)

$$PD = \frac{\ln(Nf/Ni)}{\ln 2}, \quad (1)$$

where ln equals natural logarithm, Nf equals final cell count, Ni equals initial cell count

$$Gt = \frac{t}{PD}, \quad (2)$$

t = Time in hours after cell seeding.

Average Gt value was attained by adding the obtained Gt values for different experiments divided by number of experiments.

3. Results

3.1. Derivation of Adherent Fibroblast Like Mesenchymal Stem Cells (MSCs) from Maternal Side of Human Placenta and Immunophenotypic Characterization of Human Placental MSCs. Enzyme-mediated fractionation of human termed placenta resulted in derivation of fibroblast-like cells, which are generally term placenta-derived multipotent mesenchymal stem cells (PD-MSCs). Selection for MSCs rested on the classic adhesion method on tissue culture plastic. Placental MSCs from 8 term placental samples have been established from maternal side lobules of human placenta following trypsin digestion and collagenase-I treatment following which samples were passed through the $100\,\mu$ filter and were seeded in α-MEM containing 10% FBS, and adherent cell population was then characterized for their proliferation capabilities, cell cycle, apoptosis pattern, immunophenotypic features, and differentiation capabilities. The isolated MSCs formed a homogenous monolayer of adherent spindle-shaped fibroblast-like cells. The protocol proved successful in 8 of 8 placental tissues collection. Plating of cell suspensions from the first digest with trypsin did not produce any colonies, but cell suspensions produced from final collagenase I digest of placental tissue fragments typically produced MSC colonies of variable sizes that contained outgrowing fibroblast-like cells. After initial plating of the cells, the colonies became visible after 7 days. These MSC colonies in turn started to proliferate steadily, the flask was almost 60–70% confluent and ready for splitting by day 14. Typically, approximately 5–6 × 10^4 cells were obtained within 12–14 days after plating. Following the process of initiation the flasks were subjected to trypsinization in 1:2 or 1:3 ratio. The 75 cm^2 at 1:2 splitting was subconfluent by day 3, indicating these isolated cells had very rapid proliferating capacity. Outgrowing cells when harvested and replated in higher dilutions rapidly formed secondary colonies from single cells (Figures 1(a) and 1(b)). PD-MSCs were expandable up to passage 25–30 (as far as we cultured) without any

changes in the morphological characteristics (Figures 1(c) and 1(d)) and were amenable to routine cryopreservation, thawing and differentiation protocols. The MSCs were characterized using flow-cytometry-based positive reaction for mesenchymal lineage surface markers CD29$^+$, CD73$^+$, CD90$^+$, CD105$^+$; and negative for hematopoietic marker CD34$^-$, CD45$^-$, also negative expression of CD14$^-$, HLA DR$^-$; was used to define MSCs (Figures 1(c), 1(d), and 1(e)). Flow cytometry revealed very little scatter in the phenotypic marker profile of placenta-derived isolates between all 8 cases, also population doubling time calculated were not significantly altered. The expression profile confirmed to the criteria generally defined for multipotent mesenchymal stem cells [23].

3.2. Plasticity of MSCs. Specific induction of differentiation was investigated with PD-MSCs, one early, one mid, and one late passage from all 8 subjects. This confirmed that the mesenchymal stemness profile by PD-MSC populations indeed associated with the ability to generate different mesodermal lineage cell types on their exposure to soluble growth and differentiation factors *in vitro*. At the same time, when subjected to translineage differentiation MSC shows remarkable plasticity to differentiate into ectodermal (neuronal cells, retinal cells) and endodermal lineage (pancreatic beta cells). Subconfluent culture was found critically important to maintain the stemness phenotype of PD-MSCs during expansion. The phenotypic profile of PD-MSCs when subcultured at 50–70% cell density remained unaffected, also maintained their initial marker profile and their ability to differentiate as well. MSCs can be differentiated into cells from all the three germ layers under suitable supplementary conditions *in vitro*. The figures display representative results of adipogenic (Figure 2 (a)), osteogenic (Figure 2 (b)), and chondrogenic (Figures 2 (c), and 2 (d)) differentiation assays, visualizing large lipid vacuoles, mineralized bone with calcium deposits and saffranin O positive collagen matrix respectively. These adipogenesis, osteogenesis, and chondrogenesis along with myotubule formation (Figure 2 (e)) and endothelial cells tubular assay (Figure 2 (f)) indicates the ability of the MSC to differentiate into mesodermal cell lineage. Moreover, reports are available on MSC culture in presence of the angiogenic growth factor VEGF induced expression of CD34, which is a marker of hematopoietic, as well as endothelial, precursors [35]. Figure also shows neurogenesis (Figures 2 (g), 2 (h), 2 (i), 2 (j), and 2 (k)) and retinal cell (Figure 2 (l)) differentiation which exhibits the ectodermal differentiation capacity of MSCs. Further, differentiation in pancreatic beta cells indicates (Figure 2 (m)) the endodermal differentiation capacity of placental MSCs. Also, RT-PCR amplification of calbindin2 and recoverin genes shows (Figure 2 (n)) retinal (ectodermal lineage) differentiation, and pancreatic amylase gene (Figure 2 (n)) was also amplified after pancreatic beta cell induction.

3.3. Extensively Passaged Placenta-Derived MSC Does Not Significantly Alter the Cell Cycle or Apoptotic Pattern While Maintaining the Normal Karyotype. In the next set of

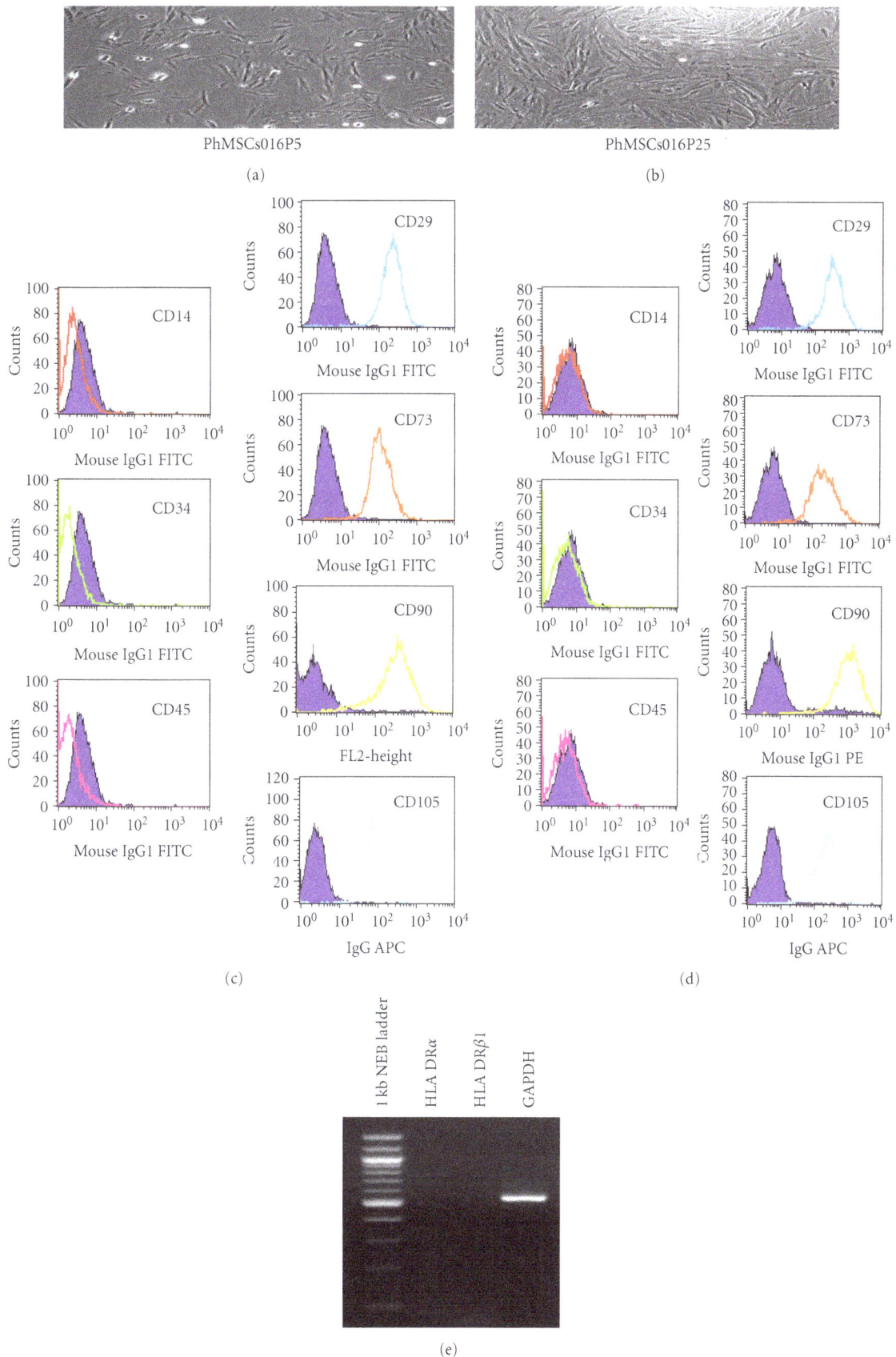

FIGURE 1: Morphology and characteristics of placental MSCs. (a) morphology of the placental MSCs at passage 5; (b) morphology of the placental MSCs at passage 25; (c) flowcytometric analysis of Placental MSCs at passage 5; (d) flowcytometric analysis of Placental MSCs at passage 25; (e) RT-PCR analysis of placental MSCs (PhMSCs 020P3) for MHC class II antigens.

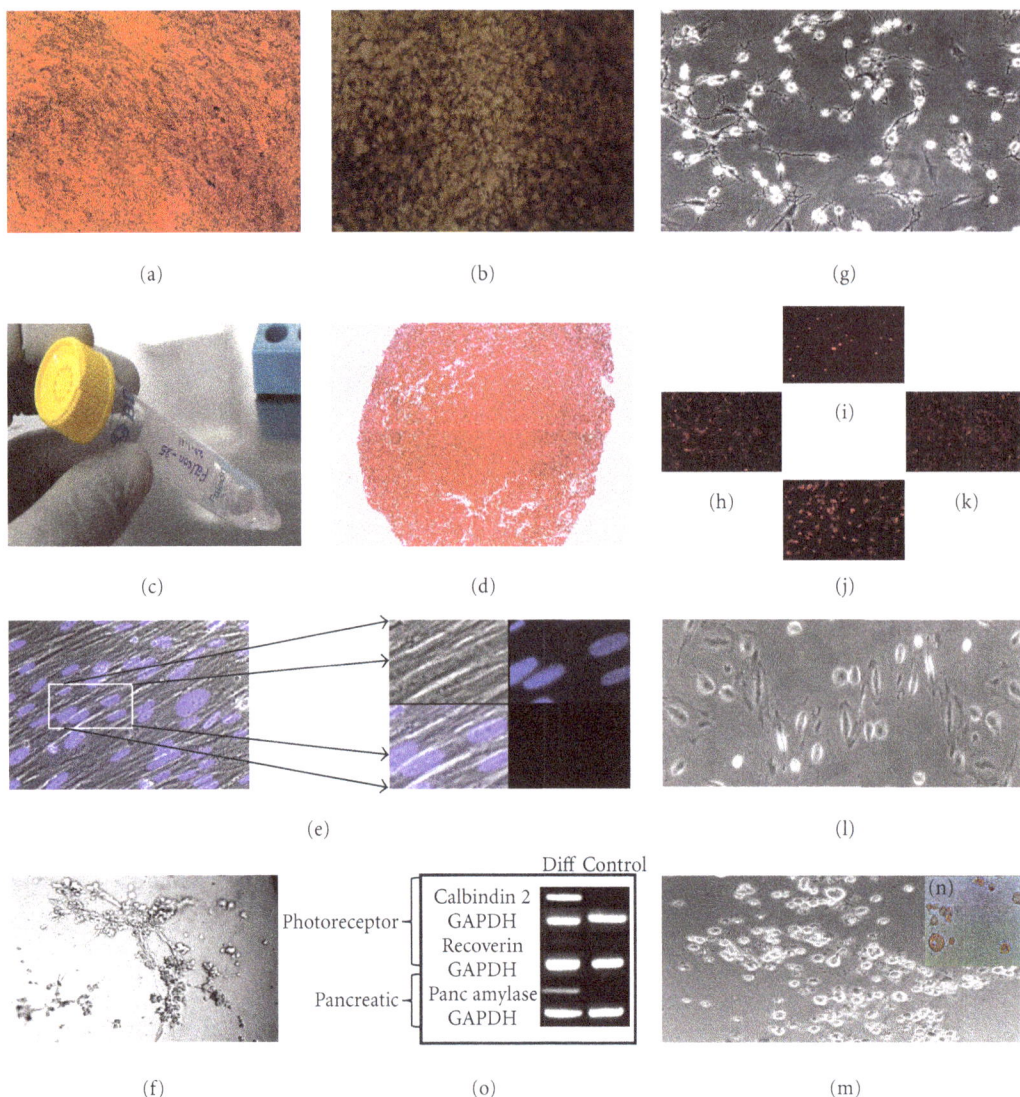

FIGURE 2: Pluripotency property of placental MSCs. (a) Oil red O staining (PhMSCsP5); (b) Von Kossa staining (PhMSCsP10); (c) "Falcon 25" static micromass cell culture system for chondrocyte differentiation; (d) saffranin O staining (PhMSCsP5); (e) hoechst 33342 staining of myotubules; (f) tubular assay; (g) neural differentiation of placental MSCs (PhMSCsP20); (h) map2 staining (PhMSCs021P15); (i) NeuN staining (PhMSCsP15); (j) GFAP staining (PhMSCs021P15); (k) Neural filament staining (PhMSCsP15); (l) Retinal cell differentiation of placental MSCs (PhMSCsP9); (m) Pancreatic progenitor cell differentiation of placental MSCs (PhMSCsP9) (n) dithizone (DTZ) positive pancreatic progenitor cells; (o) PCR analysis of ectodermal lineage (photoreceptor genes calbindin2 and recoverin) and endodermal lineage (pancreatic amylase gene).

experiments after propidium iodide staining, we tested MSC cell cycle status; Figure 3(a) shows during early and late passaging there was not significant change in the cell cycling process. As detailed in Figure 3(b), karyotypes were normal 46, XX in all test samples. Chromosome number was found normal in all analyzed PD-MSC isolates ($n = 8$). Looking at maternal origin, we found that PD-MSC isolates obtained with our isolation procedure were always of maternal origin. Also, it was important to document the apoptosis pattern of the each passage proliferating MSC; Annexin-V and 7AAD stainning did not show (Figure 3(c)) significant change in the percentage apoptotic cells (~5–7% cells).

3.4. Placental MSCs Displays Higher Endogenous Gene Expression of Oct4, Sox2 and Nanog Compared to BM-Derived MSC.
FACS analysis by Oct3/4, Stro-1 antibodies did show positive reaction. Next, we wanted to analyze the pluripotency-associated endogenous gene expression profiles of PD MSCs and bone-marrow-derived MSC (BM-MSC). Figure 4 shows data from comparative real-time qPCR, which revealed higher expression levels of Oct4, Sox2, and nanog compared to BM-MSC. Reports are also available of flow cytometry and immunocytochemistry, which revealed that PD-MSCs were positive for stage-specific embryonic antigen SSEA-3 but negative for SSEA-4 [11].

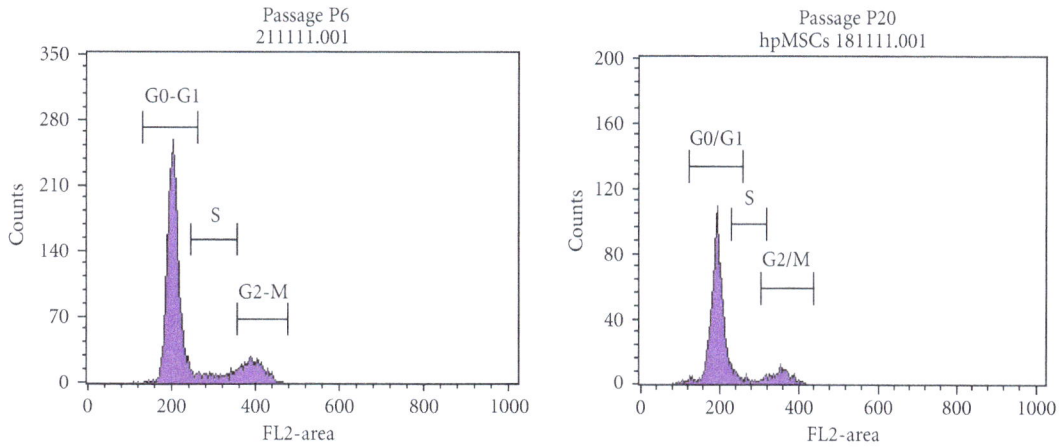

(a)

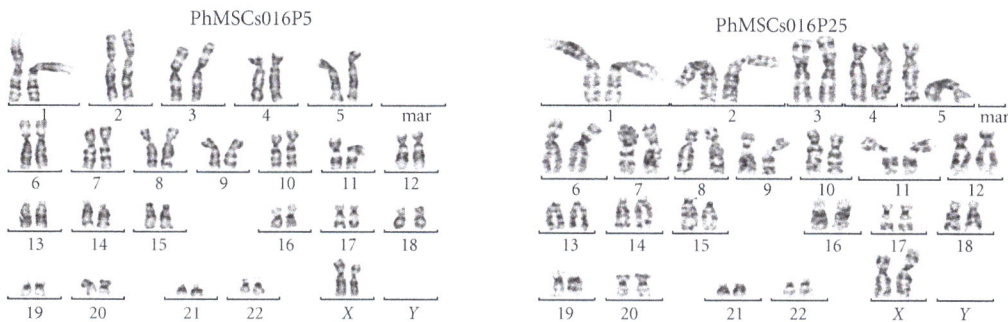

(b)

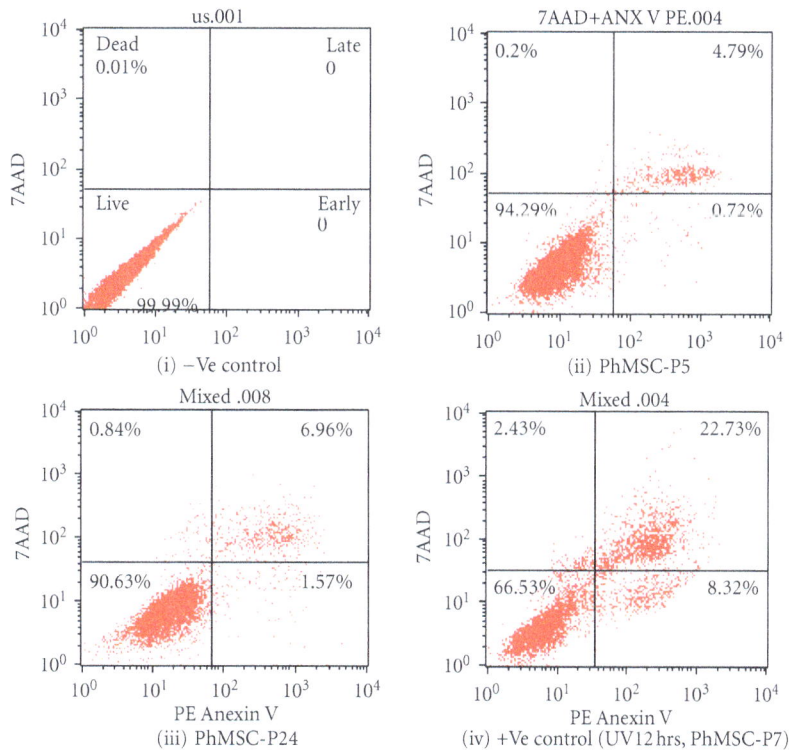

(c)

Figure 3: Cell cycle karyotype analysis: (a) cell cycle pattern of early (passage 5) and late passage (passage 20). PD-MSC were analyzed by FACS after propidim iodide staining. (b) Karyotype analysis was performed on early (passage 5) and late (passage25) passage MSC. (c) Apoptosis analysis was done by FACS using Annexin V and 7AAD. (i). negative control. (ii) Total % apoptotic MSC cells (Passage 5). (iii) % apoptotic cells (Passage 24) (iv).positive control.

QPCR analysis

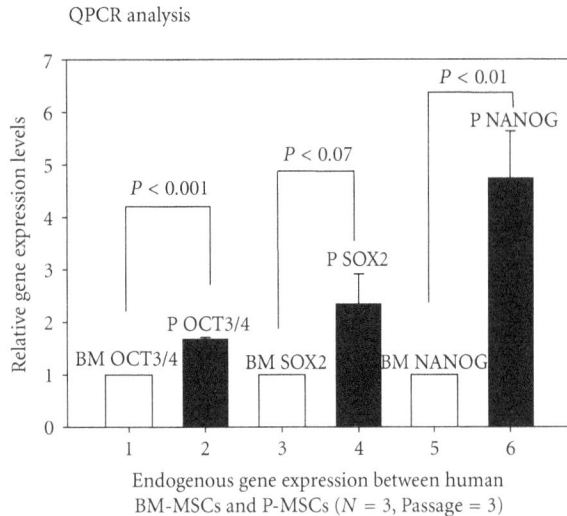

FIGURE 4: Comparative analysis of pluripotency associated endogenous gene expression between human marrow derived MSC and human placenta-derived MSC. Oct4. Sox2, and nanog gene expression profiles of bone-marrow-derived MSC and PDMSC analyzed by real-time qPCR analysis; error bars represent SE in five separate experiments.

3.5. In Vitro Tumor-Genesis Detection Assay. Placental MSCs when subjected to soft agar assay did not yield tumoroids even after 4 weeks of in vitro culture in soft agar assay (Figure 5). However, HeLa cells began to form aggregates within 7 days, and many bigger colonies were formed at the end of day 21 (Figure 5).

4. Discussion

The human embryonic stem cells (ESCs) have the potential to differentiate into all the three cell lineages [24]. However, some of the practical and ethical concerns render them in usable for day-to-day clinical applications. Nonetheless, extra embryonic tissues can be effectively used to isolate pluripotent stem cells. Placenta is one of the extra embryonic organs that has rich source of progenitor or stem cells [25]. Placenta has two sides; one is foetal side consisting of amnion and chorion and other is the maternal side consisting of deciduas [24]. Mesenchymal stem cells (MSCs) isolated from maternal side of human term-placenta represent an important cell type for stem cell research and clinical therapy not only because of their ability to differentiate into mesodermal lineage cells, such as osteocytes, chondrocytes, muscle, or endothelial cells [2], but also for their remarkable translineage differentiation capabilities like neuronal cells, retinal cells (ectodermal), and pancreatic beta cells (endodermal lineage). In addition, they secrete large amounts of proangiogenic and antiapoptotic cytokines [26] and possess remarkable immunosuppressive properties [27]. MSCs have been derived from many different organs and tissues [28]. Evidence has emerged that different parts of human placenta, umbilical cords and amniotic membrane,

as well as umbilical cord blood harbor MSC [29–32]. These tissues are normally discarded after birth, avoiding ethical concerns [23] Mechanical, as well as enzymatic, methods for MSC isolation from different regions of human placenta of different gestational ages have been reported in literature [29, 33–47]. Knowledge about vitality, average population doubling time, stable karyotype, cell cycle and apoptosis pattern, phenotype, and expandability of such placenta-derived MSC isolates is a prerequisite for therapeutic application; however, systematic investigations into reliability of this MSC source and phenotypic stability did not get that much attention. Furthermore, reports on placenta-derived MSCs often lack information about the cell cycle, apoptosis pattern, progenitor-specific endogenous gene-expression profile, and karyotype of the cell isolates. In this paper, we describe enzymatic fractionation of term-human placenta that facilitates recovery of oligo-lineage, fibroblast-like cells, which generally are termed as placenta-derived mesenchymal stem cells (PDMSCs) with high fidelity. As demonstrated by cell cycle or apoptosis analysis of cells from early as well as late passages; with average unaltered population doubling time, PD-MSC did not shows significant variations in either cell cycle or apoptosis pattern. Also, genotypic analyses of cell isolates from most of placental tissues were of maternal, not fetal, origin. Our systematic characterization of cell isolates from multiple cases showed that these cell isolates reproducibly fulfill the general definition of MSCs by both phenotypic and differentiation capabilities criteria. [24]. We demonstrate that maternally derived PD-MSCs can be greatly expanded, do not alter significantly change their cell cycle or apoptosis pattern, show pluripotency-associated endogenous gene expression, and maintain their differentiation capacity and stable phenotype displaying unaltered kayotype up to passage 25–30 passages. In these experiments, the placental MSCs were isolated from the cotyledons present in the maternal side of the placenta. Our method of cell isolation by way of sequential digestion of the trophoblast cell layer with trypsin and following digestion of remaining placental tissue with collagenase I proved very effective for obtaining PD MSCs. Outgrowth of PD-MSCs from collagenase I digests was successful in 8 of 8 placental tissues and resulted in populations with remarkably little scatter in their MSC profiles, between subjects. As for propagation, we found out that PD-MSCs must be propagated in subconfluent culture to maintain their MSC profile, because confluent culture led to gradual loss of MSC identity. With proper subconfluent passage, PDMSCs maintained their phenotypic MSC profile up to 30 passages. The flow cytometry studies indicate there is significant similarity in surface marker characteristics from passage 1 till passage 30. Microscopic observations revealed that placental MSCs proliferate rapidly till passage 30 without compromising on the morphological features and quality of the mesenchymal stem cell properties like cell cycle and apoptosis pattern, pluripotency-associated endogenous gene expression, and normal karyotype.

The characteristic data beyond passage 30 has not been tested in this study. The MSCs had spindle shaped fibroblast morphology. The absence of HLA DRα and HLA DRβ1

PhMSCs021P17

HeLa

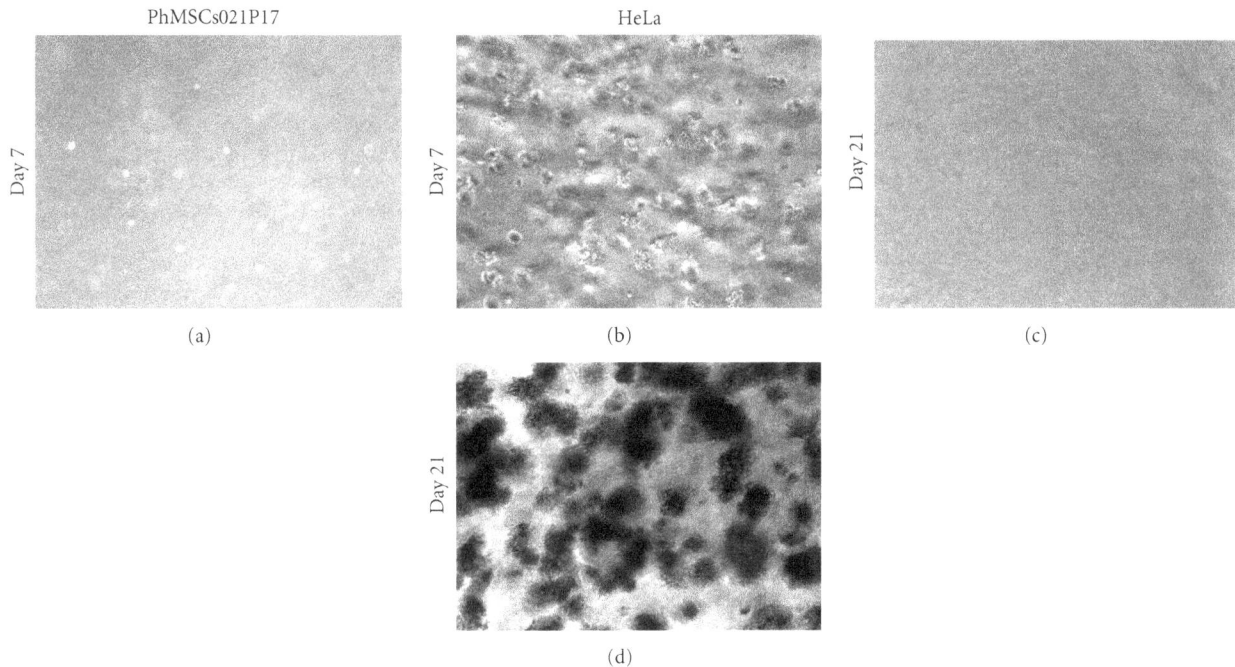

(a)

(b)

(c)

(d)

FIGURE 5: Soft agar assay. (a)Placental MSCs day 7; (b) HeLa cells day 7; (c) Placental MSCs day 21; (d) HeLa cells ay21.

expression, analyzed from RT-PCR, results indicate that placental MSCs could be effectively used for both autologous and allogenic transplantations. The rate of differentiation of MSCs is much quicker, efficient and scalable when compared to ES cells. The soft agar assay indicates that isolated placental MSCs do not possess any malignant property. Several animal as well as human trials have indicated that use of MSCs unlike ES cells does not lead to the formation of teratomas *in vivo* [24]. In addition, usage of term placental MSCs has fewer ethical concerns since they are isolated from foetal tissues that anyway would have been discarded.

5. Conclusion

The human term-placenta is relatively easily available and attracts less ethical concerns. Placental tissue constitutes a robust source of MSC. In this study, we investigated several parameters, namely, (1) chromosome number, (2) pluripotency associated gene expression, (3) maternal origin, (4) sequential enzymatic digestion (trypsin followed by collagenase) as methods of isolation, (5) cell propagation, cell cycle, and apoptosis pattern, that are important for their principal utility for cell-based therapy and could influence their proliferative, as well as differentiation, capacities. Based on the results, we conclude that the abundance of pluripotent cells, rapid proliferation, stable karyotype, plasticity and immunomodulatory property make placental MSCs ideal choice for clinical and tissue engineering applications. Nevertheless, the main drawback of using MSCs is that, a panel of surface markers are required for characterization of isolated MSCs for their homogeneity. Further, unlike the adult MSCs, where significant numbers of human clinical trials are

underway, use of placental MSCs in clinical applications is relatively new. Additional studies are required to substantiate the use of placental MSCs in medical applications.

Conflict of Interests

The authors declare no conflict of interests.

Acknowledgments

The authors appreciate encouragement and support extended by all students and staffs of CSCR and CMC in carrying out the research work successfully. they express their gratitude to Department of Biotechnology for Ramalingaswami fellowship to Sanjay Kumar and research support grant (DBT Grant no. BT/PR15420/MED/31/122/2011), Government of India.

References

[1] P. Bianco, P. G. Robey, and P. J. Simmons, "Mesenchymal stem cells: revisiting history, concepts, and assays," *Cell Stem Cell*, vol. 2, no. 4, pp. 313–319, 2008.

[2] S. Kumar, D. Chanda, and S. Ponnazhagan, "Therapeutic potential of genetically modified mesenchymal stem cells," *Gene Therapy*, vol. 15, no. 10, pp. 711–715, 2008.

[3] D. C. Ding, W. C. Shyu, and S. Z. Lin, "Mesenchymal stem cells," *Cell Transplantation*, vol. 20, pp. 5–14, 2011.

[4] J. Cohnheim, "Über entzündung und Eiterung," *Virchows Archiv für Pathologische Anatomie und Physiologie und für klinische Medizin*, vol. 40, pp. 1–79, 1867.

[5] A. Maximow, "Relation of blood cells to connective tissues and endothelium," *Physiological Reviews*, vol. 4, pp. 533–563, 1924.

[6] A. J. Friedenstein, U. F. Gorskaja, and N. N. Kulagina, "Fibroblast precursors in normal and irradiated mouse hematopoietic organs," *Experimental Hematology*, vol. 4, no. 5, pp. 267–274, 1976.

[7] Y. Miyahara, N. Nagaya, M. Kataoka et al., "Monolayered mesenchymal stem cells repair scarred myocardium after myocardial infarction," *Nature Medicine*, vol. 12, no. 4, pp. 459–465, 2006.

[8] A. Uccelli, L. Moretta, and V. Pistoia, "Mesenchymal stem cells in health and disease," *Nature Reviews Immunology*, vol. 8, no. 9, pp. 726–736, 2008.

[9] B. Parekkadan and J. M. Milwid, "Mesenchymal stem cells as therapeutics," *Annual Review of Biomedical Engineering*, vol. 12, pp. 87–117, 2010.

[10] R. Hass, C. kasper, S. Böhm, and R. Jacobs, "Different populations and scources of human Mesenchymal stem cells (MSC): a comparison of adult and neonatal tissue-derived MSC," *Cell Communication and Signaling*, vol. 9, p. 12, 2011.

[11] O. V. Semenov, S. Koestenbauer, M. Riegel et al., "Multipotent mesenchymal stem cells from human placenta: critical parameters for isolation and maintenance of stemness after isolation," *American Journal of Obstetrics and Gynecology*, vol. 202, no. 2, pp. 193.e1–193.e13, 2010.

[12] S. Kadam, S. Muthyala, P. Nair, and R. Bhonde, "Human placenta-derived mesenchymal stem cells and islet-like cell clusters generated from these cells as a novel source for stem cell therapy in diabetes," *Review of Diabetic Studies*, vol. 7, no. 2, pp. 168–182, 2010.

[13] S. Kumar and S. Ponnazhagan, "Bone homing of mesenchymal stem cells by ectopic $\alpha 4$ integrin expression," *FASEB Journal*, vol. 21, no. 14, pp. 3917–3927, 2007.

[14] Y. Zhang, Y. Chu, W. Shen, and Z. Dou, "Effect of 5-azacytidine induction duration on differentiation of human first-trimester fetal mesenchymal stem cells towards cardiomyocyte-like cells," *Interactive Cardiovascular and Thoracic Surgery*, vol. 9, no. 6, pp. 943–946, 2009.

[15] X.-Y. Hu, W.-X. Wang, M.-J. Yu et al., "Tongxinluo promotes mesenchymal stem cell tube formation in vitro," *Journal of Zhejiang University*, vol. 12, no. 8, pp. 644–651, 2011.

[16] D. Woodbury, E. J. Schwarz, D. J. Prockop, and I. B. Black, "Adult rat and human bone marrow stromal cells differentiate into neurons," *Journal of Neuroscience Research*, vol. 61, no. 4, pp. 364–370, 2000.

[17] A. Kicic, W. Y. Shen, A. S. Wilson, I. J. Constable, T. Robertson, and P. E. Rakoczy, "Differentiation of marrow stromal cells into photoreceptors in the rat eye," *Journal of Neuroscience*, vol. 23, no. 21, pp. 7742–7749, 2003.

[18] L. B. Chen, X. B. Jiang, and L. Yang, "Differentiation of rat marrow mesenchymal stem cells into pancreatic islet beta-cells," *World Journal of Gastroenterology*, vol. 10, no. 20, pp. 3016–3020, 2004.

[19] S. Şuşman, O. Soriţău, D. Rus-Ciucă, C. Tomuleasa, V. I. Pop, and C. M. Mihu, "Placental stem cell differentiation into islets of Langerhans-like glucagon-secreting cells," *Romanian Journal of Morphology and Embryology*, vol. 51, no. 4, pp. 733–738, 2010.

[20] P. Shetty, K. Cooper, and C. Viswanathan, "Comparision of proliferative and multilineage differentiation potentials of cord matix, cord blood and bone marrow Mesenchymal stem cells," *Asian Journal of Transfusion Science*, vol. 4, pp. 14–24, 2010.

[21] R. Q. Feng, L. Y. Du, and Z. Q. Guo, "*In vitro* cultivation and differentiation of fetal liver stem cells from mice," *Cell Research*, vol. 15, no. 5, pp. 401–405, 2005.

[22] W. Zhao, Z. X. Lin, and Z. Q. Zhang, "Cisplatin-induced premature senescence with concomitant reduction of gap junctions in human fibroblasts," *Cell Research*, vol. 14, no. 1, pp. 60–66, 2004.

[23] O. Parolini, F. Alviano, G. P. Bagnara et al., "Concise review: isolation and characterization of cells from human term placenta: outcome of the first international workshop on placenta derived stem cells," *Stem Cells*, vol. 26, no. 2, pp. 300–311, 2008.

[24] H. Abdulrazzak, D. Moschidou, G. Jones, and P. V. Guillot, "Biological characteristics of stem cells from foetal, cord blood and extraembryonic tissues," *Journal of the Royal Society Interface*, vol. 7, no. 6, pp. S689–S706, 2010.

[25] O. Parolini, F. Alviano, I. Bergwerf et al., "Toward cell therapy using placenta-derived cells: disease mechanisms, cell biology, preclinical studies, and regulatory aspects at the round table," *Stem Cells and Development*, vol. 19, no. 2, pp. 143–154, 2010.

[26] Y. Miyahara, N. Nagaya, M. Kataoka et al., "Monolayered mesenchymal stem cells repair scarred myocardium after myocardial infarction," *Nature Medicine*, vol. 12, no. 4, pp. 459–465, 2006.

[27] A. Uccelli, L. Moretta, and V. Pistoia, "Mesenchymal stem cells in health and disease," *Nature Reviews Immunology*, vol. 8, no. 9, pp. 726–736, 2008.

[28] G. Chamberlain, J. Fox, B. Ashton, and J. Middleton, "Concise review: mesenchymal stem cells: their phenotype, differentiation capacity, immunological features, and potential for homing," *Stem Cells*, vol. 25, no. 11, pp. 2739–2749, 2007.

[29] C. B. Portmann-Lanz, A. Schoeberlein, A. Huber et al., "Placental mesenchymal stem cells as potential autologous graft for pre- and perinatal neuroregeneration," *American Journal of Obstetrics and Gynecology*, vol. 194, no. 3, pp. 664–673, 2006.

[30] S. Ilancheran, Y. Moodley, and U. Manuelpillai, "Human fetal membranes: a source of stem cells for tissue regeneration and repair?" *Placenta*, vol. 30, no. 1, pp. 2–10, 2009.

[31] C. H. Jo, O. S. Kim, E. Y. Park et al., "Fetal mesenchymal stem cells derived from human umbilical cord sustain primitive characteristics during extensive expansion," *Cell and Tissue Research*, vol. 334, no. 3, pp. 423–433, 2008.

[32] K. Bieback, S. Kern, H. Klüter, and H. Eichler, "Critical parameters for the isolation of mesenchymal stem cells from umbilical cord blood," *Stem Cells*, vol. 22, no. 4, pp. 625–634, 2004.

[33] A. J. Marcus and D. Woodbury, "Fetal stem cells from extra-embryonic tissues: do not discard: stem cells review series," *Journal of Cellular and Molecular Medicine*, vol. 12, no. 3, pp. 730–742, 2008.

[34] V. L. Battula, S. Treml, H. Abele, and H. J. Bühring, "Prospective isolation and characterization of mesenchymal stem cells from human placenta using a frizzled-9-specific monoclonal antibody," *Differentiation*, vol. 76, no. 4, pp. 326–336, 2008.

[35] C. M. Chang, C. L. Kao, Y. L. Chang et al., "Placenta-derived multipotent stem cells induced to differentiate into insulin-positive cells," *Biochemical and Biophysical Research Communications*, vol. 357, no. 2, pp. 414–420, 2007.

[36] C. C. Chien, B. L. Yen, F. K. Lee et al., "In vitro differentiation of human placenta-derived multipotent cells into hepatocyte-like cells," *Stem Cells*, vol. 24, no. 7, pp. 1759–1768, 2006.

[37] Y. Fukuchi, H. Nakajima, D. Sugiyama, I. Hirose, T. Kitamura, and K. Tsuji, "Human placenta-derived cells have mesenchymal stem/progenitor cell potential," *Stem Cells*, vol. 22, no. 5, pp. 649–658, 2004.

[38] O. Genbacev, A. Krtolica, T. Zdravkovic et al., "Serum-free derivation of human embryonic stem cell lines on human placental fibroblast feeders," *Fertility and Sterility*, vol. 83, no. 5, pp. 1517–1529, 2005.

[39] K. Igura, X. Zhang, K. Takahashi, A. Mitsuru, S. Yamaguchi, and T. A. Takahashi, "Isolation and characterization of mesenchymal progenitor cells from chorionic villi of human placenta," *Cytotherapy*, vol. 6, no. 6, pp. 543–553, 2004.

[40] P. S. In't Anker, S. A. Scherjon, C. Kleijburg-Van Der Keur et al., "Isolation of mesenchymal stem cells of fetal or maternal origin from human placenta," *Stem Cells*, vol. 22, no. 7, pp. 1338–1345, 2004.

[41] Z. Miao, J. Jin, L. Chen et al., "Isolation of mesenchymal stem cells from human placenta: comparison with human bone marrow mesenchymal stem cells," *Cell Biology International*, vol. 30, no. 9, pp. 681–687, 2006.

[42] A. Poloni, V. Rosini, E. Mondini et al., "Characterization and expansion of mesenchymal progenitor cells from first-trimester chorionic villi of human placenta," *Cytotherapy*, vol. 10, no. 7, pp. 690–697, 2008.

[43] Z. Strakova, M. Livak, M. Krezalek, and I. Ihnatovych, "Multipotent properties of myofibroblast cells derived from human placenta," *Cell and Tissue Research*, vol. 332, no. 3, pp. 479–488, 2008.

[44] B. L. Yen, H. I. Huang, C. C. Chien et al., "Isolation of multipotent cells from human term placenta," *Stem Cells*, vol. 23, no. 1, pp. 3–9, 2005.

[45] X. Zhang, A. Mitsuru, K. Igura et al., "Mesenchymal progenitor cells derived from chorionic villi of +human placenta for cartilage tissue engineering," *Biochemical and Biophysical Research Communications*, vol. 340, no. 3, pp. 944–952, 2006.

[46] X. Zhang, Y. Soda, K. Takahashi et al., "Successful immortalization of mesenchymal progenitor cells derived from human placenta and the differentiation abilities of immortalized cells," *Biochemical and Biophysical Research Communications*, vol. 351, no. 4, pp. 853–859, 2006.

[47] S. Barlow, G. Brooke, K. Chatterjee et al., "Comparison of human placenta- and bone marrow-derived multipotent mesenchymal stem cells," *Stem Cells and Development*, vol. 17, no. 6, pp. 1095–1107, 2008.

16

Tissue Engineered Strategies for Skeletal Muscle Injury

Umile Giuseppe Longo,[1,2] **Mattia Loppini,**[1,2] **Alessandra Berton,**[1,2] **Filippo Spiezia,**[1,2]
Nicola Maffulli,[3] **and Vincenzo Denaro**[1,2]

[1] Department of Orthopaedic and Trauma Surgery, Campus Bio-Medico University, Via Alvaro del Portillo 200,
   Trigoria, 00128 Rome, Italy
[2] Centro Integrato di Ricerca (CIR) Campus Bio-Medico University, Via Alvaro del Portillo 21, 00128, Rome, Italy
[3] Centre for Sports and Exercise Medicine, Barts and The London School of Medicine and Dentistry, Mile End Hospital,
   275 Bancroft Road, London E1 4DG, UK

Correspondence should be addressed to Umile Giuseppe Longo, g.longo@unicampus.it

Academic Editor: Wasim S. Khan

Skeletal muscle injuries are common in athletes, occurring with direct and indirect mechanisms and marked residual effects, such as severe long-term pain and physical disability. Current therapy consists of conservative management including RICE protocol (rest, ice, compression, and elevation), nonsteroidal anti-inflammatory drugs, and intramuscular corticosteroids. However, current management of muscle injuries often does not provide optimal restoration to preinjury status. New biological therapies, such as injection of platelet-rich plasma and stem-cell-based therapy, are appealing. Although some studies support PRP application in muscle-injury management, reasons for concern persist, and further research is required for a standardized and safe use of PRP in clinical practice. The role of stem cells needs to be confirmed, as studies are still limited and inconsistent. Further research is needed to identify mechanisms involved in muscle regeneration and in survival, proliferation, and differentiation of stem cells.

1. Introduction

Skeletal muscle injuries are common causes of severe long-term pain and physical disability, accounting for up to 55% of all sports injuries [1]. Contusions and strains are the most frequent muscle lesions, representing more than 90% of all sports-related injuries [2]. Mechanisms of muscle lesion can be divided into direct and indirect trauma. Direct injuries include lacerations and contusions, while indirect injuries include complete or incomplete muscle strains [3]. A muscle contusion takes place when a sudden, heavy compressive force is applied to the muscle [4]. A muscle strain occurs when an excessive tensile force is applied to the muscle leading to the overstraining of the myofibers up to a rupture near the myotendinous junction [5]. Muscle injuries can also result from a combination of these mechanisms. Finally, skeletal muscle can be damaged when compartment syndromes occur because of vascular and/or neurologic impairment [3, 6]. Injuries can counter the beneficial effects of sports participation because of the residual effects. The associated morbidity, including painful contractures and muscle atrophy, can result in prolonged loss of activity and increased risk of recurrent injury [7]. In some instances, muscle injuries leads to inability of athletes to continue to practice sport.

Therefore, there is a need to improve skeletal muscle injury management. Conservative management is commonly accepted, according to the principle that "muscle injuries do heal conservatively." It follows the RICE protocol (rest, ice, compression, and elevation). Other therapies include the local application of heat and passive motion exercises. Drug therapy typically consists of nonsteroidal anti-inflammatory drugs (NSAIDs) and intramuscular corticosteroids.

Operative management is required only in selected patients, such as athletes with a large intramuscular hematoma, a complete strain of a muscle with no agonist muscles, or a partial strain when more than 50% of the muscle belly is damaged, or persisting extension pain (>6 months) in a previously injured muscle [8].

As current therapy does not seem to obtain complete restoration of preinjury status, new biological therapies could represent interesting and more effective strategies to manage muscle injuries. Biological therapies include cell therapy, tissue engineering, and the administration of growth factors with the goal of enhancing current therapies.

This paper provides an overview on current biological strategies for the management of patients with muscle injuries. The rationale behind these therapies and the best available evidence therapeutic options are reported.

2. Growth Factors

The healing process of the injured skeletal muscle is characterized by several bioactive molecules, including proinflammatory cytokines, transforming growth factor-beta (TGF-β) superfamily members, and angiogenic factors. For this reason, the growth factors and the cytokines represent a potential therapeutic option to improve the regeneration/repair process of injured skeletal muscles. These signaling molecules accelerate the regeneration of injured muscular tissue, providing a mitogenic stimulus activating myogenic precursor cells [9].

Each of these molecules shows specific biological activities. The transforming growth factor-beta (TGF-β) stimulates mesenchymal cell proliferation [10], promotes the proliferation of fibroblasts [11] and the biosynthesis of extracellular matrix, particularly type I collagen [12], regulates endothelial cell activity and angiogenesis [13], and inhibits satellite cell proliferation and differentiation [9]. Fibroblast growth factor (FGF) promotes proliferation of fibroblasts [14], stimulates satellite cells proliferation but inhibits their differentiation [15], and promotes the mitogenesis of mesenchymal cells [9]. Epidermal growth factor (EGF) stimulates fibroblasts migration and proliferation and regulates angiogenesis and extracellular matrix homeostasis [16]. The platelet-derived growth factor (PDGF) promotes the mitogenesis of mesenchymal cells and fibroblasts [17], induces proliferation of satellite cells, and inhibits the end stages of myoblast differentiation [18]. Vascular endothelial growth factor (VEGF) promotes endothelial cells mitogenesis and migration [19] and stimulates myoblast migration [20]. The neoangiogenesis plays a critical role in the healing process of muscle injuries. The new vessels sprout from the health tissue surrounding the lesion and provide the supply of oxygen, growth factor, and blood stem cell to enhance the regeneration process [21]. Thus, the restoration of vascular pattern in the injured area represents an early and necessary phase for regeneration and morphological and functional recovery of muscle tissue.

Based on the multitude of their biological effects, the clinical application of growth factors is affected by considerable side effects. An overexpression of growth factors such as TGF-β and FGF has been related to inhibition of myoblasts differentiation and muscle fiber regeneration [15]. In addition, growth factors explain their stimulatory effect on both muscle cells and fibroblasts. Particularly, TGF-β is one of the most important growth factors related to scar formation during healing, and it seems to drive the differentiation of myogenic cells into myofibroblastic cells. For this reason, muscle fiber regeneration and scar-tissue production can be considered two concomitant and competitive processes.

Also, the expression of growth factors is closely regulated by a large number of extracellular matrix (ECM) proteins, namely, the heparin sulfate proteoglycans and the small leucine-rich proteoglycans (SLRPs) [22, 23]. Several growth factors need to bind the heparan sulphate proteoglycans and the SLRPs to provide their biological effects. Thus, the application of growth factors to promote healing of the damaged muscle tissue should include the administration of these specific ECM molecules.

To date, available data from experimental settings are contradictory. Some authors did not report any beneficial effects by the administration of FGF-2 [24] or overexpression of skeletal muscle specific isoform of IGF-1 (mIGF-1) at the injured region [25]. FGF-2, IGF-1, and nerve growth factors can promote muscle healing process, increasing resistance to tensile loading when compared to untreated muscles [26, 27]. Moreover, mouse myoblasts transduced with the IGF-I gene increase their growth rate and enhance the contractile force production of skeletal muscle substitutes consisting of hydrogel and IGF-I engineered myoblasts [28].

A combination of growth factors can be used to regulate the different process of regeneration of muscle tissue and scar tissue production. Thus, the application of IGF-I combined with TGF-β allows to induce muscle regeneration, preventing the formation of a fibrous scar [29].

3. Platelet-Rich Plasma (PRP)

Platelet-rich plasma (PRP) therapy represents an interesting biological technique to provide tissue repair by inducing chemotactic, proliferative, and anabolic host cellular responses [30]. PRP is an autologous product consisting of bioactive agents derived from patients' own platelets [31–33]. Usually, PRP is administered by local injection of the PRP solution or the application of a PRP gel at the time of surgery.

Given the large amount of biological agents required for tissue repair, PRP could be an ideal biological autologous product providing a balanced combination of mediators able to improve the healing process. In clinical practice, the blood clot at the site of injury is replaced with a smaller volume of PRP solution or gel. The increased concentration of platelet at the site of lesion provides a higher concentration of healing bioactive factors than in physiological conditions. To date, PRP has been proposed for management of tendon [34–36], ligament [37, 38], muscle [39], nerve [40, 41], bone [42, 43], and joint injuries [44, 45].

The effectiveness of autologous conditioned serum (ACS) has been compared with Traumeel/Actovegin in a nonrandomized nonblinded pilot study (level III) on muscle strain injuries in professional sportsmen [39]. The ACS was obtained from whole blood, and it contained bioactive proteins including interleukin-1β (IL-1β), TNF-α, IL-7, fibroblast growth factor-2 (FGF-2), IL-1Ra, HGF, PDGF-AB, TGFβ1, and IGF-1. Traumeel is a homeopathic formulation containing both botanical and mineral ingredients in homeopathic concentrations. Actovegin is a deproteinized calf blood hemodialysate consisting of a physiological mix of amino acids. Although both treatments were safe, the ACS allowed to reduce the time to full recovery and the amount of edema and/or bleeding at MRI images.

These findings have been also confirmed in professional soccer players with muscle lesions varying for size and location [46]. Athletes were managed with activated pure PRP (P-PRP) injections. Full resumption of normal training activities was restored in half of the expected time compared to matched historical controls. The same leukocyte-free PRP preparation has been found effective to manage adductor longus strain in a professional bodybuilder [47].

ACS and PRP have been also evaluated in laboratory settings. ACS was compared with saline solution in a contusion injury model. ACS showed an earlier activation and/or recruitment of satellite cells, and an earlier fusion, with larger regenerating myofibers, compared with controls [48]. PRP increases proliferation of muscle cells, differentiation of satellite cells and synthesis of angiogenic factors in an in vitro setting [49]. PRP and leukocyte and platelet-rich plasma (L-PRP) have been also compared in a laboratory-controlled study using a muscle strain rat model. The authors demonstrated that PRP is more effective than L-PRP in terms of myogenesis enhancement and contractile function [50].

Although preliminary data are encouraging, there are some reasons of concern about PRP treatment. First of all, PRP could induce a fibrotic healing response in muscle tissues, by increasing local concentration of TGF. According to experimental data, TGF seems to be able to induce fibrosis in cultured muscle tissue [9]. Moreover, the effectiveness of PRP could be affected by leukocytes within the injected solution, because their enzymes (proteases and acid hydrolases) can damage muscle tissue [51].

Finally, several devices and systems are available for PRP preparation. Therefore, PRP products applied in several studies consist of a basic mixture of grow factors including different concentration of each single agent. Moreover, level I studies performed with adequate outcome measures and follow-up assessment are lacking.

To date, no PRP formulation has solid evidence of effectiveness to heal muscle injuries. Pilot clinical studies indicate that PRP therapies may enhance muscle repair after strain or contusion. Moreover, laboratory data indicate the ability of several growth factors to enhance myogenesis. However, at present, there is no evidence to recommend or discourage the adoption of PRP in clinical practice. Further research is required to standardize formulations (number of platelets and/or leukocytes) and administration regimens, including volume of injection and timing of treatment, to optimize PRP application for management of muscle injuries.

4. Cell Therapy

In the last decade, regenerative medicine and tissue engineering increased their role in management of musculoskeletal diseases. Transplantation of stem cells has been considered a new strategy to repair injured tissues [52–64]. Different areas of application have been explored, such as articular cartilage [65–68], bone [69–72], ligament, and tendon [73–77]. The expectations for future therapeutic strategies are great.

The idea of cell therapies for muscle regeneration has been developed from the observation that skeletal muscle has regenerative capacity [78–80]. Several studies have investigated the role of stem cells in muscle healing, showing their direct participation in tissue regeneration and their influence in healing modulation [12, 81, 82]. However, severe muscle injuries are characterized by concomitant activation of regenerative activities of the satellite cells and profibrotic activities of fibroblasts [83, 84].

The specific expression pattern of growth factors in the region of injury determines the dominant cell type in the wound healing process [12]. High levels of TGF-β3 are related to the activation of mesenchymal progenitor cells (MPCs) derived from traumatized muscle to promote wound healing after muscle injury [85]. On the other hand, high levels of TGF-β1 are related to activation of fibroblasts to produce disorganized extracellular matrix leading to fibrosis in the muscle tissue [81, 82]. The fibrotic tissue affects the ability of the satellite cells to repair the muscle tissue.

There are distinct subsets of myogenic cells. Muscle satellite cells (SCs) are localized under the basal lamina of muscle fibers [86]. They respond to regenerative stimuli by proliferating to form myoblasts which, in turn, differentiate and fuse in multinucleated myotubes [87, 88]. Their capability to renew and to produce differentiated progeny suggests that they are the adult stem-cell population of skeletal muscle [89]. They are also known as Pax7+ cells, based on their expression of the muscle-specific paired box (Pax) transcription factor Pax7 [90]. However, SCs consist of heterogeneous cell population, including Myf5+ cells (90%) and Myf5− cells (10%) [91]. The first of them are committed to the myogenic lineage because of expression of Myf5 which is an initiator of myogenic differentiation [92].

Other stem cells have been identified. They are both muscle specific, such as mesoangioblasts and pericytes, skeletal muscle precursors (SMPs), muscle stem cells (MuSCs), side-population (SP) cells, and PW1-cells, and nonspecific, such as embryonic stem (ES) cell, amniotic fluid stem (AFS) cells, mesenchymal stem cells (MSCs), and mesenchymal cells from bone marrow [93]. They are able to contribute to muscle regeneration with different myogenic potential, but their potential is still undefined. Satellite cells seem to be sufficient for the regenerative need of damaged adult skeletal muscle in vivo [94]. The MSCs present a great migration potential toward the areas of induced muscle degeneration and undergo myogenic differentiation, providing regeneration of muscle tissue. The MSC transduction with transcription factors, such as MyoD, has been also investigated to enhance their potential of myogenic differentiation [95].

The properties of the stem cells in the muscle have been analyzed using animal models of muscle dysfunctions and injuries. Improved muscular structure has been observed in mice used as Duchene Muscular Dystrophy models treated with stem cells [96–98]. Better muscle regeneration has been obtained by the use of muscle-derived stem cells (MDSCs) in models of induced skeletal muscle injury [99]. MDSCs provide an improvement of muscle healing because of their ability to recruit capillaries and nerves into the injured region [99]. They are also able to differentiate directly into endothelial cells and cell types with neuronal characteristics [100]. For these reasons, muscle regeneration seems to be more powerful with MDSCs application compared with satellite cells application.

A model of hindlimb ischemia, analogous to exercise-induced compartment syndrome, showed potential benefit of injections of marrow-derived stromal cells in term of perfusion, fibrosis development, and atrophy [101]. Results from ongoing studies on MDSCs implantation after musculoskeletal contusion are awaited [84].

The role of stem cells in musculoskeletal disease needs to be confirmed. Studies are still limited, and many questions are still unanswered. Several issues should be taken into account, such as safety and efficacy, immunogenicity, and biochemical factors involved in survival and differentiation of stem cells. Further research is needed to identify mechanisms involved in muscle regeneration to exactly understand the therapeutic potential of stem cells.

5. Scaffolds

Regenerative medicine is a multidisciplinary approach to produce living, functional substitutes for restoration, maintenance or improvement of the function of damaged tissue or organ. Tissue engineering is a specific approach included in regenerative medicine field. The tissue engineering consists of association of three main elements: cells, factors or stimuli, and biomaterials [102].

Musculoskeletal tissue engineering aims to obtain functional replacement of lost or damaged bone, cartilage, skeletal muscle, and tendon/ligament. In skeletal muscle injuries, tissue engineering represents a biological alternative for replacement of large tissue loss after severe damage.

Skeletal muscle tissue engineering could be performed by two different approaches: *in vitro* and *in vivo*. In *in vitro* tissue engineering, SCs from adult skeletal muscle are expanded and seeded on a 3D scaffold to produce a cell-biomaterial construct. After the differentiation of stem cells, the neotissue graft could be transplanted in the injured region. In *in vivo* tissue engineering, the isolated SCs are charged on a 3D scaffold carrier and promptly transplanted. Thus, the delivery of stem cells in the muscle lesion is obtained [93].

Efficient skeletal muscle regeneration is strongly related with features of biomaterials used to fabricate scaffold and with the regenerative potential of cells used for scaffold seeding. The source of cells used for scaffold seeding should be chosen based on the features of the damaged tissue. Cells can be autologous or allogeneic, including also stem cells where it is required.

The scaffold is a 3D-structure able to mimic the anatomical and biomechanical properties of the native tissue. The scaffold for muscle tissue engineering should be able to flex and stretch [103]. Moreover, they should be able to promote the alignment of myoblasts the assembly of myotubes. Nanostructured scaffolds are more efficient in promoting myotube assembly than microstructured scaffolds [104].

The biomaterials used to fabricate scaffold can be natural (like collagen) or synthetic (e.g., ceramics, polymers of lactic, and glycolic acid) and soluble or insoluble. Scaffold must have biocompatibility and biodegradability properties [105]. Biocompatibility is essential to prevent toxicity and immunogenicity biomaterial-related inducing the immune-response in the host muscle. Biodegradability allows gradual substitution of the scaffold by the newly formed muscle tissue. Moreover, the scaffold should integrate molecules or cells, providing a controlled delivery of growth factors, cytokines, plasmids, drugs, or other anabolic stimuli [106–109]. In skeletal muscle tissue engineering, biomaterials should support the myogenic process, providing a microenvironment which allows cell survival, proliferation and/or differentiation to repair, and/or regenerate the damaged tissue.

Both synthetic and natural scaffolds have been investigated for tissue engineering approaches to muscle regeneration. The polylactic-co-glycolic acid (PGA) is a synthetic biodegradable biomaterial showing appropriate rigidity and connection, appropriate for muscle tissue engineering. Constructs of myoblasts and polyglycolic acid meshes have been evaluated in a muscle regeneration rat model. Regenerate tissue-like structures have been found with aligned myoblasts along strands of polymer fibers. The PGA scaffold allowed the alignment of myoblasts and the assembly of myotubes, reproducing the organization of muscle fibres [110].

In the field of natural biodegradable biomaterials, different 3D scaffolds have been developed. Collagen scaffolds with parallel oriented pores have been used to reproduce the three-dimensional organization of skeletal muscle [111]. Permanent myogenic cells were infiltrated in these scaffolds and were cultured to induce their proliferation and differentiation [111]. The collagen scaffold with oriented pore structure showed the ability to induce skeletal muscle-like tissue regeneration with aligned multinucleated myotubes according to the orientation of pore structure [111]. In addition, cell-scaffold constructs were able to support mechanical forces generated in muscle tissue [111]. These results have been also found in an *in vitro* study in which a multilayered cultures of rat neonatal satellite cells in collagen 3D scaffolds were performed [112].

Fibrin is another natural biodegradable 3D scaffold used to obtain muscle regeneration. Three-dimensional fibrin matrix has been used as carrier to inject myoblasts in the injured muscle region of a rat model. The fibrin carrier induced no inflammatory reaction and allowed integration of myoblasts into host muscle fibers [113]. The fibrin matrix also allows to produce strained fibrin gel by applying continuous tensile strain to fibrin scaffold. The morphological features of strained fibrin gels induce the alignment of seeded myoblasts. Moreover, the aligned cells are parallel to the direction of the strain reproducing the organization of skeletal muscle tissue [114]. The fibrin matrix also allows the differentiation of myoblasts, cultured in a three-dimensional pattern, under electrical stimulation [115]. Finally, fibrin scaffolds have been also combined with adult human cells to regenerate muscle after large tissue loss in a mouse model with large defect of tibialis anterior muscle. Constructs of fibrin microthreads and adult human cells were used, showing the role of constructs in host tissue regeneration by forming skeletal muscle fibers, connective tissue, and PAX7 positive cells [116].

Another type of natural scaffold is a hyaluronan-based hydrogel that has been used to perform the delivery of either SCs or MPCs in a mice model. The construct SC-hydrogel showed more enhancement of regeneration process with a higher number of new myofibers than MPC-hydrogel or hydrogel alone. In the muscle receiving the SCs, there was a functional SC niche associated with neural and vascular networks [117].

The acellular muscle ECM has been also investigated in muscle tissue-engineering field. The acellular muscle scaffold was derived from the extensor digitorum longus muscle, and was injected with myoblasts. The constructs allowed cell survival and proliferation and showed longitudinal contractile force on electrical stimulation [118].

Each type of scaffold shows specific proprieties and peculiar advantages. The final goal of scaffold fabrication consists of promoting the proliferation of muscle stem cells, their differentiation, and parallel alignment to obtain a new skeletal muscle-like tissue. The application of scaffold for regeneration of muscle tissue could represents an interesting approach particularly in the major trauma with large loss of tissue. In the majority of muscle injuries, the role of scaffold remains unclear and maybe not as important as in bone or cartilage regeneration. In fact, the skeletal muscle is characterized by different layer of connective tissue, such as endomysium, perimysium, and epimysium, which seems to be able to drive the regeneration of new muscle fibers without the need of scaffold. Further studies are required to identify the best scaffold for skeletal muscle tissue engineering. However, the combination of available techniques could represent the right way to fabricate the ideal scaffold.

6. Conclusion

Skeletal muscle injuries are the most common injury in sport, occurring with direct and indirect mechanisms. Their effective management is a challenging issue in orthopaedic sport medicine because of the residual effects, such as severe long-term pain and physical disability. Skeletal muscle injuries cause time loss of activity and increased risk of recurrent injury. For these reasons, they constitute a health problem for athletes and an economic problem for clubs and sponsors.

In most of the instances, current therapy consists of conservative management including RICE protocol and administration of NSAIDs or intramuscular corticosteroids. However, current management of muscle injuries does

not often provide an optimal restore of preinjury status because of the fibrosis which occurs during the repair process of injured muscle. Experimental studies highlight the biological bases of muscle healing after contusion, strain, or laceration injury. This provides the rationale basis for new biological therapies, such as PRP and growth factors, cell-based therapy and tissue engineering. Biological strategies may well be more favourable to healing. Although PRP application is encouraged, reasons for concern persist in its use for muscle injury management, and its mechanism of action remains uncertain. Further research is required to allow a standardized and safety use of this product in clinical practice. Cell-based strategies have been investigated only in limited and inconsistent studies. The role of stem cells needs to be confirmed. Further research is required to identify mechanisms involved in muscle regeneration and in survival, proliferation, and differentiation of stem cells. Skeletal muscle tissue engineering represents a biological alternative for replacement of large tissue loss after severe damage, based on combination of adult or embryonic stem cells, factors or stimuli, and biomaterials. However, further studies are required to identify the best biomaterial to fabricate the ideal scaffold, the best cell source for scaffold seeding, and the role of growth factors and other stimuli used to functionalize the scaffold.

References

[1] J. M. Beiner and P. Jokl, "Muscle contusion injuries: current treatment options," *The Journal of the American Academy of Orthopaedic Surgeons*, vol. 9, no. 4, pp. 227–237, 2001.

[2] T. A. H. Järvinen, T. L. N. Järvinen, M. Kääriäinen et al., "Muscle injuries: optimising recovery," *Best Practice and Research: Clinical Rheumatology*, vol. 21, no. 2, pp. 317–331, 2007.

[3] T. A. H. Järvinen, T. L. N. Järvinen, M. Kääriäinen, H. Kalimo, and M. Järvinen, "Muscle injuries: biology and treatment," *American Journal of Sports Medicine*, vol. 33, no. 5, pp. 745–764, 2005.

[4] J. J. Crisco, P. Jokl, G. T. Heinen, M. D. Connell, and M. M. Panjabi, "A muscle contusion injury model. Biomechanics, physiology, and histology," *American Journal of Sports Medicine*, vol. 22, no. 5, pp. 702–710, 1994.

[5] W. E. Garrett, "Muscle strain injuries," *American Journal of Sports Medicine*, vol. 24, pp. S2–S8, 1996.

[6] J. L. Howard, N. G. H. Mohtadi, and J. P. Wiley, "Evaluation of outcomes in patients following surgical treatment of chronic exertional compartment syndrome in the leg," *Clinical Journal of Sport Medicine*, vol. 10, no. 3, pp. 176–184, 2000.

[7] J. Huard, Y. Li, and F. H. Fu, "Muscle injuries and repair: current trends in research," *The Journal of Bone and Joint Surgery*, vol. 84, pp. 822–832, 2002.

[8] T. A. H. Järvinen, T. L. N. Järvinen, M. Kääriäinen, H. Kalimo, and M. Järvinen, "Muscle injuries: biology and treatment," *American Journal of Sports Medicine*, vol. 33, no. 5, pp. 745–764, 2005.

[9] I. Husmann, L. Soulet, J. Gautron, I. Martelly, and D. Barritault, "Growth factors in skeletal muscle regeneration," *Cytokine and Growth Factor Reviews*, vol. 7, no. 3, pp. 249–258, 1996.

[10] A. B. Roberts, N. S. Roche, and M. B. Sporn, "Selective inhibition of the anchorage-independent growth of myc-transfected fibroblasts by retinoic acid," *Nature*, vol. 315, no. 6016, pp. 237–239, 1985.

[11] A. B. Roberts, M. A. Anzano, and L. M. Wakefield, "Type β transforming growth factor: a bifunctional regulator of cellular growth," *Proceedings of the National Academy of Sciences of the United States of America*, vol. 82, no. 1, pp. 119–123, 1985.

[12] Y. Li, W. Foster, B. M. Deasy et al., "Transforming growth Factor-β1 induces the differentiation of myogenic cells into fibrotic cells in injured skeletal muscle: a key event in muscle fibrogenesis," *American Journal of Pathology*, vol. 164, no. 3, pp. 1007–1019, 2004.

[13] M. B. Sporn, A. B. Roberts, L. M. Wakefield, and R. K. Assoian, "Transforming growth factor factor-β: biological function and chemical structure," *Science*, vol. 233, no. 4763, pp. 532–534, 1986.

[14] T. Floss, H. H. Arnold, and T. Braun, "A role for FGF-6 in skeletal muscle regeneration," *Genes and Development*, vol. 11, no. 16, pp. 2040–2051, 1997.

[15] R. E. Allen and L. K. Boxhorn, "Regulation of skeletal muscle satellite cell proliferation and differentiation by transforming growth factor-beta, insulin-like growth factor I, and fibroblast growth factor," *Journal of Cellular Physiology*, vol. 138, no. 2, pp. 311–315, 1989.

[16] B. M. Deasy, Z. Qu-Peterson, J. S. Greenberger, and J. Huard, "Mechanisms of muscle stem cell expansion with cytokines," *Stem Cells*, vol. 20, no. 1, pp. 50–60, 2002.

[17] L. T. Williams, "Signal transduction by the platelet-derived growth factor receptor," *Science*, vol. 243, no. 4898, pp. 1564–1570, 1989.

[18] R. Ross, E. W. Raines, and D. F. Bowen-Pope, "The biology of platelet-derived growth factor," *Cell*, vol. 46, no. 2, pp. 155–169, 1986.

[19] N. Ferrara, H. P. Gerber, and J. LeCouter, "The biology of VEGF and its receptors," *Nature Medicine*, vol. 9, no. 6, pp. 669–676, 2003.

[20] A. Germani, A. Di Carlo, A. Mangoni et al., "Vascular endothelial growth factor modulates skeletal myoblast function," *American Journal of Pathology*, vol. 163, no. 4, pp. 1417–1428, 2003.

[21] M. Jarvinen, "Healing of a crush injury in rat striated muscle. III. A micro angiographical study of the effect of early mobilization and immobilization on capillary ingrowth," *Acta Pathologica et Microbiologica Scandinavica Section A*, vol. 84, no. 1, pp. 85–94, 1976.

[22] J. C. Casar, C. Cabello-Verrugio, H. Olguin, R. Aldunate, N. C. Inestrosa, and E. Brandan, "Heparan sulfate proteoglycans are increased during skeletal muscle regeneration: requirement of syndecan-3 for successful fiber formation," *Journal of Cell Science*, vol. 117, no. 1, pp. 73–84, 2004.

[23] J. Villena and E. Brandan, "Dermatan sulfate exerts an enhanced growth factor response on skeletal muscle satellite cell proliferation and migration," *Journal of Cellular Physiology*, vol. 198, no. 2, pp. 169–178, 2004.

[24] C. A. Mitchell, J. K. McGeachie, and M. D. Grounds, "The exogenous administration of basic fibroblast growth factor to regenerating skeletal muscle in mice does not enhance the process of regeneration," *Growth Factors*, vol. 13, no. 1-2, pp. 37–55, 1996.

[25] T. Shavlakadze, M. Davies, J. D. White, and M. D. Grounds, "Early regeneration of whole skeletal muscle grafts is unaffected by overexpression of IGF-1 in MLC/mIGF-1 trans-genic mice," *Journal of Histochemistry and Cytochemistry*, vol. 52, no. 7, pp. 873–883, 2004.

[26] C. Kasemkijwattana, J. Menetrey, P. Bosch et al., "Use of growth factors to improve muscle healing after strain injury," *Clinical Orthopaedics and Related Research*, no. 370, pp. 272–285, 2000.

[27] J. Menetrey, C. Kasemkijwattana, C. S. Day et al., "Growth factors improve muscle healing in vivo," *Journal of Bone and Joint Surgery. Series B*, vol. 82, no. 1, pp. 131–137, 2000.

[28] M. Sato, A. Ito, Y. Kawabe, E. Nagamori, and M. Kamihira, "Enhanced contractile force generation by artificial skeletal muscle tissues using IGF-I gene-engineered myoblast cells," *Journal of Bioscience and Bioengineering*, vol. 112, no. 3, pp. 273–278, 2011.

[29] K. Sato, Y. Li, W. Foster et al., "Improvement of muscle healing through enhancement of muscle regeneration and prevention of fibrosis," *Muscle and Nerve*, vol. 28, no. 3, pp. 365–372, 2003.

[30] E. Anitua, M. Sánchez, A. T. Nurden, P. Nurden, G. Orive, and I. Andía, "New insights into and novel applications for platelet-rich fibrin therapies," *Trends in Biotechnology*, vol. 24, no. 5, pp. 227–234, 2006.

[31] F. Forriol, U. G. Longo, C. Concejo, P. Ripalda, N. Maffulli, and V. Denaro, "Platelet-rich plasma, rhOP-1 (rhBMP-7) and frozen rib allograft for the reconstruction of bony mandibular defects in sheep. A pilot experimental study," *Injury*, vol. 40, pp. S44–S49, 2009.

[32] I. Andia, M. Sanchez, and N. Maffulli, "Tendon healing and platelet-rich plasma therapies," *Expert Opinion on Biological Therapy*, vol. 10, no. 10, pp. 1415–1426, 2010.

[33] I. Andia, M. Sánchez, and N. Maffulli, "Platelet rich plasma therapies for sports muscle injuries: any evidence behind clinical practice?" *Expert Opinion on Biological Therapy*, vol. 11, no. 4, pp. 509–518, 2011.

[34] M. Sánchez, E. Anitua, J. Azofra, I. Andía, S. Padilla, and I. Mujika, "Comparison of surgically repaired Achilles tendon tears using platelet-rich fibrin matrices," *American Journal of Sports Medicine*, vol. 35, no. 2, pp. 245–251, 2007.

[35] G. Filardo, E. Kon, S. Della Villa, F. Vincentelli, P. M. Fornasari, and M. Marcacci, "Use of platelet-rich plasma for the treatment of refractory jumper's knee," *International Orthopaedics*, vol. 34, no. 6, pp. 909–915, 2010.

[36] J. C. Peerbooms, J. Sluimer, D. J. Bruijn, and T. Gosens, "Positive effect of an autologous platelet concentrate in lateral epicondylitis in a double-blind randomized controlled trial: platelet-rich plasma versus corticosteroid injection with a 1-year follow-up," *American Journal of Sports Medicine*, vol. 38, no. 2, pp. 255–262, 2010.

[37] J. R. Nin, G. M. Gasque, A. V. Azcárate, J. D. Beola, and M. H. Gonzalez, "Has platelet-rich plasma any role in anterior cruciate ligament allograft healing?" *Arthroscopy*, vol. 25, no. 11, pp. 1206–1213, 2009.

[38] M. Sánchez, E. Anitua, J. Azofra, R. Prado, F. Muruzabal, and I. Andia, "Ligamentization of tendon grafts treated with an endogenous preparation rich in growth factors: gross morphology and histology," *Arthroscopy*, vol. 26, no. 4, pp. 470–480, 2010.

[39] T. Wright-Carpenter, P. Klein, P. Schäferhoff, H. J. Appell, L. M. Mir, and P. Wehling, "Treatment of muscle injuries by local administration of autologous conditioned serum: a pilot study on sportsmen with muscle strains," *International Journal of Sports Medicine*, vol. 25, no. 8, pp. 588–593, 2004.

[40] W. Yu, J. Wang, and J. Yin, "Platelet-rich plasma: a promising product for treatment of peripheral nerve regeneration after

nerve injury," *International Journal of Neuroscience*, vol. 121, no. 4, pp. 176–180, 2011.

[41] H. H. Cho, S. Jang, S. C. Lee et al., "Effect of neural-induced mesenchymal stem cells and platelet-rich plasma on facial nerve regeneration in an acute nerve injury model," *Laryngoscope*, vol. 120, no. 5, pp. 907–913, 2010.

[42] M. Latalski, Y. A. Elbatrawy, A. M. Thabet, A. Gregosiewicz, T. Raganowicz, and M. Fatyga, "Enhancing bone healing during distraction osteogenesis with platelet-rich plasma," *Injury*, vol. 42, no. 8, pp. 821–824, 2011.

[43] S. R. Kanthan, G. Kavitha, S. Addi, D. S.K. Choon, and T. Kamarul, "Platelet-rich plasma (PRP) enhances bone healing in non-united critical-sized defects: a preliminary study involving rabbit models," *Injury*, vol. 42, no. 8, pp. 782–789, 2011.

[44] M. Sánchez, E. Anitua, J. Azofra, J. J. Aguirre, and I. Andia, "Intra-articular injection of an autologous preparation rich in growth factors for the treatment of knee OA: a retrospective cohort study," *Clinical and Experimental Rheumatology*, vol. 26, no. 5, pp. 910–913, 2008.

[45] E. Kon, R. Buda, G. Filardo et al., "Platelet-rich plasma: intra-articular knee injections produced favorable results on degenerative cartilage lesions," *Knee Surgery, Sports Traumatology, Arthroscopy*, vol. 18, no. 4, pp. 472–479, 2010.

[46] W. L. Loo, D. Y. H. Lee, and M. Y. H. Soon, "Plasma rich in growth factors to treat adductor longus tear," *Annals of the Academy of Medicine Singapore*, vol. 38, no. 8, pp. 733–734, 2009.

[47] W. L. Loo, D. Y. H. Lee, and M. Y. H. Soon, "Plasma rich in growth factors to treat adductor longus tear," *Annals of the Academy of Medicine Singapore*, vol. 38, no. 8, pp. 733–734, 2009.

[48] T. Wright-Carpenter, P. Opolon, H. J. Appell, H. Meijer, P. Wehling, and L. M. Mir, "Treatment of muscle injuries by local administration of autologous conditioned serum: animal experiments using a muscle contusion model," *International Journal of Sports Medicine*, vol. 25, no. 8, pp. 582–587, 2004.

[49] J. Alsousou, M. Thompson, P. Hulley, A. Noble, and K. Willett, "The biology of platelet-rich plasma and its application in trauma and orthopaedic surgery: a review of the literature," *Journal of Bone and Joint Surgery. Series B*, vol. 91, no. 8, pp. 987–996, 2009.

[50] B. H. Hamilton and T. M. Best, "Platelet-enriched plasma and muscle strain injuries: challenges imposed by the burden of proof," *Clinical Journal of Sport Medicine*, vol. 21, no. 1, pp. 31–36, 2011.

[51] J. W. Hammond, R. Y. Hinton, L. A. Curl, J. M. Muriel, and R. M. Lovering, "Use of autologous platelet-rich plasma to treat muscle strain injuries," *American Journal of Sports Medicine*, vol. 37, no. 6, pp. 1135–1142, 2009.

[52] E. A. Nauman and B. Deorosan, "The role of glucose, serum, and three-dimensional cell culture on the metabolism of bone marrow-derived mesenchymal stem cells," *Stem Cells International*, vol. 2011, Article ID 429187, 12 pages, 2011.

[53] S. Gavrilov, D. Marolt, N. C. Douglas et al., "Derivation of two new human embryonic stem cell lines from nonviable human embryos," *Stem Cells International*, vol. 2011, Article ID 765378, 9 pages, 2011.

[54] J. M. Gimble, B. A. Bunnell, L. Casteilla, J. S. Jung, and K. Yoshimura, "Phases I-III clinical trials using adult stem cells," *Stem Cells International*, vol. 2010, Article ID 604713, 2 pages, 2010.

[55] I. I. Katkov, N. G. Kan, F. Cimadamore, B. Nelson, E. Y. Snyder, and A. V. Terskikh, "DMSO-free programmed cryopreservation of fully dissociated and adherent human induced pluripotent stem cells," *Stem Cells International*, vol. 2011, Article ID 981606, 8 pages, 2011.

[56] C. Kelly, C. C. S. Flatt, and N. H. McClenaghan, "Stem cell-based approaches for the treatment of diabetes," *Stem Cells International*, vol. 2011, Article ID 424986, 8 pages, 2011.

[57] S.-J. Lu and E. A. Kimbrel, "Potential clinical applications for human pluripotent stem cell-derived blood components," *Stem Cells International*, vol. 2011, Article ID 273076, 11 pages, 2011.

[58] E Mansilla, V Díaz Aquino, D Zambón et al., "Could metabolic syndrome, lipodystrophy, and aging be mesenchymal stem cell exhaustion syndromes?" *Stem Cells International*, vol. 2011, Article ID 943216, 10 pages, 2011.

[59] R. T. Mitsuyasu, J. A. Zack, J. L. Macpherson, and G. P. Symonds, "Phase I/II clinical trials using gene-modified adult hematopoietic stem cells for HIV: lessons learnt," *Stem Cells International*, vol. 2011, Article ID 393698, 8 pages, 2011.

[60] H. Narimatsu, "Immune reactions following cord blood transplantations in adults," *Stem Cells International*, vol. 2011, Article ID 607569, 6 pages, 2011.

[61] A. D. Petropoulou and V. Rocha, "Risk factors and options to improve engraftment in unrelated cord blood transplantation," *Stem Cells International*, vol. 2011, Article ID 610514, 8 pages, 2011.

[62] C. Tekkatte, G. P. Gunasingh, K. M. Cherian, and K. Sankaranarayanan, ""Humanized" stem cell culture techniques: the animal serum controversy," *Stem Cells International*, vol. 2011, Article ID 504723, 14 pages, 2011.

[63] C. M. Teven, X. Liu, N. Hu et al., "Epigenetic regulation of mesenchymal stem cells: a focus on osteogenic and adipogenic differentiation," *Stem Cells International*, vol. 2011, Article ID 201371, 18 pages, 2011.

[64] T. J. Wyatt, S. L. Rossi, M. M. Siegenthaler et al., "Human motor neuron progenitor transplantation leads to endogenous neuronal sparing in 3 models of motor neuron loss," *Stem Cells International*, vol. 2011, Article ID 207231, 11 pages, 2011.

[65] F. H. Chen, K. T. Rousche, and R. S. Tuan, "Technology insight: adult stem cells in cartilage regeneration and tissue engineering," *Nature Clinical Practice Rheumatology*, vol. 2, no. 7, pp. 373–382, 2006.

[66] T. Matsumoto, S. Kubo, L. B. Meszaros et al., "The influence of sex on the chondrogenic potential of muscle-derived stem cells implications for cartilage regeneration and repair," *Arthritis and Rheumatism*, vol. 58, no. 12, pp. 3809–3819, 2008.

[67] R. Kuroda, A. Usas, S. Kubo et al., "Cartilage repair using bone morphogenetic protein 4 and muscle-derived stem cells," *Arthritis and Rheumatism*, vol. 54, no. 2, pp. 433–442, 2006.

[68] W. M. Jackson, A. B. Aragon, F. Djouad et al., "Mesenchymal progenitor cells derived from traumatized human muscle," *Journal of Tissue Engineering and Regenerative Medicine*, vol. 3, no. 2, pp. 129–138, 2009.

[69] J. Y. Lee, Z. Qu-Petersen, B. Cao et al., "Clonal isolation of muscle-derived cells capable of enhancing muscle regeneration and bone healing," *Journal of Cell Biology*, vol. 150, no. 5, pp. 1085–1099, 2000.

[70] H. Peng, V. Wright, A. Usas et al., "Synergistic enhancement of bone formation and healing by stem cell-expressed VEGF

and bone morphogenetic protein-4," *Journal of Clinical Investigation*, vol. 110, no. 6, pp. 751–759, 2002.

[71] V. J. Wright, H. Peng, A. Usas et al., "BMP4-expressing muscle-derived stem cells differentiate into osteogenic lineage and improve bone healing in immunocompetent mice," *Molecular Therapy*, vol. 6, no. 2, pp. 169–178, 2002.

[72] J. Huard, A. Usas, A. M. Ho, G. M. Cooper, A. Olshanski, and H. Peng, "Bone regeneration mediated by BMP4-expressing muscle-derived stem cells is affected by delivery system," *Tissue Engineering. Part A*, vol. 15, no. 2, pp. 285–293, 2009.

[73] Z. Ge, J. C. H. Goh, and E. H. Lee, "Selection of cell source for ligament tissue engineering," *Cell Transplantation*, vol. 14, no. 8, pp. 573–583, 2005.

[74] K. A. Hildebrand, F. Jia, and S. L. Y. Woo, "Response of donor and recipient cells after transplantation of cells to the ligament and tendon," *Microscopy Research and Technique*, vol. 58, no. 1, pp. 34–38, 2002.

[75] F. Van Eijk, D. B. F. Saris, J. Riesle et al., "Tissue engineering of ligaments: a comparison of bone marrow stromal cells, anterior cruciate ligament, and skin fibroblasts as cell source," *Tissue Engineering*, vol. 10, no. 5-6, pp. 893–903, 2004.

[76] N. Watanabe, S. L. Y. Woo, C. Papageorgiou, C. Celechovsky, and S. Takai, "Fate of donor bone marrow cells in medial collateral ligament after simulated autologous transplantation," *Microscopy Research and Technique*, vol. 58, no. 1, pp. 39–44, 2002.

[77] C. K. Kuo and R. S. Tuan, "Mechanoactive tenogenic differentiation of human mesenchymal stem cells," *Tissue Engineering. Part A*, vol. 14, no. 10, pp. 1615–1627, 2008.

[78] J. N. Walton and R. D. Adams, "The response of the normal, the denervated and the dystrophic muscle-cell to injury," *The Journal of Pathology and Bacteriology*, vol. 72, no. 1, pp. 273–298, 1956.

[79] W. E. LeGros Clark, "An experimental study of regeneration of mammalian striped muscle," *Journal of Anatomy*, vol. 80, pp. 24–36, 1946.

[80] S. Bintliff and B. E. Walker, "Radioautographic study of skeletal muscle regeneration," *American Journal of Anatomy*, vol. 106, no. 3, pp. 233–245, 1960.

[81] A. J. Cowin, T. M. Holmes, P. Brosnan, and M. W. J. Ferguson, "Expression of TGF-β and its receptors in murine fetal and adult dermal wounds," *European Journal of Dermatology*, vol. 11, no. 5, pp. 424–431, 2001.

[82] L. Lu, A. S. Saulis, W. R. Liu et al., "The temporal effects of anti-TGF-β1, 2, and 3 monoclonal antibody on wound healing and hypertrophic scar formation," *Journal of the American College of Surgeons*, vol. 201, no. 3, pp. 391–397, 2005.

[83] Y. Li and J. Huard, "Differentiation of muscle-derived cells into myofibroblasts in injured skeletal muscle," *American Journal of Pathology*, vol. 161, no. 3, pp. 895–907, 2002.

[84] A. J. Quintero, V. J. Wright, F. H. Fu, and J. Huard, "Stem cells for the treatment of skeletal muscle injury," *Clinics in Sports Medicine*, vol. 28, no. 1, pp. 1–11, 2009.

[85] W. M. Jackson, L. J. Nesti, and R. S. Tuan, "Potential therapeutic applications of muscle-derived mesenchymal stem and progenitor cells," *Expert Opinion on Biological Therapy*, vol. 10, no. 4, pp. 505–517, 2010.

[86] A. Mauro, "Satellite cell of skeletal muscle fibers," *The Journal of Biophysical and Biochemical Cytology*, vol. 9, pp. 493–495, 1961.

[87] J. E. Morgan and T. A. Partridge, "Muscle satellite cells," *International Journal of Biochemistry and Cell Biology*, vol. 35, no. 8, pp. 1151–1156, 2003.

[88] J. C. Sloper and T. A. Partridge, "Skeletal muscle: regeneration and transplantation studies," *British Medical Bulletin*, vol. 36, no. 2, pp. 153–158, 1980.

[89] A. J. Wagers and I. M. Conboy, "Cellular and molecular signatures of muscle regeneration: current concepts and controversies in adult myogenesis," *Cell*, vol. 122, no. 5, pp. 659–667, 2005.

[90] P. Seale, L. A. Sabourin, A. Girgis-Gabardo, A. Mansouri, P. Gruss, and M. A. Rudnicki, "Pax7 is required for the specification of myogenic satellite cells," *Cell*, vol. 102, no. 6, pp. 777–786, 2000.

[91] S. Kuang, K. Kuroda, F. Le Grand, and M. A. Rudnicki, "Asymmetric self-renewal and commitment of satellite stem cells in muscle," *Cell*, vol. 129, no. 5, pp. 999–1010, 2007.

[92] H. Weintraub, R. Davis, S. Tapscott et al., "The myoD gene family: nodal point during specification of the muscle cell lineage," *Science*, vol. 251, no. 4995, pp. 761–766, 1991.

[93] C. A. Rossi, M. Pozzobon, and P. De Coppi, "Advances in musculoskeletal tissue engineering: moving towards therapy," *Organogenesis*, vol. 6, no. 3, pp. 167–172, 2010.

[94] C. A. Collins, I. Olsen, P. S. Zammit et al., "Stem cell function, self-renewal, and behavioral heterogeneity of cells from the adult muscle satellite cell niche," *Cell*, vol. 122, no. 2, pp. 289–301, 2005.

[95] S. Goudenege, D. F. Pisani, B. Wdziekonski et al., "Enhancement of myogenic and muscle repair capacities of human adipose-derived stem cells with forced expression of MyoD," *Molecular Therapy*, vol. 17, no. 6, pp. 1064–1072, 2009.

[96] B. Cao, B. Zheng, R. J. Jankowski et al., "Muscle stem cells differentiate into haematopoietic lineages but retain myogenic potential," *Nature Cell Biology*, vol. 5, no. 7, pp. 640–646, 2003.

[97] Y. Torrente, J. P. Tremblay, F. Pisati et al., "Intraarterial injection of muscle-derived CD34$^+$Sca-1$^+$ stem cells restores dystrophin in mdx mice," *Journal of Cell Biology*, vol. 152, no. 2, pp. 335–348, 2001.

[98] E. Bachrach, A. L. Perez, Y. H. Choi et al., "Muscle engraftment of myogenic progenitor cells following intraarterial transplantation," *Muscle and Nerve*, vol. 34, no. 1, pp. 44–52, 2006.

[99] H. S. Bedair, T. Karthikeyan, A. Quintero, Y. Li, and J. Huard, "Angiotensin II receptor blockade administered after injury improves muscle regeneration and decreases fibrosis in normal skeletal muscle," *American Journal of Sports Medicine*, vol. 36, no. 8, pp. 1548–1554, 2008.

[100] Z. Qu-Petersen, B. Deasy, R. Jankowski et al., "Identification of a novel population of muscle stem cells in mice: potential for muscle regeneration," *Journal of Cell Biology*, vol. 157, no. 5, pp. 851–864, 2002.

[101] T. Kinnaird, E. Stabile, M. S. Burnett et al., "Local delivery of marrow-derived stromal cells augments collateral perfusion through paracrine mechanisms," *Circulation*, vol. 109, no. 12, pp. 1543–1549, 2004.

[102] R. Langer and J. P. Vacanti, "Tissue engineering," *Science*, vol. 260, no. 5110, pp. 920–926, 1993.

[103] L. A. Hidalgo-Bastida, J. J. A. Barry, N. M. Everitt et al., "Cell adhesion and mechanical properties of a flexible scaffold for cardiac tissue engineering," *Acta Biomaterialia*, vol. 3, no. 4, pp. 457–462, 2007.

[104] N. F. Huang, S. Patel, R. G. Thakar et al., "Myotube assembly on nanofibrous and micropatterned polymers," *Nano Letters*, vol. 6, no. 3, pp. 537–542, 2006.

[105] J. Tan and W. M. Saltzman, "Biomaterials with hierarchically defined micro- and nanoscale structure," *Biomaterials*, vol. 25, no. 17, pp. 3593–3601, 2004.

[106] R. R. Chen and D. J. Mooney, "Polymeric growth factor delivery strategies for tissue engineering," *Pharmaceutical Research*, vol. 20, no. 8, pp. 1103–1112, 2003.

[107] L. Y. Qiu and Y. H. Bae, "Polymer architecture and drug delivery," *Pharmaceutical Research*, vol. 23, no. 1, pp. 1–30, 2006.

[108] Y. C. Huang, K. Riddle, K. G. Rice, and D. J. Mooney, "Long-term in vivo gene expression via delivery of PEI-DNA condensates from porous polymer scaffolds," *Human Gene Therapy*, vol. 16, no. 5, pp. 609–617, 2005.

[109] E. E. Falco, M. O. Wang, J. A. Thompson et al., "Porous EH and EH-PEG scaffolds as gene delivery vehicles to skeletal muscle," *Pharmaceutical Research*, vol. 28, no. 6, pp. 1306–1316, 2011.

[110] A. K. Saxena, J. Makler, M. Benvenuto, G. H. Willital, and J. P. Vacanti, "Skeletal muscle tissue engineering using isolated myoblasts on synthetic biodegradable polymers: preliminary studies," *Tissue Engineering*, vol. 5, no. 6, pp. 525–531, 1999.

[111] V. Kroehne, I. Heschel, F. Schügner, D. Lasrich, J. W. Bartsch, and H. Jockusch, "Use of a novel collagen matrix with oriented pore structure for muscle cell differentiation in cell culture and in grafts," *Journal of Cellular and Molecular Medicine*, vol. 12, no. 5A, pp. 1640–1648, 2008.

[112] W. Yan, S. George, U. Fotadar et al., "Tissue engineering of skeletal muscle," *Tissue Engineering*, vol. 13, no. 11, pp. 2781–2790, 2007.

[113] J. P. Beier, J. Stern-Straeter, V. T. Foerster, U. Kneser, G. B. Stark, and A. D. Bach, "Tissue engineering of injectable muscle: three-dimensional myoblast-fibrin injection in the syngeneic rat animal model," *Plastic and Reconstructive Surgery*, vol. 118, no. 5, pp. 1113–1121, 2006.

[114] T. Matsumoto, J. I. Sasaki, E. Alsberg, H. Egusa, H. Yatani, and T. Sohmura, "Three-dimensional cell and tissue patterning in a strained fibrin gel system," *PLoS One*, vol. 2, no. 11, Article ID e1211, 2007.

[115] J. Stern-Straeter, A. D. Bach, L. Stangenberg et al., "Impact of electrical stimulation on three-dimensional myoblast cultures—a real-time RT-PCR study," *Journal of Cellular and Molecular Medicine*, vol. 9, no. 4, pp. 883–892, 2005.

[116] R. L. Page, C. M. Malcuit, L. Vilner et al., "Restoration of skeletal muscle defects with adult human cells delivered on fibrin microthreads," *Tissue Engineering Part A*. In press.

[117] C. A. Rossi, M. Flaibani, B. Blaauw et al., "In vivo tissue engineering of functional skeletal muscle by freshly isolated satellite cells embedded in a photopolymerizable hydrogel," *FASEB Journal*, vol. 25, no. 7, pp. 2296–2304, 2011.

[118] G. H. Borschel, R. G. Dennis, and W. M. Kuzon Jr., "Contractile skeletal muscle tissue-engineered on an acellular scaffold," *Plastic and Reconstructive Surgery*, vol. 113, no. 2, pp. 595–602, 2004.

17

Mesenchymal Stem Cells and Cardiovascular Disease: A Bench to Bedside Roadmap

Manuel Mazo, Miriam Araña, Beatriz Pelacho, and Felipe Prosper

Department of Hematology and Cell Therapy, Clínica Universidad de Navarra, Foundation for Applied Medical Research, University of Navarra, Avenida Pío XII 36, Pamplona, 31008 Navarra, Spain

Correspondence should be addressed to Felipe Prosper, fprosper@unav.es

Academic Editor: Wolfgang Wagner

In recent years, the incredible boost in stem cell research has kindled the expectations of both patients and physicians. Mesenchymal progenitors, owing to their availability, ease of manipulation, and therapeutic potential, have become one of the most attractive options for the treatment of a wide range of diseases, from cartilage defects to cardiac disorders. Moreover, their immunomodulatory capacity has opened up their allogenic use, consequently broadening the possibilities for their application. In this review, we will focus on their use in the therapy of myocardial infarction, looking at their characteristics, *in vitro* and *in vivo* mechanisms of action, as well as clinical trials.

1. Introduction

Although traditionally regarded as a health concern related particularly to the industrialized world, cardiovascular diseases are now the first cause of death worldwide [1], with myocardial infarction (MI) resulting in 12.8% of deaths. Aside from changes in ways of life associated with economic and social development, one of the main reasons is the fact that MI is an evolving disease. After the ischemic event, anaerobic conditions rapidly induce massive cell death, not only involving cardiomyocytes (CMs), but also vascular cells. Although the organism tries to exert a compensatory activity (reviewed in [2]) during the first stages of the disease and may even manage to partially restore functionality, the resulting scar is never repopulated, relentlessly leading the patient towards the setting of heart failure. Thus, though not conventionally regarded as such, cardiac disease is a degenerative affection in which lack of sufficient contractile and vascular cells leads to a decompensated neurohormonal microenvironment [3], which further impairs both organ function and cell survival.

Although the existence of stem cells has been a well-known fact for nearly half a century [4], it is in the last 15 years that the field has experienced a major boost. Their capacity for differentiation has made stem cells outstanding candidates for the treatment of degenerative diseases, substituting for cells lost during the course of the disorder. Consequently, cardiac diseases and MI have been the object of intense research [5]. Among the cell types studied, mesenchymal stem cells (MSCs) are strong candidates for success in the MI setting. In the following pages, we will discuss their capacities as well as pre- and clinical investigations in which these cells have been employed.

2. Origin, Types, and Characteristics

The studies by Friedenstein and colleagues are regarded as one of the first reports on MSC [4]. In these, the clonogenic potential of a population of bone marrow- (BM-) derived stromal cells, described as colony-forming unit fibroblasts, was examined. BM is indeed one of the best-known sources of progenitor cells, MSC being among them [6]. Although this is not entirely understood, BM-MSC are thought to act as supporters and nurturers of other cells within the marrow [7–9], possibly in a location close to blood vessels [10]. However, there is a relatively small population (0.01%–0.0001% of nucleated cells in human BM [11]), so MSC can be easily purified by plastic adherence and expanded after BM extraction. Similarly, but adding simple mechanical and enzymatic processing, a mixed cell population (called stromal vascular fraction, SVF) can be isolated from adipose depots, which, after *in vitro* culture and homogenization, gives rise to the mesenchymal progenitors from this tissue, also termed adipose-derived stem cells (ADSCs) [12]. Adipose tissue is regarded as a much richer source of progenitors, harboring 100 to 500 times the numbers seen in BM [13]. However, despite similarities in phenotype, differentiation, or growth kinetics, there are certain differences at a functional, genomic, and proteomic level [9, 14], suggesting a degree of higher commitment of BM-MSC to chondrogenic and osteogenic lineages than ADSC [15].

Adipose tissue and BM are the most widely researched sources of mesenchymal progenitors because they are easy to harvest, and owing to the relative abundance of progenitors and the lack of ethical concerns. Nevertheless, MSCs have been ubiquitously found in a variety of locations, as umbilical cord blood [16], dental pulp [17], menstrual blood [18], or heart [19], among others (reviewed in [20]). This wide variety of origins, methodologies, and acronyms prompted standardization in 2005 by the International Society for Cellular Therapy, which set the minimum requirements for MSC definition (Table 1). First, MSC must be plastic-adherent when maintained in standard culture conditions. Second, MSC must express CD105, CD73, and CD90, and lack expression of CD45, CD34, CD14 or CD11b, CD79a, or CD19 and HLA-DR surface molecules. Third, MSC must differentiate to osteoblasts, adipocytes, and chondroblasts *in vitro* [21]. Still, caution must be taken as some reports fail to meet these criteria, and MSC is often employed for "marrow stromal cell," "mesenchymal stromal cell" or "marrow stem cell." Accordingly, a clarification was published in which MSC was defined as "multipotent mesenchymal stromal Cells" [22], adding the supportive property to the required characteristics [23].

3. What Do MSCs Have to Offer to Cardiac Regeneration?

When considering the goal of cardiac tissue regeneration, the desired objective must encompass three objectives: (i) the production of a replacement myocardial mass, (ii) the formation of a functional vascular network to sustain it, and (iii) the returning of the impaired ventricle to its proper geometry. Cell therapy may theoretically affect those processes in two ways: either by direct differentiation of transplanted cells towards the desired lineages or by their production of molecules with therapeutic potential (Figure 1).

BM-MSC have shown their *in vitro* capacity to give rise to endothelial cells (ECs) [24, 25] and smooth muscle cells (SMCs) [24]. Cardiomyocyte differentiation has proved more problematic, as either demethylating agents have been employed [26], or it has been inefficient and incomplete [27, 28]. In contrast, the cardiac potential of ADSC is better documented *in vitro*, showing their capacity to give rise to CM, either by the use of DMSO [29] or CM extracts [30]. In addition, ADSC seems to harbor a progenitor subset

TABLE 1: Standardized requirements for MSC definition.

Multipotent mesenchymal stromal cells (MSE) properties
(i) Plastic adherence
(ii) Cell surface antigen expression profile
$\quad$ CD73$^+$, CD90$^+$, CD105$^+$, HLA-DR$^-$, CD11b$^-$, CD14$^-$,
$\quad$ CD19$^-$, CD34$^-$, CD45$^-$, CD79α^-
(iii) Multipotency
$\quad$ Chondroblast, Adipocyte, Osteoblast

characterized by the expression of Nkx2.5 and Mcl2v [31] and whose differentiation relies on the autocrine/paracrine activity of vascular endothelial growth factor (VEGF) [32]. SMC [33] and EC [34] have been obtained from adipose cells, yet a cautionary note must be struck, as some of these studies either rely on subpopulations of freshly isolated cells or culture them in differentiation-promoting medium before purifying the mesenchymal population [35, 36]. Finally, other mesenchymal progenitors have also been differentiated to CM or CM-like cells, such as menstrual blood-derived MSC [18] or umbilical cord blood MSC [37].

However, although it is extremely interesting, this differentiation potential must cope with two opposing factors. First, patients receiving stem cell therapy are severely diseased and usually elderly, two factors that have an outstanding impact on stem cell function. For instance, a decrease in the numbers and functionality of circulating endothelial progenitors is directly related to cardiovascular risks and smoking [38, 39] and age has also been shown to impair the angiogenic capacity of both ADSC [40] and BM-MSC [41]. Second, the small percentage of engrafted cells (see [42] for a review) coupled to the huge catastrophe caused by an MI (the loss in some cases of over 1 billion CM [43]) and the low rate of differentiation achieved even under *in vitro* controlled conditions makes the adding of such small number of cells a therapeutically inefficient approach.

Nevertheless, secretion of beneficial molecules has been demonstrated to be able to exert a positive effect, even when a few engrafted cells are left [44]. These molecules can induce a benefit either by increasing tissue perfusion, decreasing collagen deposition and fibrosis, enhancing host-cell survival, or attracting/regulating endogenous progenitors. Thus, Chen and coworkers compared the expression profile of BM-MSC and dermal fibroblasts [45], showing that mesenchymal progenitors secreted a higher amount of several molecules, including the potent proangiogenic cytokine VEGF or the chemotactic stromal derived factor-1 (SDF-1). Conditioned medium from BM-MSC induced the recruitment of EC and macrophages, and improved wound healing. Moreover, it has recently been shown that serum-deprived BM-MSC acquire EC features and increase the release of VEGF or hepatocyte growth factor (HGF), another potent angiogenic molecule [46], both of which have been reported to be secreted by ADSC [32, 47, 48]. Moreover, Dr. March's group demonstrated that ADSCs have a pericytic nature and are able to form and stabilize functional vascular networks when mixed with endothelial

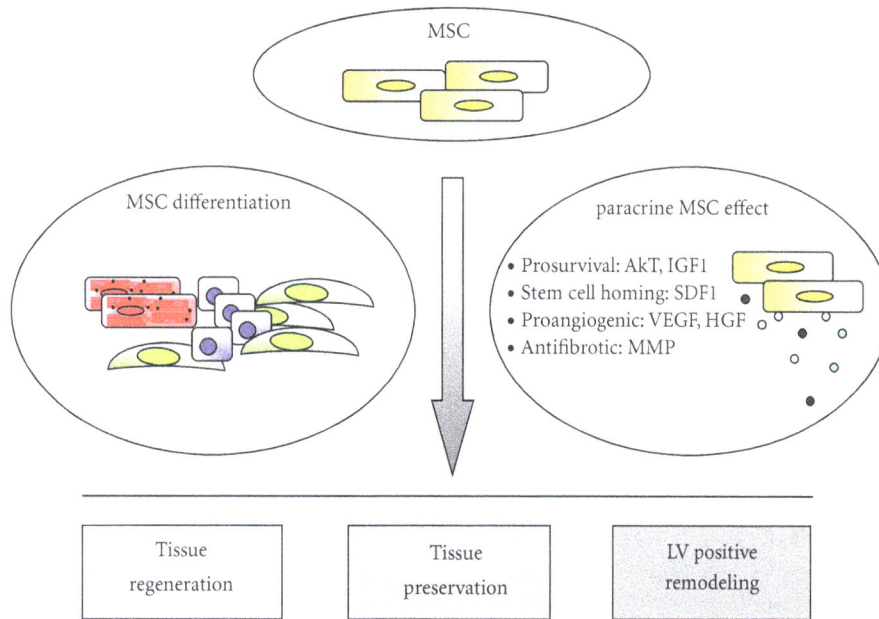

FIGURE 1: Main MSC actions on injured myocardium. Mesenchymal progenitors transplanted onto the ischemic myocardium are able to secrete a plethora of therapeutic molecules (paracrine activity) and even to differentiate towards (cardio-) vascular lineages, encouraging the healing of the damaged tissue, avoiding its transition to a scarred muscle, and regenerating the heart tissue mainly at the vascular level. Abbreviations: IGF-1: insulin-like growth factor-1; SDF-1: stromal derived factor-1; VEGF: vascular endothelial growth factor; HGF: hepatocyte growth factor; MMP: matrix metalloproteinase; LV: left ventricle.

progenitors [49]. Also, BM-MSC show a potent antifibrotic action, as their conditioned medium decreases cardiac fibroblast proliferation and expression of collagen types I and III [50, 51] and increases secretion of antifibrotic molecules such as matrix metalloproteinases (MMPs) 2, 9, and 14 [52]. These cells express five types of MMP (2, 13 and membrane type-MMP 1, 2, and 3) and are able to cross through type I collagen membranes [53], which theoretically would allow their trafficking across the infarction-derived scar. Likewise, ADSCs produce transforming growth factor- (TGF-) $\beta1$ [54], a potent regulator of fibrosis. Taken as a whole, these examples demonstrate that mesenchymal progenitors are potent paracrine mediators with a considerable capacity to impact infarct evolution.

One last noteworthy competence is the ability of BM-MSC and ADSC to modulate the immune response. Marrow-derived mesenchymal progenitors inhibit the proliferation of activated T cells and the formation of cytotoxic T cells [55], inducing an anti-inflammatory phenotype, which would allow their allogenic use and significantly broaden the scope of their applicability. However, Huang et al. reported that differentiation reduced their capacity of immunological escape [56], related to an increase of immunostimulatory molecules MHC-Ia and II and a decrease in the immuno-suppressive MHCIb. Along similar lines, McIntosh and coworkers reported that ADCS beyond passage one (and thus devoid of contaminating differentiated cells [57]) failed to elicit a response from allogenic T cells [58], but this attribute may be diminished under inflammatory stimuli, as shown *in vitro* [59].

Finally, since the onset of induced pluripotent stem cells (iPSCs) [60], mesenchymal cells have been investigated [61, 62] due to their relatively easy harvest and higher potency than other cell types (e.g., dermal fibroblasts), which show an increased efficiency, even in the absence of the oncogene c-Myc. Their supportive capacities have also made them good candidates to replace mouse cells as feeders [63, 64].

4. MSC in Animal Models of MI

However, in spite of all the positive characteristics of mesenchymal progenitors already depicted, their *in vivo* testing in animal models of the disease is compulsory. In this regard, three different settings can be found. First, the acute setting, in which cells are transplanted within hours of the MI. Here, the inflammatory microenvironment and the necrotic/apoptotic signals released from resident cells [65, 66] are the main opposing forces to the therapeutic activity of cells. Nevertheless, homing signals [67] and an antifibrotic milieu [68] may have a positive influence. Also, from a practical point of view, dealing with acute models offers the advantage of subjecting animals to only one surgery, as at the time of the MI (or minutes after it), the cells are applied, thus decreasing mortality and invasiveness. As a consequence, the majority of published reports use acute models [37, 69–84]. Most studies (with the exception of the two by van der Bogt and colleagues [74, 77]) have consistently demonstrated that the treatment induces a significant benefit for cardiac function, mainly through paracrine mechanisms that induce an increase in tissue perfusion and a decrease in the size of the scar and collagen content.

Similar results have been obtained in a second setting, the chronic one. Here, the repair processes that take place after ischemia have been completed, the scar has matured, and although a new network of blood vessels has been created, this is disorganized and inadequate [85, 86]. These facts impose a great burden upon cell survival. However, it must be taken into account that the generation of homogeneous populations as BM-MSC or ADSC needs weeks of *in vitro* culture, thus, unless used in the allogeneic setting, there is no possibility of the bedside translation of the use of mesenchymal progenitors in the acute setting. In spite of this difficulty, fewer reports deal with this issue [87–90]. Compared to results in the acute setting, mesenchymal cell therapy of chronically infarcted hearts has a positive effect upon organ contractility and histology.

As a third and intermediate position, the so-called subacute model represents a situation where angiogenic processes are still on course, either through endothelial progenitors [91] or macrophages [92], and the receding of inflammation plus the increase in fibrotic processes are also on course. As with chronic models, there are few reports in this setting [17, 18, 93, 94], but again the benefit and mechanisms appear to be consistent.

Nevertheless, analyzing in more depth the studies mentioned above, it is possible to find a fair amount of information on how mesenchymal progenitors behave when injected into the diseased heart has been gathered. Chen et al. showed that transplantation of BM-MSC into chronically infarcted rabbit hearts induced an increase in the concentration of SDF-1 that elicited the chemotaxis of host-derived BM progenitors (CD34+, CD117+, STRO1+) and was related to a functional benefit, a decrease in infarct size and improvement in tissue vascularization [89]. Li and coworkers demonstrated that the functional enhancement was accompanied by the augmented expression of the prosurvival gene Akt [95] whereas Mias and colleagues showed that the benefit upon contractility and remodeling *in vivo* was accompanied *in vitro* by a plethora of antifibrotic actions [52]. In a sheep model of MI, the group of Dr. Spinale monitored the evolution of MMP and their inhibitors, demonstrating a relationship with the number of transplanted cells [75]. Resembling their *in vitro* behavior, several publications have demonstrated the association between proangiogenic activity *in vitro* and secretion (either direct or host-derived) of angiogenic cytokines as VEGF, HGF, or insulin-like growth factor-1 (IGF-1), among others [17, 84, 93, 96, 97]. Whether these capacities are related to the claimed pericytic nature of these cells [10, 48, 49] remains to be resolved.

Immune modulation (reviewed in [98]) in theory provides the means for the allogenic use of MSCs and as an off-the-shelf product (expanded prior to the onset of the ischemia and applicable on demand). Two reports have compared the effects of allogenic versus syngenic injection of BM-MSC in rat model of MI, with conflicting results. Imanishi et al. [78] demonstrated that both autologous and allogeneic cells improved cardiac function 4 weeks after transplantation, remained in the damaged tissues, and did not stimulate rejection. Huang and coworkers conversely [56] followed animals for up to 6 months. Syngenic cells

stimulated cardiac recovery, but the effect of the allogenic treatment was transitory (significant 3 months after injection but not at 6) and BM-MSC disappeared earlier than their syngenic counterpart. However, this difference can be attributed to methodological discrepancies regarding time of transplantation (acute versus chronic resp.) or followup (1 versus 6 months). Equivalent and importantly, results from clinically relevant large animal models of MI in which allogenic cells have been employed have revealed either positive [99, 100] or no functional outcome [79]. In contrast, when autologous ADSC or BM-MSC are used [72, 83, 101, 102], reports have shown a robust and consistent functional recovery after cell transplantation. Thus, strict considerations about building up animal models must be taken into account.

5. Problems, Solutions

Despite all the optimism, stem cell therapy shows certain caveats that are amenable to improvement, namely, lack of substantial engraftment and cell persistence, high levels of death, and low *in vivo* differentiation capacity. Some approaches to try to remedy these problems have included the use of genetic manipulation and *in vitro* pretreatment of cells or biomaterials. In this sense, the CXCR4/SDF-1 axis has been greatly exploited. Ma et al. investigated the peak of cardiac SDF-1 expression [103] in rat MI, finding that injected cells at that time point (1 day postinfarction) increased cell engraftment and tissue angiogenesis. Cheng and coworkers transplanted BM-MSC engineered to overexpress the receptor CXCR4, strengthening cell homing to the injured tissue after tail vein injection [104]. The same group combined BM-MSC peripheral injection with administration of granulocyte colony-stimulating factor, which *in vitro* increased CXCR4 expression. However, although engraftment was increased, no effect of cardiac function was found [105]. Huang and associates demonstrated that overexpression of the chemokine receptor CCR1 but not CXCR2 was associated with improved survival and grafting in a mouse model of MI, which also restored functionality [106].

Cell survival in the infarcted myocardium is jeopardized by hypoxia, inflammation, or oxidative stress. Liu et al. engineered BM-MSC to overexpress angiogenin [107], which improved hypoxic resistance in culture and was translated into an increase in cell engraftment and functional and histological recovery induction. Cell overexpression of hemeoxygenase-1 through adenoviral transfection showed superior therapeutic capacity, mainly through protection from inflammation and apoptosis [108], whereas targeted Akt overproduction in MSC restored cardiac function 2 weeks after MI through paracrine actions, including protection from hypoxia-induced apoptosis, release of cytokines, and preservation of tissue metabolism [109–111]. Others have explored antioxidants, like Song et al. who published that reactive oxygen species (ROS) diminished BM-MSC adherence to the substrate, but when treated with an ROS scavenger (N-acetyl-L-cysteine), engraftment was improved and the increase in fibrosis and infarct size prevented [112].

Hsp20 overexpression also protected MSC from oxidative stress and improved their beneficial activities [97].

However, viral or genetic modification of cells implies certain risks that currently make it difficult for a devised therapy to reach the bedside. Bioengineering uses biocompatible materials to improve or direct cell therapy and either synthetic or naturally derived systems have been employed. Jin and coworkers seeded BM-MSC on poly(lactide-co-1-caprolactone) patches which when applied on a rat cryoinjury model were able to improve cardiac function and decrease infarct size [113]. Porcine small intestine submucosa, a decellularized substrate, has been employed to treat a rabbit model of chronic MI, showing a significant benefit upon contractility and histology, as well as cell migration towards the injured tissue [114]. The cell sheet technology allows increasing thickness through stacking of constructs, as shown by Chen et al. [115], where its transplantation in a rat syngenic model of cardiac ischemia improved cardiac function as well as paracrine secretion of therapeutic molecules by grafted cells. Dr. Mori's group compared the transplantation of a cell sheet seeded with ADSC versus fibroblasts, showing the superior effect of the mesenchymal progenitors [116]. Recently, autologous ADSC were transplanted along with allogenic ESC-derived CD15$^+$ cardiac progenitors in a monkey model of infarction, demonstrating the safety of the procedure, although the functional outcome was not analyzed [117].

Finally, a word of caution must be added. Animal models of the disease are a powerful tool to explore the feasibility of a certain therapy, as MSC treatment of MI, but despite positive and reproducible results, rodent and even large animal models are just oversimplifications of the more complex setting of the human disease. As above stated, animals where cell therapy is applied are not elderly, nor severely diseased, thus making any result, even if tremendously positive, just a clue or hint before proceeding to the final application to patients, where the real safety and effectiveness can be assessed.

6. Mesenchymal Progenitors and Clinical Application

Several clinical trials have been performed with autologous BM-MSC, proving their safety when transplanted in patients with either acute or chronic myocardial infarction [118–120]. Moreover, the first clinical trial designed as a randomized study showed an improvement in the cardiac function 3 months after BM-MSC intracoronary infusion in patients with acute MI [120]. In view of the encouraging results of the previous clinical trials, new phase-I/II studies have been initiated, including the transendocardial autologous cells (hMSC or hBMC) in Ischemic Heart Failure Trial (TAC-HFT; http://www.clinicaltrials.org/NCT00768066/), the Prospective Randomised study Of MSC THErapy in patients Undergoing cardiac Surgery (PROMETHEUS) trial (http://www.clinicaltrials.org/NCT00587990/), and the Percutaneous Stem Cell Injection Delivery Effects on Neomyogenesis (POSEIDON) pilot study

(http://www.clinicaltrials.org/NCT01087996/) [121], among others.

BM-MSCs from allogeneic origin have been tested as an off-the-shelf cell product. The first phase-I, randomized, double-blind, placebo-controlled, dose-escalation study was performed in 53 patients with acute MI, who intravenously received one of three doses of BM-MSCs (0.5, 1.6 or 5.0 × 10^6 BM-MSC/Kg body weight) derived from a single cell donor (Prochymal; Osiris therapeutics, Inc.) or placebo [122]. Safety of the procedure was proven, showing fewer episodes of ventricular tachycardia and even a better lung function in the cell-treated group. Also, renal, hepatic, and hematologic laboratory indexes were similar in the two groups and no patient developed tumors. Importantly, a significant increase was detected in the ejection fraction (EF) of the treated patients. In a magnetic resonance imaging substudy, cell treatment, but not placebo, increased left ventricular ejection fraction and led to a reversal of adverse remodeling after 6 months of treatment. Now, a phase-II multicentre trial of ProchymalTM has been started (http://www.clinicaltrials.org/NCT00877903/).

Furthermore, BM-MSC safety has been tested in patients with moderate-to-severe chronic heart failure in a phase-II, randomized, single-blind, placebo-controlled, dose-escalation, multicenter study. In this clinical trial, the patients received an endoventricular injection of an allogeneic BM-MSC product (Revascor, Mesoblast Ltd.) along the infarct border zone and no procedure-related complications were reported. Analysis of the data obtained after 6 months of followup (http://www.mesoblast.com/newsroom/asx-announcements/archives/) showed a significant decrease in the number of patients who developed any severe or major adverse cardiac event, such as composite of cardiac death, heart attack, or need for coronary revascularization procedures. Moreover, the first cohort in the study ($n = 20$ patients), which received the low dose of the cell treatment, showed a significantly greater increase in the EF when compared with the control group [123].

On the other hand, regarding other sources of MSC such as adipose tissue, no clinical trials have been initiated yet, despite the fact that the beneficial potential of ADSC has been preclinically demonstrated [83]. Until now, only the noncultured adipose stromal vascular fraction is being tested at the clinical level. The first study, a double-blind, placebo-controlled trial named APOLLO (http://www.clinicaltrials.org/NCT00442806/; [124]) where AMI patients received autologous adipose derived stem cells by intracoronary infusion, was proven safe. Now, a phase II/III ADVANCE trial has been initiated to evaluate their efficacy (http://www.clinicaltrials.org/NCT01216995/).

In general, the results obtained from the many clinical trials performed, either with MSC or other stem cell populations (mainly BM-derived cells and skeletal myoblasts), have taught us several important lessons that will help to design and interpret the following clinical trials. (i) Cell treatment is not equally efficacious in all the patients. In general, it seems that the worse the heart damage (meaning severely decreased postrevascularization LVEF or high degree of infarct transmurality), the better the benefit induced by the transplanted cells seems to be [125–127]. (ii) Cell dose and timing for treatment are critical. Thus, a meta-analysis of the results obtained in the most relevant clinical trials performed in acute MI patients treated with BM cells has shown a significantly greater effect in those patients that received high cell doses (10^8 cells). Also, the same study showed a greater beneficial effect when cells are infused during the first week after the infarct [128]. (iii) Autologous treatment is not necessarily the best. Until now, most of the clinical studies have been designed for autologous cell application in order to avoid the immunorejection of the transplanted cells. However, it has to be borne in mind that stem cells derived from aged patients with risk of atherosclerosis or other diseases might be defective, and thereby, treatment with them might not be as efficacious as with cells derived from young healthy donors [129–131]. In that sense, the use of MSC, which present immunomodulatory properties [132], could be of great relevance. Thus, advantages of allogeneic MSC treatment would be that, together with the putative greater paracrine effect that allogeneic cells derived from a healthy donor could exert, a fully tested clinical grade ready to use allogeneic cell product could be available for any patient. Importantly, patients with acute MI could also be eligible for such treatment. Furthermore, the logistical complexity and manufacturing costs that autologous cell preparation implies would be significantly reduced by the allogeneic application. However, caution should be taken when taking into consideration the issues related to their immune privilege explained above.

Thus, although it is mandatory to better understand the mechanisms involved in the MSC phenotype switch and to elucidate how this could affect the cells' potential benefit, it has to be considered that, in any case, because MSC would not differentiate towards cardiovascular cells and would act as a paracrine factor source [111], their permanent presence in the heart might not be necessary for therapeutic purposes. In that case, a temporarily action should be sufficient for exerting their benefit. Phase-II clinical trials are currently assessing the efficacy of the allogeneic MSC treatment, together with the long-term safety. If allogeneicity of the cells diminishes their effectiveness, several options could be considered, like temporal patient immunosuppression and/or donor-recipient HLA-II mismatch minimizing. As a consequence, the increase in the rate of engraftment of transplanted cells is so far one of the main challenges. As already indicated, the use of scaffolds could improve this factor. Interestingly, a clinical trial has been performed in 15 patients with chronic MI who were treated with a collagen scaffold previously seeded with bone marrow mononuclear cells [133]. The cellularized patch was implanted onto the pericardium and no adverse events were reported, showing the feasibility and safety of the treatment. Furthermore, a limiting effect in ventricular wall remodeling and an improved diastolic function were detected. These positive results will probably promote new larger randomized controlled trials, where mesenchymal and other stem cell populations might be tested in combination with scaffolds, thus leading to a further step in the therapeutic use of stem cells.

7. Conclusion

Mesenchymal cells have raised substantial interest in recent years due to their potential and versatility. Although we are only now starting to understand the mechanisms by which they repair or induce the repair of damaged organs, their pleiotropic activity and the technical ease of manipulation makes them good candidates for the treatment of the MI. Though waiting for randomized, double-blinded, placebo-controlled clinical trials in which large cohorts of patients could participate, the available data demonstrates the safety of the therapy and points towards a positive effect, further encouraging new investigations. The addition of the latest improvements in the field, including *in vitro* conditioning and bioengineering, will surely suppose a further step towards finding an optimized treatment. However, certain issues, mainly immunomodulatory capacity and allogenic use, need to be better understood.

Acknowledgments

This work was supported by grants to FP (FP7 INELPY, Instituto de Salud Carlos III (ISCIII-RETIC RD06/0014 (FIS)) and Ministero de Ciencia e Innovación Programa de Internacionalización CARDIOBIO) and BP (Instituto de Salud Carlos III (PI10/01621 and CP09/00333 (FIS)).

References

[1] World Health Organization, *World Health Statistics 2008*, 2008.

[2] M. Mazo, B. Pelacho, and F. Prósper, "Stem cell therapy for chronic myocardial infarction," *Journal of Cardiovascular Translational Research*, vol. 3, no. 2, pp. 79–88, 2010.

[3] N. G. Frangogiannis, "Chemokines in the ischemic myocardium: from inflammation to fibrosis," *Inflammation Research*, vol. 53, no. 11, pp. 585–595, 2004.

[4] A. J. Friedenstein, K. V. Petrakova, A. I. Kurolesova, and G. P. Frolova, "Heterotopic of bone marrow. Analysis of precursor cells for osteogenic and hematopoietic tissues," *Transplantation*, vol. 6, no. 2, pp. 230–247, 1968.

[5] B. Pelacho and F. Prosper, "Stem cells and cardiac disease: where are we going?" *Current Stem Cell Research & Therapy*, vol. 3, no. 4, pp. 265–276, 2008.

[6] C. Clavel and C. M. Verfaillie, "Bone-marrow-derived cells and heart repair," *Current Opinion in Organ Transplantation*, vol. 13, no. 1, pp. 36–43, 2008.

[7] T. Walenda, S. Bork, P. Horn et al., "Co-culture with mesenchymal stromal cells increases proliferation and maintenance of haematopoietic progenitor cells," *Journal of Cellular and Molecular Medicine*, vol. 14, no. 1-2, pp. 337–350, 2010.

[8] D. L. Jones and A. J. Wagers, "No place like home: anatomy and function of the stem cell niche," *Nature Reviews Molecular Cell Biology*, vol. 9, no. 1, pp. 11–21, 2008.

[9] W. Wagner, C. Roderburg, F. Wein et al., "Molecular and secretory profiles of human mesenchymal stromal cells and their abilities to maintain primitive hematopoietic progenitors," *Stem Cells*, vol. 25, no. 10, pp. 2638–2647, 2007.

[10] X. Cai, Y. Lin, C. C. Friedrich et al., "Bone marrow derived pluripotent cells are pericytes which contribute to vascularization," *Stem Cell Reviews and Reports*, vol. 5, no. 4, pp. 437–445, 2010.

[11] M. F. Pittenger, A. M. Mackay, S. C. Beck et al., "Multilineage potential of adult human mesenchymal stem cells," *Science*, vol. 284, no. 5411, pp. 143–147, 1999.

[12] M. Mazo, J. J. Gavira, B. Pelacho, and F. Prosper, "Adipose-derived stem cells for myocardial infarction," *Journal of Cardiovascular Translational Research*, vol. 4, no. 2, pp. 145–153, 2011.

[13] L. Casteilla, V. Planat-Benard, P. Laharrague, and B. Cousin, "Adipose-derived stromal cells: their identity and uses in clinical trials, an update," *World Journal of Stem Cells*, vol. 3, pp. 25–33, 2011.

[14] S. Kern, H. Eichler, J. Stoeve, H. Kluter, and K. Bieback, "Comparative analysis of mesenchymal stem cells from bone marrow, umbilical cord blood, or adipose tissue," *Stem Cells*, vol. 24, no. 5, pp. 1294–1301, 2006.

[15] J. M. Gimble, A. J. Katz, and B. A. Bunnell, "Adipose-derived stem cells for regenerative medicine," *Circulation Research*, vol. 100, no. 9, pp. 1249–1260, 2007.

[16] S. E. Yang, C. W. Ha, M. H. Jung et al., "Mesenchymal stem/progenitor cells developed in cultures from UC blood," *Cytotherapy*, vol. 6, no. 5, pp. 476–486, 2004.

[17] C. Gandia, A. N.A. Armiñan, J. M. García-Verdugo et al., "Human dental pulp stem cells improve left ventricular function, induce angiogenesis, and reduce infarct size in rats with acute myocardial infarction," *Stem Cells*, vol. 26, no. 3, pp. 638–645, 2008.

[18] N. Hida, N. Nishiyama, S. Miyoshi et al., "Novel cardiac precursor-like cells from human menstrual blood-derived mesenchymal cells," *Stem Cells*, vol. 26, no. 7, pp. 1695–1704, 2008.

[19] S. Carlson, J. Trial, C. Soeller, and M. L. Entman, "Cardiac mesenchymal stem cells contribute to scar formation after myocardial infarction," *Cardiovascular Research*, vol. 91, no. 1, pp. 99–107, 2011.

[20] D. C. Ding, W. C. Shyu, and S. Z. Lin, "Mesenchymal stem cells," *Cell Transplant*, vol. 20, pp. 5–14, 2011.

[21] M. Dominici, K. Le Blanc, I. Mueller et al., "Minimal criteria for defining multipotent mesenchymal stromal cells. The International Society for Cellular Therapy position statement," *Cytotherapy*, vol. 8, no. 4, pp. 315–317, 2006.

[22] E. M. Horwitz, K. Le Blanc, M. Dominici et al., "Clarification of the nomenclature for MSC: the international society for cellular therapy position statement," *Cytotherapy*, vol. 7, no. 5, pp. 393–395, 2005.

[23] B. Sacchetti, A. Funari, S. Michienzi et al., "Self-renewing osteoprogenitors in bone marrow sinusoids can organize a hematopoietic microenvironment," *Cell*, vol. 131, no. 2, pp. 324–336, 2007.

[24] T. P. Lozito, J. M. Taboas, C. K. Kuo, and R. S. Tuan, "Mesenchymal stem cell modification of endothelial matrix regulates their vascular differentiation," *Journal of Cellular Biochemistry*, vol. 107, no. 4, pp. 706–713, 2009.

[25] J. W. Liu, S. Dunoyer-Geindre, V. Serre-Beinier et al., "Characterization of endothelial-like cells derived from human mesenchymal stem cells," *Journal of Thrombosis and Haemostasis*, vol. 5, no. 4, pp. 826–834, 2007.

[26] W. Xu, X. Zhang, H. Qian et al., "Mesenchymal stem cells from adult human bone marrow differentiate into a cardiomyocyte phenotype in vitro," *Experimental Biology and Medicine*, vol. 229, no. 7, pp. 623–631, 2004.

[27] X. Yan, A. Lv, Y. Xing et al., "Inhibition of p53-p21 pathway promotes the differentiation of rat bone marrow mesenchymal stem cells into cardiomyocytes," *Molecular and Cellular Biochemistry*, vol. 354, no. 1-2, pp. 21–28, 2011.

[28] A. Armiñán, C. Gandía, J. M. García-Verdugo et al., "Cardiac transcription factors driven lineage-specification of adult stem cells," *Journal of Cardiovascular Translational Research*, vol. 3, no. 1, pp. 61–65, 2010.

[29] A. van Dijk, H. W. M. Niessen, B. Zandieh Doulabi, F. C. Visser, and F. J. Van Milligen, "Differentiation of human adipose-derived stem cells towards cardiomyocytes is facilitated by laminin," *Cell and Tissue Research*, vol. 334, no. 3, pp. 457–467, 2008.

[30] K. G. Gaustad, A. C. Boquest, B. E. Anderson, A. M. Gerdes, and P. Collas, "Differentiation of human adipose tissue stem cells using extracts of rat cardiomyocytes," *Biochemical and Biophysical Research Communications*, vol. 314, no. 2, pp. 420–427, 2004.

[31] X. Bai, K. Pinkernell, Y. H. Song, C. Nabzdyk, J. Reiser, and E. Alt, "Genetically selected stem cells from human adipose tissue express cardiac markers," *Biochemical and Biophysical Research Communications*, vol. 353, no. 3, pp. 665–671, 2007.

[32] Y. H. Song, S. Gehmert, S. Sadat et al., "VEGF is critical for spontaneous differentiation of stem cells into cardiomyocytes," *Biochemical and Biophysical Research Communications*, vol. 354, no. 4, pp. 999–1003, 2007.

[33] Y. M. Kim, E. S. Jeon, M. R. Kim, S. K. Jho, S. W. Ryu, and J. H. Kim, "Angiotensin II-induced differentiation of adipose tissue-derived mesenchymal stem cells to smooth muscle-like cells," *International Journal of Biochemistry and Cell Biology*, vol. 40, no. 11, pp. 2482–2491, 2008.

[34] V. Planat-Benard, J. S. Silvestre, B. Cousin et al., "Plasticity of human adipose lineage cells toward endothelial cells: physiological and therapeutic perspectives," *Circulation*, vol. 109, no. 5, pp. 656–663, 2004.

[35] L. J. Fischer, S. McIlhenny, T. Tulenko et al., "Endothelial differentiation of adipose-derived stem cells: effects of endothelial cell growth supplement and shear force," *Journal of Surgical Research*, vol. 152, no. 1, pp. 157–166, 2009.

[36] C. Sengenès, A. Miranville, M. Maumus, S. De Barros, R. Busse, and A. Bouloumié, "Chemotaxis and differentiation of human adipose tissue CD34 +/CD31- progenitor cells: role of stromal derived factor-1 released by adipose tissue capillary endothelial cells," *Stem Cells*, vol. 25, no. 9, pp. 2269–2276, 2007.

[37] S. A. Chang, J. L. Eun, H. J. Kang et al., "Impact of myocardial infarct proteins and oscillating pressure on the differentiation of mesenchymal stem cells: effect of acute myocardial infarction on stem cell differentiation," *Stem Cells*, vol. 26, no. 7, pp. 1901–1912, 2008.

[38] T. Kondo, M. Hayashi, K. Takeshita et al., "Smoking cessation rapidly increases circulating progenitor cells in peripheral blood in chronic smokers," *Arteriosclerosis, Thrombosis, and Vascular Biology*, vol. 24, no. 8, pp. 1442–1447, 2004.

[39] M. Vasa, S. Fichtlscherer, A. Aicher et al., "Number and migratory activity of circulating endothelial progenitor cells inversely correlate with risk factors for coronary artery disease," *Circulation research*, vol. 89, no. 1, pp. E1–7, 2001.

[40] R. Madonna, F. V. Renna, C. Cellini et al., "Age-dependent impairment of number and angiogenic potential of adipose tissue-derived progenitor cells," *European Journal of Clinical Investigation*, vol. 41, no. 2, pp. 126–133, 2011.

[41] H. Liang, H. Hou, W. Yi, G. Yang, C. Gu, W. B. Lau et al., "Increased expression of pigment epithelium-derived factor in aged mesenchymal stem cells impairs their therapeutic efficacy for attenuating myocardial infarction injury," *European Heart Journal*, In press.

[42] H. K. Haider and M. Ashraf, "Strategies to promote donor cell survival: combining preconditioning approach with stem cell transplantation," *Journal of Molecular and Cellular Cardiology*, vol. 45, no. 4, pp. 554–566, 2008.

[43] T. E. Robey, M. K. Saiget, H. Reinecke, and C. E. Murry, "Systems approaches to preventing transplanted cell death in cardiac repair," *Journal of Molecular and Cellular Cardiology*, vol. 45, no. 4, pp. 567–581, 2008.

[44] P. W. M. Fedak, "Paracrine effects of cell transplantation: modifying ventricular remodeling in the failing heart," *Seminars in Thoracic and Cardiovascular Surgery*, vol. 20, no. 2, pp. 87–93, 2008.

[45] L. Chen, E. E. Tredget, P. Y. G. Wu, Y. Wu, and Y. Wu, "Paracrine factors of mesenchymal stem cells recruit macrophages and endothelial lineage cells and enhance wound healing," *PLoS ONE*, vol. 3, no. 4, Article ID e1886, 2008.

[46] A. Oskowitz, H. McFerrin, M. Gutschow, M. L. Carter, and R. Pochampally, "Serum-deprived human multipotent mesenchymal stromal cells (MSCs) are highly angiogenic," *Stem Cell Research*, vol. 6, no. 3, pp. 215–225, 2011.

[47] G. E. Kilroy, S. J. Foster, X. Wu et al., "Cytokine profile of human adipose-derived stem cells: expression of angiogenic, hematopoietic, and pro-inflammatory factors," *Journal of Cellular Physiology*, vol. 212, no. 3, pp. 702–709, 2007.

[48] D. O. Traktuev, S. Merfeld-Clauss, J. Li et al., "A population of multipotent CD34-positive adipose stromal cells share pericyte and mesenchymal surface markers, reside in a periendothelial location, and stabilize endothelial networks," *Circulation Research*, vol. 102, no. 1, pp. 77–85, 2008.

[49] D. O. Traktuev, D. N. Prater, S. Merfeld-Clauss et al., "Robust functional vascular network formation in vivo by cooperation of adipose progenitor and endothelial cells," *Circulation Research*, vol. 104, no. 12, pp. 1410–1420, 2009.

[50] L. Li, S. Zhang, Y. Zhang, B. Yu, Y. Xu, and Z. Guan, "Paracrine action mediate the antifibrotic effect of transplanted mesenchymal stem cells in a rat model of global heart failure," *Molecular Biology Reports*, vol. 36, no. 4, pp. 725–731, 2009.

[51] S. Ohnishi, H. Sumiyoshi, S. Kitamura, and N. Nagaya, "Mesenchymal stem cells attenuate cardiac fibroblast proliferation and collagen synthesis through paracrine actions," *FEBS Letters*, vol. 581, no. 21, pp. 3961–3966, 2007.

[52] C. Mias, O. Lairez, E. Trouche et al., "Mesenchymal stem cells promote matrix metalloproteinase secretion by cardiac fibroblasts and reduce cardiac ventricular fibrosis after myocardial infarction," *Stem Cells*, vol. 27, no. 11, pp. 2734–2743, 2009.

[53] T. B. Rogers, S. Pati, S. Gaa et al., "Mesenchymal stem cells stimulate protective genetic reprogramming of injured cardiac ventricular myocytes," *Journal of Molecular and Cellular Cardiology*, vol. 50, no. 2, pp. 346–356, 2011.

[54] J. Rehman, D. Traktuev, J. Li et al., "Secretion of angiogenic and antiapoptotic factors by human adipose stromal cells," *Circulation*, vol. 109, no. 10, pp. 1292–1298, 2004.

[55] S. Aggarwal and M. F. Pittenger, "Human mesenchymal stem cells modulate allogeneic immune cell responses," *Blood*, vol. 105, no. 4, pp. 1815–1822, 2005.

[56] X. P. Huang, Z. Sun, Y. Miyagi et al., "Differentiation of allogeneic mesenchymal stem cells induces immunogenicity and limits their long-term benefits for myocardial repair," *Circulation*, vol. 122, no. 23, pp. 2419–2429, 2010.

[57] J. B. Mitchell, K. McIntosh, S. Zvonic et al., "Immunophenotype of human adipose-derived cells: temporal changes in stromal-associated and stem cell-associated markers," *Stem Cells*, vol. 24, no. 2, pp. 376–385, 2006.

[58] K. McIntosh, S. Zvonic, S. Garrett et al., "The immunogenicity of human adipose-derived cells: temporal changes in vitro," *Stem Cells*, vol. 24, no. 5, pp. 1246–1253, 2006.

[59] M. J. Crop, C. C. Baan, S. S. Korevaar et al., "Inflammatory conditions affect gene expression and function of human adipose tissue-derived mesenchymal stem cells," *Clinical and experimental immunology*, vol. 162, no. 3, pp. 474–486, 2010.

[60] K. Takahashi and S. Yamanaka, "Induction of pluripotent stem cells from mouse embryonic and adult fibroblast cultures by defined factors," *Cell*, vol. 126, no. 4, pp. 663–676, 2006.

[61] P. A. Tat, H. Sumer, K. L. Jones, K. Upton, and P. J. Verma, "The efficient generation of induced pluripotent stem (iPS) cells from adult mouse adipose tissue-derived and neural stem cells," *Cell Transplantation*, vol. 19, no. 5, pp. 525–536, 2010.

[62] N. Sun, N. J. Panetta, D. M. Gupta et al., "Feeder-free derivation of induced pluripotent stem cells from adult human adipose stem cells," *Proceedings of the National Academy of Sciences of the United States of America*, vol. 106, no. 37, pp. 15720–15725, 2009.

[63] M. K. Mamidi, R. Pal, N. A.B. Mori et al., "Co-culture of mesenchymal-like stromal cells derived from human foreskin permits long term propagation and differentiation of human embryonic stem cells," *Journal of Cellular Biochemistry*, vol. 112, no. 5, pp. 1353–1363, 2011.

[64] S. T. Hwang, S. W. Kang, S. J. Lee et al., "The expansion of human ES and iPS cells on porous membranes and proliferating human adipose-derived feeder cells," *Biomaterials*, vol. 31, no. 31, pp. 8012–8021, 2010.

[65] M. Nian, P. Lee, N. Khaper, and P. Liu, "Inflammatory cytokines and postmyocardial infarction remodeling," *Circulation Research*, vol. 94, no. 12, pp. 1543–1553, 2004.

[66] D. L. Mann, "Mechanisms and models in heart failure: a combinatorial approach," *Circulation*, vol. 100, no. 9, pp. 999–1008, 1999.

[67] M. S. Penn, "Importance of the SDF-1: CXCR4 axis in myocardial repair," *Circulation Research*, vol. 104, no. 10, pp. 1133–1135, 2009.

[68] J. P. M. Cleutjens, J. C. Kandala, E. Guarda, R. V. Guntaka, and K. T. Weber, "Regulation of collagen degradation in the rat myocardium after infarction," *Journal of Molecular and Cellular Cardiology*, vol. 27, no. 6, pp. 1281–1292, 1995.

[69] M. Ii, M. Horii, A. Yokoyama et al., "Synergistic effect of adipose-derived stem cell therapy and bone marrow progenitor recruitment in ischemic heart," *Laboratory Investigation*, vol. 91, no. 4, pp. 539–552, 2011.

[70] R. Gaebel, D. Furlani, H. Sorg et al., "Cell origin of human mesenchymal stem cells determines a different healing performance in cardiac regeneration," *PLoS ONE*, vol. 6, no. 2, Article ID e15652, 2011.

[71] X. Bai, Y. Yan, M. Coleman et al., "Tracking long-term survival of intramyocardially delivered human adipose tissue-derived stem cells using bioluminescence imaging," *Molecular Imaging and Biology*, pp. 1–13, 2010.

[72] C. Dubois, X. Liu, P. Claus et al., "Differential Effects of Progenitor Cell Populations on Left Ventricular Remodeling and Myocardial Neovascularization After Myocardial Infarction," *Journal of the American College of Cardiology*, vol. 55, no. 20, pp. 2232–2243, 2010.

[73] Y. J. Yang, H. Y. Qian, J. Huang et al., "Combined therapy with simvastatin and bone marrow-derived mesenchymal stem cells increases benefits in infarcted swine hearts,"

Arteriosclerosis, Thrombosis, and Vascular Biology, vol. 29, no. 12, pp. 2076–2082, 2009.

[74] K. E. A. van der Bogt, S. Schrepfer, J. Yu et al., "Comparison of transplantation of adipose tissue- and bone marrow-derived mesenchymal stem cells in the infarcted heart," *Transplantation*, vol. 87, no. 5, pp. 642–652, 2009.

[75] J. A. Dixon, R. C. Gorman, R. E. Stroud et al., "Mesenchymal cell transplantation and myocardial remodeling after myocardial infarction," *Circulation*, vol. 120, no. 1, pp. S220–S229, 2009.

[76] X. Bai, Y. Yan, Y. H. Song et al., "Both cultured and freshly isolated adipose tissue-derived stem cells enhance cardiac function after acute myocardial infarction," *European Heart Journal*, vol. 31, no. 4, pp. 489–501, 2010.

[77] K. E. van der Bogt, A. Y. Sheikh, S. Schrepfer et al., "Comparison of different adult stem cell types for treatment of myocardial ischemia," *Circulation*, vol. 118, no. 14, pp. S121–129, 2008.

[78] Y. Imanishi, A. Saito, H. Komoda et al., "Allogenic mesenchymal stem cell transplantation has a therapeutic effect in acute myocardial infarction in rats," *Journal of Molecular and Cellular Cardiology*, vol. 44, no. 4, pp. 662–671, 2008.

[79] S. M. Hashemi, S. Ghods, F. D. Kolodgie et al., "A placebo controlled, dose-ranging, safety study of allogenic mesenchymal stem cells injected by endomyocardial delivery after an acute myocardial infarction," *European Heart Journal*, vol. 29, no. 2, pp. 251–259, 2008.

[80] S. L. Hale, W. Dai, J. S. Dow, and R. A. Kloner, "Mesenchymal stem cell administration at coronary artery reperfusion in the rat by two delivery routes: a quantitative assessment," *Life Sciences*, vol. 83, no. 13-14, pp. 511–515, 2008.

[81] C. A. Carr, D. J. Stuckey, L. Tatton et al., "Bone marrow-derived stromal cells home to and remain in the infarcted rat heart but fail to improve function: an in vivo cine-MRI study," *American Journal of Physiology, Heart and Circulatory Physiology*, vol. 295, no. 2, pp. H533–H542, 2008.

[82] L. Cai, B. H. Johnstone, T. G. Cook et al., "IFATS collection: human adipose tissue-derived stem cells induce angiogenesis and nerve sprouting following myocardial infarction, in conjunction with potent preservation of cardiac function," *Stem Cells*, vol. 27, no. 1, pp. 230–237, 2008.

[83] C. Valina, K. Pinkernell, Y. H. Song et al., "Intracoronary administration of autologous adipose tissue-derived stem cells improves left ventricular function, perfusion, and remodelling after acute myocardial infarction," *European Heart Journal*, vol. 28, no. 21, pp. 2667–2677, 2007.

[84] B. Li, Q. Zeng, H. Wang et al., "Adipose tissue stromal cells transplantation in rats of acute myocardial infarction," *Coronary Artery Disease*, vol. 18, no. 3, pp. 221–227, 2007.

[85] J. I. Virag and C. E. Murry, "Myofibroblast and endothelial cell proliferation during murine myocardial infarct repair," *American Journal of Pathology*, vol. 163, no. 6, pp. 2433–2440, 2003.

[86] Y. Sun, M. F. Kiani, A. E. Postlethwaite, and K. T. Weber, "Infarct scar as living tissue," *Basic Research in Cardiology*, vol. 97, no. 5, pp. 343–347, 2002.

[87] H. Song, M. J. Cha, B. W. Song et al., "Reactive oxygen species inhibit adhesion of mesenchymal stem cells implanted into ischemic myocardium via interference of focal adhesion complex," *Stem Cells*, vol. 28, no. 3, pp. 555–563, 2010.

[88] M. Mazo, J. J. Gavira, G. Abizanda et al., "Transplantation of mesenchymal stem cells exerts a greater long-term effect than bone marrow mononuclear cells in a chronic myocardial

infarction model in rat," *Cell Transplantation*, vol. 19, no. 3, pp. 313–328, 2009.

[89] M. F. Chen, B. C. Lee, H. C. Hsu et al., "Cell therapy generates a favourable chemokine gradient for stem cell recruitment into the infarcted heart in rabbits," *European Journal of Heart Failure*, vol. 11, no. 3, pp. 238–245, 2009.

[90] M. Mazo, V. Planat-Bénard, G. Abizanda et al., "Transplantation of adipose derived stromal cells is associated with functional improvement in a rat model of chronic myocardial infarction," *European Journal of Heart Failure*, vol. 10, no. 5, pp. 454–462, 2008.

[91] K. Jujo, M. Ii, and D. W. Losordo, "Endothelial progenitor cells in neovascularization of infarcted myocardium," *Journal of Molecular and Cellular Cardiology*, vol. 45, no. 4, pp. 530–544, 2008.

[92] M. Nahrendorf, F. K. Swirski, E. Aikawa et al., "The healing myocardium sequentially mobilizes two monocyte subsets with divergent and complementary functions," *Journal of Experimental Medicine*, vol. 204, no. 12, pp. 3037–3047, 2007.

[93] L. Wang, J. Deng, W. Tian et al., "Adipose-derived stem cells are an effective cell candidate for treatment of heart failure: an MR imaging study of rat hearts," *American Journal of Physiology, Heart and Circulatory Physiology*, vol. 297, no. 3, pp. H1020–H1031, 2009.

[94] L. C. Amado, A. P. Saliaris, K. H. Schuleri et al., "Cardiac repair with intramyocardial injection of allogeneic mesenchymal stem cells after myocardial infarction," *Proceedings of the National Academy of Sciences of the United States of America*, vol. 102, no. 32, pp. 11474–11479, 2005.

[95] H. Li, D. Malhotra, C. C. Yeh et al., "Myocardial survival signaling in response to stem cell transplantation," *Journal of the American College of Surgeons*, vol. 208, no. 4, pp. 607–613, 2009.

[96] J. Cho, P. Zhai, Y. Maejima, and J. Sadoshima, "Myocardial injection with GSK-3β-overexpressing bone marrow-derived mesenchymal stem cells attenuates cardiac dysfunction after myocardial infarction," *Circulation Research*, vol. 108, no. 4, pp. 478–489, 2011.

[97] X. Wang, T. Zhao, W. Huang et al., "Hsp20-engineered mesenchymal stem cells are resistant to oxidative stress via enhanced activation of Akt and increased secretion of growth factors," *Stem Cells*, vol. 27, no. 12, pp. 3021–3031, 2009.

[98] K. Le Blanc, "Mesenchymal stromal cells: tissue repair and immune modulation," *Cytotherapy*, vol. 8, no. 6, pp. 559–561, 2006.

[99] K. H. Schuleri, L. C. Amado, A. J. Boyle et al., "Early improvement in cardiac tissue perfusion due to mesenchymal stem cells," *American Journal of Physiology, Heart and Circulatory Physiology*, vol. 294, no. 5, pp. H2002–H2011, 2008.

[100] L. C. Amado, K. H. Schuleri, A. P. Saliaris et al., "Multimodality noninvasive imaging demonstrates in vivo cardiac regeneration after mesenchymal stem cell therapy," *Journal of the American College of Cardiology*, vol. 48, no. 10, pp. 2116–2124, 2006.

[101] M. Rigol, N. Solanes, J. Farré et al., "Effects of adipose tissue-derived stem cell therapy after myocardial infarction: impact of the route of administration," *Journal of Cardiac Failure*, vol. 16, no. 4, pp. 357–366, 2010.

[102] Y. Zhou, S. Wang, Z. Yu et al., "Direct injection of autologous mesenchymal stromal cells improves myocardial function," *Biochemical and Biophysical Research Communications*, vol. 390, no. 3, pp. 902–907, 2009.

[103] J. Ma, J. Ge, S. Zhang et al., "Time course of myocardial stromal cell-derived factor 1 expression and beneficial effects

of intravenously administered bone marrow stem cells in rats with experimental myocardial infarction," *Basic Research in Cardiology*, vol. 100, no. 3, pp. 217–223, 2005.

[104] Z. Cheng, L. Ou, X. Zhou et al., "Targeted migration of mesenchymal stem cells modified with CXCR4 gene to infarcted myocardium improves cardiac performance," *Molecular Therapy*, vol. 16, no. 3, pp. 571–579, 2008.

[105] Z. Cheng, X. Liu, L. Ou et al., "Mobilization of mesenchymal stem cells by granulocyte colony-stimulating factor in rats with acute myocardial infarction," *Cardiovascular Drugs and Therapy*, vol. 22, no. 5, pp. 363–371, 2008.

[106] J. Huang, Z. Zhang, J. Guo et al., "Genetic modification of mesenchymal stem cells overexpressing ccr1 increases cell viability, migration, engraftment, and capillary density in the injured myocardium," *Circulation Research*, vol. 106, no. 11, pp. 1753–1762, 2010.

[107] X. H. Liu, C. G. Bai, Z. Y. Xu et al., "Therapeutic potential of angiogenin modified mesenchymal stem cells: angiogenin improves mesenchymal stem cells survival under hypoxia and enhances vasculogenesis in myocardial infarction," *Microvascular Research*, vol. 76, no. 1, pp. 23–30, 2008.

[108] B. Zeng, H. Chen, C. Zhu, X. Ren, G. Lin, and F. Cao, "Effects of combined mesenchymal stem cells and heme oxygenase-1 therapy on cardiac performance," *European Journal of Cardio-Thoracic Surgery*, vol. 34, no. 4, pp. 850–856, 2008.

[109] M. Gnecchi, H. He, L. G. Melo et al., "Early beneficial effects of bone marrow-derived mesenchymal stem cells overexpressing akt on cardiac metabolism after myocardial infarction," *Stem Cells*, vol. 27, no. 4, pp. 971–979, 2009.

[110] M. Gnecchi, H. He, N. Noiseux et al., "Evidence supporting paracrine hypothesis for Akt-modified mesenchymal stem cell-mediated cardiac protection and functional improvement," *FASEB Journal*, vol. 20, no. 6, pp. 661–669, 2006.

[111] M. Gnecchi, H. He, O. D. Liang et al., "Paracrine action accounts for marked protection of ischemic heart by Akt-modified mesenchymal stem cells," *Nature Medicine*, vol. 11, no. 4, pp. 367–368, 2005.

[112] H. Song, M. J. Cha, B. W. Song et al., "Reactive oxygen species inhibit adhesion of mesenchymal stem cells implanted into ischemic myocardium via interference of focal adhesion complex," *Stem Cells*, vol. 28, no. 3, pp. 555–563, 2010.

[113] J. Jin, S. I. Jeong, Y. M. Shin et al., "Transplantation of mesenchymal stem cells within a poly(lactide-co-ε-caprolactone) scaffold improves cardiac function in a rat myocardial infarction model," *European Journal of Heart Failure*, vol. 11, no. 2, pp. 147–153, 2009.

[114] M. Y. Tan, W. Zhi, R. Q. Wei et al., "Repair of infarcted myocardium using mesenchymal stem cell seeded small intestinal submucosa in rabbits," *Biomaterials*, vol. 30, no. 19, pp. 3234–3240, 2009.

[115] C. H. Chen, H. J. Wei, W. W. Lin et al., "Porous tissue grafts sandwiched with multilayered mesenchymal stromal cell sheets induce tissue regeneration for cardiac repair," *Cardiovascular Research*, vol. 80, no. 1, pp. 88–95, 2008.

[116] Y. Miyahara, N. Nagaya, M. Kataoka et al., "Monolayered mesenchymal stem cells repair scarred myocardium after myocardial infarction," *Nature Medicine*, vol. 12, no. 4, pp. 459–465, 2006.

[117] A. Bel, V. Planat-Bernard, A. Saito et al., "Composite cell sheets: a further step toward safe and effective myocardial regeneration by cardiac progenitors derived from embryonic stem cells," *Circulation*, vol. 122, no. 11, pp. S118–S123, 2010.

[118] S. Chen, Z. Liu, N. Tian et al., "Intracoronary transplantation of autologous bone marrow mesenchymal stem cells for ischemic cardiomyopathy due to isolated chronic occluded left anterior descending artery," *Journal of Invasive Cardiology*, vol. 18, no. 11, pp. 552–556, 2006.

[119] D. G. Katritsis, P. A. Sotiropoulou, E. Karvouni et al., "Transcoronary transplantation of autologous mesenchymal stem cells and endothelial progenitors into infarcted human myocardium," *Catheterization and Cardiovascular Interventions*, vol. 65, no. 3, pp. 321–329, 2005.

[120] S. L. Chen, W. W. Fang, F. Ye et al., "Effect on left ventricular function of intracoronary transplantation of autologous bone marrow mesenchymal stem cell in patients with acute myocardial infarction," *American Journal of Cardiology*, vol. 94, no. 1, pp. 92–95, 2004.

[121] J. M. Hare, "Translational development of mesenchymal stem cell therapy for cardiovascular diseases," *Texas Heart Institute Journal*, vol. 36, no. 2, pp. 145–147, 2009.

[122] J. M. Hare, J. H. Traverse, T. D. Henry et al., "A randomized, double-blind, placebo-controlled, dose-escalation study of intravenous adult human mesenchymal stem cells (prochymal) after acute myocardial infarction," *Journal of the American College of Cardiology*, vol. 54, no. 24, pp. 2277–2286, 2009.

[123] N. Dib, T. Henry, A. DeMaria, S. Itescu, M. M. McCarthy, and S. C. Jaggar, "The first US study to assess the feasibility and safety of endocardial delivery of allogenic mesenchymal precursor cells in patient with heart failure: three-month interim analysis," *Circulation*, vol. 120, p. S810, 2009.

[124] H. J. Duckers, J. Houtgraaf, R. J. van Geuns, B. D. van Dalen, E. Regar, and W. van der Giessen, "First-in-man experience with intracoronary infusion of adipose-derived regenerative cells in the treatment of patients with ST-elevation myocardial infarction: the apollo trial," *Circulation*, vol. 120, Article ID A12225, 2010.

[125] A. Schaefer, C. Zwadlo, M. Fuchs et al., "Long-term effects of intracoronary bone marrow cell transfer on diastolic function in patients after acute myocardial infarction: 5-year results from the randomized-controlled BOOST trial—an echocardiographic study," *European Journal of Echocardiography*, vol. 11, no. 2, pp. 165–171, 2010.

[126] J. A. Miettinen, K. Ylitalo, P. Hedberg et al., "Determinants of functional recovery after myocardial infarction of patients treated with bone marrow-derived stem cells after thrombolytic therapy," *Heart*, vol. 96, no. 5, pp. 362–367, 2009.

[127] C. Stamm, H. D. Kleine, Y. H. Choi et al., "Intramyocardial delivery of CD133+ bone marrow cells and coronary artery bypass grafting for chronic ischemic heart disease: safety and efficacy studies," *Journal of Thoracic and Cardiovascular Surgery*, vol. 133, no. 3, pp. 717–725, 2007.

[128] E. Martin-Rendon, S. J. Brunskill, C. J. Hyde, S. J. Stanworth, A. Mathur, and S. M. Watt, "Autologous bone marrow stem cells to treat acute myocardial infarction: a systematic review," *European Heart Journal*, vol. 29, no. 15, pp. 1807–1818, 2008.

[129] T. S. Li, M. Kubo, K. Ueda, M. Murakami, A. Mikamo, and K. Hamano, "Impaired angiogenic potency of bone marrow cells from patients with advanced age, anemia, and renal failure," *Journal of Thoracic and Cardiovascular Surgery*, vol. 139, no. 2, pp. 459–465, 2010.

[130] C. K. Kissel, R. Lehmann, B. Assmus et al., "Selective functional exhaustion of hematopoietic progenitor cells in the bone marrow of patients with postinfarction heart failure," *Journal of the American College of Cardiology*, vol. 49, no. 24, pp. 2341–2349, 2007.

[131] S. A. Sorrentino, F. H. Bahlmann, C. Besler et al., "Oxidant stress impairs in vivo reendothelialization capacity of endothelial progenitor cells from patients with type 2 diabetes mellitus: restoration by the peroxisome proliferator-activated receptor-γ agonist rosiglitazone," *Circulation*, vol. 116, no. 2, pp. 163–173, 2007.

[132] A. J. Nauta and W. E. Fibbe, "Immunomodulatory properties of mesenchymal stromal cells," *Blood*, vol. 110, no. 10, pp. 3499–3506, 2007.

[133] J. C. Chachques, J. C. Trainini, N. Lago et al., "Myocardial assistance by grafting a new bioartificial upgraded myocardium (MAGNUM clinical trial): one year follow-up," *Cell Transplantation*, vol. 16, no. 9, pp. 927–934, 2007.

18

Comparison of the Direct Effects of Human Adipose- and Bone-Marrow-Derived Stem Cells on Postischemic Cardiomyoblasts in an *In Vitro* Simulated Ischemia-Reperfusion Model

Mónika Szepes,[1] **Zsolt Benkő,**[1] **Attila Cselenyák,**[1] **Kai Michael Kompisch,**[2] **Udo Schumacher,**[2] **Zsombor Lacza,**[1] **and Levente Kiss**[1]

[1] *Institute of Human Physiology and Clinical Experimental Research, Semmelweis University, Tűzoltó Utca 37-47, Budapest 1094, Hungary*
[2] *Department of Anatomy and Experimental Morphology, Center for Experimental Medicine, University Hospital Hamburg-Eppendorf, Martinistraße 52, 20246 Hamburg, Germany*

Correspondence should be addressed to Levente Kiss; kiss.levente@med.semmelweis-univ.hu

Academic Editor: Shinsuke Yuasa

Regenerative therapies hold a promising and exciting future for the cure of yet untreatable diseases, and mesenchymal stem cells are in the forefront of this approach. However, the relative efficacy and the mechanism of action of different types of mesenchymal stem cells are still incompletely understood. We aimed to evaluate the effects of human adipose- (hASC) and bone-marrow-derived stem cells (hBMSCs) and adipose-derived stem cell conditioned media (ACM) on the viability of cardiomyoblasts in an *in vitro* ischemia-reperfusion (I-R) model. Flow cytometric viability analysis revealed that both cell treatments led to similarly increased percentages of living cells, while treatment with ACM did not (I-R model: $12.13\pm0.75\%$; hASC: $24.66\pm2.49\%$; hBMSC: $25.41\pm1.99\%$; ACM: $13.94 \pm 1.44\%$). Metabolic activity measurement (I-R model: 0.065 ± 0.033; hASC: 0.652 ± 0.089; hBMSC: 0.607 ± 0.059; ACM: 0.225 ± 0.013; arbitrary units) and lactate dehydrogenase assay (I-R model: 0.225 ± 0.006; hASC: 0.148 ± 0.005; hBMSC: 0.146 ± 0.004; ACM: 0.208 ± 0.009; arbitrary units) confirmed the flow cytometric results while also indicated a slight beneficial effect of ACM. Our results highlight that mesenchymal stem cells have the same efficacy when used directly on postischemic cells, and differences found between them in preclinical and clinical investigations are rather related to other possible causes such as their immunomodulatory or angiogenic properties.

1. Introduction

Regenerative therapies are representing a relatively new possibility for the treatment of diseases where functional tissue is lost. This approach is aiming to restore organ functionality either by enhancing the resident stem cell population or with substituting the damaged tissue with added cells. Various cell types—such as embryonic, induced pluripotent and adult stem cells—are used to this aim each with its respective ethical, oncological, or immunological advantages and disadvantages [1–4], but data from clinical trials are mostly available from adult stem cells, namely, bone-marrow-derived stem cells (BMSCs) and adipose-derived stem cells (ASCs) [5]. Adipose-derived stem cells have lately become an attractive pool for autologous adult stem cells because of their relatively easy harvest from patients via minimally invasive liposuction [6, 7]. The use of these cells showed promising results and sometimes great success in various situations, such as in articular cartilage regeneration [8], musculoskeletal tissue repair [9–11], and the treatment of chronic, nonhealing wounds [12]. Considering cardiovascular applications, several reports indicated a consistent and significant benefit from cell transplantation after myocardial infarction in *in vivo* animal models [13–19]. Still, the clinical trials using adult stem cell therapy in acute myocardial infarction showed significant but only modest improvements [20–22], and the relative efficacy of the different types of mesenchymal stem cells is still incompletely understood [23, 24]. In this regard, Mazo et al. showed that the transplantation of adipose-derived cells in chronic infarct provided a better left ventricular heart function, less fibrosis, and increased angiogenesis compared to bone-marrow-derived stem cells [25]. Recently, Rasmussen et al. confirmed these data using hypoxically preconditioned adipose- and bone-marrow-derived stem cells from the same patient [26]. Thus, it seems that adipose-derived stem cells are superior to mesenchymal stem cells of other origin. However, no information is provided in these papers on the direct effects of these cells on the postischemic cells. Furthermore, the exact mechanism of action of these cells is also unclear. Initial studies emphasized the role of cell fusion and differentiation as the potentially most important mechanisms of actions [27, 28], but subsequent studies questioned their importance in the beneficial effects [29, 30]. Interest, therefore, switched towards paracrine factors involving proangiogenic, antiapoptotic and anti-inflammatory pathways [31–34]. The importance of the various paracrine effects is also emphasized by the fact that improvements were found in experimental models in spite of the very limited survival of the donor cells in the hostile environment of a damaged tissue [35, 36]. Therefore, in the present study we aimed to evaluate the direct effects of human adipose- and bone-marrow-derived stem cells in a reductionist model of ischemia-reperfusion. Furthermore, we wanted to investigate if mesenchymal stem cells had any direct paracrine effect on the postischemic cells.

2. Methods

2.1. Cell Lines and Conditioned Media. H9c2 rat cardiomyoblast cell line was purchased from ATCC (Wesel, Germany). Cells were cultured in high-glucose (4.5 g/L) DMEM containing 10% fetal bovine serum, 4 mM L-glutamine, 100 U/mL penicillin, and 100 μg/mL streptomycin at 37°C in a humidified atmosphere of 5% CO_2. Cell culture media was replaced 2 times a week, and cells were passaged once they reached 70–80% confluence.

Human adipose-derived stem cells (hASCs) were isolated from liposuction samples of healthy female donors aged 22–50 years (36.4 ± 4.5 years, $n = 5$) who underwent elective cosmetic liposuction after informed consent. The isolation of hASCs from liposuction samples was performed according to an established protocol [37, 38]. Briefly, lipoaspirates were washed extensively with phosphate buffered saline (PBS) and then incubated with 0.075% collagenase at 37°C for 30 minutes. Enzyme activity was neutralized using Dulbecco's modified Eagle's medium (DMEM; Gibco/Invitrogen, Carlsbad, CA, USA) supplemented with 10% heat-inactivated fetal calf serum (FCS), 100 U/mL penicillin, 100 μg/mL streptomycin (all Gibco/Invitrogen), and 100 U/mL nystatin (Sigma-Aldrich, St. Louis, MO, USA). Samples were centrifuged

at 1500 rpm for 10 minutes, and the resulting cell pellet was plated in 75 cm²-culture flasks (Sarstedt Inc., Newton, NC, USA). Cells were cultured in a 37°C humidified 5% CO_2 atmosphere. Nonadherent cells were removed after 24 hours. Cells were grown in antimycotic culture medium for 7 days, and culture medium was changed every 2 to 3 days. After that period, hASCs were cultured in low-glucose (1.0 g/L) DMEM containing 10% fetal calf serum, 4 mM L-glutamine, 100 U/mL penicillin, and 100 μg/mL streptomycin at 37°C in a humidified atmosphere of 5% CO_2. Cell culture media was replaced 2 times a week, and cells were passaged once they reached 70–80% confluence. Cryopreservation was performed on hASCs prior to the experiments, and the revitalized cells were used in the experiments. Passage 1 cells were trypsinized and centrifuged at 1500 rpm for 10 min. Cell pellets were resuspended in CryoSafe medium (c. c. pro GmbH, Neustadt, Germany), aliquoted to cryotubes (Nalge Nunc, Roskilde, Denmark) as 1 mL samples and were stored for 40 minutes at −25°C and then transferred to −80°C for 24 hours followed by final cryopreservation in liquid nitrogen. Human adipose-derived stem cells were characterized by mesenchymal (CD90, CD105, and the stem cell antigen 1 (Sca-1) homolog CD59) and hematopoietic (CD34, CD45) markers with flow cytometry in order to confirm their lineage.

Human bone-marrow-derived stem cells (hBMSCs) were isolated from samples gathered from young patients (aged 2–20) during standard orthopedic surgical procedures with the informed consent of the patients or their parents under approved ethical guidelines set by the Ethical Committee of the Hungarian Medical Research Council. All procedures were approved by the Ethical Committee of Semmelweis University. Only such tissues were used that otherwise would have been discarded. The bone marrow was flushed into T75 flasks and diluted with low-glucose (1.0 g/L) DMEM culture medium containing 10% FCS, 100 U/mL penicillin, 100 μg/mL streptomycin, and 4 mM L-glutamine. The flasks were incubated at 37°C in fully humidified atmosphere of 5% CO_2 and 95% air for 3 days. After the incubation period, the hBMSCs adhered to the surface of the flasks and the remaining components of bone marrow were eliminated by washing with PBS. The used hBMSCs were cultured in the same conditions as hASCs. Human bone-marrow-derived stem cells were characterized by mesenchymal (CD73, CD90, CD105, and CD166) and hematopoietic (CD34, CD45) markers with flow cytometry in order to confirm their lineage. Characterization was performed on cells cultured under standard culture conditions and growing as monolayers while displaying constant cell proliferation rates over the entire culture period.

For preparing *conditioned media* (ACM) adipose-derived stem cells were used because their proliferation capabilities are much better compared to hBMSCs which helped to achieve the highest possible concentrations of paracrine molecules in the medium in the given period of time [39]. Human ASCs were seeded at 10.000 cells/cm² in 100 mm Petri dishes using 8 mL low-glucose (1.0 g/L) DMEM culture medium containing 10% FCS, 100 U/mL penicillin,

(a)

(b)

(c)

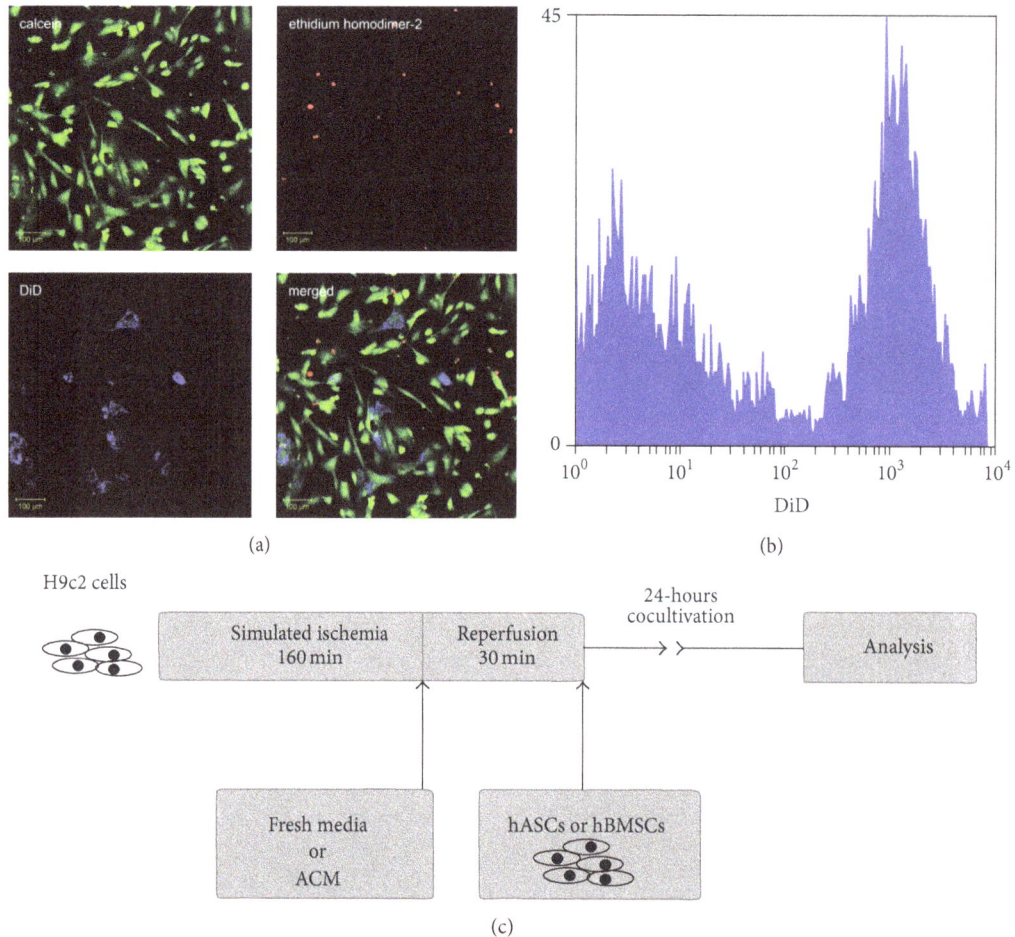

Figure 1: Ischemia-reperfusion model. (a) Representative fluorescent microscopic picture showing H9c2 cells injured with our ischemia-reperfusion model and treated with Vybrant DiD (ex/em: 644/665 nm, blue) labeled cells. The cytoplasm of the living cells is stained with calcein-AM (ex/em: 494/517 nm, green), the nuclei of the necrotic cells are ethidium homodimer-2 stained (ex/em: 536/624 nm, red). (b) Flow cytometric histogram on the distinction between stem cells and H9c2 cells based on DiD staining. (c) Schematic representation of the experimental protocol.

100 μg/mL streptomycin, and 4 mM L-glutamine. The dishes were incubated at 37°C in fully humidified atmosphere of 5% CO_2 and 95% air, and cell-free supernatants were collected for further experimental use after 48 hours.

2.2. In Vitro Ischemia-Reperfusion Model. Ischemia-reperfusion was simulated *in vitro* by oxygen and glucose deprivation as described previously in our earlier publications [40–42]. Briefly, 30.000/well H9c2 cells in 12-well plates were incubated in glucose-free DMEM in an atmosphere of 0.5% O_2 and 99.5% N_2 for 160 minutes. This procedure was performed on an established incubation system (PeCon, Erbach-Bach, Germany). After incubation, the cells were reoxygenated and glucose was provided by immediate replacement of the media with fresh high-glucose DMEM, and the cells were kept in standard cell culture conditions till further experimental actions. Representative fluorescence microscopy pictures were taken to follow the cell viability during the model using a Zeiss LSM 510 META (Carl Zeiss, Jena, Germany). We

used calcein-AM (ex/em: 494/517 nm, Invitrogen, Carlsbad, CA, USA) and ethidium homodimer-2 (ex/em: 536/624 nm, Invitrogen, Carlsbad, CA, USA) labeling to mark live/dead cells. Added mesenchymal stem cells were dyed with Vybrant DiD (ex/em: 644/665 nm, Invitrogen, Carlsbad, CA, USA) (Figure 1(a)).

2.3. Experimental Protocol. Four experimental groups were investigated in which postischemic cells received: (1) normal medium (I-R-model); (2) hASC conditioned medium (ACM); (3) hASCs; and (4) a group that received hBMSCs. Cell-treated groups were given 20.000 cells 30 minutes after the reoxygenation, and the added cells were labeled with Vybrant DiD fluorescent membrane dye to enable differentiation from the postischemic cells (Figure 1(b)). Cells were cocultivated for 24 hours in standard cell culture conditions. In the case of ACM group at the end of simulated ischemia, the glucose-free medium was changed to same volume of cell-free hASC conditioned media (Figure 1(c)).

2.4. Cell Viability Measurement with Flow Cytometry. Twenty-four hours after reoxygenation, cells were harvested by trypsinization and resuspended in 500 μL PBS containing 5 nM calcein-AM and 350 nM ethidium-homodimer-2 for flow cytometric analysis [43]. Controls were prepared as follows: for live control, cells were cultured in standard conditions; for dead control, cells were treated with 100 mM H_2O_2 for 1 hour immediately before trypsinization. For the measurements, FACSCalibur flow cytometer (Becton Dickinson, Franklin Lakes, NJ, USA) was used and the data was analyzed with the Weasel program (The Walter and Eliza Hall Institute, Parkville, VIC, Australia). Using flow cytometry, we could distinguish the therapeutically given cells from the postischemic cells on the basis of their DiD labeling, and these cells were gated in or out as appropriate for further analysis.

2.5. Metabolic Activity Measurement. For the evaluation of the metabolic activity in the groups, we used the Presto-Blue Cell Viability reagent (Invitrogen, Carlsbad, CA, USA), according to the manufacturer's instructions. Because of the relative low cell numbers used in the experiments, we chose a 24-hour incubation time in $37°C$ and measured absorbance as instructed.

In the hASC and hBMSC groups to exclude the influence of the added stem cells metabolism, we subtracted the metabolic activity value of 20.000 stem cells from the measured value. The obtained results are compared to the metabolic activity of 30.000 H9c2 cells cultured in standard cell culture conditions (control).

2.6. Lactate Dehydrogenase (LDH) Cytotoxicity Assay. The measurement was performed using LDH Cytotoxicity Kit II (PromoCell, Heidelberg, Germany) according to the manufacturer's instructions, with 30-minute incubation period and absorbance measurement at 490 nm. For the LDH measurements, the previously described experimental groups were used 24 hours after ischemia-reperfusion. The LDH enzyme level was determined in the supernatant of 30.000 H9c2 cells cultured in standard conditions (control). The absorbance results were normalized with the total cell number in each sample.

2.7. Statistics. Statistical analysis of data was carried out either with one-way analysis of variance with Newman-Keuls multiple comparison post hoc test or unpaired t-test as appropriate. All data are expressed as mean $\pm$ SEM. A P value of <0.05 was accepted as statistically significant.

3. Results

3.1. Characterization of hASCs and hBMSCs. Analyses of cell surface markers by flow cytometry demonstrated that hASCs (Figure 2(a)) were positive for the mesenchymal stromal (stem) cell markers CD90 and CD105 as well as the stem cell antigen 1 (Sca-1) homolog CD59 and were negative for the lymphohaematopoetic markers CD34 and CD45. Flow cytometry analysis of cultured bone-marrow-derived stem cells (Figure 2(b)) exhibited the lack of hematopoietic markers (CD34$^-$, CD45$^-$), but revealed mesenchymal stem cell lineage specific cell surface markers (CD73$^+$, CD90$^+$, CD105$^+$, and CD166$^+$). With respect to cell surface marker expression, our findings were consistent with previous reports [44, 45].

3.2. Flow Cytometric Viability Analysis. Our experimental results regarding the postischemic cells showed that without any treatment live cells amounted to 12.13 $\pm$ 0.75% after 24 hours. However, the percentage of live cardiomyoblasts after 24 hours was significantly increased both with hASC (24.66 $\pm$ 2.49%) and hBMSC (25.41 $\pm$ 1.99%) treatments but not with the addition of ACM (13.94 $\pm$ 1.44%). There was no significant difference between the cell-treated groups. Cell-treatments led to a significantly increased percentage of live cells compared to ACM treatment as well (Figure 3(a)).

The percentage of the dead cells in the I-R model group was 87.71 $\pm$ 0.82%, while this was significantly smaller in the hASC and hBMSC treated groups (hASC: 75.24 $\pm$ 2.49%; hBMSC: 74.62 $\pm$ 1.99%), but was not statistically different in the ACM treated group (ACM: 85.75 $\pm$ 1.57%). There was no significant difference between the hASC- and hBMSC-treated groups (Figure 3(b)).

Putting the added cells into consideration, we found that most of the stem cells were alive in both the hASC-treated group (70.30 $\pm$ 2.35%) and the hBMSC-treated group (73.30 $\pm$ 1.92%), and there was no statistically significant difference between the groups (Figure 3(c)). Furthermore, no difference was found considering the dead cell population (hASC: 29.20 $\pm$ 2.42%, hBMSC: 25.81 $\pm$ 1.89%; Figure 3(d)).

3.3. Metabolic Activity Measurement. Using the PrestoBlue colorimetric assay, we strengthened our earlier findings with the flow cytometric analysis. The reducing capability of the cells reflecting their viability was significantly higher after treatment with hASCs (0.652 $\pm$ 0.089 AU, arbitrary units) and hBMSCs (0.607 $\pm$ 0.059 AU) compared to the I-R model (0.065 $\pm$ 0.033 AU). Moreover, the treatment with ACM was also able to increase the metabolic activity of the postischemic cells (0.225 $\pm$ 0.013 AU). No difference was observed between the beneficial effects of the two different stem cell lines (Figure 4(a)).

3.4. Lactate Dehydrogenase Cytotoxicity Assay. Cellular necrosis expressed by LDH release decreased significantly compared to I-R model (0.225 $\pm$ 0.006 AU) when the postischemic cells were treated with hASC and hBMSC (hASC: 0.148 $\pm$ 0.005 AU; hBMSC: 0.146 $\pm$ 0.004 AU). Conditioned media could decrease the LDH levels only very slightly (0.208 $\pm$ 0.009 AU). In case of hASC and hBMSC treatments, the necrosis was not significantly different from the control (Figure 4(b)).

4. Discussion

We report here that human adipose- and bone-marrow-derived cells directly improve the survival of postischemic cardiomyoblasts in an *in vitro* reductionist model. Metabolic

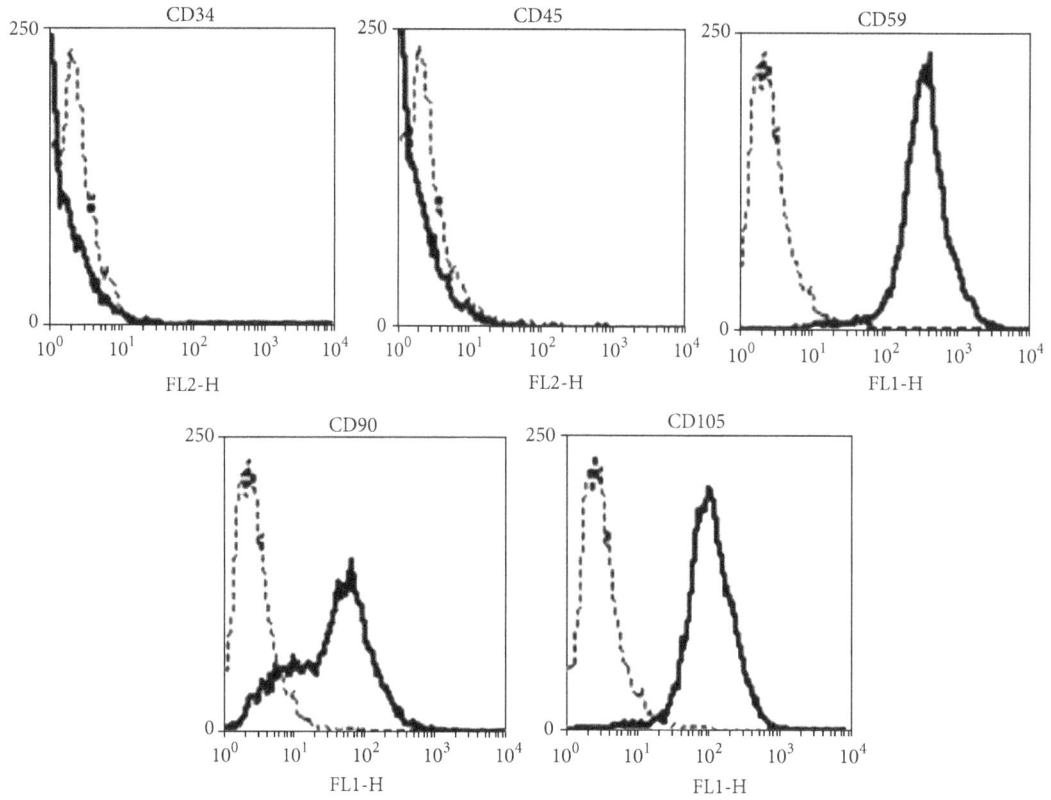

(a)

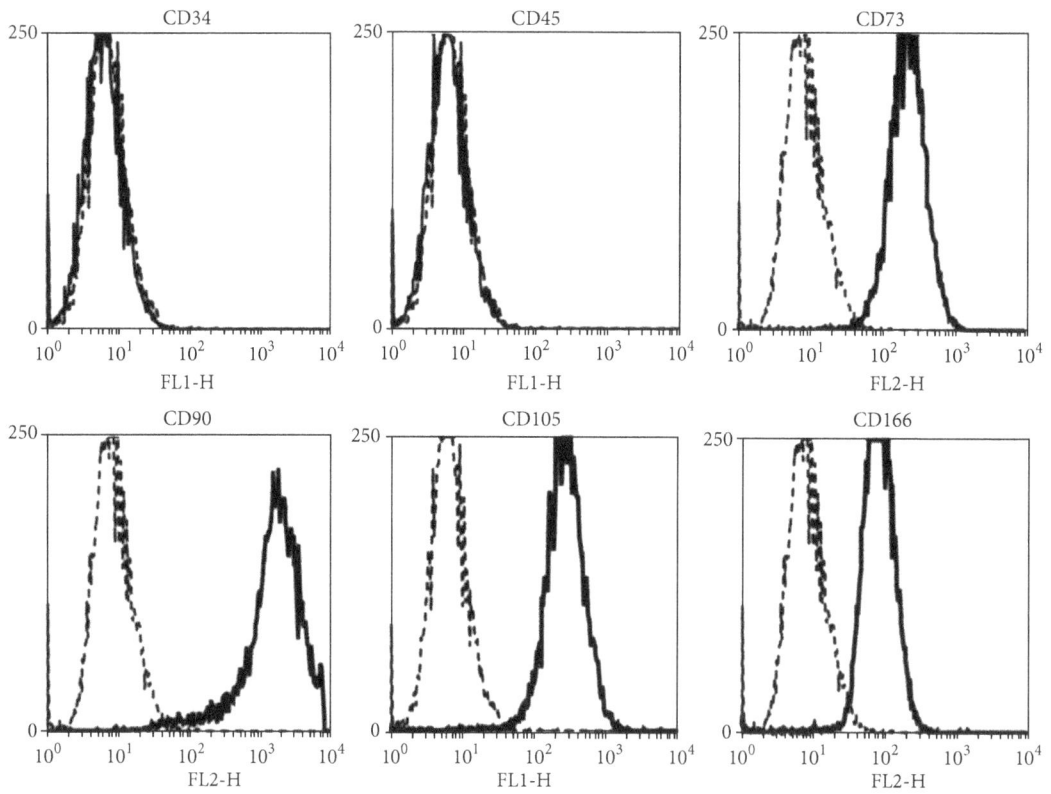

(b)

FIGURE 2: Characterization of adult stem cells. Flow cytometric analysis revealed a CD34$^-$, CD45$^-$ and CD59$^+$, CD90$^+$, CD105$^+$ pattern for hASCs (a) and a CD34$^-$, CD45$^-$ and CD73$^+$, CD90$^+$, CD105$^+$, CD 166$^+$ pattern for hBMSCs (b). The isotype controls are indicated with dashed lines.

Comparison of the Direct Effects of Human Adipose- and Bone-Marrow-Derived Stem Cells on Postischemic
Cardiomyoblasts in an In Vitro Simulated Ischemia-Reperfusion Model

179

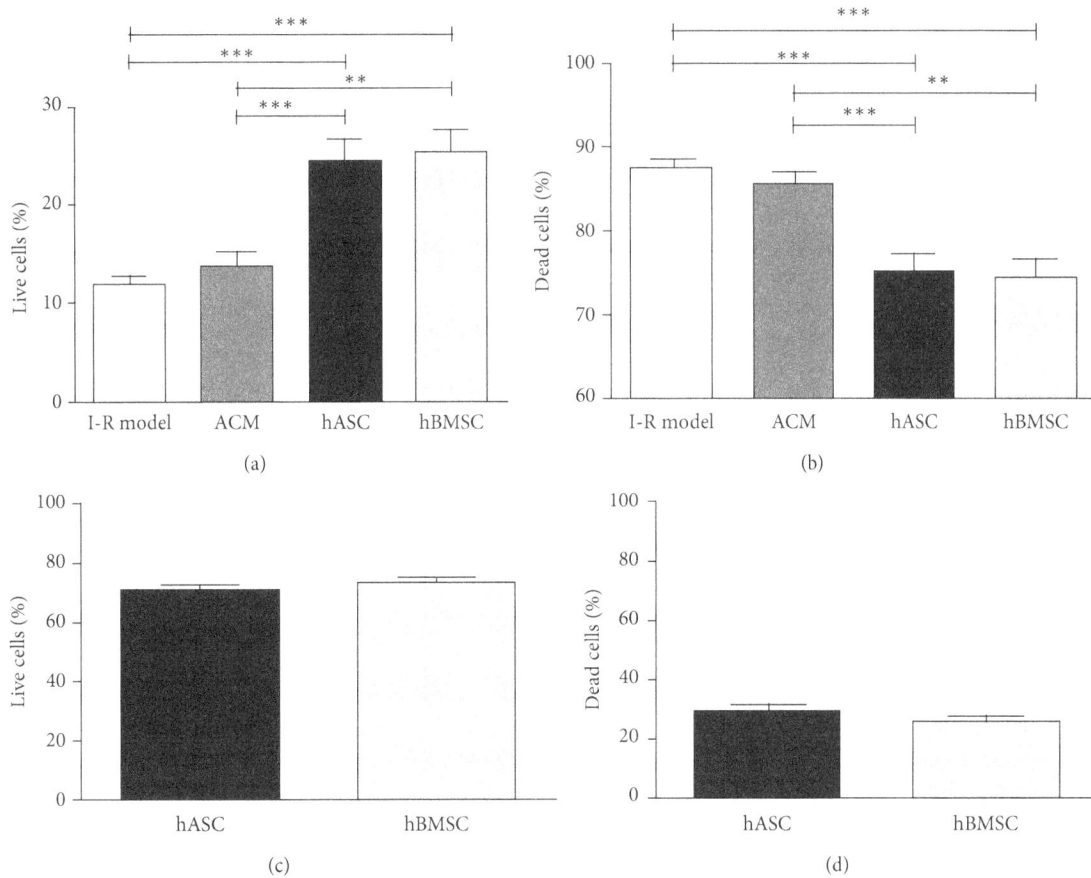

FIGURE 3: Flow cytometric analysis of the postischemic cells and the therapeutic cells after 24 hours. Flow cytometric cell death analysis of the postischemic cells revealed that cell treatment increased the percentage of live cells (a), while ACM did not (I-R model: 12.13 ± 0.75%; ACM: 13.94 ± 1.44%; hASC: 24.66 ± 2.49%; hBMSC: 25.41 ± 1.99%). (b) The percentage of dead cells decreased when therapeutic cells were added (I-R model: 87.71 ± 0.82%; ACM: 85.75 ± 1.57%; hASC: 75.24 ± 2.49%; hBMSC: 74.62 ± 1.99%). The percentages of live (c) and dead (d) cells among the therapeutically added cells were not significantly different ($n = 17$–31, $^{**}P < 0.01$, $^{***}P < 0.001$).

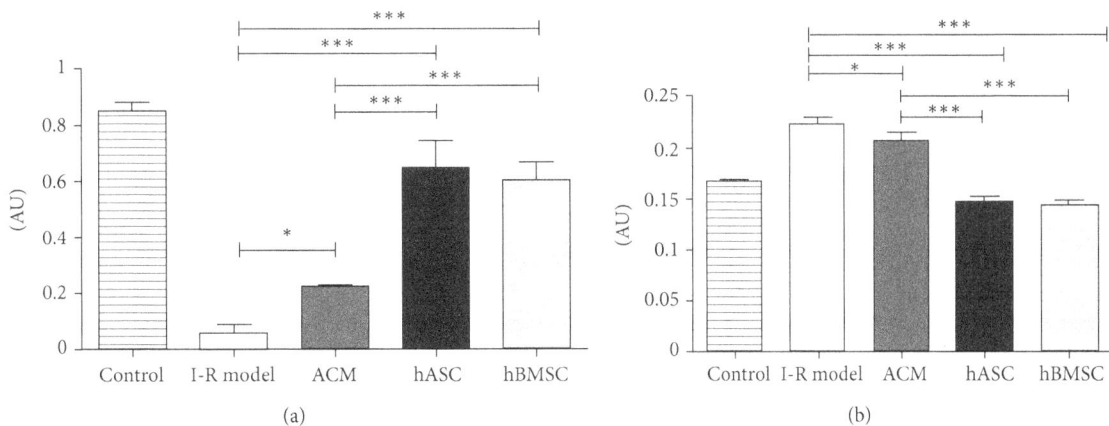

FIGURE 4: Metabolic activity measurement and LDH assay. (a) The metabolic activity measured 24 hours after the ischemia-reperfusion injury significantly decreased in the cells after the ischemic conditions compared to the control group, but the metabolic activity was enhanced with all the applied treatments (control: 0.858 ± 0.021 AU; I-R model: 0.065 ± 0.033 AU; ACM: 0.225 ± 0.013 AU; hASC: 0.652 ± 0.089 AU; hBMSC: 0.607 ± 0.059 AU; $n = 3$, $^{*}P < 0.05$, $^{***}P < 0.001$). (b) LDH levels in the cell culture supernatant were significantly lower when ACM, hASC, or hBMSC therapy was carried out (I-R model: 0.225 ± 0.006 AU; ACM: 0.208 ± 0.009 AU; hASC: 0.148 ± 0.005 AU; hBMSC: 0.146 ± 0.004 AU; $n = 3$, $^{*}P < 0.05$, $^{***}P < 0.001$). The stem cell treated groups are not significantly different from each other and also not different from the control.

activity measurement and the evaluation of necrosis strengthened the beneficial effect of cell treatment. Importantly, there was no difference in these direct effects between the adipose- and bone-marrow-derived stem cells.

Furthermore, the percentage of live mesenchymal stem cells after 24 hours was the same, so their survival properties are also likely to be similar. These observations are important because many publications indicate a better result with adipose-derived stem cells, but the underlying mechanisms of action are not clearly understood yet, and, to our knowledge, this is the first report on the comparison of the direct effects of adult stem cells on the parenchymal cells of the damaged tissue and on their survival in a standardized situation. Rasmussen et al. have shown that adipose-derived stem cells had preserved cardiac function following myocardial infarction in their animal model while bone-marrow-derived stem cells from the same source had not [26]. They reported that neither of these cell types induced angiogenesis. Thus, based on a recent report [39], they argued that the potential difference between them could be explained by differences in senescence properties of the cells. Others showed in an investigation on spinal cord injury that adipose-derived cells increased angiogenesis more than cells from other mesenchymal sources and expressed higher amounts of VEGF while having similar migration properties to the bone-marrow-derived stem cells [46]. Adipose-derived stem cells were also found to be more effective on cutaneous wounds upregulating fibroblast migration and proliferation [47]. However, this may prove to be problematic in case of myocardial regeneration due to increased possibility of scar formation. Finally, a comparative study indicated ASCs to be a more promising source because of its more favorable immunomodulatory effects [48].

We have drawn a few conclusions from our data on the possible mechanisms of actions, also. First, LDH levels decreased to control levels after cell treatment. This means that necrosis was practically blocked by the added cells, indicating that the dead cells in our study were apoptotic cells. This is beneficial as apoptotic cells were shown to be immunoregulatory, and some researchers argue that the main effect of the current cytotherapy is aspecific and is the consequence of this apoptotic pool [36]. However, it must be realized that this possibility does not explain our results on cell viability as our model is completely reductionist and contains no immune cells. Second, the conditioned medium slightly increased metabolic activity and decreased LDH levels; thus, it had an antinecrotic effect. It means that the paracrine cocktail released from mesenchymal stem cells contains substances that act directly on the ailing postischemic cells. The enhanced metabolic activity may relate to slightly better functionality of the surviving cells while the decreased LDH-levels indicate that the postischemic cells are directed from necrosis towards apoptotic cell death because the ACM had no effect on the cell viability in the flow cytometric measurements which is in accordance with our previous work using bone-marrow-derived cells in cell culture inserts [40].

In our study, the ineffectiveness of the stem cell conditioned media versus the stem cell treatment in increasing live cell numbers means either that the cell-cell contact is particularly important in the direct beneficial effect or the reached concentration of paracrine molecules is not high enough for their effect. The importance of cell-cell contact in the actions of therapeutically added cells was highlighted in earlier studies where the mechanism was related to intercellular tubular connections that potentially lead to mitochondrial exchange between the cells [40, 49]. Cell fusion is another phenomenon which can be observed in coculture studies, and in some cases it was also observed in *in vivo* animal studies of stem cell grafting [30, 50, 51]. The possibility of cell fusion in our model was addressed in our first publication and its frequency was found to be extremely low [40]. However, it must be noted that the extent of cell fusion shows extremely high variation among different culture and detection techniques, and it cannot be ruled out that extensive cell fusion is an *in vitro* artifact [28, 52, 53]. Still, recent studies suggest that despite the low frequency cell fusion may exert relevant impact on stem cell programming or reprogramming in the heart [54]. In view of the recent literature, it is more probable that the mechanism is mediated via paracrine factors, but the stem cells have to be induced by the microenvironment or by contact with injured cells to release these beneficial factors in necessary amounts. It is also possible that during the production of the conditioned media the concentration of paracrine factors in the conditioned media did not reach the levels necessary to be effective. No wonder, studies of late started to concentrate the conditioned medium to achieve higher concentrations and found promising results [55]. Our approach raises the possibility that the secreted molecules are effective only in close proximity to the affected cells where their local concentration can reach high levels. It is highly possible that only direct cell-to-cell contact can provide the necessary distance. It is interesting to note, that such "microparacrine" mechanism exists in relation of stem cells in the bone marrow, where the so-called "endosteal niche-stem-cell synapses" are formed [56]. A final, additional concern could be that conditioned media has a predominant role in angiogenesis; thus, it is ought to be ineffective in our reductionist model [26].

The relative role of the observed direct mechanism in the *in vivo* setting is difficult to measure, but it may be quite robust if we consider that we observed a doubling in the number of live cells. However, it must be realized, that in our experimental model the majority of the therapeutically added stem cells survived unlike the *in vivo* situation where most of the injected cells die soon after the transplantation [36]. Thus, the added cells had a prolonged time for exerting their effect.

At this point, it may be useful to consider some experimental points in our study. Our experimental model was devised to investigate acute effects of therapeutic stem cells on severely damaged cells to give room for the potential effects of stem cells. For this reason, we have set the length of simulated ischemia to a level where only 5–20% of cells survived without any treatment, which reflects the conditions found at the site of the injury in the heart after myocardial infarction.

Comparison of the Direct Effects of Human Adipose- and Bone-Marrow-Derived Stem Cells on Postischemic
Cardiomyoblasts in an In Vitro Simulated Ischemia-Reperfusion Model

181

We demonstrated the suitability of this model by detecting significantly elevated levels of oxidative stress and cellular necrosis after the simulation of ischemia-reperfusion in our earlier publication [42]. The effects were analyzed at 24 hours because we wanted to rule out the potential differentiation of the added stem cells, which occurs over longer time periods.

Some limitations must be accounted for considering our study. In our experiments, we used H9c2 cells which are derived from rat embryonic heart tissue. Obviously, there are differences between these cells and human adult cardiomyocytes, but H9c2 cells are frequently used in studies dealing with reperfusion injuries, and we have ample experience with these cells in our model [57–59]. Furthermore, as our aim was to analyze the direct effects of cells or media on postischemic cells, using H9c2 cultures instead of adult cardiomyocyte cell cultures we could avoid the possibility that inflammatory cells would contaminate the cultures and affect the results. Still, it has to be kept in mind that we used human cells for treatment, but as no immune functions were involved in our model this fact must not had any major effect on our results, and human therapeutic cells are widely used in the literature in animal disease models [60–62]. Also, in our experiments we used an *in vitro* approach to the much more complex issue of stem cell therapy in myocardial infarction, with all the disadvantages and advantages of such model. An *in vitro* transplantation model in a cell culture system cannot mimic the 3-dimensional tissue where cell-to-cell connections are different and it cannot reflect the complex (e.g., immunological) events taking place during and after myocardial infarction. However, a limitation of the *in vivo* models in cell treatment studies is a lack of separation between the direct effect on the treated parenchymal cells and the indirect effect caused by alteration of the environment (e.g., inactivation or reduced migration of leukocytes, angiogenesis, etc.). We believe that our model was appropriate for the scope of our study because it can focus on the direct effects of the added cells on the postischemic cells. The similar benefits achieved with hASC treatments strengthen that hASCs can be an alternative to the most commonly used hBMSCs in the emerging field of cell therapy. Subcutaneous adipose tissue is an attractive source for obtaining autologous mesenchymal stem cells as it can be harvested easily by liposuction which is performed routinely on thousands of people per year. The yield of stem cells per gram of adipose tissue is reported to be superior to that which can be achieved per milliliter of bone marrow [63], and adipose tissue can be harvested safely in much higher quantity. This is important as stem cells constitute only a small portion of cells in bone marrow and their number and differentiation capacity correlate inversely with age [64]. Similarly to hBMSCs, hASCs were shown to be able to differentiate toward osteogenic, adipogenic, myogenic, and chondrogenic lineages [6, 37, 64] and to secrete a host of paracrine factors that can increase angiogenesis and act as antiapoptotic signals [18, 31]. As their direct effects are at least as good as the effects of hBMSCs, our results strengthen the assumption that they constitute a better and more practical source for therapies using adult stem cells. No evidence is available to date, but two Phase I clinical trials have been recently completed to test the safety and feasibility of adipose-derived mesenchymal stem cell treatment in myocardial infarction and in chronic myocardial ischemia (APOLLO, NCT00442806; PRECISE, NCT00426868) [65].

5. Conclusions

Our results highlight that adipose-derived and bone-marrow-derived stem cell treatments can directly save damaged cardiomyoblasts with the same efficacy. The survival of these cells in the noxious, oxidative environment is also similar. These results may indicate that if these cells arrive to the injury site the resulting direct effect will be similar on the cardiac cells so the observed differences in efficacy found in *in vivo* experiments and in clinical trials may relate to different properties in homing, angiogenesis induction, fibroblast regulation, or immunomodulation.

Authors' Contribution

Mónika Szepes and Zsolt Benkő contributed equally to this work.

Acknowledgments

This work was supported by TÉT-SIN, TÁMOP 4.2.2-08/1/KMR-2008-0004, TÁMOP-4.2.1/B 09/1/KMR-2010-0001, OTKA 83803, and Bolyai fellowships. The authors are grateful to Gabriella Vácz for her help in the isolation of human bone-marrow-derived stem cells and to Anna Tutino, Eleni Dongó, and Áron Farkas for their kind assistance in maintaining the cell lines.

References

[1] S. Bajada, I. Mazakova, J. B. Richardson, and N. Ashammakhi, "Updates on stem cells and their applications in regenerative medicine," *Journal of Tissue Engineering and Regenerative Medicine*, vol. 2, no. 4, pp. 169–183, 2008.

[2] S. M. Wu and K. Hochedlinger, "Harnessing the potential of induced pluripotent stem cells for regenerative medicine," *Nature Cell Biology*, vol. 13, no. 5, pp. 497–505, 2011.

[3] C. Leeb, M. Jurga, C. Mcguckin et al., "New perspectives in stem cell research: beyond embryonic stem cells," *Cell Proliferation*, vol. 44, supplement 1, pp. 9–14, 2011.

[4] A. C. Brignier and A. M. Gewirtz, "Embryonic and adult stem cell therapy," *Journal of Allergy and Clinical Immunology*, vol. 125, supplement 2, no. 2, pp. S336–S344, 2010.

[5] R. Sanz-Ruiz, E. Gutiérrez Ibañes, A. V. Arranz, M. E. Fernández Santos, P. L. S. Fernández, and F. Fernández-Avilés, "Phases I-III clinical trials using adult stem cells," *Stem Cells International*, vol. 2010, Article ID 579142, 12 pages, 2010.

[6] P. A. Zuk, M. Zhu, P. Ashjian et al., "Human adipose tissue is a source of multipotent stem cells," *Molecular Biology of the Cell*, vol. 13, no. 12, pp. 4279–4295, 2002.

[7] A. Wilson, P. E. Butler, and A. M. Seifalian, "Adipose-derived stem cells for clinical applications: a review," *Cell Proliferation*, vol. 44, no. 1, pp. 86–98, 2011.

[8] F. Hildner, C. Albrecht, C. Gabriel, H. Redl, and M. van Griensven, "State of the art and future perspectives of articular cartilage regeneration: a focus on adipose-derived stem cells and platelet-derived products," *Journal of Tissue Engineering and Regenerative Medicine*, vol. 5, no. 4, pp. e36–e51, 2011.

[9] J. M. Gimble, W. Grayson, F. Guilak, M. J. Lopez, and G. Vunjak-Novakovic, "Adipose tissue as a stem cell source for musculoskeletal regeneration," *Frontiers in Bioscience*, vol. 3, pp. 69–81, 2011.

[10] S. Lendeckel, A. Jödicke, P. Christophis et al., "Autologous stem cells (adipose) and fibrin glue used to treat widespread traumatic calvarial defects: case report," *Journal of Cranio-Maxillofacial Surgery*, vol. 32, no. 6, pp. 370–373, 2004.

[11] C. M. Cowan, Y.-Y. Shi, O. O. Aalami et al., "Adipose-derived adult stromal cells heal critical-size mouse calvarial defects," *Nature Biotechnology*, vol. 22, no. 5, pp. 560–567, 2004.

[12] M. Cherubino, J. P. Rubin, N. Miljkovic, A. Kelmendi-Doko, and K. G. Marra, "Adipose-derived stem cells for wound healing applications," *Annals of Plastic Surgery*, vol. 66, no. 2, pp. 210–215, 2011.

[13] B. Léobon, J. Roncalli, C. Joffre et al., "Adipose-derived cardiomyogenic cells: *in vitro* expansion and functional improvement in a mouse model of myocardial infarction," *Cardiovascular Research*, vol. 83, no. 4, pp. 757–767, 2009.

[14] R. Sanz-Ruiz, M. E. F. Santos, M. D. Muñoa et al., "Adipose tissue-derived stem cells: the friendly side of a classic cardiovascular foe," *Journal of cardiovascular translational research*, vol. 1, no. 1, pp. 55–63, 2008.

[15] X. Bai, Y. Yan, Y.-H. Song et al., "Both cultured and freshly isolated adipose tissue-derived stem cells enhance cardiac function after acute myocardial infarction," *European Heart Journal*, vol. 31, no. 4, pp. 489–501, 2010.

[16] M. Mazo, J. J. Gavira, B. Pelacho, and F. Prosper, "Adipose-derived stem cells for myocardial infarction," *Journal of Cardiovascular Translational Research*, vol. 4, no. 2, pp. 145–153, 2011.

[17] K. Schenke-Layland, B. M. Strem, M. C. Jordan et al., "Adipose tissue-derived cells improve cardiac function following myocardial infarction," *Journal of Surgical Research*, vol. 153, no. 2, pp. 217–223, 2009.

[18] N. N. Hoke, F. N. Salloum, K. E. Loesser-Casey, and R. C. Kukreja, "Cardiac regenerative potential of adipose tissue-derived stem cells," *Acta Physiologica Hungarica*, vol. 96, no. 3, pp. 251–265, 2009.

[19] C. Valina, K. Pinkernell, Y.-H. Song et al., "Intracoronary administration of autologous adipose tissue-derived stem cells improves left ventricular function, perfusion, and remodelling after acute myocardial infarction," *European Heart Journal*, vol. 28, no. 21, pp. 2667–2677, 2007.

[20] A. Abdel-Latif, R. Bolli, I. M. Tleyjeh et al., "Adult bone marrow-derived cells for cardiac repair: a systematic review and meta-analysis," *Archives of Internal Medicine*, vol. 167, no. 10, pp. 989–997, 2007.

[21] M. J. Lipinski, G. G. L. Biondi-Zoccai, A. Abbate et al., "Impact of intracoronary cell therapy on left ventricular function in the setting of acute myocardial infarction. A collaborative systematic review and meta-analysis of controlled clinical trials," *Journal of the American College of Cardiology*, vol. 50, no. 18, pp. 1761–1767, 2007.

[22] E. Chavakis, M. Koyanagi, and S. Dimmeler, "Enhancing the outcome of cell therapy for cardiac repair: progress from bench to bedside and back," *Circulation*, vol. 121, no. 2, pp. 325–335, 2010.

[23] M. Mazo, M. Araña, B. Pelacho, and F. Prosper, "Mesenchymal stem cells and cardiovascular disease: a bench to bedside roadmap," *Stem Cells International*, vol. 2012, Article ID 175979, 11 pages, 2012.

[24] M. T. Elnakish, F. Hassan, D. Dakhlallah et al., "Mesenchymal stem cells for cardiac regeneration: translation to bedside reality," *Stem Cells International*, vol. 2012, Article ID 646038, 14 pages, 2012.

[25] M. Mazo, V. Planat-Bénard, G. Abizanda et al., "Transplantation of adipose derived stromal cells is associated with functional improvement in a rat model of chronic myocardial infarction," *European Journal of Heart Failure*, vol. 10, no. 5, pp. 454–462, 2008.

[26] J. G. Rasmussen, O. Frobert, C. Holst-Hansen et al., "Comparison of human adipose-derived stem cells and bone marrow-derived stem cells in a myocardial infarction model," *Cell Transplantation*. In press.

[27] M. Alvarez-Dolado, R. Pardal, J. M. Garcia-Verdugo et al., "Fusion of bone-marrow-derived cells with Purkinje neurons, cardiomyocytes and hepatocytes," *Nature*, vol. 425, no. 6961, pp. 968–973, 2003.

[28] J. Kajstura, M. Rota, B. Whang et al., "Bone marrow cells differentiate in cardiac cell lineages after infarction independently of cell fusion," *Circulation Research*, vol. 96, no. 1, pp. 127–137, 2005.

[29] C. E. Murry, M. H. Soonpaa, H. Reinecke et al., "Haematopoietic stem cells do not transdifferentiate into cardiac myocytes in myocardial infarcts," *Nature*, vol. 428, no. 6983, pp. 664–668, 2004.

[30] J. M. Nygren, S. Jovinge, M. Breitbach et al., "Bone marrow-derived hematopoietic cells generate cardiomyocytes at a low frequency through cell fusion, but not transdifferentiation," *Nature Medicine*, vol. 10, no. 5, pp. 494–501, 2004.

[31] J. Rehman, D. Traktuev, J. Li et al., "Secretion of angiogenic and antiapoptotic factors by human adipose stromal cells," *Circulation*, vol. 109, no. 10, pp. 1292–1298, 2004.

[32] T. P. Lozito and R. S. Tuan, "Mesenchymal stem cells inhibit both endogenous and exogenous MMPs via secreted TIMPs," *Journal of Cellular Physiology*, vol. 226, no. 2, pp. 385–396, 2011.

[33] S. Sadat, S. Gehmert, Y.-H. Song et al., "The cardioprotective effect of mesenchymal stem cells is mediated by IGF-I and VEGF," *Biochemical and Biophysical Research Communications*, vol. 363, no. 3, pp. 674–679, 2007.

[34] T. Kinnaird, E. Stabile, M. S. Burnett et al., "Marrow-derived stromal cells express genes encoding a broad spectrum of arteriogenic cytokines and promote *in vitro* and *in vivo* arteriogenesis through paracrine mechanisms," *Circulation Research*, vol. 94, no. 5, pp. 678–685, 2004.

[35] H. K. Haider and M. Ashraf, "Strategies to promote donor cell survival: combining preconditioning approach with stem cell transplantation," *Journal of Molecular and Cellular Cardiology*, vol. 45, no. 4, pp. 554–566, 2008.

[36] I. B. Copland and J. Galipeau, "Death and inflammation following somatic cell transplantation," *Seminars in Immunopathology*, vol. 33, no. 6, pp. 535–550, 2011.

[37] P. A. Zuk, M. Zhu, H. Mizuno et al., "Multilineage cells from human adipose tissue: implications for cell-based therapies," *Tissue Engineering*, vol. 7, no. 2, pp. 211–228, 2001.

[38] K. M. Kompisch, C. Lange, D. Steinemann et al., "Neurogenic transdifferentiation of human adipose-derived stem cells? A critical protocol reevaluation with special emphasis on cell

proliferation and cell cycle alterations," *Histochemistry and Cell Biology*, vol. 134, no. 5, pp. 453–468, 2010.

[39] M. A. Vidal, N. J. Walker, E. Napoli, and D. L. Borjesson, "Evaluation of senescence in mesenchymal stem cells isolated from equine bone marrow, adipose tissue, and umbilical cord tissue," *Stem Cells and Development*, vol. 21, no. 2, pp. 273–283, 2012.

[40] A. Cselenyák, E. Pankotai, E. M. Horváth, L. Kiss, and Z. Lacza, "Mesenchymal stem cells rescue cardiomyoblasts from cell death in an *in vitro* ischemia model via direct cell-to-cell connections," *BMC Cell Biology*, vol. 11, article 29, 2010.

[41] A. Cselenyák, Z. Benko, M. Szepes, L. Kiss, and Z. Lacza, "Stem cell transplantation in an *in vitro* simulated ischemia/reperfusion model," *Journal of Visualized Experiments*, no. 57, Article ID e3575, 2011.

[42] M. Szepes, Z. Janicsek, Z. Benko et al., "Pretreatment of therapeutic cells with poly(ADP-ribose) polymerase inhibitor enhances their efficacy in an *in vitro* model of cell-based therapy in myocardial infarct," *International Journal of Molecular Medicine*, vol. 31, no. 1, pp. 26–32, 2013.

[43] M. A. King, "Detection of dead cells and measurement of cell killing by flow cytometry," *Journal of Immunological Methods*, vol. 243, no. 1-2, pp. 155–166, 2000.

[44] R. de La Fuente, J. L. Abad, J. García-Castro et al., "Dedifferentiated adult articular chondrocytes: a population of human multipotent primitive cells," *Experimental Cell Research*, vol. 297, no. 2, pp. 313–328, 2004.

[45] J. Oswald, S. Boxberger, B. Jørgensen et al., "Mesenchymal stem cells can be differentiated into endothelial cells *in vitro*," *Stem Cells*, vol. 22, no. 3, pp. 377–384, 2004.

[46] X. Liu, Z. Wang, R. Wang et al., "Direct comparison of the potency of human mesenchymal stem cells derived from amnion tissue, bone marrow and adipose tissue at inducing dermal fibroblast responses to cutaneous wounds," *International Journal of Molecular Medicine*, vol. 31, no. 2, pp. 407–415, 2013.

[47] Z. Zhou, Y. Chen, H. Zhang et al., "Comparison of mesenchymal stromal cells from human bone marrow and adipose tissue for the treatment of spinal cord injury," *Cytotherapy*, vol. 15, no. 4, pp. 434–448, 2013.

[48] Z. Xishan, H. Baoxin, Z. Xinna et al., "Comparison of the effects of human adipose and bone marrow mesenchymal stem cells on T lymphocytes," *Cell Biology International*, vol. 37, no. 1, pp. 11–18, 2013.

[49] E. Y. Plotnikov, T. G. Khryapenkova, A. K. Vasileva et al., "Cell-to-cell cross-talk between mesenchymal stem cells and cardiomyocytes in co-culture," *Journal of Cellular and Molecular Medicine*, vol. 12, no. 5A, pp. 1622–1631, 2008.

[50] F. Ishikawa, H. Shimazu, L. D. Shultz et al., "Purified human hematopoietic stem cells contribute to the generation of cardiomyocytes through cell fusion," *The FASEB journal*, vol. 20, no. 7, pp. 950–952, 2006.

[51] Z. Lacza, E. Horváth, and D. W. Busija, "Neural stem cell transplantation in cold lesion: a novel approach for the investigation of brain trauma and repair," *Brain Research Protocols*, vol. 11, no. 3, pp. 145–154, 2003.

[52] J. Garbade, A. Schubert, A. J. Rastan et al., "Fusion of bone marrow-derived stem cells with cardiomyocytes in a heterologous *in vitro* model," *European Journal of Cardio-Thoracic Surgery*, vol. 28, no. 5, pp. 685–691, 2005.

[53] P. Menasché, "You can't judge a book by its cover," *Circulation*, vol. 113, no. 10, pp. 1275–1277, 2006.

[54] N. A. Kouris, J. A. Schaefer, M. Hatta et al., "Directed fusion of mesenchymal stem cells with cardiomyocytes via VSV-G facilitates stem cell programming," *Stem Cells International*, vol. 2012, Article ID 414038, 13 pages, 2012.

[55] L. Timmers, S. K. Lim, I. E. Hoefer et al., "Human mesenchymal stem cell-conditioned medium improves cardiac function following myocardial infarction," *Stem Cell Research*, vol. 6, no. 3, pp. 206–214, 2011.

[56] A. Wilson and A. Trumpp, "Bone-marrow haematopoietic-stem-cell niches," *Nature Reviews Immunology*, vol. 6, no. 2, pp. 93–106, 2006.

[57] G.-Q. Huang, J.-N. Wang, J.-M. Tang et al., "The combined transduction of copper, zinc-superoxide dismutase and catalase mediated by cell-penetrating peptide, PEP-1, to protect myocardium from ischemia-reperfusion injury," *Journal of Translational Medicine*, vol. 9, article no. 73, 2011.

[58] K. T. Keyes, Y. Ye, Y. Lin et al., "Resolvin E1 protects the rat heart against reperfusion injury," *The American Journal of Physiology*, vol. 299, no. 1, pp. H153–H164, 2010.

[59] D. K. Singla and D. E. McDonald, "Factors released from embryonic stem cells inhibit apoptosis of H9c2 cells," *The American Journal of Physiology*, vol. 293, no. 3, pp. H1590–H1595, 2007.

[60] D. Yang, W. Wang, L. Li et al., "The relative contribution of paracine effect versus direct differentiation on adipose-derived stem cell transplantation mediated cardiac repair," *PLoS One*, vol. 8, no. 3, Article ID e59020, 2013.

[61] S. Alshammary, S. Fukushima, S. Miyagawa et al., "Impact of cardiac stem cell sheet transplantation on myocardial infarction," *Surgery Today*, 2013.

[62] A. R. Williams, K. E. Hatzistergos, B. Addicott et al., "Enhanced effect of combining human cardiac stem cells and bone marrow mesenchymal stem cells to reduce infarct size and to restore cardiac function after myocardial infarction," *Circulation*, vol. 127, no. 2, pp. 213–223, 2013.

[63] J. K. Fraser, I. Wulur, Z. Alfonso, and M. H. Hedrick, "Fat tissue: an underappreciated source of stem cells for biotechnology," *Trends in Biotechnology*, vol. 24, no. 4, pp. 150–154, 2006.

[64] L. Peng, Z. Jia, X. Yin et al., "Comparative analysis of mesenchymal stem cells from bone marrow, cartilage, and adipose tissue," *Stem Cells and Development*, vol. 17, no. 4, pp. 761–773, 2008.

[65] P. Diez Villanueva, R. Sanz-Ruiz, A. Nunez Garcia et al., "Functional multipotency of stem cells: what do we need from them in the heart?" *Stem Cells International*, vol. 2012, Article ID 817364, 12 pages, 2012.

19

Histone Deacetylase Inhibitors in Cell Pluripotency, Differentiation, and Reprogramming

Androniki Kretsovali,[1] Christiana Hadjimichael,[1,2] and Nikolaos Charmpilas[2]

[1] *Institute of Molecular Biology and Biotechnology, FORTH, Heraklion, 70013 Crete, Greece*
[2] *Department of Biology, University of Crete, Heraklion, 71409 Crete, Greece*

Correspondence should be addressed to Androniki Kretsovali, kretsova@imbb.forth.gr

Academic Editor: Andras Dinnyes

Histone deacetylase inhibitors (HDACi) are small molecules that have important and pleiotropic effects on cell homeostasis. Under distinct developmental conditions, they can promote either self-renewal or differentiation of embryonic stem cells. In addition, they can promote directed differentiation of embryonic and tissue-specific stem cells along the neuronal, cardiomyocytic, and hepatic lineages. They have been used to facilitate embryo development following somatic cell nuclear transfer and induced pluripotent stem cell derivation by ectopic expression of pluripotency factors. In the latter method, these molecules not only increase effectiveness, but can also render the induction independent of the oncogenes c-Myc and Klf4. Here we review the molecular pathways that are involved in the functions of HDAC inhibitors on stem cell differentiation and reprogramming of somatic cells into pluripotency. Deciphering the mechanisms of HDAC inhibitor actions is very important to enable their exploitation for efficient and simple tissue regeneration therapies.

1. Introduction

Stem cells are distinguished from other cell types by their unique properties to self-renew and differentiate along multiple lineages [1]. These processes are regulated by extrinsic and intrinsic determinants that affect gene expression profiles, signal transduction pathways, and epigenetic mechanisms.

DNA methylation and histone modifications constitute major mechanisms that are responsible for epigenetic regulation of gene expression during development and differentiation [2–4]. Among other histone modifications, acetylation is very important in nucleosome assembly and chromatin folding. Acetylation favors an open chromatin structure by interfering with the interactions between nucleosomes and releasing the histone tails from the linker DNA. Chromatin regions that are marked by lysine acetylation catalyzed by Histone Acetyl-transferase (HATs) are generally actively transcribed, whereas regions that are bound by Histone Deacetylases (HDACs) bear deacetylated lysines and are inactive [5]. Accordingly, HATs and HDACs reside in multiprotein coactivatory or corepressory complexes, respectively. HATs and HDACs may act either in a site-specific manner, when they are recruited through binding to sequence-specific DNA binding activators or repressors, or in a broad manner whereby they function across large genomic areas.

There are up to date 18 genes coding for histone (or epsilon lysine) deacetylases in the mammalian genomes. They are grouped in four families. Group I (comprising HDACs 1, 2, 3, and 8). IIa (HDAC 4, 5, 7, 9), IIb (6, 10), III (SIRT 1–7), and IV (HDAC 11) [6]. In spite of their name, histone deacetylases have also nonhistone target proteins especially those belonging to group II which do not have histones as substrates. Class I HDACs participate in diverse repressory complexes via interaction with different cofactors such as the Sin3A, Nurd, and CoRest [7]. Contrary to their consideration as repressors, HDACs may act as coactivators of transcription as was reported in the interferon stimulated genes [8]. Genome-wide detection of HATs and HDACs of higher eukaryotic organism has revealed a highly complex situation, active genes are bound by both enzyme types, whereas inactive genes are not bound by HDACs [9]. Inactive genes that were primed for activation by H3K4 methylation were transiently bound by both HATs and HDACs [9].

HDAC inhibitors (HDACis) are natural or synthetic small molecules that can inhibit the activities of HDACs. In spite of similarities in their enzymatic activities, loss of function experiments have attributed highly specific roles to individual members of HDAC proteins in the course of development and differentiation. In addition, HDAC inhibitors that have broad specificity towards their HDAC targets have shown highly specific effects depending on the target cell type [10].

The profound events that govern stem cell differentiation and somatic cell reprogramming to pluripotency are mainly epigenetic [11]. HDACis are epigenetic modifiers that can promote efficient and temporally regulated control of gene expression. This paper will discuss the role of HDACi in stem cell pluripotency and differentiation as well as in the reprogramming of somatic cells into pluripotency.

2. The Role of HDAC Class I and II Members in Mammalian Development and Differentiation

Analysis of knockout mice lacking HDAC genes has revealed their functions during mammalian development and differentiation [10]. HDAC1 gene deletion is embryonic lethal due to cell proliferation and growth defects [12]. The same proliferation defects were reported in HDAC1-null embryonic stem (ES) cells which overexpress the cell cycle inhibitors p21 and p27 [13]. This analysis has revealed a dual role for HDAC1 in both repression and activation of gene transcription. Tissue-specific deletion of HDAC1 in mice did not have significant effect due to functional redundancy with HDAC2 [14]. However, deletion of HDAC2 was reported to cause perinatal lethality in one publication [12], whereas it resulted in a failure to reactivate fetal gene expression programme under cardiac hypertrophic stress in another study [15]. Regarding cardiac growth and development, one allele of either HDAC1 or 2 is sufficient, whereas conditional deletion of both HDAC1 and 2 is lethal due to heart development failure [12].

Similar to the cardiac differentiation, HDAC1 and 2 have essential but redundant roles in the differentiation of neuronal precursors into neurons [12]. Deletion of both enzymes results in severe brain abnormalities and lethality at postnatal day 7 [12]. The roles of individual HDACs 1, 2, and 3 have been assessed in the differentiation of cortical stem cells using dominant negative mutants [16]. Specifically, all three of them inhibit oligodentrocytic differentiation, HDAC2 inhibits astrocytic, whereas HDAC1 is required for neuronal differentiation. On the other hand, specific deletion of both HDAC1 and 2 in oligodendrocyte lineage cells resulted in Wnt pathway activation, which in turn inhibited oligodendrocyte development by repressing Olig2 expression [17]. In agreement with these data, ablation of both HDAC1 and 2 in Schwann cells caused severe myelination deficiency due to NFkB deacetylation [18].

Finally, HDAC1 and 2 have important functions in hemopoiesis [19]. HDAC1 activity is required for erythroid, whereas it blocks myeloid differentiation [20].

HDAC3 deletion is embryonic lethal due to deficient gastrulation [21–23] that is connected to failure in DNA damage repair mechanisms [23]. Conditional tissue-specific deletions of HDAC3 have pointed to an involvement in liver [22] and heart [21] function.

Although class I HDACs are widely expressed, members of the IIa group show tissue-restricted expression. HDAC4 regulates skeletogenesis and knockout mice die in the first week after birth due to excessive ossification of endochondral cartilage which interferes with breathing [24]. This effect is due to unrestricted function of MEF2 and RUNX2, two transcription factors that activate bone formation [25, 26]. RUNX2 is activated by MEF2 and both MEF2 and RUNX2 are targeted by HDAC4 [26]. HDACs 5 and 9 control, in redundant manner, cardiovascular development since single knockout mice are viable, whereas double disruption leads to lethality caused by defective cardiac development resulting from unrestricted activation of MEF2- [27], SRF-, myocardin- and Calmodulin-binding transcriptional activator 2 [28]. In addition, HDAC 4, 5, and 9 control skeletal muscle differentiation through negative regulation of MEF2, PGC1a, and NFAT in response to calcium signals [29] and motor neuron activation [30]. HDAC7 is specifically expressed in endothelial cells of the cardiovascular system [31] and HDAC7 gene deletion results in embryonic lethality due to vascular rupture and excessive hemorrhages [31]. These effects are caused by extreme activation of matrix metalloproteinase (MMP) 10 which is normaly inhibited by HDAC7 [31]. Members of the HDAC class IIb group (HDAC 6, 10) regulate cytoskeletal dynamics by controlling the acetylation of cytoskeletal proteins such as tubulin [32].

HDAC expression and activity are intimately associated with the emergence of neoplasias. In Acute Promyelocytic Leukemia (APL), fusions between Promyelocytic Leukemia (PML) and Retinoic Acid Receptor (RAR) recruit HDACs resulting in the repression of differentiation-related genes [33, 34]. In solid tumors, mutations in HATs [35] and overexpression of HDAC-associated proteins lead to relative hyperactivity of HDAC. Consequently, HDAC inhibitors are long established antitumor agents that were known before the identification of their target HDAC molecules [34, 36].

3. Inhibitors of HDACs

HDAC class I and II inhibitors (HDACi) fall into discrete structural categories such as hydroxamic acids, cyclic peptides, benzamides, benzofuranone, and sulfonamide containing molecules [37, 38]. The biological effects of HDACi result from positive or negative regulation of gene expression by induced acetylation of histones, transcription factors or other proteins. Genome-wide analyses of gene expression changes upon HDACi administration have revealed that approximately equal numbers of genes are induced and repressed [39]. The genes affected are highly dependent on the cell type and transformed cells are extremely sensitive as opposed to normal cells. Most studies have been performed with transformed cells. The antitumor activity of HDACi results from a combination of many processes involving cell cycle arrest, apoptosis, activation of mitotic cell death, and inhibition of angiogenesis. In addition, but not unrelated to the aforementioned effects on cell functions, HDACis were reported to induce differentiation of certain cancer cell types [36]. This property gains extreme importance in light of the recently established discovery of "cancer stem cells" [40], a small population of cells that are able to reproduce the tumor and possess self-renewal and pluripotency activities.

4. HDAC Inhibitors in Stem Cell Self-Renewal and Differentiation

Due to their activity in epigenetic regulation, HDACis have been widely used in order to alter the differentiation state of stem and somatic cells as shown in Table 1.

4.1. Embryonic Stem Cell Pluripotency. Differentiation is a process of gradual loss of potency that ends up to the point where specific cell fate is acquired. Embryonic stem (ES) cells are isolated from the inner cell mass of blastocysts [1, 41, 42] and are characterized by indefinite self-renewal and pluripotency, the capability to follow all potential differentiation pathways [43, 44]. Both mouse and human ES cells express networks of pluripotency transcriptional regulators exemplified by Oct4, Sox2, and Nanog [45]. They differ in the requirements for externally provided cytokines and growth factors. For instance, mouse ES cell culture requires Leukemia Inhibiting Factor (LIF) [46], whereas human ES cell culture depends on Activin/Nodal and FGF [47]. This difference is due to the developmental stages from which these two cell types were isolated. Human ES cells are derived from later stage of embryonic development compared to the mouse and are highly similar to mouse EpiSC (epiblast stem cells) [47–49]. The differentiation of stem cells is very sensitive to epigenetic changes. Therefore, application of epigenetic regulators such as inhibitors of DNA methylation (5 Azacytidine) and HDAC inhibitors may be valuable tools for stem cell interventions [50].

In accordance with their effects on the differentiation of cancer cells, HDACis are able to promote the differentiation of ES cells. Treatment with Trichostatin A (TSA) promotes morphological and gene expression changes reminiscent of differentiation even in the presence of LIF [51, 52]. Inhibition of HDAC activity accelerated the early differentiation steps of ES cells without being sufficient for commitment to a specific lineage. Genome-wide analysis revealed two gene groups that are targeted by TSA: the first one contains genes related to pluripotency that are suppressed by TSA (Sall4, Nanog, Klf4, Oct4, and Sox2), the second is required for lineage-specific differentiation and its expression is upregulated by TSA [52].

In contrast to these studies, other studies have shown that HDACis increase self-renewal and interfere with differentiation. Low doses of TSA (10 nM) reverted mouse embryoid bodies towards the undifferentiated state [53] and employment of sodium butyrate (NaBu) was reported to support human and mouse ES cells self-renewal when administered

within a narrow range of concentrations [54]. In the latter study, low doses of butyrate (and TSA) were able to substitute for FGF2 (human ES) and LIF (mouse ES). However, higher doses led to differentiation. Surprisingly, nonoverlapping transcriptional expression profile changes were observed in butyrate-treated human and mouse ES cells [54]. These findings have shown the ability of butyrate to modulate the stem cell stage pushing mouse ES forward and pulling human ES backward [54]. In agreement with these data, treatment of mouse ES with TSA was able to shift a population of epiblast-like ESC towards an ICM-like state [54, 55]. A conclusion of all these studies might be that HDACis exert an anti-differentiation effect when low doses are applied on cells that have already exited from self-renewal either as embryoid bodies [53] or epiblast-like [54, 55] cells, whereas higher doses applied on undifferentiated cells provoke differentiations [51, 52]. The same effect was observed upon HDACi treatment of two embryonic carcinoma (EC) cell lines F9 and P19. In F9 cells which belong to a less differentiated state, the expression of the pluripotency factor *Fgf4* decreased after treatment with Valproic acid (VPA) and TSA. In contrast, the same treatment of P19 cells, which are more differentiated, caused the elevation of *Fgf4* expression [56]. In agreement with this data, reactivation of pluripotency genes such as Oct4, Nanog, and Klf4 was observed in neurosphere cells treated with TSA and azacytidine, AzaC [57]. Hence, changes in the acetylation levels of stem cells result in alterations of the differentiation status in correlation with the developmental stage.

Directed differentiation of ES cells is not easy to control. Differentiation protocols generally rely either on the generation of ES cell aggregates (embryoid bodies) or on culturing on stromal cells. Effectiveness and selectivity need to be significantly improved in order for ES cell to be used as tools for cell-based therapies.

HDACi treatment was used for directed differentiation of mouse ES cells towards the cardiomyocytic lineage. TSA added on embryoid bodies between days 7 and 8 potentiated cardiac differentiation due to hyperacetylation of GATA4 [58] a master regulator of cardiogenesis. In addition, TSA induced, whereas HDAC4 overexpression inhibited, cardiomyogenesis of embryonic carcinoma P19 cells [59]. TSA was also able to facilitate the myocardial differentiation of induced pluripotent stem cells [60]. Interestingly, TSA and NaBu were reported to induce HDAC4 proteasomal degradation which in turn results in MEF2 activation and cardiac lineage commitment [61]. On the other hand, NaBu was proven effective in the induction of pancreatic and hepatic differentiation from mouse and human ES cells [62–64].

4.2. Tissue-Specific Stem Cells

4.2.1. Neural Stem Cell Differentiation. As indicated previously ablation of HDAC1 and 2 is postnatal lethal due to disorganization of brain structures [12]. However, administration of HDAC inhibitors led to the induction of neuronal and suppression of glial differentiation [65]. In addition HDAC activity is required for timing of oligodendrocyte differentiation [66].

TABLE 1: Functions of HDAC inhibitors in stem cell self-renewal or differentiation and somatic cell reprogramming to pluripotency.

Name	Chemical structure	Self-renewal	Differentiation	Reprogramming	References
Apicidin		—	—	+	[67]
m-Carboxycinnamic acid bishydroxamide (CBHA)		—	—	+	[68]
Chlamydocin		↑ HSCs			[69]
Entinostat (MS-275)		—	↑ Neuronal ↓ Oligodentrocytic	+	[70] [67]
M344		—	↑ Neuronal ↓ Oligodendrocyte	—	[70]
Oxamflatin		—	—	+	[71]
Scriptaid		—	—	+	[72]
Sodium butyrate (NaBu)		↑ hESC ↑ mESC	↓ Adipogenic, chondrogenic neurogenic ↑ Osteogenic ↑ Ductal ↑ Pancreatic and hepatic	+	[52] [52] [73] [73] [74] [60–62] [67, 75, 76]
Suberoylanilide hydroxamic acid (SAHA)		—	↑ Neuronal ↓ Oligodendrocyte	+	[70] [71]

TABLE 1: Continued.

Name	Chemical structure	Self-renewal	Differentiation	Reprogramming	References
Trichostatin A (TSA)		↑ mESC ↑ ECCs (P19) ↑ Neurosphere cells			[51] [54] [55]
			↑ ESCs ↑ NSCs Ductal Cardiomyocytic ↑ ECCs (F9) ↑ Myocardial		[49, 50] [77] [74] [78] [54] [58]
				+	[67, 79–81]
Valproic acid (VPA)		↑ ECCs (P19)			[54]
			↓ Adipogenic, chondrogenic neurogenic ↑ Osteogenic ↑ Ductal ↑ ECCs (F9) ↓ Astrocyte, oligodendrocyte ↑ Neuronal		[73] [73] [74] [54] [65] [63, 66, 82]
				+	[81, 83]

Embryonic Stem Cells (ESCs), embryonic carcinoma Cells (ECCs), hemopoietic stem cells (HSCs), and neural stem cells (NSCs).

Specifically, VPA was reported to increase neuronal differentiation of adult neural progenitor cells and inhibit astrocyte and oligodendrocyte differentiation [65]. Moreover, VPA administration inhibited the differentiation of oligodendrocyte progenitor cells in the developing rat brain [66].

The molecular mechanism of VPA function was induction of NeuroD, a neurogenic bHLH transcription factor [65]. Derepression of NeuroD and neuronal fate activation was also caused by HDAC5 nuclear exclusion [77]. In another study, VPA promoted neuronal fate commitment via activation of the ERK pathway [70]. TSA was able to increase differentiation of neural stem cells at the expense of astrocyte production [82]. Importantly, the TSA-produced nerve cells bear normal electrophysiological properties and morphological characteristics such as the extension of long dendrites with branching points. Treatment of Adult Subventricular Zone (SVZ) precursor cells with MS-275, M344, and suberoylanilide hydroxamic acid (SAHA) increased neuronal differentiation and inhibited oligodendrocyte production via induction of NeuroD cyclinD2 and B-lymphocyte translocation gene 3 [84]. VPA was reported to promote neuronal differentiation of hippocampal neural progenitor cells by induction of proneural factors Ngn1, Mash1, and p15 and histone H4 acetylation [85]. Combination of TSA with Shh, Fgf8, and Wnt1 promotes differentiation of nonmecencephalic neural stem cells to dopaminergic neurons [69]. Interestingly, the regulatory role of histone acetylation in the nervous system is evolutionarily conserved between vertebrates and invertebrates. High levels of acetylation are required for neuronal, whereas low levels are connected to the glial differentiation of Drosophila neural stem cells [86].

4.2.2. Hemopoietic Stem Cell Self-Renewal and Differentiation. Mouse and human hemopoietic stem cells (HSC) self-renewal was potentiated by chlamydocin [87]. In another study, the application of TSA with 5-AzaC increased 12.5-fold the proliferation of HSC isolated from umbilical cord HDACi [73, 74].

Mesenchymal stem cells (MSCs) from adipose tissue and umbilical cord blood were treated with two HDAC inhibitors, VPA, and NaBu [88]. Posttreatment controlled differentiation was conducted into bone, fat, cartilage, and nervous tissue. Different results were obtained depending on the cell types which were examined. VPA and NaBu attenuated the efficiency of adipogenic, chondrogenic, and neurogenic derivation. On the other hand, osteogenic differentiation was elevated after HDACi treatment. An interesting new prospect has arisen following a publication which supports that HDAC inhibitors can be used to direct pancreatic cells to a specific lineage. It was shown that NaBu and TSA promote ductal differentiation at the expense of the acinar fate [78]. Thus, cells with exocrine function are converted to endocrine cells, capable of producing hormones such as insulin and somatostatin [89].

4.2.3. Cardiomyocytic Differentiation. Cardiac side population cells isolated from rat hearts were coaxed in cardiomyocytic differentiation by TSA treatment [90]. TSA induced the expression of transcription factors Nkx2.5, GATA4, and MEF2C that play important roles in the orchestration of the events that lead to the production of cardiomyocytes, endothelial, and smooth muscle cells [90]. In another study, TSA and azacytidine treatment promoted cardiomyocytic differentiation of mesenchymal stem cells via induction of the same transcription factors GATA-4, NKx2.5, and MEF2c [91].

5. HDAC Inhibitors in Cell Reprogramming to Pluripotency

Reprogramming differentiated somatic cells to pluripotent stem cells has emerged as a way of producing patient-specific stem cells. These cells can be possible candidates for regenerative medicine after their differentiation to a specific cell fate.

A strategy used to reverse the differentiated state of cells was somatic cell nucleus transfer (SCNT) to enucleated eggs or oocytes [92, 93]. This proved in an emphatic way the fact that cell differentiation is not an irreversible process and that the nucleus of a differentiated cell can be reprogrammed to follow a dedifferentiation program. Additionally, it is a common belief that the more ancestral a cell is, the easier it is to be reprogrammed using the method of nuclear transfer. There are several reports showing that HDAC inhibitors can in fact be very helpful tools in the attempt to increase the efficiency of nuclear transfer experiments (Table 1).

Early reports have applied TSA to donor cells [94] or to the embryos following SCNT [68, 72] and shown that it improves both the in vivo and in vitro developmental rate. TSA was effective as cloning facilitating reagent for many species embryos, bovine ([95], mouse ([71, 96]), and porcine ([97]). TSA treatment caused chromatin rearrangements such as elevated histone acetylation and chromosome decondensation as well as increased rate of RNA synthesis [98]). Treatment of SCNT-generated mouse embryos with scriptaid improved the cloning efficiency for various inbred strains [96]. Moreover, scriptaid treatment resulted in higher levels of nascent mRNA transcription at the two-cell stage and this increase depended on the genotype of the mouse strain used. The cloned mice were both viable and fertile and there was a positive correlation between the increase in nascent mRNA synthesis and full-term development of cloned mice [96]. A different HDACi, CBHA, was reported to augment the developmental potential of cloned mouse embryos at both the pre- and postimplantation stages. Furthermore, CBHA treatment resulted in a statistically significant increase in the total ICM cell number, simultaneously reducing the ratio of apoptotic cells. In addition, it was shown that Oct4 expression was more abundant in the population of cells isolated from blastocysts of treated animals than untreated ones. Hence, those cells resembled ES cells as was confirmed by staining for pluripotency markers (Sox2, SSEA1, alkaline phosphatase) [71]. Finally two other HDAC I and IIa/b inhibitors suberoylanilide hydroxamic acid (SAHA) and oxamflatin could improve the development of cloned mice by reducing the apoptosis in blastocysts [99].

In a pioneer work, the group of Yamanaka [100] reprogrammed fetal and adult mouse fibroblasts to induced Pluripotent Stem (iPS) cells using four key transcription factors, namely Oct4, Sox2, c-Myc, and Klf4. A year later human fibroblasts were reprogrammed by the group of Takahasi et al. [101] and Park et al. [79], whereas the group of Thomson substituted the oncogenic factors Klf4 and c-Myc with Nanog and Lin28 [102]. The aforementioned iPS cells possess identical characteristics with ES cells, such as expression of pluripotency markers, ES cell morphology, self-renewal, and capability of teratoma formation [79, 101].

In order to improve the efficiency of reprogramming, several strategies were developed [83] using small molecules such as DNA methyltransferase inhibitors (5 AzaC, [75]), histone methylotransferase inhibitors (BIX, [76]), and HDAC inhibitors (Table 1). Important steps have been made towards the direction of replacing the oncogenic factors with chemical compounds. In particular, Valproic acid (VPA) was used to substitute for c-myc [80]. VPA and the pluripotency factors Oct4, Sox2, and Klf4 were able to reprogram primary human fibroblasts. The presence of VPA increased the number of iPS colonies by 50-fold. Produced iPS cells resemble ES cells in pluripotency and gene expression profiles [80]. In another study, Klf4 was fully dispensable [67]. The combination of Oct4, Sox2, and VPA was sufficient to reprogram somatic cells with a similar efficiency compared to three-factor reprogramming (Oct4, Sox2, and Klf4). These iPS cells exhibited several desired characteristics, such as increased levels of pluripotency markers and alkaline phosphatase activity. In addition, they seemed morphologically similar to human ES cells and were karyotypically normal. Finally, the two factor-induced human iPS cells were able to form teratomas derived from all three lineages. It is possible that VPA treatment sets somatic cells in a transition state before their complete dedifferentiation [67]. These results offer great possibilities in attaining full reprogramming with chemical reagents, a procedure both safe and practical to be used in human therapies.

In a recent study [75], human fetal fibroblasts were reprogrammed to pluripotency using human ES cell extracts with the addition of 5-azacytidine, TSA, and retinoic acid. This proves that the epigenetic state of cells has a great impact on the efficiency of reprogramming by this method. During the process, upregulation of pluripotency markers (Oct4, Sox2) and morphological changes were observed. In parallel, markers of differentiation (LAMIN A/C) were downregulated, showing a positive correlation between dedifferentiation, and increase in acetylation status of cells.

Another HDAC inhibitor NaBu used at low doses improved the generation of iPS cells by 50-fold by using retroviral or "piggyback" vectors for reprogramming human fibroblasts even in the absence of Klf4 and c-myc [81]. In another study, butyrate was reported to potentiate iPS cell generation from mouse embryonic fibroblasts in the presence of c-myc [103]. This difference might be due to differences in the endogenous c-myc levels between the human and mouse cells.

In addition to the typical iPS cells, reversion of differentiation was assisted by the addition of HDACi in other cell types. Dedifferentiation of primordial germ cells (PGC) into pluripotent embryonic germ (EG) cells was achieved using TSA to replace FGF-2 [104]. A high-throughput screen has revealed the ability of four HDAC inhibitors (NaBu, TSA, MS-275 and Apicidin) to reprogram oligodendrocyte progenitors (OPC) into multipotent neural stem-like cells that can generate both neurons and glia [105]. Finally, an intriguing new possibility emerged from a recent publication using the nematode *C. elegans* as model [106]. The researchers employed two common HDAC inhibitors (VPA and TSA) to mimic the removal of histone chaperone LIN-53 and managed to reprogram germ cells into specific neuron types. It would be interesting to examine the effect of HDAC inhibition in efforts of direct reprogramming from one type to the other in the more complex context of mammalian cells.

6. Conclusions and Perspectives

Stem cell methodologies have revolutionized modern therapeutic strategies that aim to replace damaged cells or tissues. Controlling the pluripotent stem cell fate [95] is dependent on important transcription, signaling, and epigenetic factors. Among other epigenetic regulators, Histone deacetylases have important roles in cell physiology, differentiation, developmental decisions, and tumor formation [10]. Compared to HDAC genes deletions, HDAC inhibitors elicit cell restricted, albeit pleiotropic effects. A vast collection of natural and synthetic HDAC inhibitors has shown very potent effects in embryonic stem cell differentiation pathways. They may promote either self-renewal [54, 55] or differentiation [51, 52] depending on the stem cell status and the dose employed. These effects might result from reorganization of the embryonic stem cell chromatin that is remarkably dynamic and decondensed [107]. Therefore, HDACi can reverse the repressive or activating epigenetic traits that characterize genes involved in the regulation of self-renewal or differentiation.

Most importantly, HDACis have shown considerable activity in directing the neuronal, cardiomyocytic, and hepatic lineages differentiations. In most cases where the molecular mechanism was examined, it involved the induction of differentiation-regulating transcription factors. Moreover, HDACis were used in somatic cell reprogramming processes. Treatment of donor cells before transfer or embryos following transfer resulted in facilitation of embryo cloning and improvement of embryo developmental potential. These effects were due to enhanced histone acetylation, chromatin decompaction, increase of RNA synthesis, and inhibition of apoptosis. Due to the ethical issues raised by embryo cloning, these techniques are not yet applicable to humans. Therefore, the recent achievement of iPS generation has offered great expectations in custom-specific stem cells for human health. In that field, there is increasing effort in omitting retroviral vectors, oncogenes, and—if possible—all kinds of exogenous genetic material. Substituting transcription or signaling factors with simple small molecule reagents can render the therapies both safer and simpler. For that purpose, HDAC inhibitors have shown activity to enhance reprogramming and substitute for the presence of transcription factors, importantly the oncogenes c-myc and Klf4 [67]. However, the exact molecular mechanism whereby VPA, TSA, and other HDACi function needs to be elucidated. Future researches are expected to elucidate the mechanism of HDACi action in order to design novel reagents with increased effectiveness and specificity. On the other hand, genome-wide analyses

have shown that acetylation is a modification as frequent as phosphorylation. Considering that nonhistone proteins are also targets for acetylation, it is expected that analysis of the "acetylome" [108, 109] changes in the course of stem cell differentiation will shed light on the functions and applications of HDAC inhibitors. In addition to mRNA profiling, analysis of miRNA expression changes that follow HDACi may reveal mechanisms whereby these reagents have so specific effects on different cell differentiation backgrounds. HDACis are able to potentiate both stem cell differentiation and somatic cell reprogramming to pluripotency. This may suggest that common mechanisms are involved in opposite changes of the differentiation status. Elucidation of these mechanisms is expected to open new opportunities in the interface between chemistry and stem cell biology. Combining HDAC inhibitors with other small molecule effectors and miRNAs [110] can provide valuable tools to overcome challenges due to genetic interventions and improve stem cell applications for tissue regeneration therapies.

References

[1] A. G. Smith, "Embryo-derived stem cells: of mice and men," *Annual Review of Cell and Developmental Biology*, vol. 17, pp. 435–462, 2001.

[2] E. Li, "Chromatin modification and epigenetic reprogramming in mammalian development," *Nature Reviews Genetics*, vol. 3, no. 9, pp. 662–673, 2002.

[3] B. Li, M. Carey, and J. L. Workman, "The role of chromatin during transcription," *Cell*, vol. 128, no. 4, pp. 707–719, 2007.

[4] H. Cedar and Y. Bergman, "Linking DNA methylation and histone modification: patterns and paradigms," *Nature Reviews Genetics*, vol. 10, no. 5, pp. 295–304, 2009.

[5] M. D. Shahbazian and M. Grunstein, "Functions of site-specific histone acetylation and deacetylation," *Annual Review of Biochemistry*, vol. 76, pp. 75–100, 2007.

[6] X. J. Yang and E. Seto, "The Rpd3/Hda1 family of lysine deacetylases: from bacteria and yeast to mice and men," *Nature Reviews Molecular Cell Biology*, vol. 9, no. 3, pp. 206–218, 2008.

[7] V. T. Cunliffe, "Eloquent silence: developmental functions of Class I histone deacetylases," *Current Opinion in Genetics and Development*, vol. 18, no. 5, pp. 404–410, 2008.

[8] S. Sakamoto, R. Potla, and A. C. Larner, "Histone deacetylase activity is required to recruit RNA polymerase II to the promoters of selected interferon-stimulated early response genes," *Journal of Biological Chemistry*, vol. 279, no. 39, pp. 40362–40367, 2004.

[9] H. Wang and B. W. Dymock, "New patented histone deacetylase inhibitors," *Expert Opinion on Therapeutic Patents*, vol. 19, no. 12, pp. 1727–1757, 2009.

[10] M. Haberland, R. L. Montgomery, and E. N. Olson, "The many roles of histone deacetylases in development and physiology: implications for disease and therapy," *Nature Reviews Genetics*, vol. 10, no. 1, pp. 32–42, 2009.

[11] K. Hochedlinger and K. Plath, "Epigenetic reprogramming and induced pluripotency," *Development*, vol. 136, no. 4, pp. 509–523, 2009.

[12] R. L. Montgomery, J. Hsieh, A. C. Barbosa, J. A. Richardson, and E. N. Olson, "Histone deacetylases 1 and 2 control the progression of neural precursors to neurons during brain

development," *Proceedings of the National Academy of Sciences of the United States of America*, vol. 106, no. 19, pp. 7876–7881, 2009.

[13] G. Zupkovitz, J. Tischler, M. Posch et al., "Negative and positive regulation of gene expression by mouse histone deacetylase 1," *Molecular and Cellular Biology*, vol. 26, no. 21, pp. 7913–7928, 2006.

[14] R. L. Montgomery, C. A. Davis, M. J. Potthoff et al., "Histone deacetylases 1 and 2 redundantly regulate cardiac morphogenesis, growth, and contractility," *Genes and Development*, vol. 21, no. 14, pp. 1790–1802, 2007.

[15] C. M. Trivedi, Y. Luo, Z. Yin et al., "Hdac2 regulates the cardiac hypertrophic response by modulating Gsk3β activity," *Nature Medicine*, vol. 13, no. 3, pp. 324–331, 2007.

[16] G. W. Humphrey, Y. H. Wang, T. Hirai et al., "Complementary roles for histone deacetylases 1, 2, and 3 in differentiation of pluripotent stem cells," *Differentiation*, vol. 76, no. 4, pp. 348–356, 2008.

[17] F. Ye, Y. Chen, T. Hoang et al., "HDAC1 and HDAC2 regulate oligodendrocyte differentiation by disrupting the beta-catenin-TCF interaction," *Nature Neuroscience*, vol. 12, no. 7, pp. 829–838, 2009.

[18] Y. Chen, "HDAC-mediated deacetylation of NF-kappaB is critical for Schwann cell myelination," *Nature Neuroscience*, vol. 14, no. 4, pp. 437–41, 2011.

[19] R. H. Wilting, E. Yanover, M. R. Heideman et al., "Overlapping functions of Hdac1 and Hdac2 in cell cycle regulation and haematopoiesis," *EMBO Journal*, vol. 29, no. 15, pp. 2586–2597, 2010.

[20] T. Wada, J. Kikuchi, N. Nishimura, R. Shimizu, T. Kitamura, and Y. Furukawa, "Expression levels of histone deacetylases determine the cell fate of hematopoietic progenitors," *Journal of Biological Chemistry*, vol. 284, no. 44, pp. 30673–30683, 2009.

[21] R. L. Montgomery, M. J. Potthoff, M. Haberland et al., "Maintenance of cardiac energy metabolism by histone deacetylase 3 in mice," *Journal of Clinical Investigation*, vol. 118, no. 11, pp. 3588–3597, 2008.

[22] S. K. Knutson, B. J. Chyla, J. M. Amann, S. Bhaskara, S. S. Huppert, and S. W. Hiebert, "Liver-specific deletion of histone deacetylase 3 disrupts metabolic transcriptional networks," *EMBO Journal*, vol. 27, no. 7, pp. 1017–1028, 2008.

[23] S. Bhaskara, B. J. Chyla, J. M. Amann et al., "Deletion of histone deacetylase 3 reveals critical roles in S phase progression and DNA damage control," *Molecular Cell*, vol. 30, no. 1, pp. 61–72, 2008.

[24] R. B. Vega, K. Matsuda, J. Oh et al., "Histone deacetylase 4 controls chondrocyte hypertrophy during skeletogenesis," *Cell*, vol. 119, no. 4, pp. 555–566, 2004.

[25] M. M. Cohen, "The new bone biology: pathologic, molecular, and clinical correlates," *American Journal of Medical Genetics, Part A*, vol. 140, no. 23, pp. 2646–2706, 2006.

[26] M. A. Arnold, Y. Kim, M. P. Czubryt et al., "MEF2C transcription factor controls chondrocyte hypertrophy and bone development," *Developmental Cell*, vol. 12, no. 3, pp. 377–389, 2007.

[27] S. Chang, T. A. McKinsey, C. L. Zhang, J. A. Richardson, J. A. Hill, and E. N. Olson, "Histone deacetylases 5 and 9 govern responsiveness of the heart to a subset of stress signals and play redundant roles in heart development," *Molecular and Cellular Biology*, vol. 24, no. 19, pp. 8467–8476, 2004.

[28] K. Song, J. Backs, J. McAnally et al., "The transcriptional coactivator CAMTA2 stimulates cardiac growth by opposing class II histone deacetylases," *Cell*, vol. 125, no. 3, pp. 453–466, 2006.

[29] M. S. Kim, J. Fielitz, J. McAnally et al., "Protein kinase D1 stimulates MEF2 activity in skeletal muscle and enhances muscle performance," *Molecular and Cellular Biology*, vol. 28, no. 11, pp. 3600–3609, 2008.

[30] A. Méjat, F. Ramond, R. Bassel-Duby, S. Khochbin, E. N. Olson, and L. Schaeffer, "Histone deacetylase 9 couples neuronal activity to muscle chromatin acetylation and gene expression," *Nature Neuroscience*, vol. 8, no. 3, pp. 313–321, 2005.

[31] S. Chang, B. D. Young, S. Li, X. Qi, J. A. Richardson, and E. N. Olson, "Histone deacetylase 7 maintains vascular integrity by repressing matrix metalloproteinase 10," *Cell*, vol. 126, no. 2, pp. 321–334, 2006.

[32] Y. Zhang, S. Kwon, T. Yamaguchi et al., "Mice lacking histone deacetylase 6 have hyperacetylated tubulin but are viable and develop normally," *Molecular and Cellular Biology*, vol. 28, no. 5, pp. 1688–1701, 2008.

[33] S. Minucci, C. Nervi, F. Lo Coco, and P. G. Pelicci, "Histone deacetylases: a common molecular target for differentiation treatment of acute myeloid leukemias?" *Oncogene*, vol. 20, no. 24, pp. 3110–3115, 2001.

[34] S. Minucci and P. G. Pelicci, "Histone deacetylase inhibitors and the promise of epigenetic (and more) treatments for cancer," *Nature Reviews Cancer*, vol. 6, no. 1, pp. 38–51, 2006.

[35] N. G. Iyer, H. Özdag, and C. Caldas, "p300/CBP and cancer," *Oncogene*, vol. 23, no. 24, pp. 4225–4231, 2004.

[36] O. A. Botrugno, F. Santoro, and S. Minucci, "Histone deacetylase inhibitors as a new weapon in the arsenal of differentiation therapies of cancer," *Cancer Letters*, vol. 280, no. 2, pp. 134–144, 2009.

[37] M. Yoshida, A. Matsuyama, Y. Komatsu, and N. Nishino, "From discovery to the coming generation of histone deacetylase inhibitors," *Current Medicinal Chemistry*, vol. 10, no. 22, pp. 2351–2358, 2003.

[38] P. A. Marks and R. Breslow, "Dimethyl sulfoxide to vorinostat: development of this histone deacetylase inhibitor as an anticancer drug," *Nature Biotechnology*, vol. 25, no. 1, pp. 84–90, 2007.

[39] W. S. Xu, R. B. Parmigiani, and P. A. Marks, "Histone deacetylase inhibitors: molecular mechanisms of action," *Oncogene*, vol. 26, no. 37, pp. 5541–5552, 2007.

[40] T. Reya, S. J. Morrison, M. F. Clarke, and I. L. Weissman, "Stem cells, cancer, and cancer stem cells," *Nature*, vol. 414, no. 6859, pp. 105–111, 2001.

[41] M. J. Evans and M. H. Kaufman, "Establishment in culture of pluripotential cells from mouse embryos," *Nature*, vol. 292, no. 5819, pp. 154–156, 1981.

[42] B. E. Reubinoff, M. F. Pera, C. Y. Fong, A. Trounson, and A. Bongso, "Embryonic stem cell lines from human blastocysts: somatic differentiation in vitro," *Nature Biotechnology*, vol. 18, no. 4, pp. 399–404, 2000.

[43] H. Niwa, "How is pluripotency determined and maintained?" *Development*, vol. 134, no. 4, pp. 635–646, 2007.

[44] J. Silva and A. Smith, "Capturing pluripotency," *Cell*, vol. 132, no. 4, pp. 532–536, 2008.

[45] R. Jaenisch and R. Young, "Stem cells, the molecular circuitry of pluripotency and nuclear reprogramming," *Cell*, vol. 132, no. 4, pp. 567–582, 2008.

[46] M. Boiani and H. R. Schöler, "Regulatory networks in embryo-derived pluripotent stem cells," *Nature Reviews Molecular Cell Biology*, vol. 6, no. 11, pp. 872–884, 2005.

[47] M. F. Pera and P. P. L. Tam, "Extrinsic regulation of pluripotent stem cells," *Nature*, vol. 465, no. 7299, pp. 713–720, 2010.

[48] P. J. Tesar, J. G. Chenoweth, F. A. Brook et al., "New cell lines from mouse epiblast share defining features with human embryonic stem cells," *Nature*, vol. 448, no. 7150, pp. 196–199, 2007.

[49] I. G. M. Brons, L. E. Smithers, M. W. B. Trotter et al., "Derivation of pluripotent epiblast stem cells from mammalian embryos," *Nature*, vol. 448, no. 7150, pp. 191–195, 2007.

[50] M. Shafa, R. Krawetz, and D. E. Rancourt, "Returning to the stem state: epigenetics of recapitulating pre-differentiation chromatin structure," *BioEssays*, vol. 32, no. 9, pp. 791–799, 2010.

[51] K. W. McCool, X. Xu, D. B. Singer, F. E. Murdoch, and M. K. Fritsch, "The role of histone acetylation in regulating early gene expression patterns during early embryonic stem cell differentiation," *Journal of Biological Chemistry*, vol. 282, no. 9, pp. 6696–6706, 2007.

[52] E. Karantzali, H. Schulz, O. Hummel, N. Hubner, A. K. Hatzopoulos, and A. Kretsovali, "Histone deacetylase inhibition accelerates the early events of stem cell differentiation: transcriptomic and epigenetic analysis," *Genome Biology*, vol. 9, no. 4, article no. R65, 2008.

[53] J. H. Lee, S. R. L. Hart, and D. G. Skalnik, "Histone deacetylase activity is required for embryonic stem cell differentiation," *Genesis*, vol. 38, no. 1, pp. 32–38, 2004.

[54] C. B. Ware, L. Wang, B. H. Mecham et al., "Histone deacetylase inhibition elicits an evolutionarily conserved self-renewal program in embryonic stem cells," *Cell Stem Cell*, vol. 4, no. 4, pp. 359–369, 2009.

[55] K. Hayashi, S. M. C. D. S. Lopes, F. Tang, and M. A. Surani, "Dynamic equilibrium and heterogeneity of mouse pluripotent stem cells with distinct functional and epigenetic states," *Cell Stem Cell*, vol. 3, no. 4, pp. 391–401, 2008.

[56] G. Shi, F. Gao, and Y. Jin, "The regulatory role of histone deacetylase inhibitors in Fgf4 expression is dependent on the differentiation state of pluripotent stem cells," *Journal of Cellular Physiology*, vol. 226, no. 12, pp. 3190–3196, 2011.

[57] D. Ruau, R. Ensenat-Waser, T. C. Dinger et al., "Pluripotency associated genes are reactivated by chromatin-modifying agents in neurosphere cells," *Stem Cells*, vol. 26, no. 4, pp. 920–926, 2008.

[58] T. Kawamura, K. Ono, T. Morimoto et al., "Acetylation of GATA-4 is involved in the differentiation of embryonic stem cells into cardiac myocytes," *Journal of Biological Chemistry*, vol. 280, no. 20, pp. 19682–19688, 2005.

[59] C. Karamboulas, A. Swedani, C. Ward et al., "HDAC activity regulates entry of mesoderm cells into the cardiac muscle lineage," *Journal of Cell Science*, vol. 119, no. 20, pp. 4305–4314, 2006.

[60] S. Kaichi, K. Hasegawa, T. Takaya et al., "Cell line-dependent differentiation of induced pluripotent stem cells into cardiomyocytes in mice," *Cardiovascular Research*, vol. 88, no. 2, pp. 314–323, 2010.

[61] H. P. Chen, M. Denicola, X. Qin et al., "HDAC inhibition promotes cardiogenesis and the survival of embryonic stem cells through proteasome-dependent pathway," *Journal of Cellular Biochemistry*, vol. 112, no. 11, pp. 3246–3255, 2011.

[62] L. Rambhatla, C. P. Chiu, P. Kundu, Y. Peng, and M. K. Carpenter, "Generation of hepatocyte-like cells from human embryonic stem cells," *Cell Transplantation*, vol. 12, no. 1, pp. 1–11, 2003.

[63] Q. J. Zhou, L. X. Xiang, J. Z. Shao et al., "In vitro differentiation of hepatic progenitor cells from mouse embryonic stem cells induced by sodium butyrate," *Journal of Cellular Biochemistry*, vol. 100, no. 1, pp. 29–42, 2007.

[64] M. Ren, L. Yan, C. Z. Shang et al., "Effects of sodium butyrate on the differentiation of pancreatic and hepatic progenitor cells from mouse embryonic stem cells," *Journal of Cellular Biochemistry*, vol. 109, no. 1, pp. 236–244, 2010.

[65] J. Hsieh, K. Nakashima, T. Kuwabara, E. Mejia, and F. H. Gage, "Histone deacetylase inhibition-mediated neuronal differentiation of multipotent adult neural progenitor cells," *Proceedings of the National Academy of Sciences of the United States of America*, vol. 101, no. 47, pp. 16659–16664, 2004.

[66] S. Shen, J. Li, and P. Casaccia-Bonnefil, "Histone modifications affect timing of oligodendrocyte progenitor differentiation in the developing rat brain," *Journal of Cell Biology*, vol. 169, no. 4, pp. 577–589, 2005.

[67] D. Huangfu, K. Osafune, R. Maehr et al., "Induction of pluripotent stem cells from primary human fibroblasts with only Oct4 and Sox2," *Nature Biotechnology*, vol. 26, no. 11, pp. 1269–1275, 2008.

[68] S. Kishigami, H. T. Bui, S. Wakayama et al., "Successful mouse cloning of an outbred strain by trichostatin A treatment after somatic nuclear transfer," *Journal of Reproduction and Development*, vol. 53, no. 1, pp. 165–170, 2007.

[69] R. Rossler, E. Boddeke, and S. Copray, "Differentiation of non-mesencephalic neural stem cells towards dopaminergic neurons," *Neuroscience*, vol. 170, no. 2, pp. 417–428, 2010.

[70] Y. Hao, T. Creson, L. Zhang et al., "Mood stabilizer valproate promotes ERK pathway-dependent cortical neuronal growth and neurogenesis," *Journal of Neuroscience*, vol. 24, no. 29, pp. 6590–6599, 2004.

[71] X. Dai, J. Hao, X. J. Hou et al., "Somatic nucleus reprogramming is significantly improved by m-carboxycinnamic acid bishydroxamide, a histone deacetylase inhibitor," *Journal of Biological Chemistry*, vol. 285, no. 40, pp. 31002–31010, 2010.

[72] A. Rybouchkin, Y. Kato, and Y. Tsunoda, "Role of histone acetylation in reprogramming of somatic nuclei following nuclear transfer," *Biology of Reproduction*, vol. 74, no. 6, pp. 1083–1089, 2006.

[73] H. Araki, N. Mahmud, M. Milhem et al., "Expansion of human umbilical cord blood SCID-repopulating cells using chromatin-modifying agents," *Experimental Hematology*, vol. 34, no. 2, pp. 140–149, 2006.

[74] H. Araki, K. Yoshinaga, P. Boccuni, Y. Zhao, R. Hoffman, and N. Mahmud, "Chromatin-modifying agents permit human hematopoietic stem cells to undergo multiple cell divisions while retaining their repopulating potential," *Blood*, vol. 109, no. 8, pp. 3570–3578, 2007.

[75] J. Han, P. S. Sachdev, and K. S. Sidhu, "A combined epigenetic and non-genetic approach for reprogramming human somatic cells," *PLoS One*, vol. 5, no. 8, Article ID e12297, 2010.

[76] Y. Shi, C. Desponts, J. T. Do, H. S. Hahm, H. R. Schöler, and S. Ding, "Induction of pluripotent stem cells from mouse embryonic fibroblasts by Oct4 and Klf4 with small-molecule compounds," *Cell Stem Cell*, vol. 3, no. 5, pp. 568–574, 2008.

[77] J. W. Schneider, Z. Gao, S. Li et al., "Small-molecule activation of neuronal cell fate," *Nature Chemical Biology*, vol. 4, no. 7, pp. 408–410, 2008.

[78] C. Haumaitre, O. Lenoir, and R. Scharfmann, "Histone deacetylase inhibitors modify pancreatic cell fate determination and amplify endocrine progenitors," *Molecular and Cellular Biology*, vol. 28, no. 20, pp. 6373–6383, 2008.

[79] I. H. Park, R. Zhao, J. A. West et al., "Reprogramming of human somatic cells to pluripotency with defined factors," *Nature*, vol. 451, no. 7175, pp. 141–146, 2008.

[80] D. Huangfu, R. Maehr, W. Guo et al., "Induction of pluripotent stem cells by defined factors is greatly improved by small-molecule compounds," *Nature Biotechnology*, vol. 26, no. 7, pp. 795–797, 2008.

[81] P. Mali, B. K. Chou, J. Yen et al., "Butyrate greatly enhances derivation of human induced pluripotent stem cells by promoting epigenetic remodeling and the expression of pluripotency-associated genes," *Stem Cells*, vol. 28, no. 4, pp. 713–720, 2010.

[82] V. Balasubramaniyan, E. Boddeke, R. Bakels et al., "Effects of histone deacetylation inhibition on neuronal differentiation of embryonic mouse neural stem cells," *Neuroscience*, vol. 143, no. 4, pp. 939–951, 2006.

[83] B. Feng, J. H. Ng, J. C. D. Heng, and H. H. Ng, "Molecules that promote or enhance reprogramming of somatic cells to induced pluripotent stem cells," *Cell Stem Cell*, vol. 4, no. 4, pp. 301–312, 2009.

[84] F. A. Siebzehnrubl, R. Buslei, I. Y. Eyupoglu, S. Seufert, E. Hahnen, and I. Blumcke, "Histone deacetylase inhibitors increase neuronal differentiation in adult forebrain precursor cells," *Experimental Brain Research*, vol. 176, no. 4, pp. 672–678, 2007.

[85] I. T. Yu, J. Y. Park, S. H. Kim, J. S. Lee, Y. S. Kim, and H. Son, "Valproic acid promotes neuronal differentiation by induction of proneural factors in association with H4 acetylation," *Neuropharmacology*, vol. 56, pp. 473–480, 2009.

[86] H. Flici, B. Erkosar, O. Komonyi, O. F. Karatas, P. Laneve, and A. Giangrande, "Gcm/Glide-dependent conversion into glia depends on neural stem cell age, but not on division, triggering a chromatin signature that is conserved in vertebrate glia," *Development*, vol. 138, no. 19, pp. 4167–4178, 2011.

[87] J. C. Young, S. Wu, G. Hansteen et al., "Inhibitors of histone deacetylases promote hematopoietic stem cell self-renewal," *Cytotherapy*, vol. 6, no. 4, pp. 328–336, 2004.

[88] S. Lee, J. R. Park, M. S. Seo et al., "Histone deacetylase inhibitors decrease proliferation potential and multilineage differentiation capability of human mesenchymal stem cells," *Cell Proliferation*, vol. 42, no. 6, pp. 711–720, 2009.

[89] C. Haumaitre, O. Lenoir, and R. Scharfmann, "Directing cell differentiation with small-molecule histone deacetylase inhibitors: the example of promoting pancreatic endocrine cells," *Cell Cycle*, vol. 8, no. 4, pp. 536–544, 2009.

[90] T. Oyama, T. Nagai, H. Wada et al., "Cardiac side population cells have a potential to migrate and differentiate into cardiomyocytes in vitro and in vivo," *Journal of Cell Biology*, vol. 176, no. 3, pp. 329–341, 2007.

[91] G. Yang et al., "Trichostatin A promotes cardiomyocyte differentiation of rat mesenchymel stem cells after 5-azacytidine induction or during co-culture with neonatal cardiomyocytes via a mechanism independent of histone deacetylase inhibition," *Cell Transplantation*. In press.

[92] I. Wilmut, "The first direct reprogramming of adult human fibroblasts," *Cell Stem Cell*, vol. 1, no. 6, pp. 593–594, 2007.

[93] J. B. Gurdon and D. A. Melton, "Nuclear reprogramming in cells," *Science*, vol. 322, no. 5909, pp. 1811–1815, 2008.

[94] B. P. Enright, C. Kubota, X. Yang, and X. C. Tian, "Epigenetic characteristics and development of embryos cloned from donor cells treated by trichostatin A or 5-aza-2'-deoxycytidine," *Biology of Reproduction*, vol. 69, no. 3, pp. 896–901, 2003.

[95] R. A. Young, "Control of the embryonic stem cell state," *Cell*, vol. 144, no. 6, pp. 940–954, 2011.

[96] N. van Thuan, H. T. Bui, J. H. Kim et al., "The histone deacetylase inhibitor scriptaid enhances nascent mRNA production and rescues full-term development in cloned inbred mice," *Reproduction*, vol. 138, no. 2, pp. 309–317, 2009.

[97] M. A. Martinez-Diaz, L. Che, M. Albornoz et al., "Pre- and postimplantation development of swine-cloned embryos derived from fibroblasts and bone marrow cells after inhibition of histone deacetylases," *Cellular Reprogramming*, vol. 12, no. 1, pp. 85–94, 2010.

[98] H. T. Bui, S. Wakayama, S. Kishigami et al., "Effect of trichostatin A on chromatin remodeling, histone modifications, DNA replication, and transcriptional activity in cloned mouse embryos," *Biology of Reproduction*, vol. 83, no. 3, pp. 454–463, 2010.

[99] T. Ono, C. Li, E. Mizutani, Y. Terashita, K. Yamagata, and T. Wakayama, "Inhibition of class IIb histone deacetylase significantly improves cloning efficiency in mice," *Biology of Reproduction*, vol. 83, no. 6, pp. 929–937, 2010.

[100] K. Takahashi and S. Yamanaka, "Induction of pluripotent stem cells from mouse embryonic and adult fibroblast cultures by defined factors," *Cell*, vol. 126, no. 4, pp. 663–676, 2006.

[101] K. Takahashi, K. Tanabe, M. Ohnuki et al., "Induction of pluripotent stem cells from adult human fibroblasts by defined factors," *Cell*, vol. 131, no. 5, pp. 861–872, 2007.

[102] J. Yu, M. A. Vodyanik, K. Smuga-Otto et al., "Induced pluripotent stem cell lines derived from human somatic cells," *Science*, vol. 318, no. 5858, pp. 1917–1920, 2007.

[103] G. Liang, O. Taranova, K. Xia, and Y. Zhang, "Butyrate promotes induced pluripotent stem cell generation," *Journal of Biological Chemistry*, vol. 285, no. 33, pp. 25516–25521, 2010.

[104] G. Durcova-Hills, F. Tang, G. Doody, R. Tooze, and M. A. Surani, "Reprogramming primordial germ cells into pluripotent stem cells," *PLoS One*, vol. 3, no. 10, Article ID e3531, 2008.

[105] C. A. Lyssiotis, J. Walker, C. Wu, T. Kondo, P. G. Schultz, and X. Wu, "Inhibition of histone deacetylase activity induces developmental plasticity in oligodendrocyte precursor cells," *Proceedings of the National Academy of Sciences of the United States of America*, vol. 104, no. 38, pp. 14982–14987, 2007.

[106] B. Tursun, T. Patel, P. Kratsios, and O. Hobert, "Direct conversion of *C. elegans* germ cells into specific neuron types," *Science*, vol. 331, no. 6015, pp. 304–308, 2011.

[107] E. Meshorer and T. Misteli, "Chromatin in pluripotent embryonic stem cells and differentiation," *Nature Reviews Molecular Cell Biology*, vol. 7, no. 7, pp. 540–546, 2006.

[108] S. C. Kim, R. Sprung, Y. Chen et al., "Substrate and functional diversity of lysine acetylation revealed by a proteomics survey," *Molecular Cell*, vol. 23, no. 4, pp. 607–618, 2006.

[109] M. Ocker, "Deacetylase inhibitors—focus on non-histone targets and effects," *The World Journal of Biological Chemistry*, vol. 1, no. 5, pp. 55–61, 2010.

[110] N. Miyoshi, H. Ishii, H. Nagano et al., "Reprogramming of mouse and human cells to pluripotency using mature microRNAs," *Cell Stem Cell*, vol. 8, no. 6, pp. 633–638, 2011.

20

Hippocampal Neurogenesis and the Brain Repair Response to Brief Stereotaxic Insertion of a Microneedle

Shijie Song,[1,2] **Shuojing Song,**[3] **Chuanhai Cao,**[4] **Xiaoyang Lin,**[4] **Kunyu Li,**[1]
Vasyl Sava,[1,2] **and Juan Sanchez-Ramos**[1,2,4]

[1] *Department of Neurology, University of South Florida, 13220 Laurel Drive, Tampa, FL 33612, USA*
[2] *Research Service, James A. Haley VA Medical Center, Tampa, FL 33612, USA*
[3] *Feinberg School of Medicine, Northwestern University, Chicago, IL 60611, USA*
[4] *Department of Molecular Pharmacology and Physiology, University of South Florida, Tampa, FL 33612, USA*

Correspondence should be addressed to Juan Sanchez-Ramos; jsramos@health.usf.edu

Academic Editor: Joshua J. Breunig

We tested the hypothesis that transient microinjury to the brain elicits cellular and humoral responses that stimulate hippocampal neurogenesis. Brief stereotaxic insertion and removal of a microneedle into the right hippocampus resulted in (a) significantly increased expression of granulocyte-colony stimulating factor (G-CSF), the chemokine MIP-1a, and the proinflammatory cytokine IL12p40; (b) pronounced activation of microglia and astrocytes; and (c) increase in hippocampal neurogenesis. This study describes immediate and early humoral and cellular mechanisms of the brain's response to microinjury that will be useful for the investigation of potential neuroprotective and deleterious effects of deep brain stimulation in various neuropsychiatric disorders.

1. Background

Deep brain stimulation through chronically implanted metal electrodes into specific brain regions is becoming a common therapeutic choice for medication refractory movement disorders such as Parkinson's disease (PD), tremors, and dystonia (see reviews [1–3]). More recently, DBS has been applied to psychiatric and behavioral disorders including depression, obsessive compulsive disorder, and addiction and most recently to disorders of consciousness [4–9].

Long-term implantation of a fine metal electrode, even without chronic electrical stimulation may produce unwanted effects. Neuropathological examination of brain tissue from patients with DBS revealed activated astrocytes and microglia regardless of the underlying disease [10–15]. Electrical stimulation is not required to see signs of neuroinflammation; inflammatory changes have been observed around recording electrodes used for characterizing epileptogenic tissue and around CSF fluid shunt catheters [16, 17].

To understand the earliest reactions to implantation of a metal electrode, we studied the cellular and cytokine responses over time to transient insertion of a fine needle

(maximum diameter of 200 μm) into the dorsal hippocampus of the mouse. We tested the hypothesis that the creation of a focal microlesion in hippocampus elicits self-repair mechanisms mediated by cytokines which activate microglia, promote astrocytosis, and stimulate stem/progenitor cells to proliferate and generate new neurons.

2. Materials and Methods

All procedures described here were reviewed and approved by the IACUC Committee of the University of South Florida and the Haley VA Research Service.

2.1. Animals. C57BL/6 mice, 8–10 weeks old, were purchased from Harlan Laboratories, and transgenic GFP mice (C57BL/6-Tg [ACTB-EGFP] 1Osb/J, 003291) were purchased from Jackson Laboratory (Bar Harbor, ME). Most of the experiments utilized groups of C57BL/6 mice, and one experiment utilized chimeric mice (C57BL/6 mice transplanted with green fluorescent protein expressing (GFP+) bone marrow).

2.2. Generation of Chimeric Mice. The procedure for bone marrow harvesting from tg GFP+ mice has been previously published by Sanchez-Ramos and coworkers [18, 19]. Briefly, bone marrow cells are collected from femurs and tibias of adult male GFP transgenic mice by flushing the bone shaft with PBS + 0.5% bovine serum albumin (BSA) + 2 mM ethylenediaminetetraacetic acid (EDTA) (Sigma).

To generate chimeric mice, C57BL/6J mice were lethally irradiated with 8 Gy total body irradiation (delivered in two fractions of 4 Gy, an interval of 4 hours) at dose rate of 1.03 Gy/min in a Gammacell 40 Extractor [20]. Following irradiation, the mice were given a bone marrow transplant (10×10^6 mononuclear cells) from transgenic GFP mice infused via tail vein. Bone marrow-derived cells in the rescued mice were readily tracked by virtue of their green fluorescence. Examination of blood smears from tail clippings for the presence of green monocytes confirmed successful engraftment.

2.3. Stereotaxic Insertion and Removal of Microneedle. Animals were anesthetized with sodium pentobarbital (50 mg/kg, i.p.) and placed into a stereotactic frame. Using bregma as the reference point, a trephine hole was then drilled in the skull and the needle was gently inserted into the hippocampus (AP 2.5 mm; ML 1.3 mm; DV 3.5 mm). Mice received 5-bromo-2′-deoxyuridine (BrdU) (Sigma) injections (100 mg/kg i.p. Bid, immediately after the surgery and 2 days after surgery) to label nascent cells during a 3-day period.

2.4. Tissue Preparation and Sectioning. At one, two, and four weeks after needle stimulation, mice were anesthetized with 10% chloral hydrate and a transcardial perfusion of the brain with 20 mL saline and 50 mL of 4% paraformaldehyde was done. The brain was removed and fixed for 48 hours in the same solution. After fixing, the brains were immersed overnight in 20% sucrose in PBS. Thirty μm frozen sections through the striatum, hippocampus, midbrain, and cerebellum were prepared and stored in vials containing a cryopreservation solution.

2.5. Immunohistochemistry. Brain sections were preincubated in PBS containing 10% normal serum (goat or donkey; Vector) and 0.3% Triton X-100 (Sigma) for 30 min. The sections were then transferred to a solution containing primary antibodies in 1% normal serum and 0.3% triton X-100/PBS and incubated overnight at 4°C. The specific antibodies used in each experiment were rat anti-BrdU (Serotec), 1 : 100; mouse anti-NeuN (Chemicon), 1 : 50; mouse antinestin (BD Biosciences); rabbit anti-DCX (Abcam Inc.), 1 : 1000; rabbit anti-Iba1(Wako Chemicals, USA, Inc.), 1 : 500; rabbit anti-GFAP (BioGenex), 1 : 50 in PBS containing 1 : 100 normal serum without Triton X-100. After incubation with primary antibody, the sections were washed and incubated for 1 hour with Alexa Fluor 488 goat anti-mouse IgG diluted 1 : 400 in PBS or Alexa Fluor 546 goat anti-rabbit IgG diluted 1 : 600 in PBS (Invitrogen) at room temperature. Isotype controls matching the primary antibody's host species (mouse) were used in place of the primary antibody (monoclonal to NeuN and Nestin) to check for specificity of the stain. The sections were then rinsed in PBS three times and covered with a cover glass. Some sections were stained (after all other staining) with DAPI (300 nM) for nuclear staining. Fluorescent signals from the labeled cells were visualized with fluorescence microscopy using appropriate filters or a Zeiss LSM510 confocal microscope.

2.6. Image Analysis and Cell Counts. Quantitation of microgliosis and astrogliosis was made by computerized image analysis. Images at 20x magnification were acquired as digitized tagged-image format files to retain maximum resolution using an Olympus BX60 microscope with an attached digital camera system (DP-70, Olympus). Digital images were routed into a Windows PC for quantitative analyses using ImageJ software (NIH). Images of six sections (180 μm apart) were captured from serially sectioned hippocampus. Color images were separated into green, red, and blue channels. The monochrome image for green (either Iba1 or GFAP) was then processed by setting a threshold to discriminate staining from background. Each field of interest was manually edited to eliminate artifacts. For the Iba1 (microgliosis) and GFAP (astrocytosis) burden analyses, data are reported as the percentage of labeled area captured (positive pixels) divided by the full area captured (total pixels). Bias was eliminated by analyzing each entire region of interest represented by the sampling of 6 sections per hippocampus. A total of 6–8 mice hippocampi were analyzed.

Unbiased estimates of the number of immature neurons dentate gyrus (DG) were made by counting DCX-immunoreactive cells in serially sectioned hippocampus according to the method previously described [21, 22]. Estimates of numbers of BrdU labeled microglia (Iba1-BrdU+) cells in hippocampus were also determined. Briefly, positively labeled cells were counted in every 6th section (each section separated by 180 μm) using a modification to the optical dissector method; cells on the upper and lower planes were not counted to avoid counting partial cells. The number of DCX+ cells counted in every 6th section was multiplied by 6 to get the total number of DCX cells in the DG and Iba1 cells in hippocampus. The total number of hippocampi analyzed was 3 for each time period. The unlesioned left hippocampus served as control.

2.7. Cytokine Assay. After creating a right-side hippocampus microlesion, mice were euthanized at 6, 12, 24, 48, and 72 hours ($n = 3$ mice per time interval) followed by perfusion with saline. Frontal cortex and hippocampus of the left and right brains were dissected and kept in freezer for cytokine assay. Levels of 17 cytokines were measured using Bio-Rad Bio-Plex kits (Bio-Rad, catalogue number 171F11181). Samples and standards were prepared using company protocols with the initial concentration of standards ranging from 32 ng/mL to 1.95 pg/mL. Samples were prepared for analysis by diluting 1 volume of the tissue sample with three volumes of the Bio-Plex mouse sample diluent. Using the microplate readout,

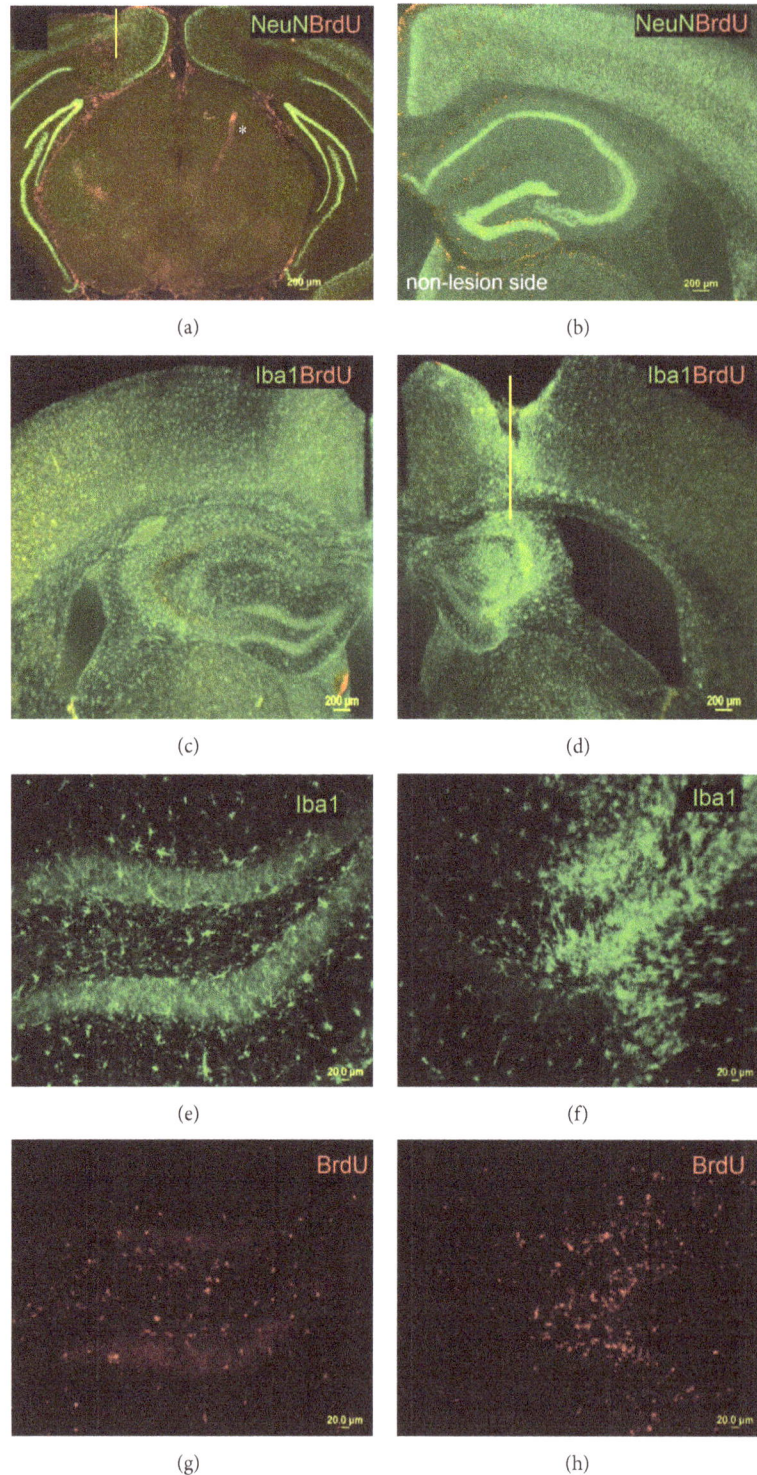

FIGURE 1: Cellular response to insertion and removal of a microneedle. (a) Low power view of cells labeled with BrdU in region of hippocampus and midbrain (BrdU = red; NeuN = green); needle was inserted on the right side of brain (yellow line). BrdU injections were given on the day of lesion and subsequent two days. Image taken one week after lesion. BrdU+ cells are found along the needle track and in the subarachnoid space and vasculature on both sides of brain. Scale bar = 200 μm for panels (a), (b), (c), and (d). (b) Hippocampus (rostral to section in (a)) from the same animal on the unlesioned side. BrdU+ cells are seen in cortex, corpus callosum, the subarachnoid space, dentate gyrus, subgranular zone, and stratum lacunosum molecular of the hippocampus (one week after lesion). (c) Nonlesioned hippocampus opposite the lesioned hippocampus in panel (d) (2 wks after lesion). (d) Site and track of needle insertion (yellow line). Two weeks after lesion. (e) Nonlesioned hippocampus at higher power (Iba1 = green scale; bar = 20 μm for panels (e), (f), (g), and (h)). (f) Iba1+ cells in lesioned hippocampus. (g) BrdU+ cells on nonlesioned side, corresponding to panel (e). (h) BrdU+ cells on lesioned side, corresponding to panel (f).

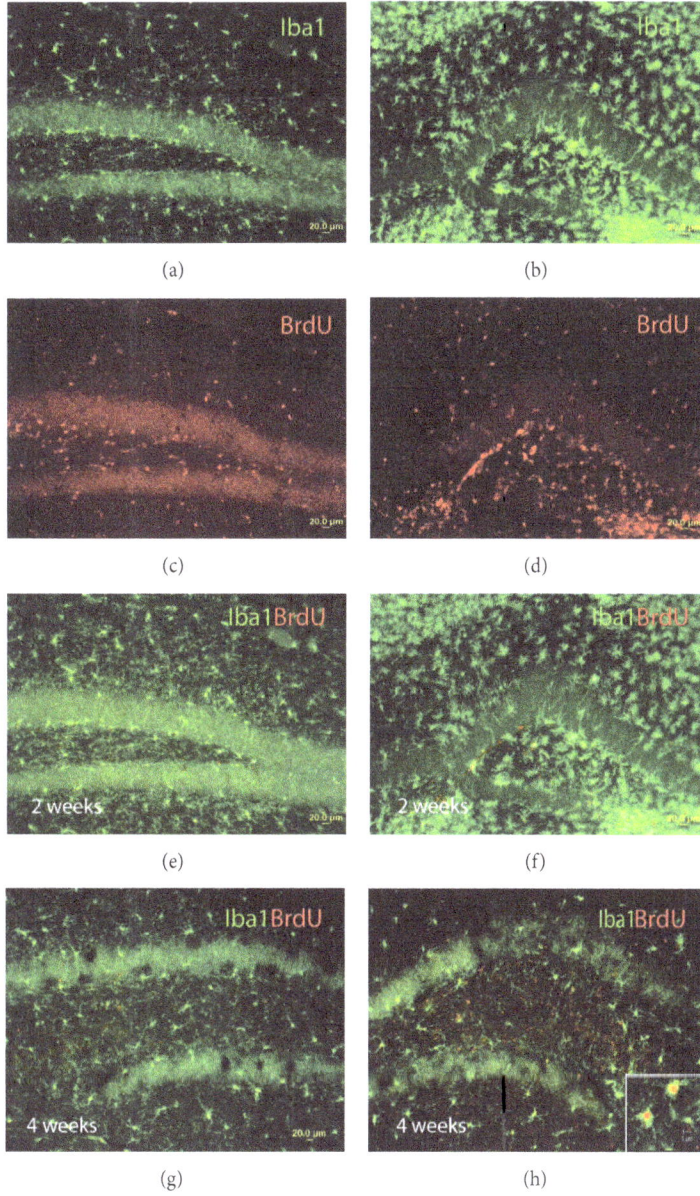

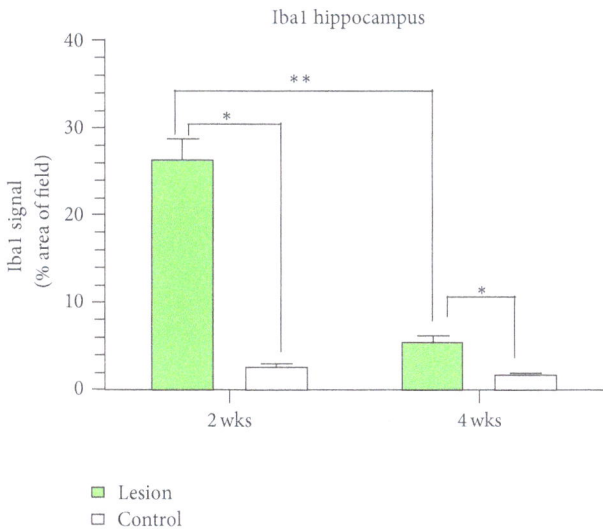

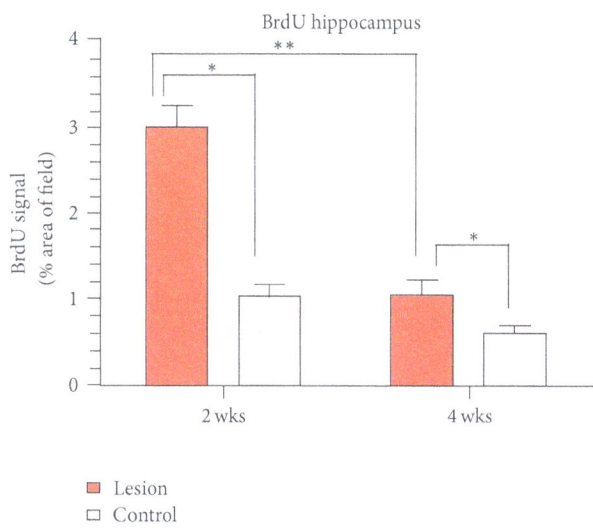

FIGURE 2: Continued.

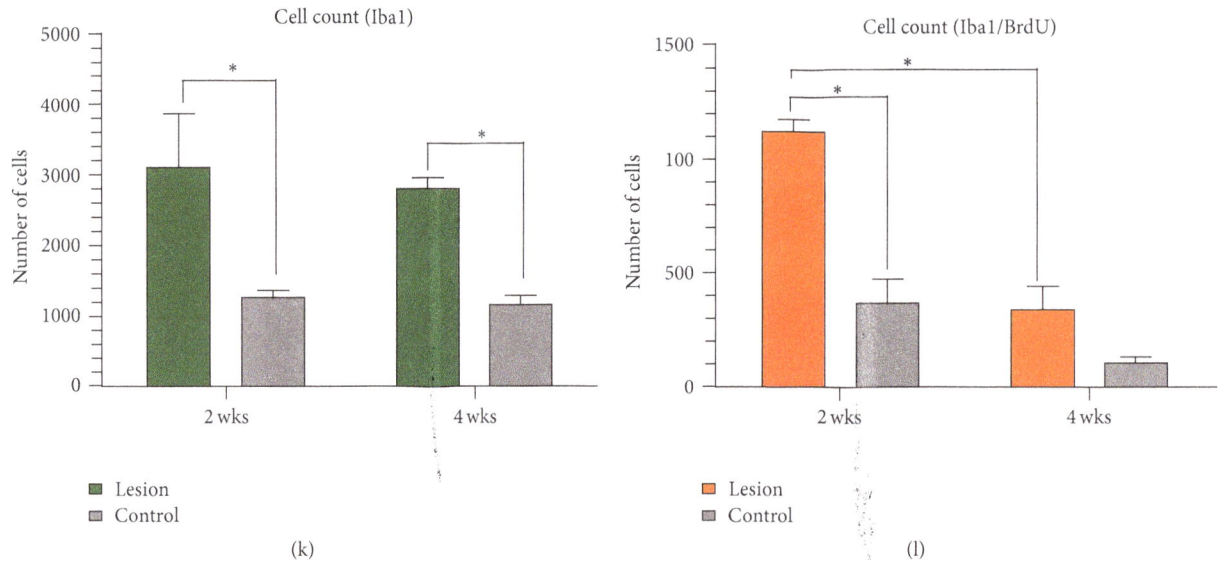

(k)

(l)

FIGURE 2: Microgliosis indicated by Iba1 immunostaining in hippocampus at 2 wks and 4 wks after microlesion. Panels on the left ((a), (c), (e), and (g)) illustrate the microglial response on the unlesioned control side, and the panels on the right ((b), (d), (f), and (h)) are the corresponding lesioned sides. Panels (a), (b) = Iba1 immunostaining; (c), (d) = BrdU+ cells corresponding to sections (a) and (b), respectively. Panels (e), (f) are merged images of Iba1-BrdU signal 2 wks after lesion. Panels (g), (h) are merged images of Iba1-BrdU signals 4 wks after lesion. Insert box shows a merged confocal microscopic image of double-labeled Iba-1-BrdU. (i) Microgliosis assessed by image analysis of Iba1 signal. y-axis = mean Iba1 signal area (as percent of hippocampal field at 20x magnification). Microglial signal was 16 times greater on the lesioned side than control at 2 wks ($^*P < 0.001$). The microglial signal on the lesioned side declined significantly after 4 wks ($^{**}P < 0.001$) but remained significantly elevated compared to the unlesioned side. (j) BrdU signal area was 3 times greater on the lesioned side at 2 wks and declined after 4 wks. (k) A number of Iba1+ cells were approximately 2.45 times greater on the lesioned hippocampus compared to the nonlesioned control at both 2 and 4 wks ($^*P < 0.01$). Notice that microglia in the lesioned hippocampus are larger than on the control side, and therefore, the total Iba1 signal area is much greater than total number of cells. (l) A number of double-labeled microglia (Iba1/BrdU) were also greater on the lesioned side than controls at both 2 wks ($^*P < 0.05$). Double-labeled microglia comprised ~36% of the total number of Iba1+ cells. Scale bar = 20 μm.

each cytokine level was calculated based on its own standard curve.

2.8. Statistical Analysis. Neurohistologic measures were expressed as mean ± SEM and statistically evaluated using 2-way ANOVA followed by Bonferroni corrections for multiple comparisons (GraphPad version 5.01). The time course of cytokines release was analyzed using 2-way ANOVA. All comparisons were considered significant at $P < 0.05$.

3. Results

Insertion and immediate removal of a fine needle to the hippocampus on one side of brain resulted in mobilization of cells along the needle track. BrdU+ cells labeled in vivo during the 3 days after placement of the lesion were found along the microinjury track through cerebral cortex to the hippocampus and to a lesser extent were observed along the corpus callosum on both sides of the brain (Figure 1). Although many of the BrdU+ cells appear to be derived from peripheral blood, any cell with proliferative capacity within brain and its lining membranes were also labeled. BrdU+ cells were found in the needle-breeched subarachnoid space and cerebrospinal fluid (CSF), from where they have access to

hippocampus by way of the CA3-dentate gyral border with the ventricle, even on the nonlesioned side (Figure 1(b)).

The labeling of tissue sections with anti-Iba1 antibodies revealed both a significant proliferation and enlargement of microglial cells (Figure 2). Two weeks after placement of the lesion, the mean Iba1 signal area per field, reflecting both size and number of cells, was 16 times the signal on the unlesioned control side (Figures 2(a), 2(b), and 2(i)). At four weeks, the signal on the lesioned side remained elevated but was decreased compared to the signal at 2 wks, suggesting a time-dependent downregulation of microgliosis in this model (Figures 2(h) and 2(i)). The mean BrdU signal area was 3 times greater on the lesioned side than the control side, but like the Iba1 signal, BrdU area decreased significantly from 2 wks to 4 wks (Figure 2(j)). The number of Iba1+ cells was approximately 2.45 times greater on the lesioned hippocampus compared to the nonlesioned control at both 2 and 4 wks (Figure 2(k)). The microglia in the lesioned hippocampus were morphologically larger than on the control side, and therefore the total Iba1 signal area is much greater than the total number of counted cells. The Iba1+ cell counts likely underestimated the true number of microglia because individual cells were difficult to distinguish in regions where the intense microgliosis resulted in clusters of Iba1+ staining. However, when Iba1+ cells that had a nucleus labeled with BrdU (Iba1/BrdU) were counted, there was clearly a significantly greater number of Iba1/BrdU+ cells on the lesioned side than in controls at 2 wks (*$P < 0.05$). Double-labeled microglia comprised ~36% of the total number of Iba1+ cells, suggesting that a significant proportion of microglia were born after the 3 days of labeling with BrdU.

The contribution of blood-derived cells (GFP+ cells in chimeric mice) to the total microglial population is shown in Figure 3. The image analysis of GFP+ and Iba1 signals on the lesioned side revealed a mean GFP+ signal equal to 26% of the total Iba1 signal (ratio of 13.4/51.6), suggesting that approximately one-fourth of the microglial signal comes from the peripheral blood (GFP+ bone marrow-derived cells). Cells counts of double-labeled Iba1/GFP cells confirm a significantly increased number of blood-derived microglia on the lesioned side compared to the unlesioned side.

The microlesion also triggered significant astrocytosis, indicated by GFAP immunoreactivity (Figure 4). GFAP signal on the lesioned side was 6 times that of the nonlesioned control side. Like the microgliosis, the GFAP signal decreased by 4 wks after the lesion (Figure 4(g)). Counts of GFAP+ cells were not done because of difficulty in discerning individual GFAP+ astrocytes in many regions of astrocytosis.

Insertion and removal of the needle stimulated neurogenesis in the subgranular zone of hippocampus, indicated by immunostaining for doublecortin (DCX), a marker of immature neurons (Figure 5). The mean DCX signal in dentate gyrus was significantly increased at 2 weeks and remained increased at 4 wks compared to the nonlesioned control side (Figure 5(d)). Unbiased estimates of cell counts of DCX-BrdU colabeled cells were also increased significantly at 2 and 4 weeks (Figure 5(e)). The total number of double-labeled cells was diminished at 4 wks compared to 2 wks, suggesting that many new neurons, born in the immediate days after lesion placement, undergo subsequent apoptosis. However, DCX+ cells, unlabeled with BrdU, were clearly maintained at approximately the same level at 2 and 4 wks, suggesting there are cytokine signals that continue to stimulate generation of new neurons beyond the time frame of BrdU injections (i.e., first 3 days of microlesioning).

The contribution of blood-born GFP+ cells to increased neurogenesis was examined (Figure 6). Rare GFP+ cells were found to coexpress nestin in the neurogenic niche (Figure 6(d)) but these cells did not express the typical fibrillary processes of neural progenitors in the subgranular zon [23]. Hence, increased neurogenesis triggered by the lesion could not be attributed to transdifferentiation of blood-derived cells.

Within 6 hrs of creating the microlesion, 3 out of 17 soluble cytokines were significantly increased in hippocampus and frontal cortex (along the path of needle insertion). Granulocyte-colony stimulating factor (G-CSF), MIP-1a, and IL12p40 were increased in both hippocampus and frontal cortex (Figure 7). G-CSF levels peaked at 6 hrs after placement of the lesion and returned to levels measured on the unlesioned control side by 24 hrs. IL12p40 concentrations peaked at 12 hrs and were back to baseline by 72 hrs. MIP-1a peaked at 12 hrs and remained elevated until 72 hrs.

4. Discussion

Simple insertion and immediate removal of a sterile fine needle into the dorsal hippocampus triggered a robust cellular response characterized by proliferation of microglia and astrocytes. The microgliosis and astrocytosis remained prominent up to 4 wks, though it declined from the maximum intensity at 2 wks after the lesion. Of the total microglial signal in hippocampus, approximately 36% of these cells were born during the 3-day period after the lesion placement (indicated by double-labeled BrdU-Iba1 cells). The contribution of blood-born cells (indicated by GFP+ cells in chimeric mice) to total microglial burden was approximately 26%. The contribution of blood monocytes to the brain population of microglia is dynamic and can change dramatically following injury, infection, or neurodegenerative processes [24–29]. As shown here, even a brief microinjury as represented by insertion and immediate removal of a fine sterile needle into brain triggers a significant infiltration and activation of blood-derived microglia.

A potentially beneficial consequence of the microlesion was the stimulation of neurogenesis in the subgranular zone of the dentate gyrus, evidenced by the significant increase in total DCX signal, a marker of immature neurons [30]. The DCX signal at 4 wks remained elevated even as the numbers of double-labeled BrdU-DCX decreased by 4 weeks. The discrepancy between total DCX and BrdU-DCX labeled cells remained high at 4 wks, but the decrease in double-labeled BrdU-DCX at 4 weeks may be explained by (a) programmed cell death of new neurons born during the immediate postlesion period and (b) continued neurogenesis in the period after BrdU injections. The contribution of blood-derived cells (GFP+) to neurogenesis in chimeric mice, as indicated by GFP-Nestin coexpression in subgranular zone, was negligible, suggesting that the source of cells for neurogenesis was within the neurogenic niche itself rather than recruitment of exogenous cells. It is notable that these GFP-Nestin expressing cells did not exhibit radial fibers typical of neural progenitors in the subgranular zone [23]. Nestin-GFP+ coexpression may also indicate development of endothelial cells from bone marrow-derived GFP+ cells.

The cascade of events that resulted in these cellular responses is complex, but the findings here identify a few salient cytokines that may contribute to the cellular mobilization. Macrophage inflammatory protein-1a (MIP-1a, also known as CCL-3) is known for its chemotactic and proinflammatory effects. Levels of MIP-1a remained elevated for 3 days and most likely played a role in the activation of microglia and astrocytes and also in the recruitment of blood-born monocytes to the site of injury. IL12-p40 (also known as cytotoxic lymphocyte maturation factor 2) is a proinflammatory cytokine with immunoregulatory properties, especially in promoting Th1 cell-mediated immune responses [31]. G-CSF is a hematopoietic cytokine that increases proliferation of blood stem stems and results in increased number of polymorphonuclear leukocytes [32]. More recently, it has been recognized as a neurotrophic factor with antiapoptotic effects and direct actions to promote neurogenesis [33]. In the present study, elevated G-CSF levels

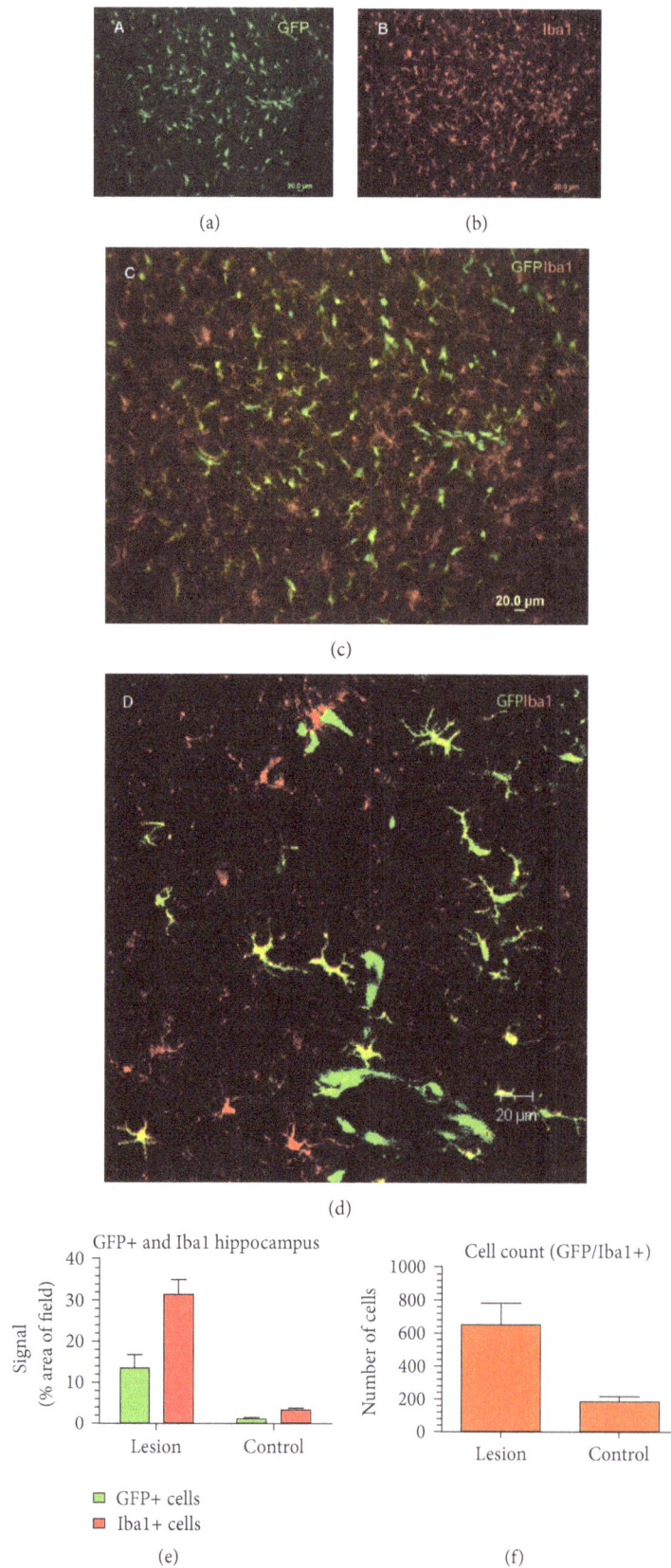

(a)

(b)

(c)

(d)

(e)

(f)

FIGURE 3: Contribution of blood-derived cells to microgliosis in chimeric mice 2 weeks after lesion placement. (a) Blood-derived GFP+ cells in hippocampal region. (b) Microgliosis two weeks after the lesion is indicated by Iba1 immunoreactivity. (c) Merged images of GFP+ (A) and Iba1+ cells (B). (d) Merged confocal image showing double-labeled microglia (yellow) at a higher magnification. (e) Mean Iba1 and GFP+ signals. On the lesioned side, the mean GFP+ signal is 26% of the total Iba1 signal (ratio of 13.4/51.6). (f) Cells count of double-labeled Iba1/GFP cells is significantly greater on the lesioned side than control.

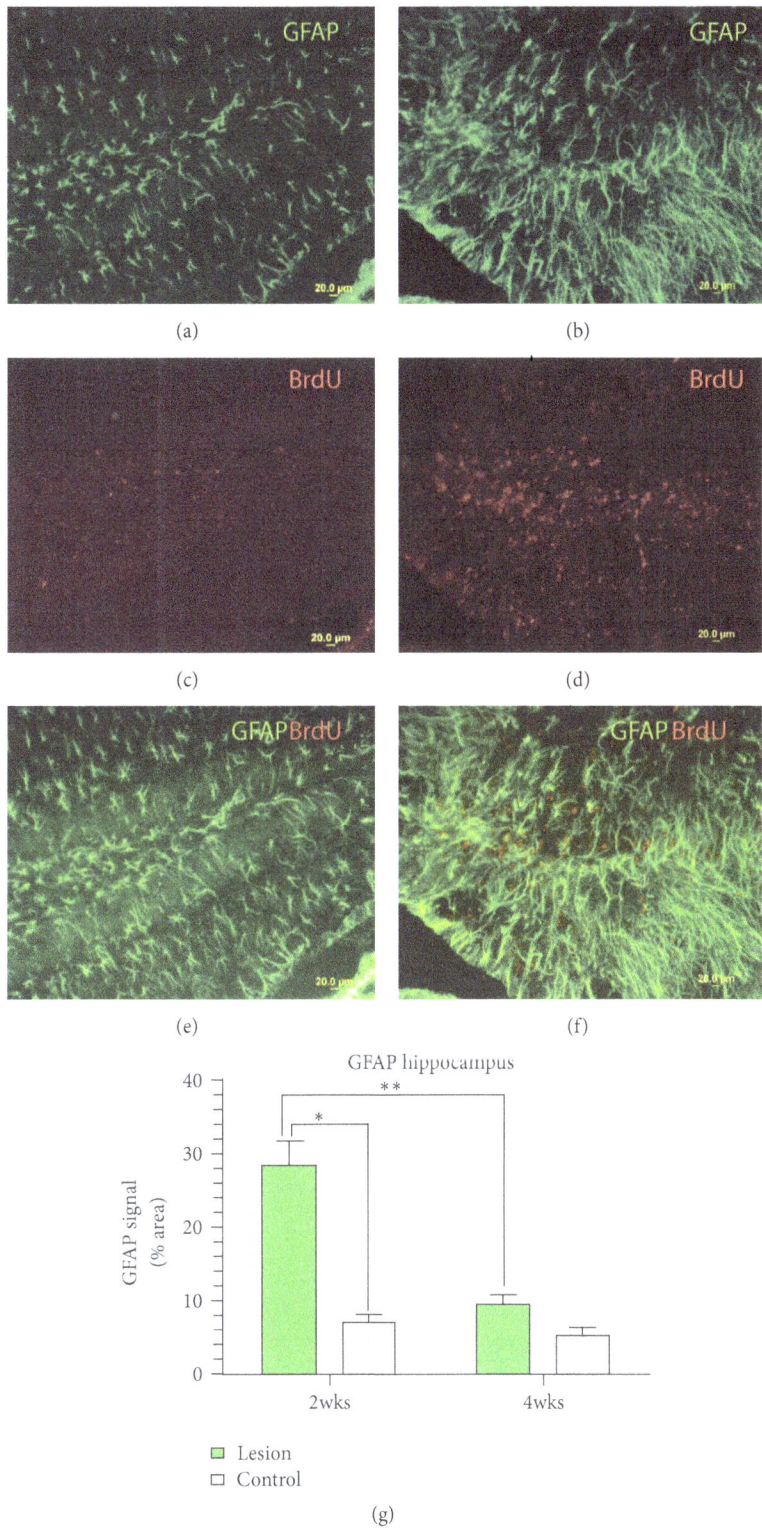

FIGURE 4: Astrocytosis in hippocampus indicated by GFAP immunoreactivity. Panels on the left ((a), (c), and (e)) depict the unlesioned control side; panels (b), (d), and (f) show the lesioned side. (a), (b) = GFAP (green channel); (c), (d) = BrdU (red channel); (e), (f) merged channels (GFAP and BrdU). (g) Astrocytosis measured as extent of GFAP immunoreactivity (mean % area of field) was increased 6 times that of control (n = 3 mice at 2 wks; 3 mice at 4 wks; 6 sections per mouse). 2-way ANOVA showed that both treatment and time contribute significantly to the variance. Signal was significantly higher on lesioned side at 2 weeks. At 4 weeks, the mean signal had declined significantly. $^{*}P < 0.001$; $^{**}P < 0.001$ using Bonferroni correction for multiple comparisons.

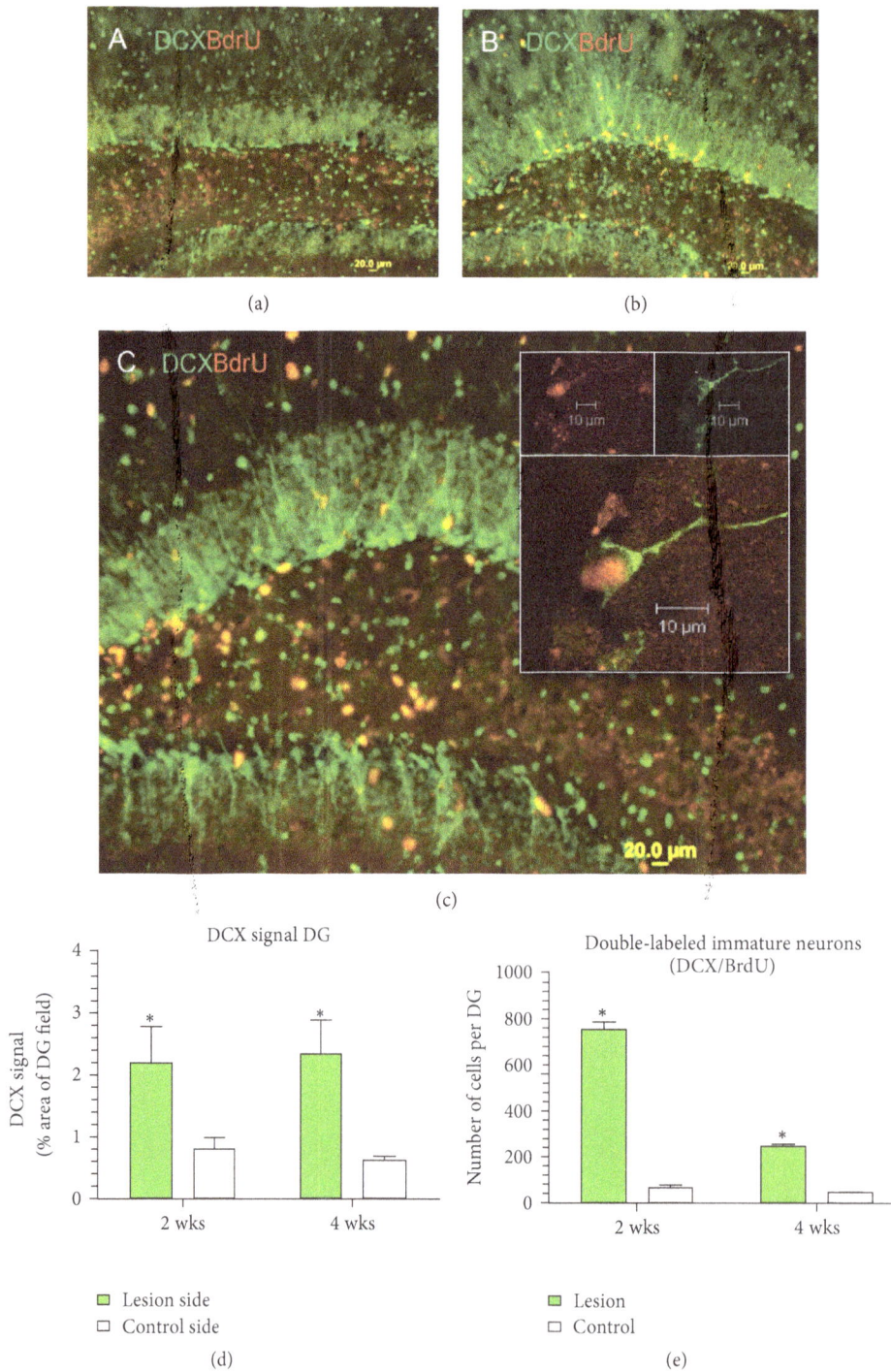

(a)

(b)

(c)

(d)

(e)

FIGURE 5: Microlesion stimulates neurogenesis. (a) Merged image of DCX and BrdU immunoreactive cells on the unlesioned control side (2 wks after the lesion). (b) Lesioned side illustrates increased DCX and BrdU (merged image). (c) Same as panel (b), but magnified; scale bar = 20 μm. Doublecortin (DCX) Immunoreactive cells in the subgranular zone of the dentate gyrus extend processes into the granular zone. The box inserted in (c) depicts confocal images of double-labeled DCX-BrdU cell at a higher power. Upper two panels are isolated for DCX (green) and BrdU (red) immunofluorescence, and the lower panel is the merged image (scale bar = 10 μm). (d) Summary data of DCX signal expressed as percent of DG field. Lesioned side exhibits a significantly increased DCX signal compared to control at both 2 and 4 wks after the microlesion. Unlike microgliosis and astrocytosis, the DCX signal does not decline after 4 wks. (e) Cell counts of double-labeled immature neurons (DCX/BrdU) born within 2 days of lesion placement. The lesion significantly increased birth of new neurons compared to unlesioned control side. $P < 0.001$. However, the number of double-labeled cells was significantly less at 4 wks than observed at 2 wks.

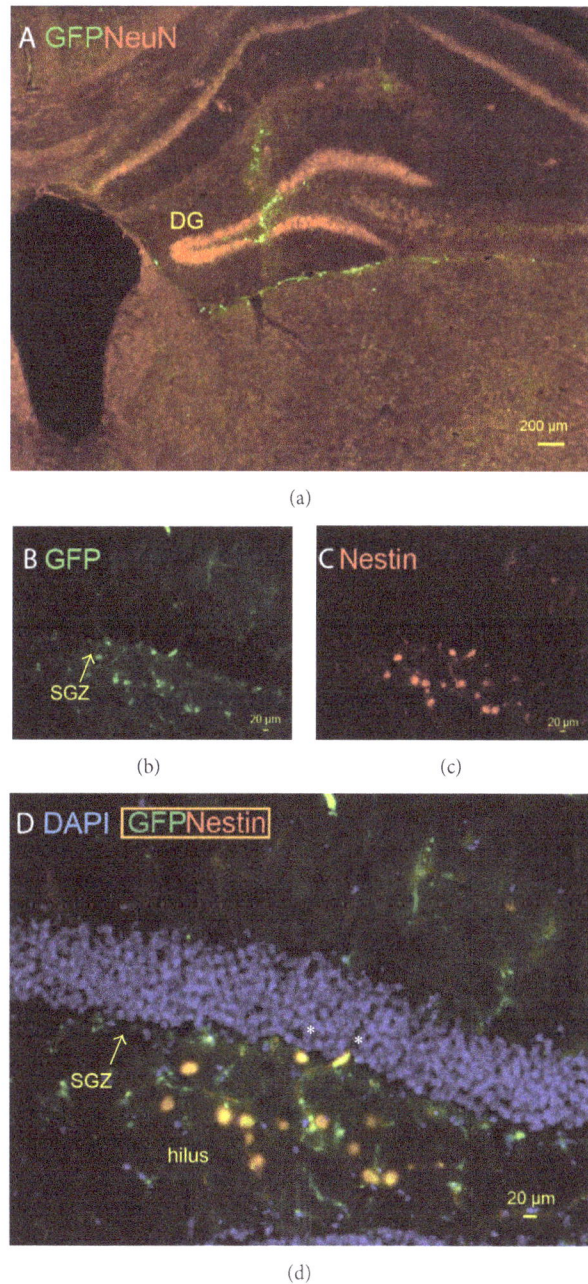

(a)

(b)   (c)

(d)

FIGURE 6: Chimeric mice stained for GFP (green) and Nestin (red). (a) GFP+ cells can be seen along the needle track and infiltrating in the sub-granular zone (SGZ) of the dentate gyrus (DG) and the CSF fluid space ventral to the hippocampus (scale bar = 200 μm). (b) GFP+ cells in the SGZ of the DG. (c) Nestin+ cells in SGZ of the DG. Most of the GFP+ cells are in the hilus (also known as CA4). (d) Merged image illustrating coexpression of GFP and nestin in two cells (asterisks) in the immediate SGZ (scale bar = 20 μm).

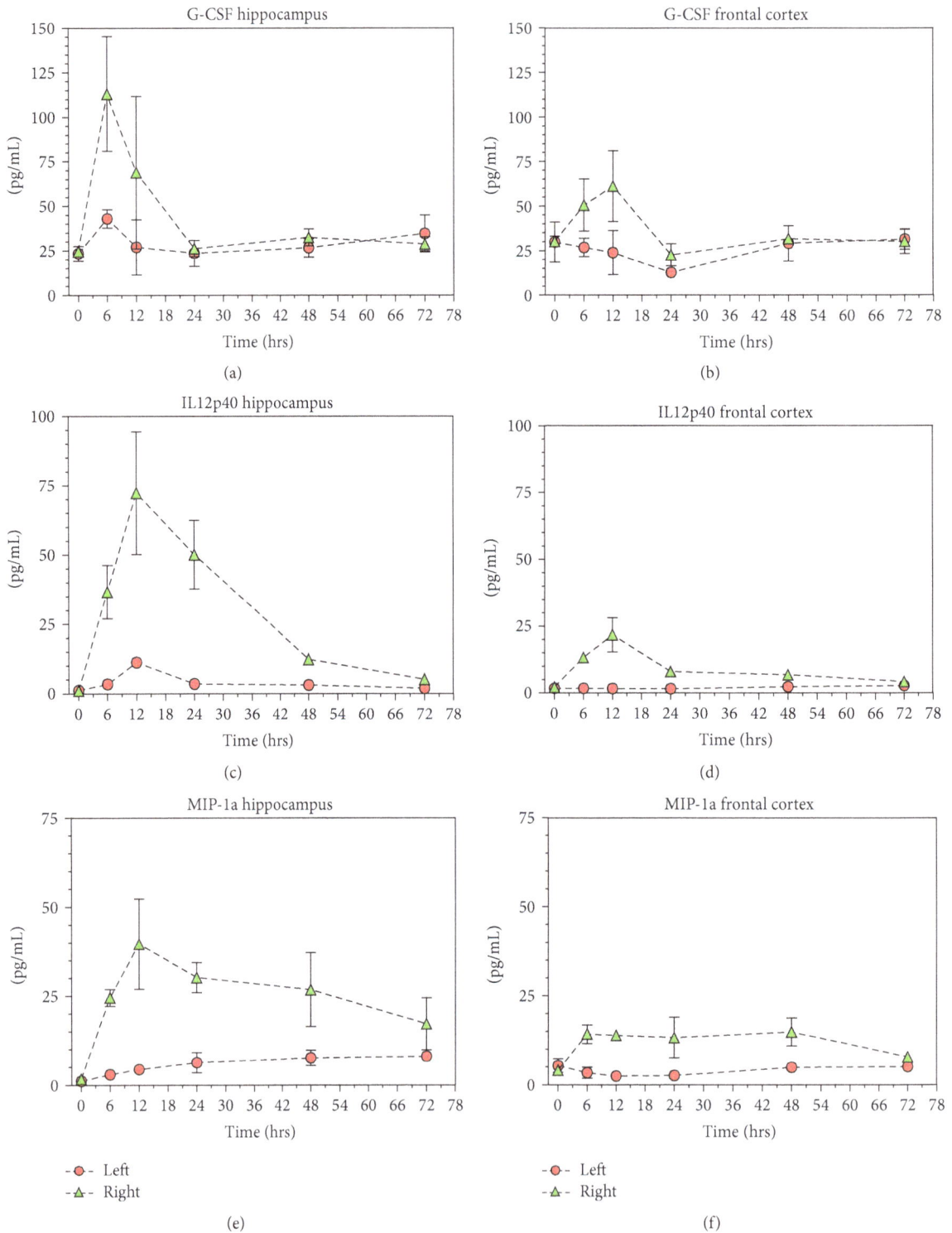

FIGURE 7: Three of the 17 cytokines measured in hippocampus and frontal cortex (path of the needle track) were significantly changed on the lesioned side compared to the control side. Each time point was determined from $n = 3$ mice (total of 18 pairs of hippocampi), and assays were run in triplicate. 2-way ANOVA (treatment versus time) revealed a significant effect ($P < 0.05$) for each of the cytokines except for G-CSF levels in frontal cortex.

may have contributed to hippocampal neurogenesis. Other cytokines were measured (including EGF, BDNF, and various pro- and anti-inflammatory cytokines) but were not found to be significantly altered. A limitation in the present study is that immediate cellular responses to microinjury (hours to several days) were not studied, and so the relationship of the acute cytokine release profile to the immediate cellular response pattern is not available. Nevertheless, the cellular responses documented here at 2 and 4 wks can be seen as a consequence of the acute humoral reaction to the microlesion. More mechanistic studies in the future will be designed to determine the effects of blocking specific cytokines on the cellular responses.

These findings may be relevant to the growing clinical practice of DBS through chronically implanted metal electrodes into specific brain regions. Electrical stimulation is not required to see signs of neuroinflammation; inflammatory changes have been observed around recording electrodes used for characterizing epileptogenic tissue and around CSF fluid shunt catheters [16, 17]. The animal literature also reveals similar activation of microglia and astrocytes following insertion of electrodes and other intracerebral implants [34–38]. Recently, a study of electrode implantation, without electrical stimulation, has revealed persistent and widespread neuroinflammation in rats, which extends beyond the electrode track in a region-selective manner [39]. Widespread neuroinflammation appears to be a general feature of the chronic implantation procedure, since it was found in rats implanted with three different types of electrodes varying in thickness and shape.

On the other hand, the enhanced hippocampal neurogenesis elicited by microlesions in young adult mice may not be completely applicable to human patients who are typically older and suffer from conditions such as AD, in which neurogenesis is impaired. However, research with transgenic mouse models of AD (tg APP/PS1) has revealed that the hippocampus retains competency to generate new neurons, especially when triggered by administration of G-CSF or when mice are provided enriched environments and exercise [18, 40].

5. Conclusions

Microinjury was produced by insertion and removal of a fine needle targeting the hippocampus on one side. The lesion caused a time-dependent increase in levels of several inflammatory and anti-inflammatory cytokines. Subsequent histological analysis at 2 and 4 weeks revealed microgliosis and astrocytosis. Microgliosis was a prominent cellular response, and though bone marrow-derived cells contributed to this population of cells, the majority of activated microglia were endogenous to the brain. The microlesion also increased hippocampal neurogenesis, indicated by the increased numbers of immature neurons (DCX+ cells) counted in the subgranular zone. Based on what is known in the literature about the cytokines (MIP-1a, IL12-p40, and G-CSF), their increased levels very likely contributed to the cellular inflammatory response around and distant from the lesion. These findings

are relevant to the growing clinical practice of DBS through chronically implanted metal electrodes into specific brain regions. Electrical stimulation is not required to see signs of neuroinflammation. G-CSF, which has neuromodulatory effects, has previously been shown to increase hippocampal neurogenesis in mice models of Alzheimer's disease, and this correlated with improved performance in a hippocampal-dependent learning task [41]. G-CSF is increasingly recognized as a neurotrophic factor that attenuates neuronal death and enhances functional recovery in various animal models of neurological disorders and is being explored in clinical trials [33, 42–45].

Acknowledgments

This paper is supported by a VA Merit Grant to S. Song. The contents of this research paper do not represent the views of the Department of Veterans Affairs or the United States Government.

References

[1] J. M. Bronstein, M. Tagliati, R. L. Alterman et al., "Deep brain stimulation for Parkinson disease an expert consensus and review of key issues," *Archives of Neurology*, vol. 68, no. 2, pp. 165–171, 2011.

[2] E. D. Flora, C. L. Perera, A. L. Cameron, and G. J. Maddern, "Deep brain stimulation for essential tremor: a systematic review," *Movement Disorders*, vol. 25, no. 11, pp. 1550–1559, 2010.

[3] P. Krack and L. Vercueil, "Review of the functional surgical treatment of dystonia," *European Journal of Neurology*, vol. 8, no. 5, pp. 389–399, 2001.

[4] L. B. Marangell, M. Martinez, R. A. Jurdi, and H. Zboyan, "Neurostimulation therapies in depression: a review of new modalities," *Acta Psychiatrica Scandinavica*, vol. 116, no. 3, pp. 174–181, 2007.

[5] A. Conca, J. Di Pauli, H. Hinterhuber, and H. P. Kapfhammer, "Deep brain stimulation: a review on current research," *Neuropsychiatrie*, vol. 25, no. 1, pp. 1–8, 2011.

[6] P. P. de Koning, M. Figee, P. van den Munckhof, P. R. Schuurman, and D. Denys, "Current status of deep brain stimulation for obsessive-compulsive disorder: a clinical review of different targets," *Current Psychiatry Reports*, vol. 13, no. 4, pp. 274–282, 2011.

[7] J. Luigjes, W. van den Brink, M. Feenstra et al., "Deep brain stimulation in addiction: a review of potential brain targets," *Molecular Psychiatry*, vol. 17, no. 6, pp. 572–583, 2012.

[8] A. N. Sen, P. G. Campbell, S. Yadla, J. Jallo, and A. D. Sharan, "Deep brain stimulation in the management of disorders of consciousness: a review of physiology, previous reports, and ethical considerations," *Neurosurgical Focus*, vol. 29, no. 2, p. E14, 2010.

[9] S. A. Shah and N. D. Schiff, "Central thalamic deep brain stimulation for cognitive neuromodulation—a review of proposed mechanisms and investigational studies," *European Journal of Neuroscience*, vol. 32, no. 7, pp. 1135–1144, 2010.

[10] P. Burbaud, A. Vital, A. Rougier et al., "Minimal tissue damage after stimulation of the motor thalamus in a case of chorea-acanthocytosis," *Neurology*, vol. 59, no. 12, pp. 1982–1984, 2002.

[11] K. L. Chou, M. S. Forman, J. Q. Trojanowski, H. I. Hurtig, and G. H. Baltuch, "Subthalamic nucleus deep brain stimulation in a patient with levodopa-responsive multiple system atrophy: case report," *Journal of Neurosurgery*, vol. 100, no. 3, pp. 553–556, 2004.

[12] J. M. Henderson, D. J. O'Sullivan, M. Pell et al., "Lesion of thalamic centromedian-parafascicular complex after chronic deep brain stimulation," *Neurology*, vol. 56, no. 11, pp. 1576–1579, 2001.

[13] M. S. Nielsen, C. R. Bjarkam, J. C. Sørensen, M. Bojsen-Møller, N. A. Sunde, and K. Østergaard, "Chronic subthalamic high-frequency deep brain stimulation in Parkinson's disease—a histopathological study," *European Journal of Neurology*, vol. 14, no. 2, pp. 132–138, 2007.

[14] J. G. Pilitsis, Y. Chu, J. Kordower, D. C. Bergen, E. J. Cochran, and R. A. E. Bakay, "Postmortem study of deep brain stimulation of the anterior thalamus: case report," *Neurosurgery*, vol. 62, no. 2, pp. E530–E532, 2008.

[15] V. Vedam-Mai, A. Yachnis, M. Ullman, S. P. Javedan, and M. S. Okun, "Postmortem observation of collagenous lead tip region fibrosis as a rare complication of DBS," *Movement Disorders*, vol. 27, no. 4, pp. 565–569, 2012.

[16] P. S. Hughes, J. P. Krcek, D. E. Hobson, and M. R. Del Bigio, "An unusual inflammatory response to implanted deep brain electrodes," *Canadian Journal of Neurological Sciences*, vol. 38, no. 1, pp. 168–170, 2011.

[17] C. L. Stephan, J. J. Kepes, K. Santacruz, S. B. Wilkinson, B. Fegley, and I. Osorio, "Spectrum of clinical and histopathologic responses to intracranial electrodes: from multifocal aseptic meningitis to multifocal hypersensitivity-type meningovasculitis," *Epilepsia*, vol. 42, no. 7, pp. 895–901, 2001.

[18] J. Sanchez-Ramos, S. Song, V. Sava et al., "Granulocyte colony stimulating factor decreases brain amyloid burden and reverses cognitive impairment in Alzheimer's mice," *Neuroscience*, vol. 163, no. 1, pp. 55–72, 2009.

[19] S. Song and J. Sanchez-Ramos, "Preparation of neural progenitors from bone marrow and umbilical cord blood," *Methods in Molecular Biology*, vol. 438, pp. 123–134, 2008.

[20] T. Furuya, R. Tanaka, T. Urabe et al., "Establishment of modified chimeric mice using GFP bone marrow as a model for neurological disorders," *NeuroReport*, vol. 14, no. 4, pp. 629–631, 2003.

[21] T. J. Shors, G. Miesegaes, A. Beylin, M. Zhao, T. Rydel, and E. Gould, "Neurogenesis in the adult is involved in the formation of trace memories," *Nature*, vol. 410, no. 6826, pp. 372–376, 2001.

[22] T. J. Shors, D. A. Townsend, M. Zhao, Y. Kozorovitskiy, and E. Gould, "Neurogenesis may relate to some but not all types of hippocampal-dependent learning," *Hippocampus*, vol. 12, no. 5, pp. 578–584, 2002.

[23] J. M. Encinas and G. Enikolopov, "Identifying and quantitating neural stem and progenitor cells in the adult brain," *Methods in Cell Biology*, vol. 85, pp. 243–272, 2008.

[24] A. R. Simard, D. Soulet, G. Gowing, J. P. Julien, and S. Rivest, "Bone marrow-derived microglia play a critical role in restricting senile plaque formation in Alzheimer's disease," *Neuron*, vol. 49, no. 4, pp. 489–502, 2006.

[25] T. M. Malm, M. Koistinaho, M. Pärepalo et al., "Bone-marrow-derived cells contribute to the recruitment of microglial cells in response to β-amyloid deposition in APP/PS1 double transgenic Alzheimer mice," *Neurobiology of Disease*, vol. 18, no. 1, pp. 134–142, 2005.

[26] M. Djukic, A. Mildner, H. Schmidt et al., "Circulating monocytes engraft in the brain, differentiate into microglia and contribute to the pathology following meningitis in mice," *Brain*, vol. 129, no. 9, pp. 2394–2403, 2006.

[27] E. Kokovay and L. A. Cunningham, "Bone marrow-derived microglia contribute to the neuroinflammatory response and express iNOS in the MPTP mouse model of Parkinson's disease," *Neurobiology of Disease*, vol. 19, no. 3, pp. 471–478, 2005.

[28] A. Mildner, H. Schmidt, M. Nitsche et al., "Microglia in the adult brain arise from Ly-6ChiCCR2+ monocytes only under defined host conditions," *Nature Neuroscience*, vol. 10, no. 12, pp. 1544–1553, 2007.

[29] R. Tanaka, M. Komine-Kobayashi, H. Mochizuki et al., "Migration of enhanced green fluorescent protein expressing bone marrow-derived microglia/macrophage into the mouse brain following permanent focal ischemia," *Neuroscience*, vol. 117, no. 3, pp. 531–539, 2003.

[30] S. S. Magavi, B. R. Leavitt, and J. D. Macklis, "Induction of neurogenesis in the neocertex of adult mice," *Nature*, vol. 405, no. 6789, pp. 951–955, 2000.

[31] L. Bao, J. U. Lindgren, P. Van Der Meide, S. W. Zhu, H. G. Ljunggren, and J. Zhu, "The critical role of IL-12p40 in initiating, enhancing, and perpetuating pathogenic events in murine experimental autoimmune neuritis," *Brain Pathology*, vol. 12, no. 4, pp. 420–429, 2002.

[32] A. D. Ho, D. Young, M. Maruyama et al., "Pluripotent and lineage-committed CD34+ subsets in leukapheresis products mobilized by G-CSF, GM-CSF vs. a combination of both," *Experimental Hematology*, vol. 24, no. 13, pp. 1460–1468, 1996.

[33] A. Schneider, C. Krüger, T. Steigleder et al., "The hematopoietic factor G-CSF is a neuronal ligand that counteracts programmed cell death and drives neurogenesis," *The Journal of Clinical Investigation*, vol. 115, no. 8, pp. 2083–2098, 2005.

[34] G. C. McConnell, T. M. Schneider, D. J. Owens, and R. V. Bellamkonda, "Extraction force and cortical tissue reaction of silicon microelectrode arrays implanted in the rat brain," *IEEE Transactions on Biomedical Engineering*, vol. 54, no. 6, pp. 1097–1107, 2007.

[35] B. K. Leung, R. Biran, C. J. Underwood, and P. A. Tresco, "Characterization of microglial attachment and cytokine release on biomaterials of differing surface chemistry," *Biomaterials*, vol. 29, no. 23, pp. 3289–3297, 2008.

[36] P. Stice, A. Gilletti, A. Panitch, and J. Muthuswamy, "Thin microelectrodes reduce GFAP expression in the implant site in rodent somatosensory cortex," *Journal of Neural Engineering*, vol. 4, no. 2, pp. 42–53, 2007.

[37] M. Lenarz, H. H. Lim, T. Lenarz et al., "Auditory midbrain implant: histomorphologic effects of long-term implantation and electric stimulation of a new deep brain stimulation array," *Otology and Neurotology*, vol. 28, no. 8, pp. 1045–1052, 2007.

[38] R. Biran, D. C. Martin, and P. A. Tresco, "The brain tissue response to implanted silicon microelectrode arrays is increased when the device is tethered to the skull," *Journal of Biomedical Materials Research A*, vol. 82, no. 1, pp. 169–178, 2007.

[39] Y. K. Hirshler, U. Polat, and A. Biegon, "Intracranial electrode implantation produces regional neuroinflammation and memory deficits in rats," *Experimental Neurology*, vol. 222, no. 1, pp. 42–50, 2010.

[40] B. J. Catlow, A. R. Rowe, C. R. Clearwater, M. Mamcarz, G. W. Arendash, and J. Sanchez-Ramos, "Effects of environmental enrichment and physical activity on neurogenesis in transgenic PS1/APP mice," *Brain Research*, vol. 1256, pp. 173–179, 2009.

[41] J. Sanchez-Ramos, S. Song, V. Sava et al., "Granulocyte colony stimulating factor decreases brain amyloid burden and reverses

cognitive impairment in Alzheimer's mice," *Neuroscience*, vol. 163, no. 1, pp. 55–72, 2009.

[42] W. R. Schäbitz and A. Schneider, "New targets for established proteins: exploring G-CSF for the treatment of stroke," *Trends in Pharmacological Sciences*, vol. 28, no. 4, pp. 157–161, 2007.

[43] L. Tonges, J. C. Schlachetzki, J. H. Weishaupt, and M. Bahr, "Hematopoietic cytokines—on the verge of conquering neurology," *Current Molecular Medicine*, vol. 7, no. 2, pp. 157–170, 2007.

[44] Y. Nishio, M. Koda, T. Kamada et al., "Granulocyte colony-stimulating factor attenuates neuronal death and promotes functional recovery after spinal cord injury in mice," *Journal of Neuropathology and Experimental Neurology*, vol. 66, no. 8, pp. 724–731, 2007.

[45] T. Duning, H. Schiffbauer, T. Warnecke et al., "G-CSF prevents the progression of structural disintegration of white matter tracts in amyotrophic lateral sclerosis: a pilot trial," *PLoS ONE*, vol. 6, no. 3, Article ID e17770, 2011.

Permissions

The contributors of this book come from diverse backgrounds, making this book a truly international effort. This book will bring forth new frontiers with its revolutionizing research information and detailed analysis of the nascent developments around the world.

We would like to thank all the contributing authors for lending their expertise to make the book truly unique. They have played a crucial role in the development of this book. Without their invaluable contributions this book wouldn't have been possible. They have made vital efforts to compile up to date information on the varied aspects of this subject to make this book a valuable addition to the collection of many professionals and students.

This book was conceptualized with the vision of imparting up-to-date information and advanced data in this field. To ensure the same, a matchless editorial board was set up. Every individual on the board went through rigorous rounds of assessment to prove their worth. After which they invested a large part of their time researching and compiling the most relevant data for our readers. Conferences and sessions were held from time to time between the editorial board and the contributing authors to present the data in the most comprehensible form. The editorial team has worked tirelessly to provide valuable and valid information to help people across the globe.

Every chapter published in this book has been scrutinized by our experts. Their significance has been extensively debated. The topics covered herein carry significant findings which will fuel the growth of the discipline. They may even be implemented as practical applications or may be referred to as a beginning point for another development. Chapters in this book were first published by Hindawi Publishing Corporation; hereby published with permission under the Creative Commons Attribution License or equivalent.

The editorial board has been involved in producing this book since its inception. They have spent rigorous hours researching and exploring the diverse topics which have resulted in the successful publishing of this book. They have passed on their knowledge of decades through this book. To expedite this challenging task, the publisher supported the team at every step. A small team of assistant editors was also appointed to further simplify the editing procedure and attain best results for the readers.

Our editorial team has been hand-picked from every corner of the world. Their multi-ethnicity adds dynamic inputs to the discussions which result in innovative outcomes. These outcomes are then further discussed with the researchers and contributors who give their valuable feedback and opinion regarding the same. The feedback is then collaborated with the researches and they are edited in a comprehensive manner to aid the understanding of the subject.

Apart from the editorial board, the designing team has also invested a significant amount of their time in understanding the subject and creating the most relevant covers. They scrutinized every image to scout for the most suitable representation of the subject and create an appropriate cover for the book.

The publishing team has been involved in this book since its early stages. They were actively engaged in every process, be it collecting the data, connecting with the contributors or procuring relevant information. The team has been an ardent support to the editorial, designing and production team. Their endless efforts to recruit the best for this project, has resulted in the accomplishment of this book. They are a veteran in the field of academics and their pool of knowledge is as vast as their experience in printing. Their expertise and guidance has proved useful at every step. Their uncompromising quality standards have made this book an exceptional effort. Their encouragement from time to time has been an inspiration for everyone.

The publisher and the editorial board hope that this book will prove to be a valuable piece of knowledge for researchers, students, practitioners and scholars across the globe.

List of Contributors

Gaskon Ibarretxe, Olatz Crende, Maitane Aurrekoetxea, Victoria Garcıa-Murga, Javier Etxaniz and Fernando Unda
Department of Cell Biology and Histology, Faculty of Medicine and Dentistry, University of the Basque Country (UPV/EHU), 48940 Bizkaia, Leioa, Spain

Gisela Velez
Department of Ophthalmology, University of Massachusetts Medical School, Worcester, MA 01605, USA
Department of Ophthalmology, Harvard Medical School, Boston, MA 02115, USA
The Schepens Eye Research Institute, Massachusetts Eye and Ear, Boston, MA 02114, USA

Alexa R. Weingarden
The Schepens Eye Research Institute, Massachusetts Eye and Ear, Boston, MA 02114, USA

Budd A. Tucker, Andrius Kazlauskas, Hetian Lei and Michael J. Young
Department of Ophthalmology, Harvard Medical School, Boston, MA 02115, USA
The Schepens Eye Research Institute, Massachusetts Eye and Ear, Boston, MA 02114, USA

Maria G. Roubelakis, Ourania Trohatou and Nicholas P. Anagnou
Laboratory of Biology, University of Athens School of Medicine, 115 27 Athens, Greece
Cell and Gene Therapy Laboratory, Centre of Basic Research II, Biomedical Research Foundation of the Academy of Athens (BRFAA), 115 27 Athens, Greece

Jing Yang, Jinmei Wang, X. Joann You and Henry Klassen
Department of Ophthalmology, Ophthalmology Research Laboratories, The Gavin Herbert Eye Institute, University of California, Irvine, CA 92697, USA

Ping Gu
Department of Ophthalmology, Ophthalmology Research Laboratories, The Gavin Herbert Eye Institute, University of California, Irvine, CA 92697, USA
Department of Ophthalmology, Shanghai Ninth People's Hospital, School of Medicine, Shanghai Jiaotong University, Shanghai 200011, China

Sunghoon Jung, Krishna M. Panchalingam and Leo A. Behie
Pharmaceutical Production Research Facility (PPRF), Schulich School of Engineering, University of Calgary, Calgary, AB, Canada T2N 1N4

Lawrence Rosenberg
Department of Surgery, McGill University, Montreal, QC, Canada H3G 1A4

Natasha Kekre
Blood and Marrow Transplant Program, Division of Hematology, Department of Medicine, University of Ottawa, 501 Smyth Rd., Box 704, Ottawa, ON, Canada K1H8L6

Jennifer Philippe and Susan Smith
One Match Stem Cell and Marrow Network, Canadian Blood Services, 40 Concourse Gate, Ottawa, ON, Canada K2E 8A6

Ranjeeta Mallick
Clinical Epidemiology Program, Ottawa Hospital Research Institute, 501 Smyth Rd., Ottawa, ON, Canada K1H 8L6

David Allan
Blood and Marrow Transplant Program, Division of Hematology, Department of Medicine, University of Ottawa, 501 Smyth Rd., Box 704, Ottawa, ON, Canada K1H8L6
One Match Stem Cell and Marrow Network, Canadian Blood Services, 40 Concourse Gate, Ottawa, ON, Canada K2E 8A6
Regenerative Medicine Program, Ottawa Hospital Research Institute, 501 Smyth Rd., Ottawa, ON, Canada K1H 8L6

Olivier Liard, Emmanuel Sagui, Andre Nau, Aurelie Pascual and Thierry Fusai
Unite de Chirurgie et Physiologie Experimentale (UCPE), Institut de Medecine Tropicale, 58 boulevard Charles Livon, 13007 Marseille, France

Stephanie Segura and Emmanuel Moyse
Unite Physiologie de la Reproduction et des Comportements, UMR 85, Centre INRA de Tours, 37380 Nouzilly, France

Melissa Cambon
Laboratoire d'Ecologie fonctionnelle, Batiment 4R3, 118 route de Narbonne, 31062 Toulouse cedex 9, France

Jean-Luc Darlix
Unite de Retrovirologie, U421 INSERM, Ecole Normale Superieure de Lyon, 46 Allee d'Italie, 69364 Lyon cedex 07, France

Ming Li and Susumu Ikehara
Department of Stem Cell Disorders, Kansai Medical University, Moriguchi, Osaka 570-8506, Japan

Lucıa Calatrava-Ferreras, Rafael Gonzalo-Gobernado, Antonio S. Herranz and Diana Reimers
Servicio de Neurobiologıa, Instituto Ramon y Cajal de Investigacion Sanitaria (IRYCIS), 28034 Madrid, Spain

Teresa Montero Vega
Servicio de Bioquımica, Instituto Ramon y Cajal de Investigacion Sanitaria (IRYCIS), 28034 Madrid, Spain

Adriano Jimenez-Escrig
Servicio de Neurologıa, Hospital Universitario Ramon y Cajal, 28034 Madrid, Spain

Luis Alberto Richart Lopez
Centro de Transfusiones de la Comunidad de Madrid, Valdebernardo, 28030 Madrid, Spain

Eulalia Bazan
Servicio de Neurobiologıa, Instituto Ramon y Cajal de Investigacion Sanitaria (IRYCIS), 28034 Madrid, Spain
Servicio de Neurobiologıa - Investigacion, Hospital Ramon y Cajal, Carretera de Colmenar Km. 9, 1, 28034 Madrid, Spain

Chuck C.-K. Chao, Feng-Chun Hung and Jack J. Chao
Department of Biochemistry and Molecular Biology and Institute of Biomedical Sciences, College of Medicine, Chang Gung University, Taoyuan 333, Taiwan

Sally K. Mak, Y. Anne Huang, Shifteh Iranmanesh, Malini Vangipuram, Ramya Sundararajan, Loan Nguyen, J. William Langston and Birgitt Schule
Basic Research Department, The Parkinson's Institute, 675 Almanor Ave, Sunnyvale, CA 94085, USA

Solomon O. Ugoya and Jian Tu
Australian School of Advanced Medicine, Macquarie University, 2 Technology Place, North Ryde, Sydney, NSW 2109, Australia

Daniil Simanov and Imre Mellaart-Straver
Hubrecht Institute, KNAW, University Medical Center Utrecht, 3584 CT Utrecht, The Netherlands

Irina Sormacheva
Institute of Cytology and Genetics SB RAS, 630090 Novosibirsk, Russia

Eugene Berezikov
Hubrecht Institute, KNAW, University Medical Center Utrecht, 3584 CT Utrecht, The Netherlands
European Research Institute for the Biology of Ageing and University Medical Center Groningen, University of Groningen, 9713 AV Groningen, The Netherlands

Umile Giuseppe Longo, Stefano Petrillo, Edoardo Franceschetti, Alessandra Berton and Vincenzo Denaro
Department of Orthopaedic and Trauma Surgery, Campus Bio-Medico University, Via Alvaro del Portillo 200, Trigoria, 00128 Rome, Italy
Centro Integrato di Ricerca (CIR), Universita Campus Bio-Medico, Via Alvaro del Portillo, 21, 00128, Rome, Italy

Nicola Maffulli
Centre for Sports and Exercise Medicine, Barts and The London School of Medicine and Dentistry, Mile End Hospital, 275 Bancroft Road, London E1 4DG, UK

Vikram Sabapathy, Saranya Ravi and Sanjay Kumar
Center for Stem Cell Research, Christian Medical College, Bagayam, Vellore 632002, India

Vivi Srivastava
Department of Cytogenetics, Christian Medical College, Bagayam, Vellore 632002, India

Alok Srivastava
Center for Stem Cell Research, Christian Medical College, Bagayam, Vellore 632002, India
Department of Hematology, Christian Medical College, Bagayam, Vellore 632002, India

Umile Giuseppe Longo, Mattia Loppini, Alessandra Berton, Filippo Spiezia and Vincenzo Denaro
Department of Orthopaedic and Trauma Surgery, Campus Bio-Medico University, Via Alvaro del Portillo 200, Trigoria, 00128 Rome, Italy
Centro Integrato di Ricerca (CIR) Campus Bio-Medico University, Via Alvaro del Portillo 21, 00128, Rome, Italy

Nicola Maffulli
Centre for Sports and Exercise Medicine, Barts and The London School of Medicine and Dentistry, Mile End Hospital, 275 Bancroft Road, London E1 4DG, UK

Manuel Mazo, Miriam Arana, Beatriz Pelacho and Felipe Prosper
Department of Hematology and Cell Therapy, Clinica Universidad de Navarra, Foundation for Applied Medical Research, University of Navarra, Avenida Pio XII 36, Pamplona, 31008 Navarra, Spain

Mónika Szepes, Zsolt Benky, Attila Cselenyák, Zsombor Lacza and Levente Kiss
Institute of Human Physiology and Clinical Experimental Research, Semmelweis University, Tuzolto Utca 37-47, Budapest 1094, Hungary

Kai Michael Kompisch and Udo Schumacher
Department of Anatomy and Experimental Morphology, Center for Experimental Medicine, University Hospital Hamburg-Eppendorf, Martinistraße 52, 20246 Hamburg, Germany

Androniki Kretsovali
Institute of Molecular Biology and Biotechnology, FORTH, Heraklion, 70013 Crete, Greece

Nikolaos Charmpilas
Department of Biology, University of Crete, Heraklion, 71409 Crete, Greece

Christiana Hadjimichael
Institute of Molecular Biology and Biotechnology, FORTH, Heraklion, 70013 Crete, Greece
Department of Biology, University of Crete, Heraklion, 71409 Crete, Greece

Kunyu Li
Department of Neurology, University of South Florida, 13220 Laurel Drive, Tampa, FL 33612, USA

Shijie Song and Vasyl Sava
Department of Neurology, University of South Florida, 13220 Laurel Drive, Tampa, FL 33612, USA
Research Service, James A. Haley VA Medical Center, Tampa, FL 33612, USA

Juan Sanchez-Ramos
Department of Neurology, University of South Florida, 13220 Laurel Drive, Tampa, FL 33612, USA
Research Service, James A. Haley VA Medical Center, Tampa, FL 33612, USA
Feinberg School of Medicine, Northwestern University, Chicago, IL 60611, USA

Shuojing Song
Feinberg School of Medicine, Northwestern University, Chicago, IL 60611, USA

Chuanhai Cao and Xiaoyang Lin
Department of Molecular Pharmacology and Physiology, University of South Florida, Tampa, FL 33612, USA